Principles and Practice of
Clinical Trial Medicine

Principles and Practice of Clinical Trial Medicine

Richard Chin and Bruce Y. Lee

AMSTERDAM • BOSTON • HEIDELBERG • LONDON • NEW YORK • OXFORD
PARIS • SAN DIEGO • SAN FRANCISCO • SINGAPORE • SYDNEY • TOKYO
Academic Press is an imprint of Elsevier

Academic Press is an imprint of Elsevier
84 Theobald's Road, London WC1X 8RR, UK
Radarweg 29, PO Box 211, 1000 AE Amsterdam, The Netherlands
30 Corporate Drive, Suite 400, Burlington, MA 01803, USA
525 B Street, Suite 1900, San Diego, CA 92101-4495, USA

First edition 2008

British Library Cataloguing in Publication Data
A catalogue record for this book is available from the British Library

Library of Congress Cataloging-in-Publication Data
A catalog record for this book is available from the Library of Congress

ISBN: 978-0-12-373695-6

Typeset by Charon Tec Ltd., A Macmillan Company.
(www.macmilliansolutions.com)

For information on all Academic Press publications
visit our website at books.elsevier.com

Dedication

This endeavor would not have been possible had we not met as classmates (and dormitory mates) at Harvard Medical School. This book is dedicated to our families, whose support and encouragement made the endeavor possible. We also would like to thank everyone at Elsevier for their hard work and invaluable help and making the process an exciting and enjoyable one.

RYC and BYL

Contents

About the Authors   ix

Introduction   xi

Section I: Overview   **1**
Chapter 1: Overview of Clinical Research Medicine   3
Chapter 2: Ethical, Legal, and Regulatory Issues   17

Section II: The General Structure of Clinical Trials and Programs   **41**
Chapter 3: Introduction to Clinical Trial Statistics   43
Chapter 4: Measures and Variables   61
Chapter 5: Study Groups   79
Chapter 6: Periods, Sequences, and Trial Design   95

Section III: Key Components of Clinical Trials and Programs   **119**
Chapter 7: Endpoints   121
Chapter 8: Economics and Patient Reported Outcomes   145
Chapter 9: Patient Selection and Sampling   167
Chapter 10: Dosing and Intervention   181
Chapter 11: Epidemiology, Decision Analysis, and Simulation   213

Section IV: Conduct of the Study   **231**
Chapter 12: Study Execution   233
Chapter 13: Site Selection and Patient Recruitment   283

Section V: Analysis of Results   **301**
Chapter 14: Assessing Data Quality and Transforming Data   303
Chapter 15: Analysis of Data   325
Chapter 16: Data Interpretation and Conclusions   361

Appendices
Appendix A: FDA Internal Compliance Manuals   389
Appendix B: Medwatch Form   409
Appendix C: FDA Reviewer Guidance on Safety Review   411
Appendix D: Common Terminology Criteria for Adverse Events (CTCAE)   461
Appendix E: Sample Investigational New Drug Application Form   535
Appendix F: Statement of Investigator Form 1572   537

Index   539

About the Authors

Richard Chin, MD
San Francisco, California, USA

Dr. Chin is a Harvard trained, Board Certified internist with drug development across a wide range of specialties, including oncology, immunology, ophthalmology, neurology, endocrinology, and cardiovascular medicine, among others. He has been responsible for over 40 Investigational New Drug (IND) Applications and 8 New Drug Applications (NDAs)/ Biologic License Applications (BLAs). Some of the drugs Dr. Chin has overseen include ranibizumab, natalizumab, tenecteplase, bapineuzumab, ziconotide, and omalizumab. He has both US and international experience, and has overseen a wide variety of functions, including Clinical Development, Regulatory, Biostatistics, Quality Assurance/Compliance, Chemistry Manufacturing, and Control, Safety and Medical Affairs.

Dr. Chin is currently President and CEO of a NASDAQ-listed biotechnology company. Previously, he was Senior Vice President and Head of Global Development for Elan Corporation, and before that served as the Head of Clinical Research for the Biotherapeutics Unit at Genentech. Dr. Chin holds an M.D. from Harvard Medical School. He received the equivalent of a J.D. with honors from Oxford University, England under a Rhodes Scholarship. He graduated with a B.A. in Biology, *magna cum laude*, from Harvard University. He previously served on the adjunct clinical faculty at Stanford Medical School. Dr. Chin may be contacted at richardchin@clinicaltrialist.com.

Bruce Y. Lee, MD, MBA
University of Pittsburgh
Pittsburgh, Pennsylvania, USA

Dr. Lee is currently an Assistant Professor of Medicine and Biomedical Informatics, and Epidemiology at the University of Pittsburgh. He is also Core Faculty in the Section for Decision Sciences and Clinical Systems Modeling, the Center for Research in Health Care, and the RAND-University of Pittsburgh Health Institute. He is a Co-Investigator for the National Institutes of Health (NIH) Modeling of Infectious Diseases Agent Study (MIDAS) research and informatics network, and a Co-Investigator for a Bill & Melinda Gates Foundations Grant on the evaluation of candidate vaccine technologies using computational models.

His previous positions include serving as Senior Manager at Quintiles Transnational, working in biotechnology equity research at Montgomery Securities, and co-founding Integrigen, a biotechnology company. His consulting experience includes a large variety of clients, ranging from large and small pharmaceutical, biotechnology, and medical device companies.

Dr. Lee has authored three books, as well as numerous research publications, review articles, and book chapters.

Dr. Lee received his B.A. from Harvard University, M.D. from Harvard Medical School, and M.B.A. from the Stanford Graduate School of Business. He is board-certified in Internal Medicine, having completed his residency training at the University of California, San Diego.

Introduction

While we may not recognize it, we all use the skills necessary to conduct and interpret "clinical trials" every single day. Sampling and comparing one restaurant, article of clothing, television show, fitness club, vacation location, date, job candidate, or client to another is effectively conducting a clinical trial. Evidence and results from these mini-trials guide your choices and decisions throughout the day. Should you buy that swimsuit? Is it better than the one in the other store? Are the Philadelphia Eagles or the Pittsburgh Steelers a better football team? Which sushi restaurant has the best salmon? What job will provide the best experience? Where should you live and what house should you buy? Is it better to hire Job Candidate #1 or Job Candidate #2? Faulty "trial" design, data, or interpretation leads to inaccurate assessments and perhaps poor decisions. For example, using the wrong criteria will result in hiring the wrong person for a job. We all have suffered from that impulse buy, that forehead-slapping wrong decision, or that bad choice of friend, employee, or significant other.

Formal and informal clinical trials are a large part of our lives. If you use, produce, study, purchase, invest in, or conduct research in drugs, medical devices, or any type of health care intervention, understanding the science and operations of formal clinical trials can only help. Today, even understanding many major news items requires at least some knowledge of clinical trials. Whenever a drug or medical device is recalled, a medical intervention is debunked, or a new therapy hits the market, clinical trial design, conduct, or analysis is at the heart of the evidence or the controversy. Health care is such a major business that even seemingly unrelated industries and professions can be dramatically affected by a successful or unsuccessful clinical trial. Flaws in a clinical trial that force a major drug or device to be pulled from the market can alter many lives and rock the economy.

Therefore, during our planning stages for *Principles and Practices of Clinical Trial Medicine*, confining the book's audience was difficult. Should this book be geared toward just physicians? Pharmaceutical industry professionals? Statisticians? Academics? Clinical research specialists? Regulatory professionals? Ethicists? Medical students? Nursing students? Medicine residents? Graduate students? Post-doctoral fellows? Epidemiologists? Engineers? Pharmacologists? Pharmacists? Biologists? Pharmaceutical or medical device executives? The more we thought about it, the more we realized that the audience could be quite broad. Both of our career journeys have taken us through a variety of functions and domains in industry, academics, and business. We have seen the investment, research, technical, management, teaching, writing, consulting, and clinical practice realms of the health care industry. In the end, while each area may have different jargon, cultures, personalities, and perspectives, the guiding principles are the same. A good clinical trial at an academic institution is a good one in industry and vice-versa.

Therefore, we wrote this book with a broad audience in mind, trying to minimize the jargon and explain any important terminology in the process. The goal was to write a book that could be easily understood regardless of your background, especially since people from so many different backgrounds are involved in clinical trials. In fact, in many professions, understanding the jargon and terminology is half the battle.

Moreover, regardless of your interest and function in the clinical research world, knowing the general concepts of all aspects of clinical trials can be very advantageous. In many ways, the clinical research world has become far too specialized. Many individuals stay ensconced within their areas of knowledge and expertise. But the best clinical researchers or trialists have broad knowledge bases that span statistics, regulatory affairs, ethics, clinical medicine, science, basic probability, data management, and trial and personnel management. The ones that stand out, are most marketable, and do the best work cannot afford to say, "I do not need to know that because it is not in my area."

Designing, conducting, and analyzing a clinical trial is like designing, building, and using a house. Recognizing a house's design and construction helps you realize its potential use. For example, a thin-walled house may cause problems during the winter. Very cramped rooms may not facilitate hosting a party. At the same time, anticipating the house's use aids its design and construction. Your design of a beach house likely will differ significantly from your design of a farm house or a city dwelling.

The building a house analogy helps illustrate the general organization of our book. *The Principles and Practices of Clinical Trial Medicine* contains five sections. Section I introduces the field of clinical research with Chapter 1 delineating some general theory and Chapter 2 covering important legal, ethical, and regulatory issues. The materials in this section are analogous to all of the rules and regulations that govern the construction of a house: ranging from general engineering and architectural principles to zoning laws and building codes. Just as you can't build any kind of house anywhere you choose (e.g., Igloos do not belong in Philadelphia or San Francisco), you must understand general clinical research theory and comply with legal, ethical, and regulatory principles when designing and conducting a trial.

Section II focuses on the general design of clinical trials. If you imagine a clinical trial to be a house, statistics (Chapter 3) are the tools used to build the house. The final design of the house depends heavily on the tools that you have at your disposal. Sure you can rely on others to choose and wield the tools… but to be truly competent at clinical research, you have to know your tools, even if you have specialists to employ them. Measures and Variables (Chapter 4) are the construction materials for the house. Construction materials help determine the house's appearance and utility. Building a house resistant to harsh elements may be difficult without good quality bricks or cinder blocks. Similarly, studying heart disease may be challenging without accurate echocardiograms, electrocardiograms, and blood pressure measurements. Study Groups (Chapter 5) and Periods, Sequences and Design (Chapter 6) are the rooms and corridors of the house. Changing these will dramatically change the house's functionality and purpose. Having no kitchen makes cooking and hosting dinner parties difficult. An indoor garage allows you to shield your car from the elements. Similarly, comparing two medical interventions normally requires employing at least two different study groups. Seeing the long-term effects of a drug necessitates patients being on the drug for a long period of time.

Section III takes a closer look at an array of important elements in clinical trial design. Endpoints (Chapter 7) are special measures and variables that serve as the outcomes of the trial. So, continuing our building analogy, endpoints are the key construction materials that determine the worth, strength, and utility of the house. Chapter 8 (Economics and Patient Reported Outcomes) discusses some special types of endpoints,

Chapter 9 (Patient Selection and Sampling) reviews considerations when choosing patients for your trial; and Chapter 10 (Dosing and Intervention) analyzes how medical interventions should be administered to patients. All of these are as important factors and parameters to clinical trials as ceiling height, room size, lighting, house temperature, and other features are to house construction. Chapter 11 (Epidemiology, Decision Analysis and Simulation) offers additional tools that may help in the planning and analysis of trials, and is analogous to the model building and roughing-in phase of house building, where you visualize how a house might look.

Section IV covers practical logistical issues involved in conducting a trial. This is analogous to concerns that arise when actually building the house. For example, from where do you procure building materials? Which forms should you complete when ordering such materials? Which nails should you use? Where should you place the beams? How do you select and supervise the contractor? All of these types of issues discussed in Chapter 12 (Study Execution). Recruiting Patients and Choosing Trial Locations (Chapter 13) are such an important part of conducting trials that a separate chapter is devoted to the topic.

Finally, Section V discusses how to analyze the results of clinical trial. In our building analogy, this is similar to using and inhabiting the house. Data is the output of a clinical trial, just as a house is the end product of house construction. Chapter 14 (Assessing Data Quality and Transforming Data) is akin to inspecting the house and making the final adjustments and reworking anything that needs to be reworked. If the stairs are not to code, they need to be redone, and if the painters overpainted the moldings, they need to be repainted. Data similarly need to be cleaned and transformed, to ameliorate missing or unreliable data points.

Chapter 15 (Analysis of Data) is akin to decorating the house and moving the furniture into the appropriate rooms. You manipulate the data that has been gathered and prepared. This allows you to then interpret the data, which is the subject of Chapter 16 (Data Interpretation and Conclusions). This is akin to moving into the house and living in it. This is the acid test. No matter how well-built or well-decorated the house is, if you don't enjoy living in it, all has been for naught. Similarly, the ultimate end product of a clinical trial is a conclusion that is actionable for the treatment of future patients.

So whether you are new to the world of clinical trials or have been conducting clinical research for many years, we hope that this book serves you well. The importance and use of clinical trials will only continue to grow in the future. Concomitantly, trial design and conduct will face increasing scrutiny. In many cases, lives of innumerable patients and significant amounts of time and resources will be riding on them. Will you be ready?

Richard Chin, MD
Bruce Y. Lee, MD, MBA

Chapter 1

Overview of Clinical Trial Medicine

1.1 CLINICAL TRIAL MEDICINE

1.1.1 Definition of Clinical Trial Medicine

Let us begin by defining the science that is the focus of this book. We call this science clinical trial medicine (CTM) and define it as the science of designing, conducting, and interpreting clinical trials. Its goal is to understand and improve methods for determining whether an intervention, such as a drug, a device, or a procedure, improves clinical outcome in patients. For example, it might address a question such as, "How can one determine whether or not angiotensin converting enzyme (ACE) inhibitors slow the progression of renal disease?" Or it might answer a question such as, "How can one determine whether or not patients with angina benefit from coronary artery bypass surgery?" CTM is a broad field that addresses issues such as types of patients to enroll in a trial, appropriate size of a trial, and ways of maximizing the amount and quality of information elicited from a trial.

Put another way, a clinical trial is concerned with finding therapies not for an individual person but rather for a group of patients with a disease. This is different from clinical practice where the goal is to treat individual patients. As an illustration, a question for a practicing clinician treating a patient may be, "Will administration of ibuprofen to Mr. X who has pain in his knee improve his symptoms?" In a clinical trial, the question may be, "Will administering ibuprofen to patients with arthritis decrease their symptoms?" It is not sufficient that ibuprofen improves knee pain in Mr. X; the goal of a clinical trial is whether as a group, most (or a sufficient proportion) of patients with knee pain of a certain type benefit. Clinical trials can eventually lead to improved therapies for a large group of patients if the treatment is demonstrated to be effective.

CTM is primarily a methodological science, in that it is primarily concerned with *how* to best answer such questions, not *what* the specific answer is. In other words, CTM is concerned not with the answer to questions such as, "Do ACE inhibitors slow the progression of renal disease?" Regardless of the answer, if the results are definitive, then CTM has served its purpose. Nor is it concerned with *which* clinical questions to study or how to apply the results to specific patients. Rather, it is concerned with determining what is the best way to design trials to answer such questions.

To put it another way, the goal of CTM is not to be able to declare, "ACE inhibitors slow the progression of renal disease." Its goal is to be able to say, "A double-blind, placebo-controlled study using measured creatinine as an endpoint at 6 months will answer the question, but a single arm study using calculated creatinine at 4 weeks will not." As an analogy, CTM is to clinical medicine what an architect is to the house builder, or what a coach is to an athlete.

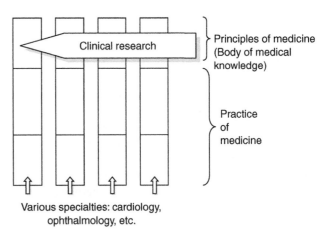

FIGURE 1.1 Technical research medicine in context.

In this way, CTM is more similar to other methodological fields such as statistics, education, or epistemology than to most other branches of medicine.

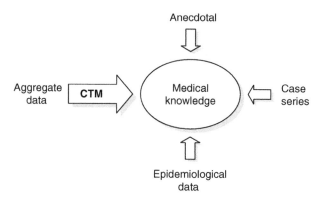

FIGURE 1.2   Sources of medical knowledge.

CTM as Methodological Science

The body of data generated by CTM is usually added to specific disciplines such as cardiology, oncology, and gastroenterology. Only the methodological advances are added to the body of CTM knowledge. For example, the answer to the question, "Does administering ACE inhibitors to patients with diabetes slow the progression of renal disease?" would enter the body of knowledge for nephrology. The answer to the question, "What is the best way to answer questions of this type where disease progression is slow, and surrogate markers are only partially validated?" would enter the body of knowledge for CTM.

1.1.2 Epistemology of Medicine

As was previously mentioned, CTM is only one of several possible ways of generating medical knowledge. Indeed, knowledge acquired through clinical trials, especially prospective, randomized, controlled clinical trials, is the exception rather than the rule in medicine. Historically – and even today – much of the body of medical knowledge was based on other types of evidence, such as personal experience, historical knowledge, case reports, and observational studies (Figure 1.2). Commonly, intuition and pathophysiological rationale have also played important roles in shaping medical thinking. Habits and practice patterns based on informal knowledge have been handed down from one generation of physicians to the next, usually without formal verification or validation.   .

In many instances, traditional methods worked adequately, and even now, clinical trials are not always necessary. For much of medicine, particularly those branches not concerned with intervention, traditional sources of knowledge are acceptable. These include branches such as diagnosis, prognosis, education, and monitoring. Even for interventions, CTM is not always the most rigorous nor the most practical way of generating data. In cases where it is impossible to blind treatments, in cases where it would be unethical to randomize patients, and in cases of extremely rare diseases, formal, rigorous clinical trials may not be the best option. As an example, for advanced colon cancer, where the survival is less than 5% at 5 years, efficacy of a drug that achieves 100% survival at 10 years can be established even without a controlled clinical trial. A small case series may be sufficient to establish efficacy.

Evidence-Based Medicine

It is often thought that "evidence-based medicine" is a modern development. This term is often used with the implication physicians in the past practiced medicine without relying on evidence. This is inaccurate. Our forbearers in medicine practiced a form of evidence-based medicine, but the sources of evidence were different. They did not have the luxury of basing their decisions on aggregate data from large trials – they had little access to such data. They relied on anecdotal data and small case series.

The new paradigm of modern evidence-based medicine is different mostly in that it asserts a hierarchy of evidence, placing randomized controlled clinical trials at the top and others below that. This hierarchy is appropriate in most instances, since in most cases, data generated from randomized, prospective clinical trials is more robust than anecdotal data. It is however not always appropriate, as will be discussed.

Clinical trials are expensive, difficult to conduct, and suffer from some significant validity flaws. Conducting clinical trials for every therapy is neither practical nor prudent, and knowledge generated from other methods is not infrequently both necessary and helpful. However, for many diseases, a clinical trial is the most reliable tool for establishing a causal relationship between intervention and outcome. It may sometime be the only way of establishing effectiveness of a new therapy and developing a new treatment. This is because of randomization, prospective treatment assignment, and large aggregate data sets that characterize well-designed clinical trials (Figure 1.3).

Unlike anecdotal data or small case series, where patient histories can be individually studied and understood, clinical trials have too many patients to allow analysis on an individual level. Rather, they require that aggregate data be analyzed. Large sample size is a major strength of CTM but analysis of aggregate data is neither easy nor intuitive, and fraught with cognitive illusions and intellectual fallacies. In order to avoid inaccurate or spurious conclusions, clinical

	CTM	Anecdotal data	Case series	Epidemiology
Prospective?	Yes	Yes	Sometimes	Sometimes
Active intervention?	Yes	Yes	No	No
Assigned, unbiased intervention?	Yes	No	N/A	N/A
Aggregate data?	Yes	No	Sometimes	Yes
Blinded?	Yes	No	No	No
Representative of clinical practice?	No	Yes	Yes	Yes
Unbiased, random sample?	No	No	Sometimes	Sometimes

FIGURE 1.3   Characteristics of different sources of medical knowledge.

trials must be designed, executed, and analyzed in a rigorous way. CTM provides the tools to accomplish this.

1.1.3 Case Studies, Personal Observations, and Case Series

As noted above, most medical knowledge has been generated through accumulation of anecdotal data by individual physicians over time, and passed down through generations. Informal experience, such as personal observations, historical knowledge, case studies, and case series are effective ways of accumulating, clarifying, and disseminating such knowledge. In many instances, this type of knowledge is invaluable, and has been critical in advancement of medical care. Some examples include case series of Wegener's Granulomatosis and retrospective analysis of Reye's syndrome. In addition, the intellectual tools required to observe, describe, and assimilate such knowledge usually come readily to an average physician because they draw upon the arts of physical examination and diagnosis. These are skills used in daily practice.

The drawback to this approach is that the number of cases any individual physician or even an institution encounters is usually small. It is also difficult to enlarge the data set by pooling the experience of multiple physicians. Data collected by different persons, under different conditions, documented in different ways, can be difficult to collate and interpret. In addition, knowledge obtained this way is commonly fraught with confounding factors. In short, the probability of inaccurate conclusions based on these types of sources tends to be higher than conclusions drawn from randomized, controlled clinical trials.

Many treatments that were supported by conventional wisdom, and many practices based on knowledge distilled from thousands of physician-years of expert experience have subsequently been demonstrated to be erroneous. A classic example is the digoxin and cardioversion. Digoxin had previously enjoyed general acceptance as being efficacious for cardioversion of atrial fibrillation until well-designed

controlled randomized clinical trials were performed. The trials conclusively demonstrated that digoxin is ineffective in inducing cardioversion.

1.1.4 Epidemiology and Observational Data

One formal – as opposed to anecdotal – source of knowledge is epidemiology. This discipline relies on surveys, close recording of aggregate data, retrospective studies, registries, and prospective nonrandomized studies. Unlike case histories, epidemiology relies on a quantitative data set collected in a consistent enough manner to allow mathematical and statistical analysis.

Example: Matches and Lung Cancer

Correlation does not establish causation. A classic demonstration of this is the relationship between matches and lung cancer. There is a strong correlation between carrying of matches and risk of lung cancer, but matches do not cause cancer. Rather, many people who carry matches do so because they smoke, and smoking causes lung cancer. A randomized trial that assigned one group to carry matches and another not to carry matches would find that there was no difference in lung cancer rates between the two groups.

Epidemiology is a sister discipline of CTM. The two disciplines are similar to each other, particularly with respect to the inferential method of drawing conclusions. However, epidemiology, unlike clinical trials, does not involve an active intervention and therefore does not normally lead to causal inferences. It can establish correlations between patient characteristics or therapies and outcome, but correlations do not establish causation in and of themselves.

Formal observational knowledge can come from cross-sectional surveys, case-controlled studies, and cohort studies.

A cross-sectional study is a survey that collects risk factors and outcome data in a group at one point of time and examines the data for correlations. A case-controlled study compares a group of patients with a disease to a group without, and explores risk factors in the past. A cohort study examines a group with a risk factor and one without and follows them prospectively for the disease.

Note: Epidemiology and Safety Data

As an aside, one aspect of CTM that overlaps with epidemiology is the monitoring and analysis of safety data. This branch of CTM relies heavily on epidemiology, as will be discussed in a later section of this book.

1.2 RATIONALE FOR CLINICAL TRIALS

1.2.1 Scientific Rationale

As noted above, there are multiple paths to medical knowledge. Reliable medical knowledge, particularly about efficaciousness of interventions, is difficult to glean for most diseases and most interventions. There are several reasons for this, and a modern randomized, controlled, prospective clinical trial can address most of these factors.

The first reason is the difficulty of determining whether an outcome represents a true signal or just background noise. For example, administering a new compound to one patient (or even to 10) and observing that the patient recovers from pneumonia doesn't establish that the drug cured the infection. This is because most diseases have variable outcome; anecdotal evidence is subject to tremendous biases and confounding factors; and most drugs only work partially. The patient could have spontaneously recovered from pneumonia, as many patients do.

There is great variability in the onset, course, and outcome of many common diseases. For example, only a few of the patients exposed to *M. leprae* contract leprosy; only a fraction of the patients who harbor *H. pylori* develop ulcers; and only some of the patients who experience a myocardial infarction develop lethal arrhythmias. There is also great variability in response to many therapies. Statins prevent cardiovascular events in only a fraction of patients who receive them; infliximab induces a response in only a fraction of rheumatoid arthritis patients; and aspirin relieves headache in only some patients, some of the time.

As another example, psoriasis is a disease with a waxing and waning course. Most drugs for the disease work in some patients but only sporadically, and in other patients never. Small uncontrolled series or trials in psoriasis often will yield misleading results because some drugs will seem to work when in fact they have no effect. Just by chance, some patients' symptoms will spontaneously regress.

Clinical trials, with (usually) large aggregate data sets, randomization, and blinding, can often overcome these issues of variability and noise.

The second argument against relying on informal observations or nonrandomized studies is the difficulty in distinguishing between a result due to a bias vs. a result due to a real effect. For example, when a patient and/or the treating physician know that a therapy is being administered, there may be a placebo effect. For another, a physician conducting a psoriasis trial might under-report the area of body affected by psoriasis when he or she is measuring the response.

Another potential source of bias is imbalance between the treatment groups. The group receiving the intervention, for example, may be younger and healthier than the one not receiving it. The outcome in that group may be better than the control group, not because of the intervention but because they were healthier to begin with. In addition, there can be regression to the mean in waxing and waning diseases, in that any therapy administered during flares will seem to improve symptoms in some patients, just due to the natural history of the disease.

Clinical trials can ameliorate or eliminate these biases and issues. Blinding can reduce the placebo effect and randomization can reduce imbalances in patient characteristics between the groups.

The third argument against informal observations as the sole source of medical knowledge is the hazards of multiple *post hoc* analyses. Given any set of data, and given sufficient numbers of analysis of subgroups and endpoints, it is possible to link almost any therapeutic intervention to an outcome. In other words, if the data is analyzed enough times in enough different ways, one can often find a convincing association between therapy and outcome. For example, it is often possible to find correlations between even patently trivial characteristics such as zodiac signs and response rate. On average, looking at the data in 20 different ways can be expected to yield one spurious association with a p value of 0.05 or less.

Prospective clinical trials prespecify one primary endpoint. This minimizes the risk of spurious results. By convention, a randomized, prospective clinical trial that demonstrates a difference between a treated group and an untreated group for the prespecified primary endpoint with a p value of less than 0.05 is accepted as having established a causal relationship. This convention does not eliminate the possibility of spurious results, but does make it much less likely, and establishes a common language and common ground for decisions on whether an intervention was effective.

The fourth and most important rationale for limiting reliance on informal knowledge, especially knowledge based on retrospective data, is the need to establish causation. Although in some special cases, it is possible to establish causation – for example, that a drug can treat or cure a disease – purely based on anecdotal or informal knowledge, this is the exception. In most cases, it is not possible to establish causation without randomized intervention. For example, patients who ingest aspirin might be found to have low incidence of cardiovascular events. Based on that information alone, it is possible to postulate that aspirin lowers the risk of cardiovascular events, but other possible explanations cannot be ruled out. An alternate reason might be that patients who exercise more tend to injure their knees more and tend to take aspirin for their aching joints. Or, it may be that a diet low in fat is more likely to cause dental caries and patients therefore take more aspirin to relieve the dental pain.

The opposite is also true: confounding may mask causal association. As an example, myocardial infarction patients who appear to be sicker might be more likely to receive thrombolytics than ones who appear less sick. Those patients who received thrombolytics would have different characteristics from those who did not. As a result, the group receiving the intervention may not do better than the one not receiving it, despite the intervention being effective. Of course, multivariate analysis can tease out some of the effects due to differences in the patient population, but such analysis has significant limitations, not the least of which is that multivariate modeling can only adjust for measured confounders.

Therefore, a clinical trial – ideally, a randomized prospective clinical trial – is the optimal (or sometimes the only) way of establishing clear causation. In a randomized prospective trial, the assignment to treatment groups is arbitrary and uninfluenced by preferences or characteristics of the patient and the physician. And the intervention precedes the clinical outcome. Only by randomizing patients to intervention groups in a prospective fashion, with the intervention assigned independent of patient or physician characteristics and occurring prior to outcome, can causation be definitely established.

In summary, the advantages of a rigorous, randomized, well-controlled clinical trial is that it can establish causation, limit the placebo effect, avoid spurious conclusions, and yield reliable information.

1.2.2 Regulatory Rationale

The second major reason for performing randomized clinical trials is that new drugs and therapies must demonstrate efficacy in such a trial before it can be registered. This reason is related to the scientific reason, in that the scientific rationale drives the regulatory requirements. Regulatory approvals of new therapies generally require clear evidence of efficacy and safety. These usually can come only from well-designed and well-conducted randomized prospective clinical trials.

1.3 LIMITATIONS OF CLINICAL TRIALS

Although the randomized, prospective clinical trials constitute the gold standard for investigating interventions, they are imperfect and have important limitations. The two most critical limitations are generalizability and effectiveness. In addition, there are several less critical, though still important, limitations regarding some fundamental assumptions behind clinical trials and analysis of aggregate biological data. These assumptions are sometimes inappropriate. Furthermore, data from clinical trials can only be one of the considerations that go into a medical decision.

Generalizability refers to the appropriateness of extrapolating the results from a study to the general patient population as a whole. Clinical trials normally enroll a sample or a subset of patients with a disease. For example, there might be millions of patients with multiple sclerosis worldwide, but a clinical trial might enroll only a thousand of the patients. The data from the thousand patients might be used to guide treatment of all other multiple sclerosis patients. This is appropriate only if the results of the study are generalizable.

In order for a clinical trial to be truly generalizable, it ought to enroll a random sample of patients with a disease, the patient population should reflect the patient population at large, and it should manage the patients in a way similar to the way they would be managed by a typical physician in clinical practice. Otherwise, the likelihood that the overall patient population will respond to the intervention in the same way as the patients in the clinical trial is diminished.

None of these conditions is fully fulfilled in a typical clinical trial. Enrollment is never at random, inclusion and exclusion criteria often define a patient population somewhat different from the patient population at large, and the patients in a clinical trial receive different types of care than the patient population at large.

Closely related to generalizability is effectiveness. Clinical trials test efficacy, not effectiveness, of a drug. The goal of a clinical trial is usually to determine the true difference between a drug and placebo. In order to accomplish this goal, many artificial restrictions and atypical processes are common in clinical trials. This includes frequent visits to the physician, extra attention by the health care staff, processes to maximize compliance, prohibition of concomitant medications, and so on.

Frequently, results of clinical trial may be an overestimate or underestimate of the effect likely to be seen in true clinical practice. For example, overestimation may occur since compliance tends to be higher in well-run clinical trials. On the other hand, clinical trial results are often analyzed with rigorous methodologies imputing worst possible outcome against the drug arm for missing data, and therefore conclusions may underestimate the effectiveness of the drug.

The question of how much clinical benefit a drug will deliver in community-based clinical practice is a different question from whether the drug can improve outcome in a tightly controlled clinical trial. Sometimes called external validity, effectiveness is influenced by factors such as compliance in real life, interaction with other medications, benefit from placebo effect, etc.

In addition to the above two limitations, there are some assumptions and approximations that are implicit in clinical trials. These include assumption of linearity of biological phenomena, assumption of a normal distribution for patient and outcome parameters, assumption that environmental factors (e.g., bacterial resistance patterns) and clinical practice patterns remain stable over time, and so on. These assumptions are usually reasonable but never completely accurate. Assumption of linearity, for example, is necessary in order for mean blood pressure to be calculable. The difference between 95 mmHg and 100 mmHg (of 5 mmHg) is assumed to be equivalent to the difference between 120 mmHg and 125 mmHg. Otherwise, adding and subtracting blood pressure to derive mean blood pressure would be meaningless. An assumption that practice patterns and patient characteristics remain constant from the first patient to the last patient is a prerequisite required to aggregate clinical trial data for analysis in a meaningful way.

In some cases, these assumptions are clearly inappropriate. For example, leprosy rates have decreased over time, *H. pylori* is nearing extinction in some populations, and asthma rates are increasing rapidly in industrialized countries. And practice patterns and patients certainly change over time. If a trial lasts for a long time, the consistency of patient and clinical treatment characteristics over time cannot be guaranteed.

Also, there are inherent assumptions about definition of diseases and patient groups. For example, all trials must define inclusion and exclusion criteria that rely on assumptions about whether and which patients can be grouped together – whether to distinguish, for example, between patients with different genotypes or from different geographies. The assumptions about the group of patients enrolled, that they share similar pathophysiology and response to therapy, are usually but not always appropriate. For example, grouping patients with ST elevation myocardial infarctions with patients with non-ST elevation myocardial infarctions may be appropriate for a trial of bivalirudin but not for thrombolytics, since thrombolytics do not appear to benefit the non-ST elevation myocardial infarction patients. Grouping patients with myocardial infarctions with patients undergoing bypass surgery may be appropriate for a trial of antiplatelet agent but not for a trial of anti-inflammatory agent.

Ideally, conducting a trial in a highly homogeneous population, or within the smallest subcategorization of patients, would yield the highest likelihood that the results can be generalizable to that population, but there are not enough resources to conduct clinical trial, with current methodologies, in each niche indication. It is not practical, for example, to do a study just on patients with anterior myocardial infarctions, with ST elevation greater than 2 mm, who have had symptoms for 4–6 hours. Instead, the category of enrollable patients might be patients with anterior or inferior myocardial infarctions, with ST elevation greater than 1 mm, who have had symptoms for 0–12 hours.

Another limitation is the practical limitation on the amount of data that can be collected. Given the finite number of patients that can be enrolled in a clinical trial, and finite length of follow-up, it is often impossible to collect the amount of data one would like. Estimation of rare safety events can be particularly difficult, because rare events may not appear in even a large database. Also, demonstrating an effect on a rarely occurring endpoint can be difficult, and sometimes surrogates are required.

There are also some fundamental assumptions about drugs themselves that are sometimes not appropriate. For example, a common assumption is that the drug dose can be reproduced from pill to pill and batch to batch. It is assumed that 100 mg of a drug will always have the same exact amount of drug and consistent amount of other ingredients and contaminants. For biologics, this assumption can be particularly tenuous, and it is sometimes necessary to test the biologics that come from several different batches and have a range of characteristics such as molecular weight, *N*-terminal modifications, and glycosylation patterns in the patients to verify that the differences don't affect the outcome.

Similarly, there are often constraints on the way that the patients are treated with regard to dosing frequency, compliance, and other characteristics that may be in conflict with the assumptions of clinical trials. These limitations will be discussed later in this book.

Finally, much of medical treatment is driven by art rather than science. Even in instances where data regarding intervention and outcome are available, it is sometimes overshadowed by nonscientific considerations such as tradition, patient preference, and practical considerations. For example, many physicians often base medical decisions not solely on data and teleological considerations but also on deontological factors such as practice guidelines or knowledge of what their peers are doing in a particular situation – standard of care, in other words. For example, they may prescribe IV nitroglycerin to myocardial infarction patients because other physicians in the city do so, while in another city, different practice may prevail.

Often, physicians also base interventions on the philosophy that making the patients feel better through comfort, reassurance, and education is as important as or more important than whether the clinical outcome is improved. Of course, patients' preferences, family and caregivers' preferences, and logistic constraints such as cost and availability of therapy (particularly in less affluent societies) also play an important role.

1.4 CHARACTERISTICS AND PERFORMANCE CRITERIA OF CTM

1.4.1 Characteristics of Clinical Trial Medicine

As was previously noted, the goal of a clinical trial is not directly to maximize benefit to the patients in the trial but rather to discover whether a treatment is effective and safe. Viewed another way, the goal of the clinical trial is to render causal conclusions between the treatment and outcome, both efficacy outcome and safety outcome. In order to accomplish this, the trials are designed, conducted, and analyzed along specific principles, and share particular characteristics. This set of principles and characteristics make up CTM. For example, CTM relies on statistical inference and aggregate data that are collected in a quantitative manner to render causal conclusions.

Perhaps the most salient characteristic of CTM is that it is a stochastic science: it is a probabilistic science. This is because, as was previously mentioned, unlike some other scientific fields, there is tremendous variability in the subject matter when it comes to clinical trials. Patients are heterogeneous, may be taking different concomitant medications, be subject to different practice patterns, and so on.

Of course, there are many branches of science where the outcome is variable and the effects of intervention are also variable. In these cases, there are several traditional approaches to elucidating cause and effect. The most common method is the reductionist one. Classical physics provides a good example. In physics, complex phenomena are broken down into basic elements, such as mass, speed, inertia, etc. and basic laws have been elucidated to describe and predict behavior of objects. In physics, if mass and velocity are known, then momentum can be calculated with certainty. Reductionist approaches are helpful when the scientific problem can be broken down into small pieces, each piece investigated separately, and then a fuller understanding achieved by reassembling the pieces. For example, each part of a metabolic cycle might be studied in isolation and knowledge of the overall metabolic cycle built up one step at a time.

In rare cases, the variability in clinical trials can be addressed by classic reductionist methods – for example, by enrolling a very homogeneous patients population or a population that has a specific genetic marker. Perhaps some day in the future, pathogenesis of diseases and variability among patients will be understood well enough so that a reductionist approach can be generally applied to medicine. However, the current state of medical knowledge is such that this is not possible. There are too many independent variables in diseases, patients, and interventions. It is not possible for example to identify all genes, all environmental factors, and other factors to predict with certainty how a patient will respond to a therapeutic intervention. (In a small number of cases, the contributing effect of one factor, such as tumor or sepsis is so overwhelming that the outcome is highly predictable, but as previously mentioned, these examples are rare.)

Instead of a reductionist method, clinical trials rely on collecting aggregate data. The problem of variability is addressed via repeated measurements on multiple patients. Rather than using a reductionist approach utilizing deterministic methods, clinical trials are conducted and analyzed with statistical methods (apart from a few specific corners of CTM, such as metabolism and pharmacokinetics/pharmacodynamics).

Note: Stochasticism vs. Determinism

Traditional science is based on deductive reasoning: linear conclusion based on assumptions and logic. CTM is a probabilistic science, and relies on induction and inference for conclusions (but based on strict conventions relating to standards for accepting such inferences, such as p value <0.05).

Indeed, statistical analysis on aggregate data lies at the heart of CTM. CTM is an inferential science. It is not possible to draw any conclusions from clinical trials with absolute certainty. From clinical trials, it is only possible to infer that something is likely or unlikely. This type of science, probabilistic science, is called stochasticism, and it is very different from deductive or deterministic science.

In general, a clinical trial is concerned with testing a hypothesis, generally with the requirement that the results have less than 5% likelihood of occurring by chance if the null hypothesis were true. Its goal is to determine whether an intervention has an effect on outcome.

However, a clinical trial is sometimes concerned with determining the mechanism of action, such as "will a non-steroidal anti-inflammatory drug (NSAID) improve arthritis," and sometimes it is concerned with diagnostics, such as "will response to ibuprofen predict the likelihood of responding to other NSAID or the likelihood of worsening symptoms over the next 5 years." But these tend to be the exceptions rather than the rule. CTM is an applied science, not basic science, and the goal is to discover actionable knowledge that can be used by clinicians.

Also, a clinical trial is a scientific experiment, and like other scientific experiments, the goal is to keep all variables constant except for one – in this case the intervention – and to measure whether there is a difference in outcome between the group that received the intervention and the one that did not. For example, in a trial of a new drug for knee pain, it would not be prudent to have some patients receive acetaminophen and some not, to have some patients rest their knee and others run marathons, and to put all the acute knee pain in one treatment group and chronic in the other. While there are various techniques to compensate for imbalances, such as matching, multivariate analysis, etc., the most effective way to minimize imbalance between the treatment groups is through prospective randomization.

A clinical trial assigns patients prospectively to a treatment group. Usually, the assignment is via randomization. This is necessary in order to establish causation. This is in contrast to an observational study where the physician or patient selects the treatment. It prescribes an intervention.

A clinical trial assesses outcome with a quantitative measurement that can be applied across many patients by many assessors. This is in contrast to qualitative assessments or assessments that are so highly operator dependent as to make aggregation of data meaningless.

A clinical trial also involves people. As such, there are strict constraints on how a trial is conducted. For example, Phase I trials are usually conducted in a dose escalation manner. Nonparallel dosing groups violate a cardinal rule in clinical trial design, but parallel dosing is not possible in most first-in-man trials because of patient safety issues, which obviously trump all other considerations.

Finally, CTM relies on aggregate, quantitative data, not qualitative data. Clinicians utilize two types of data: qualitative and quantitative. Qualitative data consists of descriptive, nonaggregate data such as a case history. The details of an individual's past medical history, the doses of medication, the physical examination on each visit, etc. can be evaluated in rich detail, and a conclusion drawn from it. The conclusions are usually based on pattern recognition and qualitative associations, such as, "every patient I've seen in the last 10 years with a particular distinctive rash and arthritis turned out to have a particular infection that resolved with treatment with a certain antibiotic, therefore this particular patient with the same rash and arthritis may respond to the antibiotic." Typically, in clinical practice, this is the type of data that physicians rely upon.

Qualitative data interpretation is often also utilized for evaluation of safety data which involves looking at individual case characteristics such as concomitant medications, the specific characteristics of the outcome, etc. The outcome is not necessarily a proof but rather the purpose of the analysis is signal detection. For safety data, this is useful because for potential safety issues, a nondefinitive signal is often enough to impact course of action.

The heart of CTM, though, is interpretation of quantitative aggregate data, stripped of some of the details but standardized in such a way that aggregate analysis is possible.

Example: A Typical Clinical Trial

Let's trace the steps in experimental design that leads from a noncausal associative knowledge to well-controlled prospective randomized trial. As an example, let's discuss how one might investigate the question, "What should Mr. X do when he has an episode of knee pain?" The first step might be to review things in the past that might have helped his pain, such as hot bathes, ibuprofen, massages, etc. In this way, we might establish a correlation between improvement in pain and an intervention, but it is almost impossible to establish causation. For example, there might be a good correlation between massages and relief of pain, but it may be that Mr. X received massages only when the pain lasted more than a week, and it just happened that the maximum duration of this particular type of pain was no more than 10 days.

The simplest example of a prospective clinical trial might be to give Mr. X some randomimab the next time he has knee pain, and to determine whether the pain improves. This is a clinical trial in its simplest form – an unblinded, uncontrolled, nonrandomized, prospective clinical trial.

In order to do this, though, it would be necessary to define what improvement means, and how to measure the improvement, is it sufficient if Mr. X feels better, or would objective signs such as swelling need to improve?

Also, it is not possible to determine from one experiment whether randomimab was the cause of his relief. It might have been a fluke.

So one might try giving Mr. X randomimab for his knee on several occasions when he has knee pain. This would prove reproducibility, but then the next question would be whether the natural history of his knee pain was such that it would spontaneously improve on its own.

The next refinement of the clinical trial might be to alternate or use some random sequence or treatment. He might receive randomimab on some occasions and nothing on others. If there were a correlation between randomimab and relief, this would be stronger evidence. The next question then becomes whether there is placebo effect.

A better method might be to alternate randomimab with placebo. This would help establish a causal relationship between randomimab and relief, if one were to assume certain things, such as: the knee pain is same type of pain in each occurrence, the patient remained blinded, etc. By causal relationship, we mean the conclusion that if Mr. X were to receive randomimab for his knee pain in the future, then his pain would improve.

These sets of experiments however, would not necessarily lead to the conclusion that if other patients with knee pain were to receive randomimab then they would improve as well. In order to establish that, a group of patients with knee pain would need to be tested. Also, in many diseases, such as stroke, it is not possible to repeat multiple trials of a medicine on the same patient because the patient does not return to baseline, or only has one or few episodes of the symptoms in his or her life. Because of these and other reasons, clinical trials are generally conducted in a group of patients with a disease. It is of course important to define which disease population of patients to test. Fortunately, often, clinical practitioners have defined groups of patients into "diseases" and it is often useful to use these categories. However, these should just be a starting point.

1.4.2 The Practice of CTM

Although CTM is largely a methodological discipline, it has important practical aspects. It is methodological in that like the field of statistics, CTM is largely concerned with the theoretical issues, such as what kind of data to collect, in what fashion, and what kind of conclusions to draw from the data. It has a practical aspect in that there are logistics, real-world issues and constraints that must be addressed in order to collect and verify the data. The practice of CTM (as opposed to the principles or theory of CTM) can be divided into a clinical and a nonclinical aspect.

The primary clinical aspect is protection of patient safety. In the course of a clinical trial, clinical knowledge has to be brought to bear real-time in order to assess safety events, understand them, and collate them; and in some cases, alter the conduct of the study in response to safety signals. In the design of a clinical protocol, clinical judgment is required to ensure that the dose and other aspects of the trial protect patient safety.

It is because of this aspect of CTM that it is a branch of medicine, and more importantly, why the most important principle of CTM is the same as in any branch of medicine: do no harm.

After a drug is marketed, there is additional safety surveillance responsibility that is part of CTM where clinical judgment and practice is required.

The nonclinical practical aspect of CTM includes assurance of quality, Good Clinical Practice (GCP), and other practical aspects of running a trial and assuring data integrity.

1.5 TYPES OF CLINICAL STUDIES

1.5.1 Types of Therapies

Although CTM is most commonly used for investigating efficacy and safety of drugs, its scope spans across a wide variety of therapies. They include all of the following (non-exhaustive list):

1. Drugs
   - Small molecules
     - Enzyme inhibitors
     - Nutrients/Vitamins
     - Antibiotics
     - Receptor antagonists
   - Biologics
     - Proteins and peptides
     - Antibodies and antibody mimetics
     - Blood and blood products
     - Therapeutic vaccines
     - Viruses
     - Probiotics
   - Oligonucleotides
     - Antisense RNA
     - siRNA, miRNA
2. Prophylactic vaccines
   - DNA vaccines
   - Protein vaccines
   - Killed or attenuated organisms
3. Gene therapies
4. Devices
   - Electronic devices
   - Monitoring devices
   - Drug delivery devices
   - Stents
   - Photo and UV therapies
5. Drug/Delivery Combinations
6. Psychotherapy
7. Surgical procedures

Regardless of therapeutic modality, the principles outlined in this book can be applied across the entire spectrum listed above. The key requirements are that the therapeutic modality is intended to affect clinical outcome or a surrogate outcome, that the therapy can be applied a large number of patients in an assigned or randomized fashion, and that the therapy can be applied consistently so that the results can be aggregated and compared.

1.5.2 Descriptive vs. Hypothesis Testing Trials

There are multiple ways to categorize clinical trials, but one of the most important distinctions is between descriptive trials and hypothesis-testing trials.

Descriptive trials are trials such as open label safety trials and pharmacokinetic/pharmacodynamic studies, in which the goal is to characterize a clinical or laboratory phenomenon after an intervention. They do not test hypothesis and do not establish causation between intervention and clinical outcome. Nonetheless, they are often important for hypothesis generation, efficacy characterization, safety characterization, establishment of risk–benefit, and guidance of therapy. Phase I studies are usually descriptive trials.

Descriptive trials can sometimes be confused with historically controlled trials, but the distinction between the two is important. Descriptive trials are not intended to establish correlation and causation. Studies that are called uncontrolled trials are often actually historical controlled, and are intended to establish causation. For example, a trial that describes the long-term survival rate after administration of a chemotherapeutic agent can be descriptive if the primary endpoint of short-term survival has already been established, and the long-term survival is meant to collect additional information to guide use of the drug. It may be an uncontrolled trial if its goal is to establish initial efficacy, there is good historical control data, and the anticipated benefit is far greater than historical controls – for instance, if the survival rate is 0% after 1 year and the drug is expected to result in 80% survival.

Descriptive trials are important, but at the heart of CTM are trials that test hypothesis. This is because the main goal of CTM is to determine whether an intervention improves outcome. A randomized, controlled, prospective clinical trial is usually the most definitive way to obtain this information. This book is mostly concerned with design of such trials, and methods for optimizing such trials.

Of course, most hypothesis-testing trials usually include multiple descriptive secondary endpoints that are ancillary to the primary endpoint. In a sense, almost all studies have descriptive components. Strictly speaking, it would be more correct to classify endpoints rather than trials as hypothesis-testing or descriptive. But by convention, if a study has a primary endpoint that is testing a hypothesis, the study is considered to be hypothesis-testing, and if not, descriptive. The critical difference between the descriptive and hypothesis-testing endpoints is establishment of causal relationships.

Within the category of hypothesis-testing trials, the archetypical trial is the randomized, prospective, parallel-group, placebo-controlled, two-arm trials (Figure 1.4). Essentially all clinical trials are prospective, since it is otherwise almost impossible to establish causation, but the other typical characteristics of hypothesis-testing trials are variable.

Most trials are randomized because randomization is usually the most rigorous way to assign treatment. All hypothesis-testing trials assign patients to treatment in some fashion, even if it is an assignment method other than randomization. Without assignment, it is not possible to establish causation in a rigorous fashion, because this is the only way to make certain that the treatment choice has not been influenced by a factor associated with the outcome. For example, if the treatment choice is left up to the physician, he might consciously or subconsciously select the sickest patients to receive the drug and less sick to receive placebo.

Most hypothesis-testing trials are parallel group, because it is usually the cleanest way to compare groups, but several other temporal sequencing schemes exist, including dose-escalation and crossover. These are discussed in chapters 6 and 10.

Clinical trials most often have two arms, and almost always test for superiority of one arm over the other. However, multiple arms are possible, and nonequivalence and noninferiority trials are possible. Nonequivalence trials are multiple dose trials where the goal is to determine whether one arm is different from the others. In noninferiority trials, the goal is to demonstrate that the two arms are relatively similar. In all cases, however, there is at least one control group.

Most trials also tend to be directed toward treating rather than preventing disease. However, there are multiple other types of trials. There are trials in patient with a disease where the goal is to reverse the disease, such as antibiotic trials in patients with pneumonia; trials in patients with a disease where the goal is to prevent worsening of the disease, such as chemotherapy in cancer patients; trials in patients at risk for a disease where the goal is to prevent the disease, such as varicella vaccine in young children. Even for the same disease, such as psoriasis, there can be several different potential types of trials, such as trials to induce remission or to maintain remission.

In addition, there are multiple additional degrees of freedom in clinical trial design, such as fixed dose vs. weight-based dose vs. dose titrated to effect. This book addresses these and other topics.

1.6 PERFORMANCE CRITERIA FOR WELL-DESIGNED CLINICAL TRIALS

1.6.1 Criteria

The criteria that distinguish well-designed trials from poorly designed ones are multiple. A clinical trial is a scientific endeavor, so the first criterion is, "are the results accurate"? In other words, does it render an accurate answer to the hypothesis? This is sometimes referred to as internal validity.

Furthermore, it is an applied science, so the second criterion is, are the results of the study useful? Usefulness can be divided into three parts. In most cases, positive results are more useful than negative result, so is the study optimized for likelihood of positive result? However, positive results are only useful if the question that is being posed does an adequate job of capturing the manifestations of the disease – it is not useful to improve one symptom of a disease while worsening another. So, is the question being posed by the trial well-formed? Also, is the study designed so that the results are applicable to real-life patients, and will they be of use to the practicing clinician? This is sometimes referred to as external validity.

A clinical trial is different from most applied sciences in that the subjects are human, so the third criterion, and a criterion that is more important than all others, is, does the trial protect patient safety and is it ethical? Does it limit risk to subjects by involving the fewest number of patients

Invariant requirement of hypothesis-testing clinical trials	Variable properties of hypothesis-testing clinical trials
Prospective intervention	Randomization vs. other ways of assignment
Assignment to treatment groups	Number of treatment groups
At least one control group	Superiority vs. other testing
Null hypothesis	Type of outcome being tested

FIGURE 1.4   Propeties of hypothesis-testing clinical trials.

necessary? Finally, clinical trials are expensive and difficult to carry out, so the fourth criterion is, "is the trial efficient and feasible to carry out?" These criteria are discussed below.

Are the Results Accurate?

The most important goal of a well-designed clinical trial is to render clear and accurate answer to the hypothesis. In other words, it must yield the correct answer to the question being asked, which is usually whether the drug candidate is effective. The result of a clinical trial can be classified into three categories: accurate result, inaccurate result, and uninterpretable result.

Accurate result: A well-designed clinical trial will maximize the likelihood that a trial will yield accurate result: positive result (statistically significant) when the drug works, and negative result (lack of significance) when the drug does not. Even a well-designed trial will not guarantee an accurate result, but it will maximize the likelihood.

Inaccurate result: Statistical fluke or a fundamental design flaw(s) can lead to an inaccurate result: positive result when the drug does not actually work, and negative result when it does work.

Uninterpretable result: Worse than an inaccurate result, and unfortunately seen nearly as frequently are uninterpretable results. This can be due to insufficient data, for example because the study was underpowered, did not test a high enough dose, or was terminated too early. It may also be due to poor quality data, missing data, patient dropouts, unreliable measurements, etc. It may also be due to failure to minimize bias such that the results are not reliable. All of these flaws can lead to results being unreliable and/or not robust to sensitivity analysis.

Bias

In order for a study to draw valid conclusions, it must be free of bias – that is, systematic error that will make one treatment or another appear superior when in fact there is no difference between the two. The goal of a clinical trial is usually to determine whether difference in a single factor – presence or absence of the intervention or drug – can causally alter the outcome. In other words, all other factors should be identical, including patient population, concomitant treatment, assessment, follow-up, etc.

Any difference in any of the factors between the two groups can create bias, and greater the bias, the more difficult it is to attribute any difference in outcome to the intervention alone.

There are natural imperfections in the trials. There might be too many dropouts. There are issues of imputation. There might be inadvertent unblinding. There might be regression to the mean. There might be too much inter-observer variability. There might be training effects and other biases introduced by the study itself.

Also, like all scientific experiments, clinical trials are conducted in controlled settings. The patients are homogeneous; they receive regular medical attention; etc. This in itself can introduce biases. There are multiple challenges in keeping the trial free of biases, both systematic and random.

Good clinical trial design minimizes the likelihood of these, and makes the analysis plan robust to errors as much as possible. In other words, a well-designed clinical trial has internal validity: the results indicate a causal relationship between the intervention and outcome when such a relationship really exists and vice versa.

Bias can be classified into several categories.

Systematic bias is a systematic error that affects both the control and active arms equally. Examples include training effect, better health care due to patients being in the study, and time bias. All of these can affect the generalizability of the study, but because they affect both control and treated arms equally, do not usually affect the ability to draw conclusions regarding the differences between the arms (internal validity). In some cases, there can be an interaction – for example, results of a complicated surgical or interventional procedure may only be applicable to tertiary care centers with highly advanced staff – but this is the exception. This topic is discussed in depth in a later section.

Differential bias is error that affects one arm more than the other and does represent a threat to internal validity of a study because such biases affect the apparent efficacy of the treatment. One important differential bias is differences in baseline characteristics. These can clearly introduce bias. Randomization, stratification, and in some cases, multivariate adjustment, can address the bias due to imbalances in baseline characteristics.

The other differential bias is differences occurring not at the initiation of the study but during the course of the study, including differences in how the patients are assessed, differential placebo effect, differences in dropout rates, etc. Some of the differences arise as a result of the drug itself – such as differences in efficacy and safety that result in patients being treated differently – but more commonly, they arise because knowledge of treatment arm can lead to different treatments.

There are several other sources of bias: biased selection of patients into the groups, biased assignment of treatment groups, and biased response by the patient due to placebo effect. It is important to minimize bias from all the potential sources.

Is the Study Question Well Formed?

Is the Study Designed to Maximize Likelihood of a Positive Result?

In most instances, a safe and effective therapy is more useful to the clinician than one that is not. Therefore, demonstrating that a therapy is safe and effective for a disease is more desirable than demonstrating that it isn't, except for cases where an ineffective therapy is already in wide use. Therefore a clinical trial design should maximize the likelihood of positive study results. This is different from the question of whether the results are accurate. A study that is well-designed, in addition to yielding accurate results, also poses the right question. For example, a study looking at the impact on 30-day mortality of administering 100 mg of a certain drug in severe sepsis patients may yield an accurate result that it has no impact. However, it may be that 200 mg of the drug in moderate sepsis patients has a beneficial impact on 60-day mortality. Selecting the right patient population, the right dose, and the right endpoint make a crucial difference on the likelihood of success.

Does the Study Question Address the Appropriate Issues?

It is important that the question has construct validity. For instance, if the purpose of the study is to determine whether a thrombolytics has beneficial effect on myocardial infarction patients, including the incidence of re-ischemia and congestive heart failure without including death as part of a composite endpoint might lead to inappropriate conclusions. This is because congestive heart failure and re-ischemia rates might increase even when the therapy is providing a benefit. Patient who would have died might live but with congestive heart failure. Similarly, measuring myelitis without accounting for renal failure in lupus patients may yield erroneous conclusion that the drug is beneficial when in fact it just shifts one manifestation of the disease to another.

Are the Results Generalizable?

As was previously mentioned, the goal of a clinical trial is to generate knowledge about whether an intervention can help patients with a disease. As was also previously mentioned, CTM is a methodological science, but it is used to construct experiments that fall into the realm of applied science, and the end results must be such that they are useful in clinical practice – that is, the knowledge must be generalizable (have external validity and be actionable). It must have external validity in that the types of patients who are enrolled should not be so specific and homogeneous that the results seen in those patients would be different from those in clinical practice. The characteristics of the patients, intervention, and outcome, must be close enough to clinical practice in order to be transferable to everyday practice.

In addition, the results of the clinical trial must be actionable in that the drug should be given in a fashion that would be practicable in the real world. The patients must be treated in a similar fashion as they would be in real practice. For example, administration of a drug 6 times a day would not be practicable in clinical practice.

Early Phase Studies

Of course, for Phase I or II studies that will be followed by a Phase III study, the performance criteria are somewhat different. For example, practicability and generalizability are less important, since both of these generally will be addressed in Phase III. Early phase studies should be to enable later phase studies, to provide clear evidence when a drug candidate is unlikely to ultimately succeed in Phase III, to validate new measurement instruments for Phase III, to provide information to allow appropriate dose selection, and to allow accurate sample size calculation.

Are Patient Safety and Rights Protected?

The most important constraint – and the most important guiding principle in clinical trial design and conduct – is: do no harm. The key guiding principle should be to protect patient safety. And as was previously mentioned, clinical trials are not conducted for the direct benefit of the enrolled patients. Clinical trials, by definition, are primarily directed toward answering a scientific or clinical question that will benefit the broad group of patients with a disease. The patients in the trial may benefit ultimately, but the trials are in general not designed to maximize the direct benefit to the patients in the trial. Therefore, they must be designed to minimize any potential harm to the patients.

Even the best-designed clinical trials expose patients to risks they would not otherwise have faced; so the scientific and clinical justification for the study must be pristine. There must be scientific equipoise. The lowest (or safest) reasonable dose of the drug, given the goals of the study, must be used. Informed consent must be complete and comprehensible. The monitoring of the study must be close and thorough. Alternate treatment, if withheld, must be withheld only when absolutely necessary and opportunity for rescue medication must be provided.

Is the Study Parsimonious? Is It Feasible?

In addition, a well-designed study yields not just the right answer but also the maximum quantity and quality of data while utilizing the least amount of resources. CTM is an applied science, and parsimony is an important goal. A well-designed clinical trial enrolls the fewest number of patients necessary to answer the scientific question or hypothesis being tested. In this way, fewest patients are exposed to risk inherent in all clinical trials. Parsimony is achieved by selecting the right group of patients, selecting the appropriate endpoint (for example, sensitive to the treatment effect), and utilizing appropriate statistical analysis.

This is not to say that no data apart from the primary endpoint should be collected. For example, data that identifies any important subgroups that might have a different risk–benefit profile compared to the overall tested patient population would be important. This type of data collection should be distinguished from indiscriminate collection of information – this is often wasteful if it is not hypothesis driven, and is often not a good return on the resource used.

The clinical trial should also be feasible. It should be designed so that it can be enrolled, the patients can be compliant, the measurement can be taken, and so on. Sometimes the protocol will have unreasonably narrow inclusion criteria, specify very difficult requirements (such as prohibition of common concomitant medications), or require logistically difficult procedures (such as FACS analysis within 12 hours of blood collection). In such cases, the trial will often need to be amended or in some cases terminated early. In either case, the validity of the study is affected. Even in cases that don't require an amendment, the study can become plagued with errors and protocol violations. There are also logistic considerations – for example, it may become prohibitively expensive because of the procedures required.

1.7 CRITICAL PARAMETERS IN CLINICAL TRIAL DESIGN

1.7.1 Design Principles

As was enumerated in the previous section, a well-designed study has to achieve multiple goals: it must have internal and external validity, maximize the likelihood of a positive result, protect patient safety, and be feasible and practicable. In many cases, these priorities are competing, and appropriate trade-offs must be made. For example, making the trial patient population homogeneous might make a positive result more likely and make the study smaller, but it might lessen generalizability and might make enrollment more difficult.

In addition to making appropriate trade-offs, the second major challenge is minimization of biases. This is important in achieving internal validity. For example, the blinding process must be highly rigorous. If there are reactions to the drug administration, side effects, or laboratory parameters that might lead to unblinding, then an appropriate placebo, a blinded assessor, or special blinding procedures are necessary.

Biases can come from outside the study as well. For example, a competing trial enrolling a subset of the patients in question can affect the patient population enrolled. For example, for a myocardial infarction trial taking all comers, if there is a competing trial enrolling only anterior myocardial infarction patients, the resulting enrollment may consist mostly of inferior myocardial infarction patients even though the intent was to enroll a representative group of myocardial infarction patients.

Clinical trial hygiene is a critical and difficult aspect of designing and conducting clinical trials. Poor hygiene, such as changing a major inclusion or exclusion criteria in the middle of a study, can lead to major, gross bias in the study.

The third challenge is to make sure that the assumptions behind the clinical trial are valid. All clinical trials make assumptions – for example, most trials operate under the assumptions that patients respond independently, that they remain blinded, that dropouts are random, and that clinical practice pattern remains unchanged over time. Making wrong assumptions can lead to failure. For example, if the placebo rate is expected to be 20% on the basis of previous clinical trials, and it turns out to be 30%, then the study may be underpowered to demonstrate a benefit. A common mistake is to assume that the degree of benefit seen in Phase II will be replicated in Phase III. Because of regression to the mean, the effect seen in Phase III will often be less impressive than that seen in Phase II. This is particularly true for escalating dose studies. As another example, if the measurement tool used to assess the endpoint is assumed to have linear response, and if the response turns out to be nonlinear, then the statistical analysis methods may need to be modified.

The fourth, and often the greatest, challenge is to ensure that the right question is being asked. No matter how well the trial is designed – even if it does a laudable job of randomization, has appropriate statistical tests, and minimizes other biases – if it asks the wrong question then the study may fail. Each clinical trial is an instance of a particular patient population being treated with a particular dose(s) of the drug, with a particular outcome being measured. If the wrong patient(s)/indication, wrong dose, or wrong endpoint is selected, then the results will be negative, misleading, and/or not generalizable.

1.7.2 Critical Design Variables

In designing a clinical trial, there are multiple trade-offs and many degrees of freedom. The critical parameters in clinical trial design are the appropriate patient population, the appropriate endpoint, and the appropriate dose. There are other subtleties of clinical trial design that are important, including sample size, blinding, comparator arms, boundaries for accepting or rejecting the hypothesis, etc. that are discussed in the following chapters, but these three factors have the greatest impact, and the design choices regarding these are the greatest because there are infinite permutations of patients/doses/endpoints and only a few permutations can be tested.

Implicit in the goal of clinical trials is the assumption that there is a group of subjects who have an undesirable condition (disease) or are at risk of developing an undesirable condition. This brings us to the first step in designing a clinical trial: defining the target and sample populations for the trial. In rare instances, the target population is everyone in the world, such as the target population for the polio vaccine. More typically, it will be necessary to define a group of patients with a set of characteristics and conditions who constitute the target population for the trial. This is the population to whom the results of the study will be generalized or applied. In addition, a group that will be a representative sample drawn from the target population will need to be defined. This is the sample population.

The choice of population, particularly the sample population, is critical. It will determine the likelihood of the intervention showing an effect: if patients whose disease is not responsive to the intervention are included, they could dilute the effect of the intervention. It will determine the ultimate risk–benefit analysis: sicker the group of patients, greater the magnitude of safety issues that can be accepted. The right population will also have an important effect on the practicability of the trial. Narrowing the inclusion criteria, for example, might make internal validity easier to achieve, and might make statistical power greater, but this is often at the expense of generalizability. The appropriate patient population includes patients who are likely to respond to the drug, who will be compliant with therapy, who are homogeneous, and who have an unmet medical need.

Also implicit in clinical trials is the assumption that the difference between the treatment groups can be compared and contrasted. In order to compare the results, at least with the quantitative and statistical tools, it is necessary to measure the outcome. CTM is not a branch of aesthetics. The conclusions are based on manipulation of aggregate data measured and collated in a consistent manner. Therefore, the second critical aspect of clinical trial design is endpoints.

The choice of an appropriate endpoint is perhaps one of the most difficult aspects of clinical trial design. The endpoint must be clinically significant, be responsive to therapy, have low variability, and be representative of the disease status as a whole. Choosing an endpoint that is simple and reductionist might make it easier to determine whether drug exerts an effect on the primary endpoint, but such an endpoint may ignore other clinical parameters and might make generalizability more difficult.

Also implicit in the goal is the assumption that the two comparison groups are two separate groups, uninfluenced by each other. It would make no sense to compare a group to itself. In addition, the assumption is that although the groups are separate, they are groups of similar patients. This is necessary because if there were major underlying differences in the groups, it would be difficult to compare the outcome in the two groups. The groups must be similar enough so that the outcome in the two groups would be similar in the absence of intervention. That way, when there is a difference in outcome, the conclusion can be that the intervention caused the difference. Randomization and blinding are two of the ways that this is achieved.

Finally, selection of the appropriate intervention and dose is critical to the success of the trial. Each group of patients should receive a consistent dose or dosing regimen. Comparison between groups would otherwise be impossible. Careful consideration of the dose must be given. Too high of a dose will result in safety issues, and too low of a dose will result in lack of efficacy. Issues such as whether to adjust based on weight, the route of administration, whether to monitor pharmacokinetics/pharmacodynamics, etc. are all critical questions. These issues are addressed in the subsequent chapters of this book.

Chapter 2

Ethical, Legal, and Regulatory Issues

2.1 RULES AND REGULATIONS

2.1.1 The Reasons for Regulations

Never let your sense of morals prevent you from doing what's right.
Isaac Asimov

There would be a lot more scientific breakthroughs if it weren't for those darn ethics and laws.
Anonymous former business school student

A big part of clinical research is dealing with and conforming to the seemingly innumerable ethical, legal, and regulatory requirements. These requirements can add significant time, cost, and paperwork to your study and even may prevent you from doing the most scientifically rigorous and accurate study. Many people involved in clinical research and drug or device development has at one time or another cursed the administrative hassles associated with executing a study. So it is easy to forget why many rules and regulations are in place.

Seemingly unreasonable rules emerge whenever someone somewhere decides to do something outrageous. It often does not matter if the majority of people would never think of doing something so extreme. Think back to your grade school days. Whenever one kid in your class did something egregious, the entire class suffered. The teacher might have let you bring pets into the classroom until that one day when someone brought in a skunk. After that incident, no more pets were allowed. Chewing gum might have been acceptable until Billy decided to stick a wad of gum into Stephanie's hair. After that incident, no more gum was allowed in the classroom. What happens in grade school also happens in the grown-up world. Governing bodies can operate in a reactive way, and often will revoke privileges from everyone once someone abuses the privileges.

Therefore, to understand the rules and regulations of clinical research and medical product development, you have to understand some of the underlying ethical principles.

While these principles may seem obvious, not everyone knows or heeds them. Knowing the specific ethical principles is important, even if there's little chance that you will consciously violate them. Well-meaning investigators can accidentally overlook some ethical principles. Sometimes you have to explain how or prove that your study conforms to these principles.

Even when individuals try their best to remain ethical, their environments or organizations can lead them down the wrong path. There are several ways this can happen:

- *Disengagement*: Individuals may be too far removed from the effects of their decisions to see, understand, or be affected by the ethical violations. (For example, someone in marketing makes incorrect claims about the safety of a medication. Several years down the road, some patients die from the medication. By then, the marketer is working for another company and does not have to deal with the problems).
- *Competing pressures*: The pressures to publish, get a drug approved, obtain grant money, get promoted, continue earning a paycheck, feed the family, put kids through school, or satisfy supervisors can goad people into doing the wrong thing. Such pressures can be so consuming that individuals see no other options or fail to realize the implications of their actions. (For example, if an investigator fails to get positive results on a study, he will lose his job, his spouse, and not be able to provide for his family. What might he do?)
- *Peer pressure and groupthink*: Sometimes *groupthink* (i.e., everyone going with the entire group and subverting individual thought) can influence the actions of the entire group. Individuals may be loath to go against the prevailing thoughts and be seen as a whistle-blower (i.e., someone who rats on everyone else).
- *Stressful environments and time pressure*: Stressful environments can cloud an individual's judgment. When an individual is in survival mode, he or she can overlook

details that may be problematic. When supervisors mistreat subordinates, the subordinates may lose motivation and consciously or unconsciously be lax (e.g., a physician who is overworked is more likely to make mistakes and be rude to patients).

Science, medicine, and ethics sometimes can be at odds. What is scientifically or medically the right thing to do may not be the most ethical thing to do. Here are some examples:

- You cannot find enough children in your study because it involves injections from a large needle. The only way to accumulate a large enough population is to coerce children to participate. Coercion, of course, is unethical. However, without enough participants, you cannot complete the study.
- A patient has a terminal illness. The only way to save her is to try an unapproved and potentially dangerous medication.
- A study involves half of the patients receiving a medication and the other half not getting any treatment. You feel uncomfortable about patients not receiving treatment.

2.1.2 Brief History of Human Experimentation

What do you think of when you hear the words "human experimentation"? After all, clinical research in effect is human experimentation. At their best, human experimentation can yield valuable information, advance science, and eventually benefit thousands and even millions of people. At their worst, human experimentation can treat people like guinea pigs, causing physical and psychological torture (even death), and violate many ethical principles.

Human experimentation has been around ever since the dawn of humankind. Anytime a person tested something on his or her or someone else's body, it's clinical research. A cave person who stuck his or her hand into a fire for the first time to see what happened conducted a clinical study. The only way anyone could have determined what to eat was to have run multiple "clinical studies," each time either trying to eat something or observing what happened when others ate different things. Undoubtedly many adverse events occurred during these "trials." Many people accidentally died or suffered bad side effects to slowly add to the body of knowledge that we have today. We don't eat dirt (at least most of us do not) and wear clothes made out of poison ivy because of some of these early clinical studies.

Until the twentieth century, clinical research was relatively unregulated. Scientists would often try new discoveries on themselves or whoever happened to be closest or available. Dr. Jekyll and Mr. Hyde are a classic fictional example of self-experimentation. Family members and close friends often became testing subjects. Many of history's most famous physicians/scientists used themselves as test subjects. Without these heroic self-experimenters, we may not have the body of knowledge and medical interventions that we have today. Of course, for every impromptu human experiment that led to medical breakthroughs, undoubtedly many resulted in bad consequences. We do not know how many people suffered or died from such experiments.

Recruitment for clinical studies often occurred in manners that would be considered unethical today. Slaves, children, students, soldiers, and other subordinates often were pressured into being subjects. Many times they had no choice. Sometimes these *vulnerable populations* were unaware that they were the subjects of experiments. There are incidences of researchers covertly disseminating diseases or experimental interventions among unaware populations. Undoubtedly, there are countless documented and undocumented cases of prisoners, slaves, and other subordinates suffering horrible consequences from odious and torturous experiments.

Human experiments did not always have a clear purpose. At times, researchers would conduct an experiment just to see what happens. They could not predict the risk and benefits of the experiment and were not even sure what they were trying to find or prove. This haphazard "scientific" method would sometimes lead to surprises such as unexpected debilitation and death.

Researchers would offer significant inducements to participate and not reveal the risks of the studies to their participants. For example, when American physician Walter Reed studied Yellow Fever, he offered American soldiers large amounts of money to be bitten by infected mosquitoes and severely understated the risks of participating.

A landmark event in clinical research ethics occurred following World War II. During the war, German Nazi scientists conducted gruesome and reprehensible experiments on concentration camp prisoners causing torture, mutilation, and death. The experiments involved appalling dismemberment and disfigurement of a defenseless population. Many of these experiments did not even have any clear scientific rationale. After the defeat of the Nazi empire, the ensuing trial of the war criminals in Nuremberg addressed this horrendous experimentation. From the trials arose the Nuremberg Code in 1946, a set of ethical principles guiding human experimentation. Figure 2.1 shows the Nuremberg Code.

The Code outlined many of the ethical principles of clinical research. The key tenets of the Code is that subject participation in a clinical study should be completely voluntary, the researcher should make every effort to protect the subject, the researcher should be qualified to conduct the experiment, the design should be scientifically sound, and the experiment should have a justifiable purpose. The Nuremberg Code helped increase dialog about clinical research ethics but failed to address some important issues and did little to eliminate some of the questionable practices that continued to occur throughout the world including the United States.

NUREMBERG CODE

1. The voluntary consent of the human subject is absolutely essential. This means that the person involved should have legal capacity to give consent; should be so situated as to be able to exercise free power of choice, without the intervention of any element of force, fraud, deceit, duress, overreaching, or other ulterior form of constraint or coercion; and should have sufficient knowledge and comprehension of the elements of the subject matter involved as to enable him to make an understanding and enlightened decision. This latter element requires that before the acceptance of an affirmative decision by the experimental subject there should be made known to him the nature, duration, and purpose of the experiment; the method and means by which it is to be conducted; all inconveniences and hazards reasonable to be expected; and the effects upon his health or person which may possibly come from his participation in the experiment.

   The duty and responsibility for ascertaining the quality of the consent rests upon each individual who initiates, directs, or engages in the experiment. It is a personal duty and responsibility which may not be delegated to another with impunity.
2. The experiment should be such as to yield fruitful results for the good of society, unprocurable by other methods or means of study, and not random and unnecessary in nature.
3. The experiment should be so designed and based on the results of animal experimentation and a knowledge of the natural history of the disease or other problem under study that the anticipated results will justify the performance of the experiment.
4. The experiment should be so conducted as to avoid all unnecessary physical and mental suffering and injury.
5. No experiment should be conducted where there is an *a priori* reason to believe that death or disabling injury will occur; except, perhaps, in those experiments where the experimental physicians also serve as subjects.
6. The degree of risk to be taken should never exceed that determined by the humanitarian importance of the problem to be solved by the experiment.
7. Proper preparations should be made and adequate facilities provided to protect the experimental subject against even remote possibilities of injury, disability, or death.
8. The experiment should be conducted only by scientifically qualified persons. The highest degree of skill and care should be required through all stages of the experiment of those who conduct or engage in the experiment.
9. During the course of the experiment the human subject should be at liberty to bring the experiment to an end if he has reached the physical or mental state where continuation of the experiment seems to him to be impossible.
10. During the course of the experiment the scientist in charge must be prepared to terminate the experiment at any stage, if he has probable cause to believe, in the exercise of the good faith, superior skill and careful judgment required of him that a continuation of the experiment is likely to result in injury, disability, or death to the experimental subject.

From the National Institutes of Health

FIGURE 2.1   Nuremberg Code.

First developed in 1964 by the World Medical Association, the Declaration of Helsinki augmented the principles set forth by the Nuremberg Code. Figure 2.2 shows the Declaration of Helsinki. This Declaration has undergone several subsequent revisions. As you can see, the Declaration of Helsinki is more detailed and addresses some issues not tackled by the Nuremberg Code.

The Nuremberg Code and Declaration of Helsinki were statements and not laws. As a result, a number of clinical researchers ignored their tenets. Without legal consequences, some researchers continued to conduct studies with abandon. No significant oversight was present until two major developments: a New England Journal article by Henry K. Beecher in 1966 and the revelation of the Tuskegee experiment in 1970. The Beecher article listed multiple cases of human subjects being given life-threatening interventions without being adequately informed and without offering consent. Although Beecher was roundly criticized by the medical establishment for this article, the article helped motivate change.

The Tuskegee Experiment is one of the most notorious cases of ethics violations in clinical research. Commenced in the 1930s, the experiment continued until 1970 when the details of the experiment were uncovered, causing an uproar. Researchers followed 400 African American men with syphilis and kept them from receiving treatment so that they could observe the natural course of the disease. This experiment had two major problems. Firstly, the researchers denied the subjects available treatment for a major disease for so long. Secondly, the researchers were Caucasian and the subjects were African Americans. There was no scientific reason why all the subjects had to be African Americans. The experiment appeared to be a case of one race experimenting on another.

These developments prompted action from the major governing bodies in the United States. For the first time, clinical researchers were no longer allowed to regulate themselves. The violations had demonstrated that oversight was needed. The National Institutes of Health (NIH) began requiring that each institution conducting clinical research have an Institutional Review Board (IRB) to review and approve clinical study protocols. The Food and Drug Administration (FDA) followed suite by strengthening its drug and medical device rules and regulations. In 1973, the U.S. Congress assembled the 11-member National Commission for the Protection of Human Subjects of Biomedical and Behavioral Research, which issued the Belmont Report in 1979. Figure 2.3 shows the Belmont

WORLD MEDICAL ASSOCIATION DECLARATION OF HELSINKI

Ethical Principles for Medical Research Involving Human Subjects
Adopted by the 18th WMA General Assembly, Helsinki, Finland, June 1964, and amended by the
29th WMA General Assembly, Tokyo, Japan, October 1975
35th WMA General Assembly, Venice, Italy, October 1983
41st WMA General Assembly, Hong Kong, September 1989
48th WMA General Assembly, Somerset West, Republic of South Africa, October 1996 and the 52nd WMA General Assembly, Edinburgh, Scotland, October 2000
Note of Clarification on Paragraph 29 added by the WMA General Assembly, Washington 2002
Note of Clarification on Paragraph 30 added by the WMA General Assembly, Tokyo 2004

INTRODUCTION

1. The World Medical Association has developed the Declaration of Helsinki as a statement of ethical principles to provide guidance to physicians and other participants in medical research involving human subjects. Medical research involving human subjects includes research on identifiable human material or identifiable data.
2. It is the duty of the physician to promote and safeguard the health of the people. The physician's knowledge and conscience are dedicated to the fulfillment of this duty.
3. The Declaration of Geneva of the World Medical Association binds the physician with the words, "The health of my patient will be my first consideration," and the International Code of Medical Ethics declares that, "A physician shall act only in the patient's interest when providing medical care which might have the effect of weakening the physical and mental condition of the patient."
4. Medical progress is based on research which ultimately must rest in part on experimentation involving human subjects.
5. In medical research on human subjects, considerations related to the well-being of the human subject should take precedence over the interests of science and society.
6. The primary purpose of medical research involving human subjects is to improve prophylactic, diagnostic, and therapeutic procedures, and the understanding of the aetiology and pathogenesis of disease. Even the best proven prophylactic, diagnostic, and therapeutic methods must continuously be challenged through research for their effectiveness, efficiency, accessibility, and quality.
7. In current medical practice and in medical research, most prophylactic, diagnostic, and therapeutic procedures involve risks and burdens.
8. Medical research is subject to ethical standards that promote respect for all human beings and protect their health and rights. Some research populations are vulnerable and need special protection. The particular needs of the economically and medically disadvantaged must be recognized. Special attention is also required for those who cannot give or refuse consent for themselves, for those who may be subject to giving consent under duress, for those who will not benefit personally from the research and for those for whom the research is combined with care.
9. Research investigators should be aware of the ethical, legal, and regulatory requirements for research on human subjects in their own countries as well as applicable international requirements. No national ethical, legal, or regulatory requirement should be allowed to reduce or eliminate any of the protections for human subjects set forth in this Declaration.

B. BASIC PRINCIPLES FOR ALL MEDICAL RESEARCH

10. It is the duty of the physician in medical research to protect the life, health, privacy, and dignity of the human subject.
11. Medical research involving human subjects must conform to generally accepted scientific principles, be based on a thorough knowledge of the scientific literature, other relevant sources of information, and on adequate laboratory and, where appropriate, animal experimentation.
12. Appropriate caution must be exercised in the conduct of research which may affect the environment, and the welfare of animals used for research must be respected.
13. The design and performance of each experimental procedure involving human subjects should be clearly formulated in an experimental protocol. This protocol should be submitted for consideration, comment, guidance, and where appropriate, approval to a specially appointed ethical review committee, which must be independent of the investigator, the sponsor, or any other kind of undue influence. This independent committee should be in conformity with the laws and regulations of the country in which the research experiment is performed. The committee has the right to monitor ongoing trials. The researcher has the obligation to provide monitoring information to the committee, especially any serious adverse events. The researcher should also submit to the committee, for review, information regarding funding, sponsors, institutional affiliations, other potential conflicts of interest, and incentives for subjects.
14. The research protocol should always contain a statement of the ethical considerations involved and should indicate that there is compliance with the principles enunciated in this Declaration.
15. Medical research involving human subjects should be conducted only by scientifically qualified persons and under the supervision of a clinically competent medical person. The responsibility for the human subject must always rest with a medically qualified person and never rest on the subject of the research, even though the subject has given consent.
16. Every medical research project involving human subjects should be preceded by careful assessment of predictable risks and burdens in comparison with foreseeable benefits to the subject or to others. This does not preclude the participation of healthy volunteers in medical research. The design of all studies should be publicly available.

FIGURE 2.2 World Medical Association Declaration of Helsinki.

17. Physicians should abstain from engaging in research projects involving human subjects unless they are confident that the risks involved have been adequately assessed and can be satisfactorily managed. Physicians should cease any investigation if the risks are found to outweigh the potential benefits or if there is conclusive proof of positive and beneficial results.

18. Medical research involving human subjects should only be conducted if the importance of the objective outweighs the inherent risks and burdens to the subject. This is especially important when the human subjects are healthy volunteers.

19. Medical research is only justified if there is a reasonable likelihood that the populations in which the research is carried out stand to benefit from the results of the research.

20. The subjects must be volunteers and informed participants in the research project.

21. The right of research subjects to safeguard their integrity must always be respected. Every precaution should be taken to respect the privacy of the subject, the confidentiality of the patient's information, and to minimize the impact of the study on the subject's physical and mental integrity and on the personality of the subject.

22. In any research on human beings, each potential subject must be adequately informed of the aims, methods, sources of funding, any possible conflicts of interest, institutional affiliations of the researcher, the anticipated benefits and potential risks of the study, and the discomfort it may entail. The subject should be informed of the right to abstain from participation in the study or to withdraw consent to participate at any time without reprisal. After ensuring that the subject has understood the information, the physician should then obtain the subject's freely given informed consent, preferably in writing. If the consent cannot be obtained in writing, the nonwritten consent must be formally documented and witnessed.

23. When obtaining informed consent for the research project the physician should be particularly cautious if the subject is in a dependent relationship with the physician or may consent under duress. In that case the informed consent should be obtained by a well-informed physician who is not engaged in the investigation and who is completely independent of this relationship.

24. For a research subject who is legally incompetent, physically or mentally incapable of giving consent, or is a legally incompetent minor, the investigator must obtain informed consent from the legally authorized representative in accordance with applicable law. These groups should not be included in research unless the research is necessary to promote the health of the population represented and this research cannot instead be performed on legally competent persons.

25. When a subject deemed legally incompetent, such as a minor child, is able to give assent to decisions about participation in research, the investigator must obtain that assent in addition to the consent of the legally authorized representative.

26. Research on individuals from whom it is not possible to obtain consent, including proxy or advance consent, should be done only if the physical/mental condition that prevents obtaining informed consent is a necessary characteristic of the research population. The specific reasons for involving research subjects with a condition that renders them unable to give informed consent should be stated in the experimental protocol for consideration and approval of the review committee. The protocol should state that consent to remain in the research should be obtained as soon as possible from the individual or a legally authorized surrogate.

27. Both authors and publishers have ethical obligations. In publication of the results of research, the investigators are obliged to preserve the accuracy of the results. Negative as well as positive results should be published or otherwise publicly available. Sources of funding, institutional affiliations, and any possible conflicts of interest should be declared in the publication. Reports of experimentation not in accordance with the principles laid down in this Declaration should not be accepted for publication.

C. ADDITIONAL PRINCIPLES FOR MEDICAL RESEARCH COMBINED WITH MEDICAL CARE

28. The physician may combine medical research with medical care, only to the extent that the research is justified by its potential prophylactic, diagnostic, or therapeutic value. When medical research is combined with medical care, additional standards apply to protect the patients who are research subjects.

29. The benefits, risks, burdens, and effectiveness of a new method should be tested against those of the best current prophylactic, diagnostic, and therapeutic methods. This does not exclude the use of placebo, or no treatment, in studies where no proven prophylactic, diagnostic, or therapeutic method exists.

30. At the conclusion of the study, every patient entered into the study should be assured of access to the best proven prophylactic, diagnostic, and therapeutic methods identified by the study.

31. The physician should fully inform the patient which aspects of the care are related to the research. The refusal of a patient to participate in a study must never interfere with the patient–physician relationship.

32. In the treatment of a patient, where proven prophylactic, diagnostic, and therapeutic methods do not exist or have been ineffective, the physician, with informed consent from the patient, must be free to use unproven or new prophylactic, diagnostic, and therapeutic measures, if in the physician's judgment it offers hope of saving life, reestablishing health or alleviating suffering. Where possible, these measures should be made the object of research, designed to evaluate their safety and efficacy. In all cases, new information should be recorded and, where appropriate, published. The other relevant guidelines of this Declaration should be followed.

Note: Note of clarification on paragraph 29 of the WMA Declaration of Helsinki

The WMA hereby reaffirms its position that extreme care must be taken in making use of a placebo-controlled trial and that in general this methodology should only be used in the absence of existing proven therapy. However, a placebo-controlled trial may be ethically acceptable, even if proven therapy is available, under the following circumstances:

- where for compelling and scientifically sound methodological reasons its use is necessary to determine the efficacy or safety of a prophylactic, diagnostic, or therapeutic method; or
- where a prophylactic, diagnostic, or therapeutic method is being investigated for a minor condition and the patients who receive placebo will not be subject to any additional risk of serious or irreversible harm.

All other provisions of the Declaration of Helsinki must be adhered to, especially the need for appropriate ethical and scientific review.

FIGURE 2.2 Continued.

The Belmont Report

Ethical Principles and Guidelines for the protection of human subjects of research

The National Commission for the Protection of Human Subjects of Biomedical and Behavioral Research April 18, 1979

AGENCY: Department of Health, Education, and Welfare.

ACTION: Notice of Report for Public Comment.

SUMMARY: On July 12, 1974, the National Research Act (Pub. L. 93-348) was signed into law, thereby creating the National Commission for the Protection of Human Subjects of Biomedical and Behavioral Research. One of the charges to the Commission was to identify the basic ethical principles that should underlie the conduct of biomedical and behavioral research involving human subjects and to develop guidelines which should be followed to assure that such research is conducted in accordance with those principles. In carrying out the above, the Commission was directed to consider: **(i)** the boundaries between biomedical and behavioral research and the accepted and routine practice of medicine, **(ii)** the role of assessment of risk–benefit criteria in the determination of the appropriateness of research involving human subjects, **(iii)** appropriate guidelines for the selection of human subjects for participation in such research and **(iv)** the nature and definition of informed consent in various research settings.

The Belmont Report attempts to summarize the basic ethical principles identified by the Commission in the course of its deliberations. It is the outgrowth of an intensive 4-day period of discussions that were held in February 1976 at the Smithsonian Institution's Belmont Conference Center supplemented by the monthly deliberations of the Commission that were held over a period of nearly 4 years. It is a statement of basic ethical principles and guidelines that should assist in resolving the ethical problems that surround the conduct of research with human subjects. By publishing the Report in the Federal Register, and providing reprints upon request, the Secretary intends that it may be made readily available to scientists, members of Institutional Review Boards, and Federal employees. The two-volume Appendix, containing the lengthy reports of experts and specialists who assisted the Commission in fulfilling this part of its charge, is available as DHEW Publication No. (OS) 78-0013 and No. (OS) 78-0014, for sale by the Superintendent of Documents, U.S. Government Printing Office, Washington, D.C. 20402.

Unlike most other reports of the Commission, the Belmont Report does not make specific recommendations for administrative action by the Secretary of Health, Education, and Welfare. Rather, the Commission recommended that the Belmont Report be adopted in its entirety, as a statement of the Department's policy. The Department requests public comment on this recommendation.

National Commission for the Protection of Human Subjects of Biomedical and Behavioral Research

Members of the Commission

Kenneth John Ryan, M.D., Chairman, Chief of Staff, Boston Hospital for Women.

Joseph V. Brady, Ph.D., Professor of Behavioral Biology, Johns Hopkins University.

Robert E. Cooke, M.D., President, Medical College of Pennsylvania.

Dorothy I. Height, President, National Council of Negro Women, Inc.

Albert R. Jonsen, Ph.D., Associate Professor of Bioethics, University of California at San Francisco.

Patricia King, J.D., Associate Professor of Law, Georgetown University Law Center.

Karen Lebacqz, Ph.D., Associate Professor of Christian Ethics, Pacific School of Religion.

*** David W. Louisell, J.D., Professor of Law, University of California at Berkeley.

Donald W. Seldin, M.D., Professor and Chairman, Department of Internal Medicine, University of Texas at Dallas.

Eliot Stellar, Ph.D., Provost of the University and Professor of Physiological Psychology, University of Pennsylvania.

*** Robert H. Turtle, LL.B., Attorney, VomBaur, Coburn, Simmons & Turtle, Washington, D.C.

*** Deceased.

Ethical Principles & Guidelines for Research Involving Human Subjects

Scientific research has produced substantial social benefits. It has also posed some troubling ethical questions. Public attention was drawn to these questions by reported abuses of human subjects in biomedical experiments, especially during the Second World War. During the Nuremberg War Crime Trials, the Nuremberg code was drafted as a set of standards for judging physicians and scientists who had conducted biomedical experiments on concentration camp prisoners. This code became the prototype of many later codes (1) intended to assure that research involving human subjects would be carried out in an ethical manner.

The codes consist of rules, some general, others specific, that guide the investigators or the reviewers of research in their work. Such rules often are inadequate to cover complex situations; at times they come into conflict, and they are frequently difficult to interpret or apply. Broader ethical principles will provide a basis on which specific rules may be formulated, criticized, and interpreted.

Three principles, or general prescriptive judgments, that are relevant to research involving human subjects are identified in this statement. Other principles may also be relevant. These three are comprehensive, however, and are stated at a level of generalization that should assist scientists, subjects, reviewers, and interested citizens to understand the ethical issues inherent in research involving human subjects. These principles cannot always be applied so as to resolve beyond dispute particular ethical problems. The objective is to provide an analytical framework that will guide the resolution of ethical problems arising from research involving human subjects.

FIGURE 2.3   Belmont Report.

This statement consists of a distinction between research and practice, a discussion of the three basic ethical principles, and remarks about the application of these principles.

Part A: Boundaries Between Practice & Research

A. Boundaries Between Practice and Research

It is important to distinguish between biomedical and behavioral research, on the one hand, and the practice of accepted therapy on the other, in order to know what activities ought to undergo review for the protection of human subjects of research. The distinction between research and practice is blurred partly because both often occur together (as in research designed to evaluate a therapy) and partly because notable departures from standard practice are often called "experimental" when the terms "experimental" and "research" are not carefully defined.

For the most part, the term "practice" refers to interventions that are designed solely to enhance the well-being of an individual patient or client and that have a reasonable expectation of success. The purpose of medical or behavioral practice is to provide diagnosis, preventive treatment, or therapy to particular individuals. (2) By contrast, the term "research" designates an activity designed to test an hypothesis, permit conclusions to be drawn, and thereby to develop or contribute to generalizable knowledge (expressed, e.g., in theories, principles, and statements of relationships). Research is usually described in a formal protocol that sets forth an objective and a set of procedures designed to reach that objective.

When a clinician departs in a significant way from standard or accepted practice, the innovation does not, in and of itself, constitute research. The fact that a procedure is "experimental," in the sense of new, untested or different, does not automatically place it in the category of research. Radically new procedures of this description should, however, be made the object of formal research at an early stage in order to determine whether they are safe and effective. Thus, it is the responsibility of medical practice committees, for example, to insist that a major innovation be incorporated into a formal research project. (3)

Research and practice may be carried on together when research is designed to evaluate the safety and efficacy of a therapy. This need not cause any confusion regarding whether or not the activity requires review; the general rule is that if there is any element of research in an activity, that activity should undergo review for the protection of human subjects.

Part B: Basic Ethical Principles

B. Basic Ethical Principles

The expression "basic ethical principles" refers to those general judgments that serve as a basic justification for the many particular ethical prescriptions and evaluations of human actions. Three basic principles, among those generally accepted in our cultural tradition, are particularly relevant to the ethics of research involving human subjects: the principles of respect of persons, beneficence, and justice.

1. *Respect for persons* – Respect for persons incorporates at least two ethical convictions: first, that individuals should be treated as autonomous agents, and second, that persons with diminished autonomy are entitled to protection. The principle of respect for persons thus divides into two separate moral requirements: the requirement to acknowledge autonomy and the requirement to protect those with diminished autonomy.

An autonomous person is an individual capable of deliberation about personal goals and of acting under the direction of such deliberation. To respect autonomy is to give weight to autonomous persons' considered opinions and choices while refraining from obstructing their actions unless they are clearly detrimental to others. To show lack of respect for an autonomous agent is to repudiate that person's considered judgments, to deny an individual the freedom to act on those considered judgments, or to withhold information necessary to make a considered judgment, when there are no compelling reasons to do so.

However, not every human being is capable of self-determination. The capacity for self-determination matures during an individual's life, and some individuals lose this capacity wholly or in part because of illness, mental disability, or circumstances that severely restrict liberty. Respect for the immature and the incapacitated may require protecting them as they mature or while they are incapacitated.

Some persons are in need of extensive protection, even to the point of excluding them from activities which may harm them; other persons require little protection beyond making sure they undertake activities freely and with awareness of possible adverse consequence. The extent of protection afforded should depend on the risk of harm and the likelihood of benefit. The judgment that any individual lacks autonomy should be periodically reevaluated and will vary in different situations.

In most cases of research involving human subjects, respect for persons demands that subjects enter into the research voluntarily and with adequate information. In some situations, however, application of the principle is not obvious. The involvement of prisoners as subjects of research provides an instructive example. On the one hand, it would seem that the principle of respect for persons requires that prisoners not be deprived of the opportunity to volunteer for research. On the other hand, under prison conditions they may be subtly coerced or unduly influenced to engage in research activities for which they would not otherwise volunteer. Respect for persons would then dictate that prisoners be protected. Whether to allow prisoners to "volunteer" or to "protect" them presents a dilemma. Respecting persons, in most hard cases, is often a matter of balancing competing claims urged by the principle of respect itself.

2. *Beneficence* – Persons are treated in an ethical manner not only by respecting their decisions and protecting them from harm, but also by making efforts to secure their well-being. Such treatment falls under the principle of beneficence. The term "beneficence" is often understood to cover acts of kindness or charity that go beyond strict obligation. In this document, beneficence is understood in a stronger sense, as an obligation. Two general rules have been formulated as complementary expressions of beneficent actions in this sense: **(1)** do not harm and **(2)** maximize possible benefits and minimize possible harms.

FIGURE 2.3   Continued.

The Hippocratic maxim "do no harm" has long been a fundamental principle of medical ethics. Claude Bernard extended it to the realm of research, saying that one should not injure one person regardless of the benefits that might come to others. However, even avoiding harm requires learning what is harmful; and, in the process of obtaining this information, persons may be exposed to risk of harm. Further, the Hippocratic Oath requires physicians to benefit their patients "according to their best judgment." Learning what will in fact benefit may require exposing persons to risk. The problem posed by these imperatives is to decide when it is justifiable to seek certain benefits despite the risks involved, and when the benefits should be foregone because of the risks.

The obligations of beneficence affect both individual investigators and society at large, because they extend both to particular research projects and to the entire enterprise of research. In the case of particular projects, investigators and members of their institutions are obliged to give forethought to the maximization of benefits and the reduction of risk that might occur from the research investigation. In the case of scientific research in general, members of the larger society are obliged to recognize the longer term benefits and risks that may result from the improvement of knowledge and from the development of novel medical, psychotherapeutic, and social procedures.

The principle of beneficence often occupies a well-defined justifying role in many areas of research involving human subjects. An example is found in research involving children. Effective ways of treating childhood diseases and fostering healthy development are benefits that serve to justify research involving children – even when individual research subjects are not direct beneficiaries. Research also makes it possible to avoid the harm that may result from the application of previously accepted routine practices that on closer investigation turn out to be dangerous. But the role of the principle of beneficence is not always so unambiguous. A difficult ethical problem remains, for example, about research that presents more than minimal risk without immediate prospect of direct benefit to the children involved. Some have argued that such research is inadmissible, while others have pointed out that this limit would rule out much research promising great benefit to children in the future. Here again, as with all hard cases, the different claims covered by the principle of beneficence may come into conflict and force difficult choices.

3. *Justice* – Who ought to receive the benefits of research and bear its burdens? This is a question of justice, in the sense of "fairness in distribution" or "what is deserved." An injustice occurs when some benefit to which a person is entitled is denied without good reason or when some burden is imposed unduly. Another way of conceiving the principle of justice is that equals ought to be treated equally. However, this statement requires explication. Who is equal and who is unequal? What considerations justify departure from equal distribution? Almost all commentators allow that distinctions based on experience, age, deprivation, competence, merit, and position do sometimes constitute criteria justifying differential treatment for certain purposes. It is necessary, then, to explain in what respects people should be treated equally. There are several widely accepted formulations of just ways to distribute burdens and benefits. Each formulation mentions some relevant property on the basis of which burdens and benefits should be distributed. These formulations are **(1)** to each person an equal share, **(2)** to each person according to individual need, **(3)** to each person according to individual effort, **(4)** to each person according to societal contribution, and **(5)** to each person according to merit.

Questions of justice have long been associated with social practices such as punishment, taxation, and political representation. Until recently these questions have not generally been associated with scientific research. However, they are foreshadowed even in the earliest reflections on the ethics of research involving human subjects. For example, during the nineteenth and early twentieth centuries the burdens of serving as research subjects fell largely upon poor ward patients, while the benefits of improved medical care flowed primarily to private patients. Subsequently, the exploitation of unwilling prisoners as research subjects in Nazi concentration camps was condemned as a particularly flagrant injustice. In this country, in the 1940s, the Tuskegee syphilis study used disadvantaged, rural black men to study the untreated course of a disease that is by no means confined to that population. These subjects were deprived of demonstrably effective treatment in order not to interrupt the project, long after such treatment became generally available.

Against this historical background, it can be seen how conceptions of justice are relevant to research involving human subjects. For example, the selection of research subjects needs to be scrutinized in order to determine whether some classes (e.g., welfare patients, particular racial and ethnic minorities, or persons confined to institutions) are being systematically selected simply because of their easy availability, their compromised position, or their manipulability, rather than for reasons directly related to the problem being studied. Finally, whenever research supported by public funds leads to the development of therapeutic devices and procedures, justice demands both that these should not provide advantages only to those who can afford them and that such research should not unduly involve persons from groups unlikely to be among the beneficiaries of subsequent applications of the research.

Part C: Applications

C. Applications

Applications of the general principles to the conduct of research lead to consideration of the following requirements: informed consent, risk/benefit assessment, and the selection of subjects of research.

1. *Informed consent* – Respect for persons requires that subjects, to the degree that they are capable, be given the opportunity to choose what shall or shall not happen to them. This opportunity is provided when adequate standards for informed consent are satisfied.

While the importance of informed consent is unquestioned, controversy prevails over the nature and possibility of an informed consent. Nonetheless, there is widespread agreement that the consent process can be analyzed as containing three elements: information, comprehension, and voluntariness.

Information. Most codes of research establish specific items for disclosure intended to assure that subjects are given sufficient information. These items generally include: the research procedure, their purposes, risks and anticipated benefits, alternative procedures (where therapy is involved), and a statement offering the subject the opportunity to ask questions and to withdraw at any time from the research. Additional items have been proposed, including how subjects are selected, the person responsible for the research, etc.

FIGURE 2.3 Continued.

However, a simple listing of items does not answer the question of what the standard should be for judging how much and what sort of information should be provided. One standard frequently invoked in medical practice, namely the information commonly provided by practitioners in the field or in the locale, is inadequate since research takes place precisely when a common understanding does not exist. Another standard, currently popular in malpractice law, requires the practitioner to reveal the information that reasonable persons would wish to know in order to make a decision regarding their care. This, too, seems insufficient since the research subject, being in essence a volunteer, may wish to know considerably more about risks gratuitously undertaken than do patients who deliver themselves into the hand of a clinician for needed care. It may be that a standard of "the reasonable volunteer" should be proposed: the extent and nature of information should be such that persons, knowing that the procedure is neither necessary for their care nor perhaps fully understood, can decide whether they wish to participate in the furthering of knowledge. Even when some direct benefit to them is anticipated, the subjects should understand clearly the range of risk and the voluntary nature of participation.

A special problem of consent arises where informing subjects of some pertinent aspect of the research is likely to impair the validity of the research. In many cases, it is sufficient to indicate to subjects that they are being invited to participate in research of which some features will not be revealed until the research is concluded. In all cases of research involving incomplete disclosure, such research is justified only if it is clear that **(1)** incomplete disclosure is truly necessary to accomplish the goals of the research, **(2)** there are no undisclosed risks to subjects that are more than minimal, and **(3)** there is an adequate plan for debriefing subjects, when appropriate, and for dissemination of research results to them. Information about risks should never be withheld for the purpose of eliciting the cooperation of subjects, and truthful answers should always be given to direct questions about the research. Care should be taken to distinguish cases in which disclosure would destroy or invalidate the research from cases in which disclosure would simply inconvenience the investigator.

Comprehension. The manner and context in which information is conveyed is as important as the information itself. For example, presenting information in a disorganized and rapid fashion, allowing too little time for consideration or curtailing opportunities for questioning, all may adversely affect a subject's ability to make an informed choice.

Because the subject's ability to understand is a function of intelligence, rationality, maturity, and language, it is necessary to adapt the presentation of the information to the subject's capacities. Investigators are responsible for ascertaining that the subject has comprehended the information. While there is always an obligation to ascertain that the information about risk to subjects is complete and adequately comprehended, when the risks are more serious, that obligation increases. On occasion, it may be suitable to give some oral or written tests of comprehension.

Special provision may need to be made when comprehension is severely limited – for example, by conditions of immaturity or mental disability. Each class of subjects that one might consider as incompetent (e.g., infants and young children, mentally disable patients, the terminally ill, and the comatose) should be considered on its own terms. Even for these persons, however, respect requires giving them the opportunity to choose to the extent they are able, whether or not to participate in research. The objections of these subjects to involvement should be honored, unless the research entails providing them a therapy unavailable elsewhere. Respect for persons also requires seeking the permission of other parties in order to protect the subjects from harm. Such persons are thus respected both by acknowledging their own wishes and by the use of third parties to protect them from harm.

The third parties chosen should be those who are most likely to understand the incompetent subject's situation and to act in that person's best interest. The person authorized to act on behalf of the subject should be given an opportunity to observe the research as it proceeds in order to be able to withdraw the subject from the research, if such action appears in the subject's best interest.

Voluntariness. An agreement to participate in research constitutes a valid consent only if voluntarily given. This element of informed consent requires conditions free of coercion and undue influence. Coercion occurs when an overt threat of harm is intentionally presented by one person to another in order to obtain compliance. Undue influence, by contrast, occurs through an offer of an excessive, unwarranted, inappropriate or improper reward, or other overture in order to obtain compliance. Also, inducements that would ordinarily be acceptable may become undue influences if the subject is especially vulnerable.

Unjustifiable pressures usually occur when persons in positions of authority or commanding influence – especially where possible sanctions are involved – urge a course of action for a subject. A continuum of such influencing factors exists, however, and it is impossible to state precisely where justifiable persuasion ends and undue influence begins. But undue influence would include actions such as manipulating a person's choice through the controlling influence of a close relative and threatening to withdraw health services to which an individual would otherwise be entitled.

2. *Assessment of risks and benefits* – The assessment of risks and benefits requires a careful arrayal of relevant data, including, in some cases, alternative ways of obtaining the benefits sought in the research. Thus, the assessment presents both an opportunity and a responsibility to gather systematic and comprehensive information about proposed research. For the investigator, it is a means to examine whether the proposed research is properly designed. For a review committee, it is a method for determining whether the risks that will be presented to subjects are justified. For prospective subjects, the assessment will assist the determination whether or not to participate.

The nature and scope of risks and benefits. The requirement that research be justified on the basis of a favorable risk/benefit assessment bears a close relation to the principle of beneficence, just as the moral requirement that informed consent be obtained is derived primarily from the principle of respect for persons. The term "risk" refers to a possibility that harm may occur. However, when expressions such as "small risk" or "high risk" are used, they usually refer (often ambiguously) both to the chance (probability) of experiencing a harm and the severity (magnitude) of the envisioned harm.

The term "benefit" is used in the research context to refer to something of positive value related to health or welfare. Unlike, "risk," "benefit" is not a term that expresses probabilities. Risk is properly contrasted to probability of benefits, and benefits are properly contrasted with harms rather than risks of harm. Accordingly, so-called risk/benefit assessments are concerned with the probabilities and

FIGURE 2.3 Continued.

magnitudes of possible harm and anticipated benefits. Many kinds of possible harms and benefits need to be taken into account. There are, for example, risks of psychological harm, physical harm, legal harm, social harm, and economic harm and the corresponding benefits. While the most likely types of harms to research subjects are those of psychological or physical pain or injury, other possible kinds should not be overlooked.

Risks and benefits of research may affect the individual subjects, the families of the individual subjects, and society at large (or special groups of subjects in society). Previous codes and federal regulations have required that risks to subjects be outweighed by the sum of both the anticipated benefit to the subject, if any, and the anticipated benefit to society in the form of knowledge to be gained from the research. In balancing these different elements, the risks and benefits affecting the immediate research subject will normally carry special weight. On the other hand, interests other than those of the subject may on some occasions be sufficient by themselves to justify the risks involved in the research, so long as the subjects' rights have been protected. Beneficence thus requires that we protect against risk of harm to subjects and also that we be concerned about the loss of the substantial benefits that might be gained from research.

The systematic assessment of risks and benefits. It is commonly said that benefits and risks must be "balanced" and shown to be "in a favorable ratio." The metaphorical character of these terms draws attention to the difficulty of making precise judgments. Only on rare occasions will quantitative techniques be available for the scrutiny of research protocols. However, the idea of systematic, nonarbitrary analysis of risks and benefits should be emulated insofar as possible. This ideal requires those making decisions about the justifiability of research to be thorough in the accumulation and assessment of information about all aspects of the research, and to consider alternatives systematically. This procedure renders the assessment of research more rigorous and precise, while making communication between review board members and investigators less subject to misinterpretation, misinformation, and conflicting judgments. Thus, there should first be a determination of the validity of the presuppositions of the research; then the nature, probability, and magnitude of risk should be distinguished with as much clarity as possible. The method of ascertaining risks should be explicit, especially where there is no alternative to the use of such vague categories as small or slight risk. It should also be determined whether an investigator's estimates of the probability of harm or benefits are reasonable, as judged by known facts or other available studies.

Finally, assessment of the justifiability of research should reflect at least the following considerations: **(i)** Brutal or inhumane treatment of human subjects is never morally justified. **(ii)** Risks should be reduced to those necessary to achieve the research objective. It should be determined whether it is in fact necessary to use human subjects at all. Risk can perhaps never be entirely eliminated, but it can often be reduced by careful attention to alternative procedures. **(iii)** When research involves significant risk of serious impairment, review committees should be extraordinarily insistent on the justification of the risk (looking usually to the likelihood of benefit to the subject – or, in some rare cases, to the manifest voluntariness of the participation). **(iv)** When vulnerable populations are involved in research, the appropriateness of involving them should itself be demonstrated. A number of variables go into such judgments, including the nature and degree of risk, the condition of the particular population involved, and the nature and level of the anticipated benefits. **(v)** Relevant risks and benefits must be thoroughly arrayed in documents and procedures used in the informed consent process.

3. *Selection of subjects* – Just as the principle of respect for persons finds expression in the requirements for consent, and the principle of beneficence in risk/benefit assessment, the principle of justice gives rise to moral requirements that there be fair procedures and outcomes in the selection of research subjects.

Justice is relevant to the selection of subjects of research at two levels: the social and the individual. Individual justice in the selection of subjects would require that researchers exhibit fairness: thus, they should not offer potentially beneficial research only to some patients who are in their favor or select only "undesirable" persons for risky research. Social justice requires that distinction be drawn between classes of subjects that ought, and ought not, to participate in any particular kind of research, based on the ability of members of that class to bear burdens and on the appropriateness of placing further burdens on already burdened persons. Thus, it can be considered a matter of social justice that there is an order of preference in the selection of classes of subjects (e.g., adults before children) and that some classes of potential subjects (e.g., the institutionalized mentally infirm or prisoners) may be involved as research subjects, if at all, only on certain conditions.

Injustice may appear in the selection of subjects, even if individual subjects are selected fairly by investigators and treated fairly in the course of research. Thus injustice arises from social, racial, sexual, and cultural biases institutionalized in society. Thus, even if individual researchers are treating their research subjects fairly, and even if IRBs are taking care to assure that subjects are selected fairly within a particular institution, unjust social patterns may nevertheless appear in the overall distribution of the burdens and benefits of research. Although individual institutions or investigators may not be able to resolve a problem that is pervasive in their social setting, they can consider distributive justice in selecting research subjects.

Some populations, especially institutionalized ones, are already burdened in many ways by their infirmities and environments. When research is proposed that involves risks and does not include a therapeutic component, other less burdened classes of persons should be called upon first to accept these risks of research, except where the research is directly related to the specific conditions of the class involved. Also, even though public funds for research may often flow in the same directions as public funds for health care, it seems unfair that populations dependent on public health care constitute a pool of preferred research subjects if more advantaged populations are likely to be the recipients of the benefits.

One special instance of injustice results from the involvement of vulnerable subjects. Certain groups, such as racial minorities, the economically disadvantaged, the very sick, and the institutionalized may continually be sought as research subjects, owing to their ready availability in settings where research is conducted. Given their dependent status and their frequently compromised capacity for free consent, they should be protected against the danger of being involved in research solely for administrative convenience, or because they are easy to manipulate as a result of their illness or socioeconomic condition.

FIGURE 2.3   Continued.

(1) Since 1945, various codes for the proper and responsible conduct of human experimentation in medical research have been adopted by different organizations. The best known of these codes are the Nuremberg Code of 1947, the Helsinki Declaration of 1964 (revised in 1975), and the 1971 Guidelines (codified into Federal Regulations in 1974) issued by the U.S. Department of Health, Education, and Welfare Codes for the conduct of social and behavioral research have also been adopted, the best known being that of the American Psychological Association, published in 1973.

(2) Although practice usually involves interventions designed solely to enhance the well-being of a particular individual, interventions are sometimes applied to one individual for the enhancement of the well-being of another (e.g., blood donation, skin grafts, organ transplants) or an intervention may have the dual purpose of enhancing the well-being of a particular individual, and, at the same time, providing some benefit to others (e.g., vaccination, which protects both the person who is vaccinated and society generally). The fact that some forms of practice have elements other than immediate benefit to the individual receiving an intervention, however, should not confuse the general distinction between research and practice. Even when a procedure applied in practice may benefit some other person, it remains an intervention designed to enhance the well-being of a particular individual or groups of individuals; thus, it is practice and need not be reviewed as research.

(3) Because the problems related to social experimentation may differ substantially from those of biomedical and behavioral research, the Commission specifically declines to make any policy determination regarding such research at this time. Rather, the Commission believes that the problem ought to be addressed by one of its successor bodies.

FIGURE 2.3 Continued.

Report. This report clearly defined concepts such as autonomy, informed consent, beneficence, and justice. It included guidelines on weighing the risks and benefits of a study and subject selection.

The most recent major U.S. document regarding clinical study conduct was Part 46 ("Protection of Human Subjects") of the Code of Federal Regulations, Title 45, last revised in 1991. This document (which is too lengthy to include here) defined *exempt* (not covered by regulations) and *nonexempt* (covered by regulations) research. Exempt research includes research for certain educational purposes, involving publicly available data in which individual identities cannot be identified, to evaluate public benefit or service programs, and to evaluate food quality. The document also discussed the requirements and roles of IRBs (which we discuss later in this chapter) and stated that each institution engaged in research activities involving human experimentation have an approved Assurance of Compliance on file. It also included additional provisions to protect the welfare of research subjects.

Although all of these developments have provided more protection for clinical research subjects, clinical research and ethics are continually evolving. There will always be individuals pushing the limits for various reasons. Moreover, science and technology will continue to grow rapidly at a faster pace than laws and regulations.

2.2 ETHICAL PRINCIPLES

2.2.1 Beneficence and Maleficence

Beneficence (do good) and *maleficence* (do no harm) must be central to any clinical study. While all clinical studies have the potential to harm patients, you must take reasonable steps to protect patients. Similarly, while there's no guarantee that a study will help patients, you should do what you can within the confines of the study to keep patients comfortable and well. These principles emphasize that the patient is central to the study. All other parties and motivations should come after the patient. Never sacrifice the patient's well-being for any other gain.

A clinical study's potential benefits always should outweigh the risks. You should carefully examine and predict the risks and benefits before attempting the study. When the potential benefits are too small or the risks are too high, do not do the study (e.g., using a highly toxic substance to remove acne).

Note that nonmaleficence is distinct from *nonmalevolence*. Nonmalevolence means that you should not *intend* to do harm. Nonmalevolence is the intent; nonmaleficence is the result. Accidentally injuring a patient preserves nonmalevolence but violates nonmaleficence.

In some real-life situations, maintaining both beneficence and maleficence can be nearly impossible. Doing good may require doing harm. This is especially true when resources are limited, and tough decisions must be made. For example, whenever the government shifts money from one endeavor to another, the population that loses funding suffers (e.g., cutting medical research funding to allot more money to transportation). When food or medications are in short supply (e.g., in an underserved location), decision makers must choose who should receive these resources and whom should be denied.

If possible, such scenarios should not be part of a clinical study. Never sacrifice members of your study population for the benefit of other members (e.g., shifting resources to those patients who seem to be benefiting from the study intervention). Do not commence a clinical study if you think resources will be too limited.

2.2.2 Informed Consent

A subject provides *informed consent* when he or she fully understands the risks and benefits of the clinical study and agrees to participate. Participation in the study must be completely voluntary. The subject must be *competent* to provide informed consent (i.e., be able to comprehend all the relevant facts about the study). When you try to obtain informed consent, make sure you clearly describe and explain all the relevant facts about the study. Give the patient an opportunity to ask questions. Make sure the patient understands what you are saying. Informed consent is a legal agreement and therefore must be in writing (i.e., the patient must sign an informed consent form that includes relevant information about the study). You should let the patient keep a copy of the signed form.

A patient cannot give informed consent if he or she is:

- *Underage*: Only legal adults can give informed consent. Legally children do not have enough experience to decide on their own to participate in a study. A child's legal guardian must provide consent as well.
- *Chemically impaired*: Never accept informed consent from intoxicated patients, even though they believe or act as if they can consent.
- *Mentally impaired*: Patients who are temporarily or permanently mentally impaired may not be able to appreciate and understand the implications of joining a study. Remember that some diseases or medications can cloud someone's judgment.
- *Does not understand the language of the consent form*: For example, a patient who can speak only Spanish should be given a form written in Spanish.

Determining mental competence can be challenging. Some studies will involve patients who are at high risk of not being mentally competent (e.g., psychiatric patients, substance abusers, or heavily medicated patients). When in doubt, perform a mental status exam (i.e., a series of questions that determine the clarity of a patient's thinking) or enlist a psychiatrist to make an assessment.

Informed consent is never permanent or absolute. Patients at any time can refuse to participate in any or all of the study's activities and requirements. Even after giving informed consent, patients are never obligated to explain why they do not want to participate.

Never coerce patients to participate or remain in a study. *Coercion* is any technique that may force patients against their free will. Coercive techniques can be overt (e.g., threatening the patient in any way physically, emotionally, psychologically, or financially) or subtle (e.g., using peer pressure). You must emphasize to the patient that participation is completely *voluntary*.

2.2.3 Justice and Access

Clinical studies should exhibit *justice* or fairness to all patients in the study population. In other words, no patient should be disadvantaged when compared to others. The principle of justice implies that those who are weaker or worse off should receive more attention, help, and care to bring them back on par with everyone else. In other words, patients should have equal opportunity. So a patient's financial situation, location, ethnicity, gender, or personality should not prevent him or her from participating, unless such factors matter scientifically (e.g., a man cannot participate in a study on vaginal yeast infections). Patients have equal access to study resources, as long as it is scientifically allowed (e.g., a patient assigned to the no treatment group should not get the study treatment).

Another tenet of justice is to protect and not exploit *vulnerable populations*. As we discussed earlier, human experimentation often occurred on individuals who were not able to decline participation (e.g., prisoners, indigent, students, subordinates, or slaves). A vulnerable population is any group of people over which the researcher has undue influence. This influence may be financial, social, professional, physical, and/or psychological. The vulnerable population may fear repercussions if they do not participate and comply with the clinical study. The stated or unstated threat of retribution amounts to coercion. So, for example, a teacher who wants his students to participate in a clinical study must make it crystal clear that refusing to participate will in no way affect their grades. Similarly a supervisor cannot imply in any way that lack of compliance with a clinical study will affect a person's job status.

You can also exploit a vulnerable population when you withhold something that they want unless they participate in the study. Examples of coercive inducements include offering significant money to an indigent population, entry into a particular social group, promises of job promotions or good grades, freedom for a prisoner or servant, or promises of cure for a disease. Of course, many patients will participate in a trial because they are seeking a cure for their ailment. Promising a cure and not mentioning alternative treatments is coercion. Clearly stating the risks and benefits of participating and making no promises is not coercion.

A clinical study should provide *open access* to all qualifying patients. In other words, you should allow any scientifically appropriate patient to enroll in your study so long as they meet the study inclusion and exclusion criteria. Only scientific reasons should keep a patient from participating in a trial. Showing favoritism or nepotism when enrolling patients is unethical. This is important since clinical studies may be the only way patients can receive experimental but potentially effective medications.

2.2.4 Patient Autonomy and Human Dignity

Respect a patient's *autonomy*, that is, his or her right to make independent choices and take independent actions.

Remember that different patients have different beliefs, motivations, and perspectives. You cannot decide their lives for them. Respecting autonomy implies obtaining informed consent and never using coercion. Health care providers often act too *paternalistic*, believing that they know (more than anyone else including the patients) what's best for their patients. Truly respecting patient autonomy involves providing an environment that engenders freedom of choice. Patients may need time alone in a stress-free location when making decisions.

Respecting a patient's autonomy does not necessarily mean always accomodating the patient. Although a patient should be free to leave the study or, in general, refuse treatment, you do not have to comply with every patient's demand. Patient autonomy is not always absolute. Other moral considerations can override patient autonomy. If the patient is endangering the safety of others, you may take action to restrain or restrict the patient.

Do whatever you can to preserve *human dignity*. This means that every patient deserves the appropriate amount of respect. Do not treat patients as objects or things without feelings, family, friends, or pride. Every human being has intrinsic worth. Every human being has many rights, including the right to privacy, knowledge, and good care. Some common violations of human dignity include denying them adequate clothing, food, clean quarters, and other basic comforts. Of course, insulting or abusing patients is never acceptable.

2.2.5 Privacy and Confidentiality

Maintaining human dignity includes respecting their privacy and confidentiality of sensitive information. We will discuss this issue in greater detail later in this chapter when we cover the Health Insurance Portability and Accountability Act.

2.2.6 Tolerance and Acceptance

Patients must have *freedom of religion and beliefs*, that is, they can espouse any religion, belief system, or moral standards as long as they don't harm or endanger others. Except for scientific reasons, you cannot exclude a patient from a study because of his or her beliefs. You should be *tolerant* of views, cultures, and behaviors different from your own.

You and your study personnel should be *accepting* of people from different cultural, ethnic, racial, or gender backgrounds. Many patients may have lifestyles (e.g., different sexual orientations or practices) that you find unusual. Unless there are scientific reasons, never discriminate against certain patients.

2.2.7 Scientific Rationale and Equipoise

There must be good scientific rationale for the study, and there must be equipoise. Equipoise means that the results of the study is not already known in advance.

2.3 PROTECTING PATIENTS RIGHTS AND WELFARE

2.3.1 Institutional Review Board (IRB)/ Independent Ethics Committee (IEC)

An IRB [or independent ethics committee (IEC), as IRBs are referred to outside the United States and Canada] is a group officially responsible for reviewing and monitoring biomedical research involving human subjects and imbued with the power to approve, require alterations in, or disapprove clinical studies. The primary purpose of the IRB is to safeguard the rights and welfare of human subjects. Clinical studies cannot commence without IRB approval (or the IRB indicating that formal approval is not necessary). The IRB will not only review study protocols before studies begin but also periodically monitor clinical research as it progresses.

An institution does not have to have an IRB to engage in research. If you do not belong to an institution with an IRB, you can establish formal relationships with an outside independent IRB (e.g., community hospital, university, independent IRB, or government agency) to oversee your research activities. If you cannot find an outside IRB, you can contact the FDA for assistance. If your study is rejected by an independent IRB, you have the right to submit it to another IRB but must provide the documentation from the first IRB that rejected your study (including the reasons for rejecting your study protocol). However, you may not have this recourse if your study is rejected by your institution's IRB.

Remember the primary purpose of an IRB is to protect study subjects, not the institution or the investigator. An IRB should not reject a study just to protect the reputation of the institution (e.g., a study showing the number of medical mistakes occurring in a hospital) or accept a study simply because it may bring positive publicity for the institution.

A researcher may be part of an IRB but may not review any studies for which he or she may have a conflicting interest (e.g., the researcher's study or a potential competitor). The IRB should have a reasonable amount of diversity (e.g., gender, race, ethnicity, scientific disciplines, and professional backgrounds) and consist of both scientists and nonscientists. While IRB members may be paid for their services, payment cannot in any way be tied to their decisions. Since members will not always be available, the

IRB should formally appoint adequate alternates to fill in whenever an IRB member cannot attend a meeting.

When your clinical study involves minimal risk to its subjects, you may request an *expedited review*, that is, the chairperson or certain designated members of the IRB may review and approve the study protocol without convening a formal meeting. This reviewer (or reviewers) has (or have) all the power of the IRB except the right to reject a study protocol (the full committee must meet to do so). Minor changes in an existing IRB-approved study protocol also may qualify for expedited review.

The IRB has the right to observe (or designate someone else to observe) any part of your research process (e.g., the subject recruitment and informed consent process). You should notify your IRB of patient adverse events and any significant change in your study protocol or procedures. The IRB must review and approve all amendments to the study protocol before the changes are implemented, unless an emergent protocol change is needed to protect patients from imminent danger. You should inform patients of any changes that may affect their desire to participate in the study and give them the opportunity to withdraw from the study if they choose.

2.3.2 Data Safety Monitoring Boards

The IRB determines the level of independent oversight that a study needs. Small studies that pose little or no apparent risk to patients usually do not require much monitoring from a third party. However, the larger the study population, the greater the number of study sites, the more dangerous the treatments and procedures, and the sicker the study population, the more monitoring is needed. A study may require a *Data Safety Monitoring Board (DSMB)*, that is, an independent committee specifically assembled to closely observe the study data throughout the duration of the study and look for any signs of scientific or ethical irregularities. A DSMB should consist of relevant clinical and scientific experts, statistical experts, and lay representatives; the majority of a DSMB's members should come from outside the organization conducting the study.

2.3.3 Health Insurance Portability and Accountability Act

Enacted in 1996, the *Health Insurance Portability and Accountability Act (HIPAA)* helps ensure that electronic patient health, administrative and financial data is standardized, individuals, employers, health plans, and health care providers have unique identifying codes, and patient health information is secure and protected. As a result, anyone with access to or uses patient information must comply with the security standards. Noncompliance with the security standards can result in substantial penalties. Keep in mind that more stringent state or local regulations may supersede HIPAA.

As a result of HIPAA, the Department of Health and Human Services (DHHS) issued the Standards for Privacy of Individually Identifiable Health Information, otherwise known as the *Privacy Rule*. The Privacy Rule defined *protected health information (PHI)* as patient data that can be used or disclosed only under certain circumstances. PHI is a type of individually identifiable health information (i.e., any data that may somehow be linked to specific individuals). When you remove the identifying information (e.g., patient names, social security numbers, or addresses) from such data, it becomes *de-identified information*. (Note PHI does not include educational or employee records.) A "covered entity" is an organization, such as health plans, health care providers, or health care clearinghouses that electronically transmit patient information for transactions that have a standard developed by the DHHS (e.g., billing and payment for services or insurance coverage). The Privacy Rule applies to "covered entities" as well as researchers who work for or receive data from covered entities. (Note that the Privacy Rule does not apply to organizations that are not covered entities or researchers working with such organizations.)

So how does the Privacy Rule apply to researchers? First of all, de-identified health information is not PHI and therefore does not fall under the purview of the Privacy Rule. So if someone else (e.g., an *honest broker* who is a third party not involved in your research project) removes all identifying information from the data so that you cannot decipher the identity of the patients, you may use the data without obtaining permission from the patients. Second, patients may provide you with written *authorization* to use their PHI for a specific research project. The authorization must specify the research project and applies only to that research project. Third, you may use PHI when the IRB grants you a waiver of the authorization requirement. This is because obtaining authorization from the patient may not be practical or possible. For example, the patient may no longer be alive, or you may only need a limited PHI data set to prepare for a research project. A *limited data set* is defined as one that does not have any of 16 categories of direct identifiers. Using the limited data set does not require authorization from the patients as long as you enter into a *data use agreement* (which specifies how the limited data set will be used and protected) with the covered entity.

The Privacy Rule grants patients a set of rights regarding their PHI. Patients must be able to access their PHI. They have a right to know what, how, and why data is being collected and used. When patients grant you authorization to use their PHI, they may withdraw this authorization at any time without explanation. You should also be aware that in countries outside the U.S. there are often different set of privacy rules, some of which may be much more strict than U.S. regulations. European Union, for example, has extremely stringent privacy regulations.

2.4 CLINICAL RESEARCH AND MANUFACTURING STANDARDS

2.4.1 International Conference on Harmonization and Good Clinical Practices

In the 1970s and 1980s standards on how to perform clinical research proliferated. Different countries had different regulations. The US FDA, European Union, and Japan each had its own Code of Regulations. As the scope of clinical research grew and multi-national studies were becoming the norm, it became increasingly clear that having a multitude of different standards could wreak havoc with clinical studies. As a result, attempts were made to achieve some consensus over the different components and conduct of clinical research.

In 1990, the first International Conference on Harmonization (ICH) convened in Brussels, Belgium, with the goal of defining standards for medical product development. Industry, academic, and governmental representatives from the United States, the European Union, and Japan attended the ICH and generated a variety of important documents, including the ICH Good Clinical Practices (GCP) guideline. Since its first draft in 1990 (referred to as Step 1), the ICH GCP has undergone several revisions

(Step 2, Step 3, Step 4, and Step 5) with the latest dated January 1997.

The ICH GCP guideline consists of eight sections:

- *Glossary*: This defines important terms in clinical research.
- *The principles of ICH GCP*: This is the 13 basic tenets of the ICH GCP (Figure 2.4).
- *IRBs/IECs*: This describes the roles, composition, and responsibilities of IRB/IEC.
- *Investigators*: This describes the roles and responsibilities of the investigator.
- *Sponsor*: This describes the roles and responsibilities of sponsor.
- *Clinical trial protocol*: Requirements for a clinical trial protocol.
- *Investigator's brochure.*
- *Essential documents for the conduct of a clinical trial.*

2.4.2 Good Manufacturing Practices

Good Manufacturing Practices (GMP) are a set of regulations for manufacturers, processors, and packagers of drugs, medical devices, certain types of food, and blood to ensure the safety, purity, and effectiveness of these products. Without such GMP regulations, even well-designed drugs and medical devices may become ineffective and unsafe from defects, contamination, mislabeling, and other errors.

Different types of GMP regulations exist throughout the world. The FDA has a set of GMP regulations for the

1. Clinical trials should be conducted in accordance with the ethical principles that have their origin in the Declaration of Helsinki, and that are consistent with GCP and the applicable regulatory requirement(s).
2. Before a trial is initiated, foreseeable risks and inconveniences should be weighed against the anticipated benefit for the individual trial subject and society. A trial should be initiated and continued only if the anticipated benefits justify the risks.
3. The rights, safety, and well-being of the trial subjects are the most important considerations and should prevail over interests of science and society.
4. The available nonclinical and clinical information on an investigational product should be adequate to support the proposed clinical trial.
5. Clinical trials should be scientifically sound, and described in a clear, detailed protocol.
6. A trial should be conducted in compliance with the protocol that has received prior institutional review board (IRB)/independent ethics committee (IEC) approval/favorable opinion.
7. The medical care given to, and medical decisions made on behalf of, subjects should always be the responsibility of a qualified physician or, when appropriate, of a qualified dentist.
8. Each individual involved in conducting a trial should be qualified by education, training, and experience to perform his or her respective task(s).
9. Freely given informed consent should be obtained from every subject prior to clinical trial participation.
10. All clinical trial information should be recorded, handled, and stored in a way that allows its accurate reporting, interpretation, and verification.
11. The confidentiality of records that could identify subjects should be protected, respecting the privacy and confidentiality rules in accordance with the applicable regulatory requirement(s).
12. Investigational products should be manufactured, handled, and stored in accordance with applicable good manufacturing practice (GMP). They should be used in accordance with the approved protocol.
13. Systems with procedures that assure the quality of every aspect of the trial should be implemented.

FIGURE 2.4   The 13 Principles of the International Conference on Humanization Good Clinical Practice (ICH GCP).

United States. Japan, Singapore, Australia, the European Union, and many other countries have their own GMP requirements. The World Health Organization's (WHO's) GMP regulations apply in many countries that do not have their own GMP requirements.

Each country has a particular agency or organization that enforces GMP regulations. In the United States, the FDA enforces GMP regulations. Australia has the Therapeutical Goods Administration (TGA). The United Kingdom has the Medicines and Healthcare Products Regulatory Agency (MHRA). These agencies and organizations conduct routine and surprise inspections of manufacturing facilities. In fact, Pre-Approval Inspections (PAI) are standard before a drug or medical device is approved for marketing. Noncompliance with GMP regulations can lead to forfeiture of rights to continue manufacturing the goods, recall of products from the market, seizure of the goods, fines, and jail time.

GMP regulations address all aspects of manufacturing, packaging, and labeling including cleanliness and sanitation, equipment function and use, recordkeeping, personnel, operations and processes, product testing, and addressing errors and complaints. Manufacturers must document clearly procedure and process, and have quality assessment and control measures in place. Testing and validation (i.e., does the process or equipment do what it is supposed to do) of equipment and operations is essential. Processes must be reliable (i.e., produce the same result every time) with minimal variation. Equipment, techniques, and processes must be up-to-date (which is why GMP is also frequently referred to as "CGMP," with the "C" standing for current). What worked 20, 10, or even a few years ago may not be adequate today.

2.5 US PHARMACEUTICAL APPROVAL PROCESS

2.5.1 Overview

The long and winding road …

The Beatles

Drug development is indeed a very long, complicated, and unpredictable road, taking an average of 8½ years from concept to the market. Drug development is also very expensive and resource-intensive. Figure 2.5 presents an overview of the process. The FDA's Center for Drug Evaluation and Research (CDER) regulates the drug development and approval process. Most drugs fail at some point along the developmental process. The failure rate is highest near the beginning of the whole process. However, making it to clinical studies is no guarantee. The odds are still against a drug succeeding through the gauntlet of clinical trials.

2.5.2 Pre-clinical Studies

For every compound that ends up being tested in humans, hundreds or perhaps even thousands of compounds end up stalling somewhere in pre-clinical testing. Pre-clinical development includes identifying appropriate molecular targets for the compound, finding how different compounds interact with and affect the target cells, and devising ways to synthesize and purify the compound so that it may act as a drug. By the time a compound reaches human testing, it usually has gone through countless modifications and

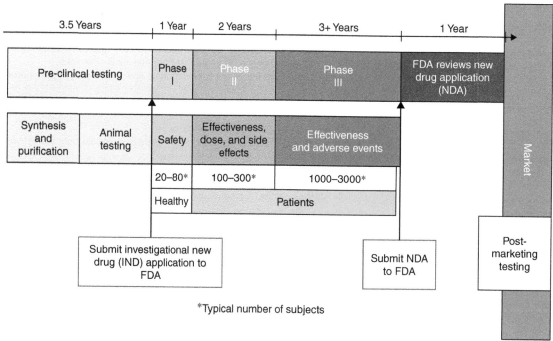

FIGURE 2.5   An Overview of Typical Drug Development Timeline.

adjustments. Frequently, the final compound appears nothing like the original compound.

Drug development can take a variety of different routes. In some cases, scientists attempt to find a solution for a specific need or disease. In other cases, scientists identify an interesting mechanism, process, or technique and then attempt to find an application for it. In general, developing and testing drug compound begin in the test tube (i.e., assays), proceed to cells (i.e., *in vitro* testing using cultured cells), and then perhaps microorganisms (e.g., fungal, viral, or bacterial cultures). Nowadays, computers can play a major role in testing and planning modifications in compounds.

After enough *in vitro* data has been generated, *in vivo* (i.e., in animal) testing may commence. The challenge of animal testing is generating enough data while minimizing the number of animals used and the discomfort and injury caused to the animals. Usually, at least two different animal species are necessary, since drugs can behave differently in different species. Animal testing should measure the effects, distribution, metabolism, and toxicity of the drug. Animal testing should include short-term testing (2 weeks to 3 months) and long-term testing (few weeks to several years), as some effects manifest rather quickly while others take a while to develop (e.g., cancer-causing effects or birth defects). Sometimes human testing raises questions that additional animal testing may address (e.g., new unexpected side effects are found in humans).

The FDA mandates that at the conclusion of pre-clinical studies you should have at a minimum:

- developed a pharmacological profile of the drug;
- determined the acute toxicity of the drug in at least two species of animals; and
- conducted short-term toxicity studies ranging from 2 weeks to 3 months, depending on the proposed duration of the use of the substance in the proposed clinical studies.

Not all drugs in clinical trials come directly from pre-clinical studies. The drug may already be in the market in another country, and the goal of the clinical trial is to get the drug approved in the United States. Alternatively, the drug may be in the market in the United States for a different indication, and the clinical trial will be testing the drug for a new indication. In these cases, performing pre-clinical studies before starting clinical studies may not be necessary. Instead of pre-clinical study data, you may submit clinical data to the FDA to prove that the drug will be safe for human testing.

2.5.3 Investigational New Drug Application

Before testing a medication in humans for the first time, you must submit an investigational new drug (IND) application. The *applicant* or *sponsor* is the person or organization (e.g., pharmaceutical company or medical center) who submits the IND and ultimately will be responsible for complying with FDA regulations. Although Federal law prohibits anyone from shipping a non-FDA approved drug across state borders, a successful IND application exempts the sponsor from this federal law, allowing the sponsor to transport drugs to different study sites.

The IND application requires evidence that the drug will be reasonably safe for testing in humans. This entails presenting data to support the following:

- *Your drug is safe in animals*: Your data from animal toxicology and pharmacology studies should show that the drug is safe in animals.
- *Your drug is stable and consistent*: Your data on the composition, stability, and manufacturing of the medication must prove that the drug is stable enough to be transported and administered to patients and that the manufacturing process can generate consistent doses with consistent activity. Wildly fluctuating drug composition and activity will be unpredictable and potentially dangerous in humans.
- *Your clinical trial protocol will be safe*: Your clinical study protocols should include appropriate safeguards for patients and not expose patients to unreasonable risks. After all, even stable drugs with low toxicity can be dangerous in certain trial designs.
- *Your clinical trial design will generate useful results*: The design of your clinical study should be able to provide adequate efficacy and safety information. Running a trial that yields useless data will put patients through unnecessary risks.
- *Your study personnel are qualified to run the trial*: A relatively safe, stable drug in the wrong hands can be dangerous even in a well-designed trial.

Figure 2.6 provides an overview of the IND process. As you can see, the first stage of the FDA's review of an IND entails a medical review (conducted by medical/clinical reviewers or medical officers, who are usually physicians), a chemistry review (conducted by chemistry reviewers, i.e., chemists), a pharmacology/toxicology review (conducted by pharmacologists and toxicologists), and a statistical review (conducted by statisticians).

Once you submit an IND, CDER has 30 days to decide whether to put a *clinical hold* on your trial. A clinical hold is an order to either immediately halt (or not initiate) a clinical study because of safety concerns (i.e., the patients may be unreasonably endangered). CDER will contact you by phone and in writing and describe their concerns. To remove the hold, you will have to adequately address the concerns. CDER will then review your response and determine whether to lift the clinical hold. In general, reviewers will scrutinize the safety aspects of your data and trial design more stringently than the efficacy aspects.

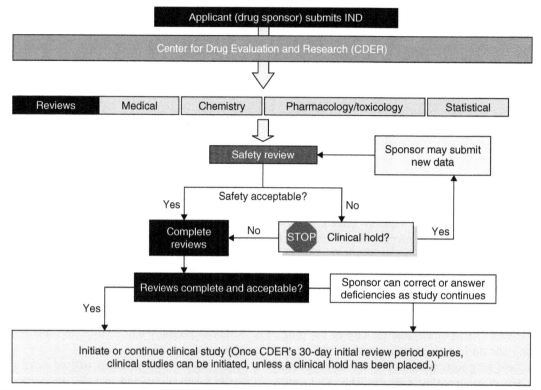

FIGURE 2.6   An overview of the Investigational New Drug (IND) application process.

Significant safety concerns almost always will prompt reviewers to order a clinical hold. By contrast, questionable effectiveness alone is not a reason to place a clinical hold. If you have not heard anything from CDER 31 days after submitting the IND, it is reasonable to commence the clinical trial as planned.

There are several different types of IND applications. A *commercial IND* is for sponsors who ultimately want to market the drug (e.g., pharmaceutical or biotechnology company). A *Noncommercial IND* is for anyone who will not be the one marketing the drug (e.g., academic physician). The typical noncommercial IND application is an *Investigator-Initiated IND*, submitted by the physician who will initiate and conduct the trials. The Investigator-Initiated IND is very similar to a commercial IND in that it allows the investigator to start Phase I clinical trials. By contrast, an *Emergency Use IND* and a *Treatment IND* are noncommercial INDs for an experimental drug that is desperately needed by very ill patients (e.g., advanced AIDS) who have no viable alternatives. An Emergency Use IND will allow a physician to treat one patient for one time only with an experimental drug. The Emergency Use IND will not allow you to use the drug to conduct human research. A Treatment IND will permit you to initiate Phase I clinical trials on the drug, but unlike a regular IND, will make the drug available to patients in need before the drug is approved for marketing (i.e., less evidence is needed before the drug can be used to treat certain patients).

2.5.4 Clinical Studies

Once the IND is approved, you can proceed to clinical studies. Clinical studies consist of several steps:

- *Phase I clinical studies*: Phase I are the so-called first in man studies. Study subjects are usually healthy volunteers but occasionally may be patients with the targeted disease. Typically Phase I studies are relatively small (20–80 subjects) compared to future Phase studies. Phase I studies help determine how the human body will handle the drug (e.g., drug absorption, distribution, metabolism, and excretion), how the drug will behave within the human body (e.g., mechanism of action) and what doses to use for Phase II clinical studies (e.g., side effects associated with increasing doses).
- *Phase II clinical studies*: Unlike Phase I studies, Phase II studies use patients (usually several hundred) with the disease or condition that the drug intends to treat. Phase II studies, which are typically well-controlled, generate early data on the drug's efficacy and safety while being used to treating the particular disease.
- *Sponsor/FDA meetings (end of Phase II)*: Following Phase II studies, you usually will meet with the FDA to determine whether to proceed to Phase III studies and the general design of these studies. Working closely with FDA can save you considerable time, efforts, and money.

- *Phase III clinical studies*: Phase III studies are the so-called pivotal trials: the trial will determine whether a new drug is inferior, equivalent, or superior to the standard treatment. Usually consisting of hundreds to thousands of patients, Phase III studies aim to prove a drug's effectiveness and safety (i.e., do the benefits of the drug outweigh the risks). These studies will help predict how the drug may behave in the general population and establish the information that will appear on the drug label.

Drug development can stall or halt at any of these steps. You may decide to abandon the drug when results are not promising or you run out of resources. The FDA may put on clinical hold at any stage if evidence suggests that the drug may not be safe.

2.5.5 New Drug Application

In order to commercialize or market a drug, you must submit a *new drug application* (*NDA*) to CDER. An NDA must contain comprehensive information from the drug's preclinical and clinical trials. Although the exact information differs depending on the type of drug and indication, some common sections of an NDA include Index; Summary; Chemistry, Manufacturing, and Control; Samples, Methods Validation Package, and Labeling; Nonclinical Pharmacology and Toxicology; Human Pharmacokinetics and Bioavailability; Microbiology (for anti-microbial drugs only); Clinical Data; Safety Update Report; Statistical; Case Report Tabulations; Case Report Forms; Patent Information; Patent Certification; and Other Information.

The NDA must demonstrate that a drug's:

- benefits outweigh its risks;
- labeling is justified and appropriate;
- manufacturing processes and controls are adequate to preserve the drug's identity, strength, quality, and purity.

Table 2.1 shows CDER's number and letter codes for type of NDA.

Prior to the NDA-submission, sponsors may have a *pre-NDA meeting* with CDER to discuss and help plan the application. Presenting a summary of the clinical data and the tentative format of the submission at the meeting will help reveal and address any potential stumbling blocks, familiarize the reviewers with the information, and in general facilitate the review.

Once CDER has received the application, they will first determine if the application is "fileable," that is, is all the information necessary present? If the application is deemed incomplete, CDER will issue a refuse-to-file letter to the applicant. If the application is fileable, the NDA review will commence. Relevant specialists will conduct reviews in multiple different areas such as medical, biopharmaceutical, pharmacology/toxicology, statistics, chemistry,

TABLE 2.1 Type of NDA

Code	Type of drug
1	New molecular entity
2	New salt of previously approved drug (not a new molecular entity)
3	New formulation of previously approved drug (not a new salt OR a new molecular entity)
4	New combination of two or more drugs
5	Already marketed drug product
6	New indication (claim) for already marketed drug (includes switch in marketing status from prescription to OTC)
7	Already marketed drug product
	Review priority
S	Standard review for drugs similar to currently available drugs
P	Priority review for drugs that represent significant advances over existing treatments

manufacturing, and microbiology (if relevant). Before approval, CDER may request an inspection of your manufacturing facilities and clinical trial sites to verify statements in the NDA and determine if the manufacturing process complies with Current Good Manufacturing Practices (CGMPs). CDER may also collect and analyze drug samples. According to the FDA, inspection is particularly likely for:

- drugs that are new chemical or molecular entities;
- drugs with narrow therapeutic ranges;
- first-time applicants;
- applicants with a history of CGMP violations;
- applicants that have not had CGMP inspections recently.

In order to have broad range of opinions and input, CDER often employs *advisory committees* composed of experts from outside the FDA to make nonbinding recommendations. These advisory committees can assist in approval decisions, labeling information, and drug use guidelines. Through the course of the review, CDER may find and inform you about "easily correctable deficiencies in the NDA" (e.g., errors in filling out the application or the need for more data or information). During the review, you may submit additional relevant information that will be considered amendments to your NDA and may extend the review process.

Following the review, CDER may issue one of the three possible action letters:

- *Not approvable*: Explains why the NDA cannot be approved.

- *Approvable*: The drug can be approved if you address and correct certain minor deficiencies (e.g., labeling changes). When these deficiencies are addressed, an approval letter ensues.
- *Approval*: The drug is approved. You may begin marketing the drug in the United States.

You have the option of participating in an "end of review conference" with CDER to discuss the deficiencies in an NDA and how they may be addressed. For a biologic (a drug that is composed of peptides or proteins), a biologic license application (BLA) is filed and is subject to a similar process as an NDA.

Drug Label Review

A drug that is commercialized must have a label that includes the components shown in Table 2.2. Scientific data and evidence must support every claim made on the label. Label approval is an iterative process that may involve significant negotiation. Many times a label will not be finalized and approved until multiple revisions have occurred.

2.5.6 Special Mechanisms

Several special mechanisms can accelerate the drug development process for specific situations:

- *Treatment IND*: This mechanism (which we mentioned earlier) makes experimental drugs available to desperately ill patients while the drug is still in clinical trials (usually during Phase III studies).
- *Accelerated development/review*: This highly specialized mechanism aims to reduce the time to market for very promising drugs for serious or life-threatening illnesses that currently do not have adequate treatments. According to the FDA, "accelerated development/review can be used under two special circumstances: when approval is based on evidence of the product's effect on a 'surrogate endpoint,' and when the FDA determines that safe use of a product depends on restricting its distribution or use." With this mechanism, testing of the drug to prove its effectiveness must continue even after the drug is approved and are on the market, otherwise the FDA may withdraw the drug from the market.
- *Parallel track*: AIDS patients whose conditions prevent them from participating in controlled clinical trials may receive experimental drugs that have promising early clinical trial results.

Signed into law on January 4, 1983, the *Orphan Drug Act* aims to stimulate research and development of drugs to treat rare diseases (i.e., drugs that will have small focused markets). An "orphan drug" is a drug aiming to treat a disease afflicting fewer than 200,000 Americans. The Act offers a sponsor of an orphan drug exclusive rights to market the drug for 7 years after approval, tax incentives, research study design assistance from the FDA's Office of

TABLE 2.2 Components of a Drug Label

Component	FDA definition
Description	Proprietary and established name of drug; dosage form; ingredients; chemical name; and structural formula.
Clinical pharmacology	Summary of the actions of the drug in humans; *in vitro* and *in vivo* actions in animals if pertinent to human therapeutics; pharmacokinetics.
Indications and Usage	Description of use of drug in the treatment, prevention, or diagnosis of a recognized disease or condition.
Contraindications	Description of situations in which the drug should not be used because the risk of use clearly outweighs any possible benefit.
Warnings	Description of serious adverse reactions and potential safety hazards, subsequent limitation in use, and steps that should be taken if they occur.
Precautions	Information regarding any special care to be exercised for the safe and effective use of the drug. Includes general precautions and information for patients on drug interactions, carcinogenesis/mutagenesis, pregnancy rating, labor and delivery, nursing mothers, and pediatric use.
Adverse reactions	Description of undesirable effect(s) reasonably associated with the proper use of the drug.
Drug abuse/dependence	Description of types of abuse that can occur with the drug and the adverse reactions pertinent to them.
Overdosage	Description of the signs, symptoms, and laboratory findings of acute overdosage and the general principles of treatment.
Dosage/administration	Recommendation for usage dose, usual dosage range, and, if appropriate, upper limit beyond which safety and effectiveness have not been established.
How supplied	Information on the available dosage forms to which the labeling applies.

Orphan Products Development, and eligibility for special research grant funding.

2.6 US MEDICAL DEVICE APPROVAL PROCESS

2.6.1 Definition of Medical Device

What exactly is a medical device? Defining a "medical device" is more difficult than defining a drug. The spectrum of what can qualify as a medical device is incredibly broad. Implantable cardiac defibrillators and vascular stents are obviously medical devices, but so are hearing aids, bandages, MRI machines, blood pressure cuffs, crutches, intrauterine devices, and certain wash basins. Many items that appear on late night infomercials advertised as exercise or health items are borderline medical devices. Even lab tests that never enter or contact a patient's body, such as pregnancy tests, are medical devices.

According to the Medical Device Amendments to the Federal Food, Drug, and Cosmetic Act Section 201(h), a medical device is: "an instrument, apparatus, implement, machine, contrivance, implant, *in vitro* reagent, or other similar or related articles, including any component, part, or accessory, which is:

- recognized by the official National Formulary, or the U.S. Pharmacopoeia (USP), or any supplement to them;
- intended for use in the diagnosis of disease or other conditions, or in the cure, mitigation treatment, or prevention of disease, in a man or other animals;
- intended to affect the structure or any function of the body of a man or other animals, and which does not achieve any of its principal intended purposes through chemical action within or on the body of a man or other animals and which is not dependent on being metabolized for the achievement of its principal intended uses."

An item's *intended use* or *indication for use* is very important and determines the rigor with which it is regulated. For example, a metal container used to hold shredded paper would not be a medical device. The same metal container used to soak a person's injured foot may be a medical device. An item's function or physiological purpose, the condition that the item will diagnose or treat, and the population that item will target determine the required approval and monitoring process.

In the United States, two FDA centers regulate medical devices:

- *Center for Biologics Evaluation and Research (CBER)*: This center regulates any medical device that helps manufacture, collect (e.g., needles and syringes), process, test (e.g., HIV tests), and administer (e.g., blood transfusion machines and catheters) blood, blood components, and cellular products.
- *Center for Devices and Radiological Health (CDRH)*: All other medical devices fall under the purview of the CDRH (e.g., surgical instruments, imaging equipment, and laboratory tests). The CDRH also regulates any electronic product that emits radiation, including those used for nonmedical functions (e.g., microwave ovens and televisions).

2.6.2 Routes to Approval

The FDA classifies medical devices depending on their potential risk that they may pose. When attempting to get your device cleared or approved, you can either identify the class of your device or formally request the FDA to identify an appropriate class. Table 2.3 shows these three classes: Class I (low risk), Class II (moderate risk), and Class III (high risk). Each medical device marketed in the United States must conform with a certain level of "controls," depending on the class of the device. As Table 2.3 shows, most Class I devices require only *general controls*.

TABLE 2.3 FDA Classification of Medical Devices

Class	General controls	Special controls	Pre-market notification (510(k))	Pre-market approval (PMA)	Description	Examples
I	X		X		Minimal risk and often simpler in design	Elastic bandages, examination gloves, and hand-held surgical instruments
II	X	X	X		Moderate risk	Powered wheelchairs, infusion pumps, and surgical drapes
III				X	Support/sustain human life, prevent health impairment, or pose significant risk	Artificial heart valves, breast implants, and brain stimulators

For general controls, you have to register the company that plans to manufacture and distribute the device with the FDA, list the device with the FDA as a device to be marketed, manufacture your device in compliance with the Quality Systems regulation (GMPs), label your devices properly per FDA regulations, and submit a pre-market notification 510(k) before marketing a device. In addition to general controls, Class II devices require *special controls*, that is, special labeling requirements, mandatory and voluntary performance standards and post-market surveillance. With some exceptions, Class III devices usually necessitate *pre-market approval (PMA)*. General and special controls alone are not sufficient.

In general, medical devices can take one of three routes to the market.

Pre-market Notification 510(k)

For this route, you only have to prove your device has *substantial equivalence*. This less rigorous standard is appropriate for most low- to moderate-risk devices (usually Class I or II devices, but some older, pre-amendment Class III devices may sometimes qualify). The standard entails demonstrating that your device has the same intended use, characteristics, safety, and efficacy as a *predicate device* (i.e., a device already on the market). You can choose the predicate device for comparison but ultimately the FDA decides whether the comparison is appropriate. Meeting this standard gives device FDA "clearance" rather than FDA "approval."

A 510(k) is required when you:

- want to commercially manufacture and distribute a device for the first time;
- would like to introduce a new use for a currently marketed device;
- change a currently marketed device in a way that may substantially alter its safety or effectiveness.

A 510(k) is not required when you will:

- not market or commercially distribute the device;
- distribute or import a device that is manufactured by someone else who obtained the necessary clearance or approval.

Additionally, some devices are exempt from the 510(k) requirement. For example, a *pre-amendment device* (legally on the market before May 28, 1976, has not undergone significant change or modification, and does not require a PMA application) is a "grandfathered" device and does not require a 510(k).

Often, 510(k) does not need true clinical study data. Although clinical study data is preferable, you may demonstrate substantial equivalence by just showing that the device performs in a similar fashion to the predicate under a similar set of circumstances. Traditionally a 510(k) includes information about the device's performance under specific relevant conditions, design, components, packaging and labeling, nonclinical and clinical studies that support the device performance characteristics, means by which users can assess the quality of the device, and information about any computer software or additional or special equipment needed.

Following its review, the FDA may:

- deem the device substantially equivalent and issue a clearance letter;
- deem the device not substantially equivalent (NSE) and issue an NSE letter, which prohibits marketing of the device;
- request additional information (with the final clearance decision pending review of that information).

Pre-market Approval

Obtaining a PMA involves demonstrating that your device is *safe and effective*, which is a more rigorous standard than "substantial equivalence." Meeting this standard results in medical device "approval" (instead of just "clearance"). You must provide scientific evidence (e.g., animal studies and human studies) that the benefits of the device outweigh the risks for the device's intended use. Additionally, a PMA entails giving detailed information on the device's design, components, manufacturing (including inspection of the manufacturing facility and processes), instructions, packaging, and labeling. Like the pharmaceutical approval process, the FDA may convene advisory committees for advice and suggestions.

Humanitarian Device Exemption

The FDA defines a Humanitarian Use Device (HUD) as a "medical device intended to benefit patients in the treatment or diagnosis of a disease or condition that affects or is manifested in fewer than 4000 individuals in the United States per year." A HUD can reach the market through a *Humanitarian Device Exemption (HDE)*, which is similar to a PMA but without the same effectiveness requirements.

Keep in mind that you can market a medical device *only for its cleared or approved use*. You cannot add uses or indications or change the device's design or manufacturing process without at least filing a supplement to the original application. You cannot use an unapproved device in a clinical study without an *Investigational Device Exemption (IDE)*, which allows you to ship the device for use in the clinical study.

2.7 POST-APPROVAL

2.7.1 Expanding Indications and Labeling

Clinical research does not end once a product or intervention has hit the market. Manufacturers, researchers, and

---

Post-market Surveillance of Medical Devices

(from the FDA)

FDA may order a manufacturer to conduct post-market surveillance of a medical device under Section 522 of the Food, Drug and Cosmetic Act (act). FDA has the authority to order post-market surveillance of any class II or class III medical device, including a device reviewed under the licensing provisions of Section 351 of the Public Health Service Act that meets any of the following criteria:

(a) failure of the device would be reasonably likely to have serious adverse health consequences;
(b) the device is intended to be implanted in the human body for more than 1 year; or
(c) the device is intended to be used to support or sustain life and to be used outside a user facility.

Post-market surveillance means the active, systematic, scientifically valid collection, analysis, and interpretation of data or other information about a marketed device. The data can reveal unforeseen adverse events, the actual rate of anticipated adverse events, or other information necessary to protect the public health. Title 21 CFR 822, Post-market Surveillance, provides procedures and requirements for post-market surveillance.

FIGURE 2.7   Post-market surveillance of medical devices (from the U.S. FDA).

health care providers are continuously expanding the *indications* (i.e., the uses) of drugs and devices. It may be as simple as demonstrating whether a treatment works for a different segment of the population or more or less severe cases of the disease. They may want to combine treatments or treat closely related diseases.

In fact, in the real world, a large percentage of drug and medical device use is *off-label*, that is, use for purposes or in ways that do not appear on the product's label. Such a practice is legal unless the treatment is a *controlled substance*, that is, a highly regulated substance (e.g., narcotics) that may be used only for specific purposes. Once a drug or device is approved and on the market, the FDA allows physicians to use their discretion about how to use different treatments, as long as the use is not overtly abusive or unacceptably dangerous.

A *Phase IV study* is a clinical trial of an already approved and marketed drug. A Phase IV trial can provide more information on the drug's effectiveness and safety in more real-life conditions and either confirm or add indications to a drug's label. Such studies can examine different drug doses and study populations (e.g., varying ages, ethnic groups, disease severity, or disease presentation) from those used in Phase I through III studies. Phase IV studies can also employ varying designs and measures (e.g., economic or quality of life).

2.7.2 Post-market Surveillance

As we have seen in recent years, passing through the gauntlet of FDA approval does not guarantee that a drug or device will not have future problems. Clinical trial settings are idealized situations and settings. Frequently a

drug or device behaves quite differently in the real world. Moreover, as time passes, we continue to learn more and more about different drugs and devices. Look at some of the high profile drugs that have been pulled from the U.S. market for serious adverse drug reactions: Baycol (cerivastatin) for rhabdomyolysis, Propulsid (cisapride) and Seldane (terfenadine) for abnormal heart rhythms, and Rezulin (troglitazone) for liver failure. Even with the best intentions, the clinical development of drugs, devices, and other medical interventions is far from perfect.

As a result, the need for *post-market surveillance* continues to grow. Post-market surveillance is the monitoring of drugs and devices after they have been approved and are on the market. Post-market surveillance is important not only to catch drugs and devices that are not working or unsafe but also to identify situations where supplies are not meeting the demands (e.g., a drug is not being manufactured quickly enough to treat all patients with a disease). Moreover, post-marketing surveillance may find misleading or unjustified claims in product labeling or advertising.

Manufacturers, researchers, or regulatory bodies may perform post-market surveillance. For example, the FDA has the right to order manufacturers of Class II or Class III devices to conduct post-market surveillance studies if any of their devices meet any of the criteria listed in Figure 2.7. Many manufacturers prefer to be proactive and perform pharmacovigilance and pharmacosurveillance, two terms that mean monitoring drug safety. *Pharmacosurveillance* sometimes implies a more proactive look for adverse events and problems (e.g., running case control or cohort clinical studies) while *pharmacovigilance* may imply putting systems in place that can detect adverse events or other problems should they emerge.

Chapter 3

Introduction to Clinical Trial Statistics

3.1 INTRODUCTION

3.1.1 Types of Statistics

The American Heritage Dictionary of the English Language defines statistics as follows:

> **sta·tis·tics (st-tstks) n.**
> 1. (used with a sing. verb) The mathematics of the collection, organization, and interpretation of numerical data, especially the analysis of population characteristics by inference from sampling.
> 2. (used with a pl. verb) Numerical data.

Like it or not, if you are involved in clinical research, understanding statistics is very important. Statistics affect the design, execution, and interpretation of clinical trials. While this may appear daunting to mathematics-phobes and numero-phobes, it really should not be. The goal should not be to memorize how to calculate each and every statistical formula but rather to understand the logic behind different statistical tests and assumptions.

Depending on how you use them, statistics can be a powerful beacon or dangerous charlatan. Properly used, statistics can shed light on important associations and cause-and-effect relationships. Improperly used, statistics can suggest associations and cause-and-effect relationships that are not really present. Some cynics suggest that you can use statistics to draw any type of conclusion you want to draw. As a famous quote says:

There are three kinds of lies: lies, damned lies, and statistics.
Benjamin Disraeli

Despite the potential weaknesses, statistics can serve a variety of purposes. You can classify statistics into three major categories as follows based on how they are used:

Descriptive Statistics

Descriptive statistics paint a picture of a situation, providing a concise numerical or graphical summary. We use descriptive statistics every day to help communicate a phenomenon or situation to other people. People often view descriptive statistics as being more objective than nonnumerical descriptions. Say your friends want you to describe a party that you attended last night. A nonnumerical description could be: The party had lots of attractive and interesting people with lots of dating potential. A set of descriptive statistics may be as follows: 75 people, the average age was 35 years old, the range of ages from 21 to 47, 65% female and 35% male, 80% were college graduates and 20% had advanced degrees, 30% were from out of state, and 20% had black hair, 20% had blonde hair, 50% had brown hair, and 10% had red hair. As you can see, descriptive statistics provide hard numbers against which each person can compare his or her personal benchmarks.

Comparative Statistics

Simple descriptive statistics without a proper context or comparison may not be useful. Is a party with 80% college graduates good or bad? How good or bad is a 35% to 65% male-to-female ratio? Remember very few things are inherently good or bad. It all depends on comparisons. A party with 65% women may not be good for a man who is used to attending social gatherings with 80% women. However, a man who has been living and working among only men for several years may be elated to find a party with any women.

A more sophisticated type of descriptive statistics, *comparative statistic* serves to compare in a numerical or graphical fashion one situation with another (or multiple other situations). People rely on comparative statistics every day to make evaluations and decisions:

- *Should you go to this party?* How many men or women will be there? How does this compare with other parties? What will be the average age and age range? What will be their intellectual, social, and professional backgrounds (e.g., average education and professional levels)?

- *Is that football player good and worth drafting?* What are his average yards per reception, median touchdowns per year, and range of yards per carry or game compared to other players?
- *Should you go to this college?* What are the students' median test scores, the male:female ratio, the range of student ages, the average number of parties per week, and the median income of graduates compared to other schools?
- *Are you doing well socially and professionally?* How does your income, number of friends, family size, and house value compare to local and national averages or medians?

In fact, people tend to overuse comparative statistics. Just because your income, family size, and house value are lower than local or national averages or medians does not mean you are not doing well. A finite number of statistics cannot fully capture a situation. Moreover, statistics cannot adequately represent many important characteristics (e.g., having a loving spouse, enjoyable hobbies, or supportive friends). Comparative statistics are useful but you need to understand their limitations.

Inferential Statistics

Inferential statistics suggests explanations for a situation or phenomenon. It allows you to draw conclusions based on extrapolations, and is in that way fundamentally different from descriptive statistics that merely summarize the data that has actually been measured. Let us go back to our party example. Say comparative statistics suggest that parties hosted by your friend Sophia are very successful (e.g., the average number of attendees and the median duration of her parties are greater than those of other parties). Your next questions may be: Why are her parties so successful? Is it the food she serves, the size of her social network, the prestige of her job, the number of men or women she knows, her physical attractiveness, the alcohol she provides, or the location and size of her residence? Inferential statistics may help you answer these questions. Finding that less well-attended parties had on average fewer drinks served would suggest that your friend Sophia's drinks might be the important factor. The differences in attendance and drinks served between her parties and other parties would have to be large enough to draw any conclusions.

Note that the inferential statistics usually suggest but cannot absolutely prove an explanation or cause-and-effect relationship. Inferential comes from the word infer. To infer is to conclude or judge from premises or evidence (American Heritage Dictionary) and not to prove. Often, inferential statistics help to draw conclusions about an entire population by looking at only a sample of the population. Inferential statistics frequently involves estimation (i.e., guessing the characteristics of a population from a sample of the population)

and hypothesis testing (i.e., finding evidence for or against an explanation or theory).

Statistics describe and analyze variables. We discuss measures and variables in greater detail in Chapter 4. A variable is a measured characteristic or attribute that may assume different values. A variable may be quantitative (e.g., height) or categorical (e.g., eye color). Variables may be *independent* (the value it assumes is not affected by any other variables) or *dependent* (the value it assumes is pre-determined by other variables). Variables are not inherently independent or dependent. An independent variable in one statistical model may be dependent on another. For example, assume that we have a statistical model to identify the cause of heart disease. Independent variables would be risk factors for heart disease: cigarettes smoked per day, drinks per day, and cholesterol level. The presence of heart disease would be a dependent variable. The risk factor variables affect the presence of heart disease.

Statistical methods can analyze one variable at a time (i.e., *univariate analysis*) or more than one variable together at the same time (i.e., *multivariate analysis*). *Bivariate analysis* analyzes two variables together. An example of a univariate analysis would be simply looking at the death rate (mortality) in different countries. An example of a bivariate analysis would be analyzing the relationship between alcoholism and mortality.

3.1.2 Samples

A *population* is an entire group of people, animals, objects, or data that meet a specific set of criteria. So the human female population of the United States consists of every woman and girl in the United States. The European golf ball population is every golf ball located in Europe. The population of New York City heart attack cases in year 2000 includes every incidence of a heart attack in New York City in that year.

A population may be real or hypothetical. A hypothetical population could be the patients with decreased cardiac ejection fractions due to a certain heart procedure if it were instituted among patients in France. The heart procedure is not in use yet, and the resulting population is only a guess or prediction.

A *sample* is a portion or subset of a population. When populations are very large, observing or testing every single member of the population becomes impractical. Therefore, observing or testing a portion of the population often is more realistic. Lack of time and resources force us to rely on samples nearly every day to draw conclusions and to make decisions. Peeking at the traffic outside your office may help you estimate your commute time, even though this sample of traffic does not necessarily represent rest of the commute traffic.

Choosing an appropriate sample is very important. Over-reliance on poorly constructed samples can even be a source of stereotyping and prejudice. For example, a person's experience with a few members of a certain race may influence his perception of all members of that race. If those few members were rude, he may erroneously conclude that all people of that race are rude. If those few members were meek, he may erroneously conclude that all people of that race are meek. The person's sample did not reflect the true diversity of the entire population.

Therefore, in order to generate conclusions about a population, your sample must be reasonably *representative* of the overall population. In other words, the sample must have a similar diversity of all relevant characteristics as the total population. For example, Jackie Chan action movies are not a representative sample of Hong Kong movies. A representative sample would have to at minimum include dramas, comedies, documentaries, and horror movies. Jackie Chan action movies would be a *biased sample*, an overrepresentation of certain characteristics or members of the population. Biased samples often lead to improper conclusions. Inferential statistics can generate reasonable and useful conclusions about the population only if the sample is representative.

Usually, samples must be *random* to be representative of the population. Choosing a *simple random sample* is equivalent to putting every member of the population in a hat or large container and blindly selecting a specified number of members. Every member of a population has an equal chance of being selected for a simple random sample. Selecting a *stratified random sample* involves first dividing the population into different relevant categories or strata (e.g., men and women or under 21 years old and 21 years and older) and then selecting random samples from each category. Creating a nonrandom sample that is truly representative of the population is very difficult since a population has so many different characteristics. How can you make sure that your sample has a similar distribution of every single important characteristic? How do you know which characteristics are important and which are irrelevant? Using random samples makes it more likely that by chance the sample's distribution of characteristics will be similar to that of the overall population.

Going back to the Hong Kong movie analogy, how would a representative sample of movies be constructed? Should every style of movie be included? Should every major actor and actress be represented? Who would be considered a major actor or actress? What about movies from different time periods? Should our sample have an equal distribution of short and long, bad and good, black and white and color movies? Such an endeavor would be unbelievably time consuming and require a lot of subjective decision making. Instead, dumping every single Hong Kong movie ever made in a bin (it would have to be a very large bin) and then randomly drawing movies may be easier and perhaps more effective.

The *study population* is a group of patients who are part of a clinical study. Usually the study population is a sample of the total population. The goal of a clinical study is to use descriptive, comparative, or inferential statistics to portray or draw conclusions about the study population that are applicable to the total population. For example, to determine if a drug works on patients with congestive heart failure, testing the drug on everyone with congestive heart failure would be unfeasible and unethical. Instead, you may test the drug on a sample of patients with congestive heart failure and use statistics to determine whether the drug may be effective for the total population of congestive heart failure patients.

Distinguishing between parameters and statistics is important. A *parameter* is a numerical value that measures, represents, or describes some aspect of a *population*. Frequently, Greek letters represent parameters. Examples of parameters would be the population mean (μ), the population standard deviation (σ), the proportion (π) of population, or the correlation (ρ) in population. Frequently, the values of parameters are not known. By contrast, a *statistic* is a numerical value calculated from a *sample of the population*. Roman letters designate statistics. So the sample mean (M), the sample standard deviation (s), proportion (p) of a sample, and the correlation (r) in a sample would be statistics. You use statistics to guess the parameters. If the sample is representative of the population then the statistics may be good approximations of the parameters.

A statistic will vary among different samples from the same population. For example, if you take 50 different random samples of 10,000 people from New York City, the mean incomes of each of those samples will be different. The *sampling fluctuation* is the extent to which the statistics vary. The *efficiency* of a statistic is its relative constancy from sample to sample. A highly efficient statistic will have the same or very similar values in different samples from the same population. An inefficient statistic will fluctuate significantly.

3.2 STATISTICS AND PARAMETERS

3.2.1 Central Tendency

The *central tendency* of a variable is the "middle" or "typical" values of the variable in a sample of population. Measures of the central tendency provide a single number answer to the question: What is the typical value of that variable in your sample or population? People who want to "go along with the crowd" are most interested in central tendencies. Table 3.1 lists the common measures of central tendencies.

Your choice of the central tendency measure depends on the situation and the distribution of the data. The *arithmetic mean (average)* is the most common measure of the central tendency since it is easy to calculate, accounts for every value in the sample (i.e., every value in the sample influences the mean), and is appropriate for normal distributions (which we discuss later). However, extreme values can significantly distort the mean (e.g., if Bill Gates, Warren Buffet, or some other billionaire were to move next door to you, your town's mean income would rocket

TABLE 3.1 Measure of Central Tendency

Measure	Definition	Advantages	Disadvantages	Calculation
Arithmetic mean (average)	Sum of values divided by number of different values	Good for symmetric distributions	Affected by extreme values; bad for skewed distributions	Population mean $\mu = \Sigma X/N$ Sample mean M = $\Sigma X/N$
Geometric mean	nth root of product of n scores	Less affected by extreme values; useful for some positively skewed distributions	Cannot use if any of values is less than zero	$\left(\prod_{i=1}^{n} a_i \right)^{1/n}$ $= (a_1 a_2 a_3 a_4 \ldots a_n)^{1/n}$
Harmonic mean	Number of values divided by sum of reciprocals of values	Good when need average of rates	Useful in only specific situations	$N_h = k/[(1/n_1) + (1/n_2) + \ldots (1/n_k)]$
Median	*Middle of distribution*: value at which half of values are greater and half of values are lesser	Compared to mean, less affected by extreme values or significant skewed distributions	Does not adequately reflect data values above or below median	*Odd number of values*: median = middle number *Even number of values*: median = mean of two middle numbers
Mode	Most frequently occurring value	Easy to understand; can use with nominal data	Greatly subject to sample fluctuations; may be greater than one mode ("multi modal")	Count the frequency of each variable value and choose one with highest frequency
Trimean	Weighed average of median and quartiles	Resistant to extreme scores; *in extremely skewed distributions*: less subject to sampling fluctuation	Less efficient than mean for normal distributions	TM = $(Q_1 + 2Q_2 + Q_3)/4$ Q_1 = 25th percentile Q_2 = 50th percentile Q_3 = 75th percentile
Trimmed mean	Discards a percentage of outliers before calculating arithmetic average	Less susceptible to extreme scores; *in extremely skewed distributions*: less susceptible to sampling fluctuation	*Normal distributions*: less efficient than mean	x% trimmed mean = mean of sample after discarding largest x% and smallest x% of sample

skywards). Moreover, highly skewed distributions (which we discuss later) can significantly inflate or deflate the mean. The *median* is the next most common measure of the central tendency. Extreme values or skewed distributions do not significantly affect the median. However, the median offers no inkling of how many different values may be present (e.g., the median of 6 and 8 would be the same as the median of 1, 2, 2, 7, 100, 433, and 2,700). Although useful, the *mode* on its own does not provide enough information about sample as a whole. Moreover, there can be multiple modes in a sample or population (e.g., What is the mode of the body weight in the U. S. population?) In a normal distribution, the values of the mean, median, and mode are very similar or equivalent. A mean trimmed by 100% is essentially the median and a mean trimmed by 0% is essentially the average.

3.2.2 Spread (Dispersion or Variability)

The *spread* (*dispersion or variability*) measures how different values of a variable are from each other. So the spread of height and weight may be a lot less among gymnasts than among the general population. Spread is akin to diversity. The greater the diversity of values, the greater the spread is. Table 3.2 lists the common measures of spread.

Each measure of spread has its advantages and disadvantages, but the standard deviation is by far the most commonly used measure. The *standard deviation*, which is the square root of the *variance*, provides the most valuable information for normal distributions. When the distribution of a variable's values is normal, approximately 68% of the values fall within one standard deviation of the mean and 95% fall within two standard deviations. Since extreme values dramatically affect the *range* (e.g., Bill Gates moving into your neighborhood will dramatically increase the range of incomes in your town), the range alone is not a sufficient measure of spread. The *semi-interquartile range* is more resistant to sampling fluctuations in highly skewed distributions and extreme values than the standard deviation so may be useful as an adjunct measure of spread.

3.2.3 Shape

Knowing the central tendency and the spread of data does not necessarily give you enough information. Two different

TABLE 3.2 Measure of Spread

Measure	Definition	Comments	Calculation
Range	Span of the entire set of data	Easily understood. Sensitive to extreme scores	Range = maximum − minimum
Semi-interquartile range	Range between 1st and 3rd quartiles	Not affected by extreme scores	IQR = $(Q_3 − Q_1)/2$ Q_1 = 25th percentile Q_3 = 75th percentile
Variance	Spread of values around the mean	Accounts for the mean; subject to sampling fluctuation	Population variance $(\sigma^2) = \Sigma(x−\mu)^2/N$ Sample variance $(s^2) = \Sigma(x−M)^2/(N − 1)$
Standard deviation	Square root of the variance	Same as variance	Population standard deviation = $\sqrt{\sigma^2}$ Sample standard deviation = $\sqrt{s^2}$

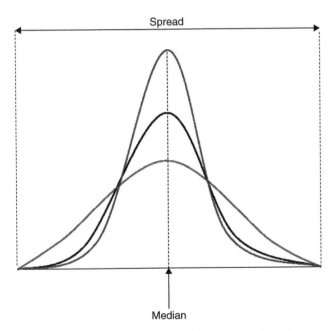

FIGURE 3.1 Examples of curves with the same central tendency but different spreads.

sets of data could have equivalent measures of the central tendency and spread but be very different (Figure 3.1). Therefore, knowing the *distribution* of the variable's values is very helpful. The distribution is the shape of the curve generated if you were to plot the frequencies of each value of the variable.

The two common measures of shape are skew and kurtosis. Skew is the degree to which a curve is "bent" toward one direction. The skew is:

- *Positive (Right skewed)*: If the curve's right tail is longer than its left and most of the distribution is shifted to the left. The mean is usually (but not always) greater than the median (Figure 3.2a).

- *Negative (Left skewed)*: If the curve's left tail is longer than its right and most of the distribution is shifted to the right. The mean is usually (but not always) less than the median (Figure 3.2b).

- *Zero (No skew)*: If the right and left tails are of equal length and most of the distribution is in the center of the curve. The normal distribution has a skew of zero. The mean and the median are usually (but not always) equal (Figure 3.2.c).

The following formula measures skew:

$$\text{Skew} = \sum \frac{(X − \mu)^3}{N\sigma^3}$$

where μ is the mean and σ is the standard deviation.

The *kurtosis* is the degree to which a curve is peaked or flat. The greater the kurtosis, the more "peaked" a curve is. The less the kurtosis, the flatter the curve is. The following formula measures kurtosis:

$$\text{Kurtosis} = \sum \frac{(X − \mu)^4}{N\sigma^4 − 3}$$

where μ is the mean and σ is the standard deviation.

The kurtosis may be:

- *Zero (mesokurtic or mesokurtotic)*: Normal distributions have zero kurtosis (Figure 3.3a).

- *Positive (leptokurtic or leptokurtotic)*: Compared to a normal curve, these curves have a more acute, taller peak at the mean (i.e., a greater number of values close to the mean) and "fatter" tails (i.e., a greater number of extreme values) at the more extreme (Figure 3.3b).

- *Negative (platykurtic or platykurtotic)*: Compared to a normal curve, these curves have a flatter, lower peak at the mean (i.e., a smaller number of values close to the mean) and "thinner" tails (i.e., fewer extreme values) (Figure 3.3c).

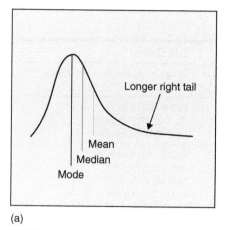
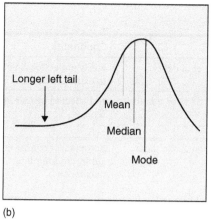
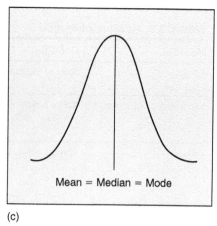

(a)   (b)   (c)

FIGURE 3.2   Different types of skew: (a) Positive (right) skew; (b) negative (left) skew; and (c) zero (no) skew.

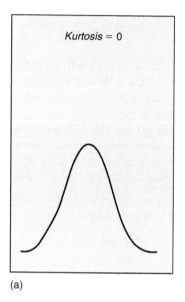
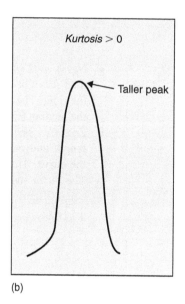
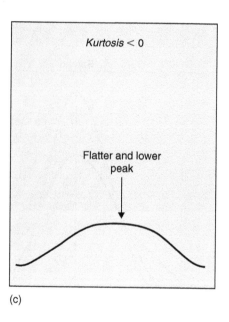

(a)   (b)
                                                                  (c)

FIGURE 3.3   Different types of kurtosis: (a) Mesokurtic ; (b) leptokurtic; and platykurtic.

3.3 NORMAL DISTRIBUTION

3.3.1 The Importance of Normal Distributions

Normal distributions, also known as *bell-shaped curves* or *Gaussian distributions*, have the same general shape: symmetric and unimodal (i.e., a single peak) with tails that appear to extend to positive and negative infinity. In a normal curve, approximately 68% of the values fall within one standard deviation of the mean, 95% fall within two standard deviations, and 99.7% fall within three standard deviations.

The following formula describes a normal curve:

$$Y = [1/\sqrt{(2\pi\sigma^2)}]\exp[-(X - \mu)^2/2\sigma^2]$$

where π is the 3.14159 and σ is the standard deviation.

Figure 3.4 shows examples of a normal distribution. Normal curves can differ in spread. Like most distributions, the normal distribution has a mean (μ) and a standard deviation (σ).

Understanding the normal distribution is important. Interestingly, many biological, psychological, sociological, economical, chemical, and physical variables exhibit normal distributions. A classic example is that educational test scores tend to follow a bell curve: most students score close to the mean and much fewer have very high or very low scores. In fact, when the distribution of a variable is unknown, you frequently assume that it is normal until proven otherwise. Many statistical tests are based on normal distributions. Violations of normal distributions, in fact, may invalidate some of these tests, although many statistical tests still function reasonably well with other types of distributions.

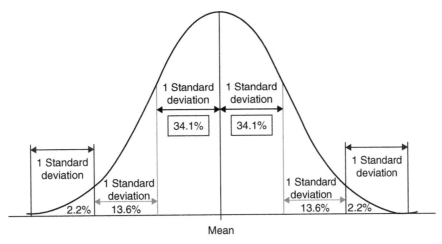

FIGURE 3.4 Normal distribution.

- *Step 1*: Determine the Z-score using the following formula: $Z = (X-\mu)/\sigma$
- *Step 2*: Using a Z-table, look up the percentile rank that corresponds to that Z-score.
- *Step 3*: This percentile rank will be the percentage of values that the value is higher than.
- *Step 4*: Subtracting the percentile rank from 1 (=1-percentile rank) gives you the percentage of values that are higher than the value.

FIGURE 3.5 Converting a value into a percentile rank.

3.3.2 Standard Normal Distribution

The *standard normal (or Z-) distribution* is a special normal distribution that has a mean of 0 and a standard deviation of 1. If you know the mean and standard deviation of a normal distribution, you can transform it into a standard normal distribution by the following formula:

$$Z = \frac{X - \mu}{\sigma}$$

Z is the standard normal value, X is the original value, μ is the mean and σ is the standard deviation.

Z represents the number of standard deviations a value is away from the mean. So a Z-score of 1.0 corresponds to the value being one standard deviation away from the mean. A Z-score of 2.0 corresponds to the value being two standard deviations away from the mean.

Transforming a normal distribution into the standard normal distribution is analogous to converting foreign money into known domestic currency. You may not know the foreign currency well but are very familiar with the relative worth of domestic currency. So you would prefer performing any financial transaction in domestic currency.

Once your normal distribution is transformed into a standard normal distribution, it is easy to determine the *percentile rank* of a given value. The percentile rank is where a given value falls compared to the rest of the values. Is the value in the top 5%, top 10%, bottom 25%, or bottom 1% of all values? A value in the top 5% means that it is higher than at least 95% of the other values. If you know the Z-score equivalent of a value, standard normal (or Z-) tables translate every Z-score into a percentile rank (Figure 3.5). For example, a Z-score of 1.0 means that the value is 1 standard deviation above the mean, which implies that the value is higher than 84.13% of the other values. A Z-score of 2.0 means that the value is 2 standard deviations above the mean, which implies that the value is higher than 97.72% of the other values. A Z-score of -1.0 means that the value is 1 standard deviation below the mean, which implies that the value is higher than only 15.87% of the other values. A positive Z-score means that the value is higher than the mean. A negative Z-score means that it is lower than the mean.

You can also go in the reverse direction and convert a percentile rank into a value (Figure 3.6).

3.3.3 The *t*-Distribution

While large samples have a distribution close to the normal distribution (i.e., the larger the sample, the more normal the distribution), small samples do not. Moreover, many times

- *Step 1*: Using a Z-table, find the Z-score that corresponds to the percentile rank.
- *Step 2*: Multiply the Z-score by the standard deviation (σ) for your normal distribution.
- *Step 3*: Add the result from Step 2 to the mean of your normal distribution.

FIGURE 3.6   Converting a percentile rank into a value.

the population standard deviation is unknown, requiring you to use the sample standard deviation to estimate the population standard deviation. Whenever you have a small sample or do not know the population standard deviation, using a *t-distribution* may be more appropriate than using a normal distribution.

t-Distributions are similar to (i.e., symmetrical and bell shaped) but flatter (leptokurtic) than the standard normal distribution. Unlike the normal distribution, the *t*-distribution has a special additional parameter, *degrees of freedom (df)*, that can be any real number greater than zero and changes the *t*-distribution curve's shape. Curves with smaller df have more of their area under their tails and are therefore flatter than curves with higher degrees of freedom. As df increase, the *t*-distribution becomes more and more like the standard normal distribution. In fact, when df = ∞, the *t*-distribution becomes the standard normal curve.

The following example illustrates the concept of degrees of freedom. Knowing the average income of a group of 10 people and the actual incomes of 9 of the people, allows you to calculate the income of the 10th person. Thus, the income for the 10th person is "pre-determined" (i.e., it is not "free" to assume any value) by the mean and the incomes of the other 9 people. In this situation, only 9 values are completely "free," and we say that there are 9 degrees of freedom.

So, when using a single sample to estimate a mean or proportion, the degrees of freedom (i.e., the number of independent observations) is equal to the sample size minus one. A sample size of 5 would have 4 degrees of freedom, and a sample size of 50 would have 49 degrees of freedom. (*Note*: The formula for degrees of freedom is not always $n-1$ and is different for other situations.)

The *t*-score (or *t*-statistic) is to the *t*-distribution what the Z-score is to the normal distribution. Use the following formula to calculate a *t*-score:

$$t = \frac{(\text{Mean of sample}) - (\text{Presumed mean of population})}{(\text{Standard deviation of sample})/\sqrt{(\text{Sample size})}}$$

Knowing the df allows you to use a *t*-score table to convert the *t*-score into a percentile rank or probability.

3.4 SAMPLING DISTRIBUTIONS

3.4.1 Standard Error

Remember that the mean of a sample is an approximation of the population mean. Different samples from the same population will have different means. Some sample means will be closer to and other sample means will be farther from the true population mean (e.g., say the true population mean is 7, the mean of one sample may be 6.9, the mean of another sample may be 7.1, and the mean of a third sample may be 7.3). Ultimately calculating many different sample means will give you a distribution of sample means, which we call a *sampling distribution of the mean*. The larger the sample size, the more likely a sample mean will be close to the true population mean.

As with any distribution, we can calculate the mean and standard deviation of the sampling distribution of the mean. If the true population mean is μ, the true population standard deviation is σ, and the sample size is n then:

$$\text{Mean of the sampling distribution}$$
$$\text{of the mean } (\mu_M) = \mu$$
$$\text{Standard deviation of the sampling}$$
$$\text{distribution of the mean } (\sigma_M) = \text{standard}$$
$$\text{error of the mean} = \sigma/\sqrt{n}$$

As you can see, the larger n becomes, the smaller the standard error of the mean (and in turn, the spread of the sampling distribution of the mean) becomes. This makes intuitive sense. The mean incomes of 500 person random samples from New York City will fluctuate a lot more dramatically than the mean incomes of 10,000 person samples from New York City. The standard error of the mean gives you an idea of the sampling fluctuation of the sample means.

Other statistics have sampling distributions and *standard errors* as well. Table 3.3 shoes how to calculate these.

3.4.2 Central Limit Theorem

According to the *central limit theorem*, the distribution of a sample (with a mean μ and variance σ^2) becomes more and

TABLE 3.3 Standard Errors	
Statistic	Standard Error
Mean	$\sigma_M = \sigma/\sqrt{n}$
Median	$\sigma_{Median} = 1.253 \times \sigma/\sqrt{n}$
Standard deviation	$\sigma_S = 0.71 \times \sigma/\sqrt{n}$
Difference between independent means	$\sigma_{Md} = \sqrt{[(\sigma_1^2/n_1) + (\sigma_2^2/n_2)]}$

more like a normal distribution (with a mean μ and a variance σ^2/N) as the sample size N increases, regardless of the shape of the original distribution. So, the distribution of a variable in an infinite number of 10,000 person samples will look more like a normal distribution than that of an infinite number of 500 person samples. As the sample size N increases, the spread of the sampling distribution decreases (e.g., the distribution from the 10,000 person samples will be narrower than that of the 500 person samples).

As a result of the central limit theorem, we can use statistical tests that assume a normal distribution to evaluate sampling distributions. For example, if we know the population mean and standard deviation, we can calculate the probability of a sample mean being a certain value.

This tendency toward a normal distribution comes in handy when trying to compare two different populations. Say you have two arms in a clinical trial. Study Arm A (with 15 patients) receives the study intervention that is designed to improve a patient's functional score. The mean functional score for patients in Study Arm A is 70 with a variance of 21. Study Arm B (with 11 patients) does not receive the intervention and has a mean functional score of 60 with a variance of 17. It appears that the intervention improves the functional score by 10 points.

The mean of the sampling distribution of the difference between the means of Study Groups A and B then is $\mu_{Md} = \mu_A - \mu_B = 70 - 60 = 10$. The standard error of this sampling distribution (of the difference between the means of Study Groups A and B) then is $\sigma_{Md} = \sqrt{[(\sigma_A^2/n_A) + (\sigma_B^2/n_B)]} = \sqrt{[(21/15) + (17/11)]} = 1.72$. Knowing this we can ask questions such as, What is the probability that the study intervention will result in a 15 point increase in functional score? Calculating the Z-statistic will help answer this question:

$$Z = \frac{X - \mu}{\sigma} = \frac{15 - 10}{1.72} = 2.91$$

The Z-table shows that 2.91 corresponds to a 0.998 percentile rank. In other words, 0.998 of the time the difference between the means of Study Group A and Study Group B should be less than 15. Therefore, there is only a 0.002 chance that the difference between the two means will be 15 or larger.

3.5 CORRELATION

3.5.1 Pearson's Correlation

The *correlation* between two variables is the way and degree to which one variable changes when the other variable changes. If two variables are *highly correlated*, then changing one variable will almost certainly change the other variable. In sports, the amount of practice and game performance are very highly correlated. Practice more and you will play better during games. Practice less and you probably will play worse. Two variables are *poorly correlated* when they appear to be unrelated. The number of toilet paper rolls in your closet and the number of cars you have are probably poorly correlated (i.e., they have no relationship with each other).

Two variables are *positively correlated* when they change in the same direction (i.e., increasing one variable increases the other while decreasing one variable decreases the other) and *negatively correlated* when they change in opposite directions (i.e., increasing one variable decreases the other). Examples of positively correlated variables include income and house size; education and income; number of cars and weekly gas consumption; and daily calorie intake and body weight. Examples of negatively correlated variables include exercise frequency and body fat percentage; number of children and amount of free time; and number of skunks owned and frequency of dates.

When two variables are *linearly correlated*, changing one variable by a given amount changes the other by a fixed constant amount. For example, if the number of skunks owned and the frequency of dates are perfectly linearly (and negatively) correlated, every additional skunk you purchase results in a decrease in two dates each month. Buy three more skunks and you will have six fewer dates per month.

The *Pearson Product Moment Correlation* (otherwise known as *Pearson's correlation*) is the best known measure of linear correlation. You can calculate the Pearson's correlation in an entire population (rho or ρ) or a sample (r or "Pearson's r"). The Pearson's correlation measures the direction and degree of correlation and ranges from -1 (perfect negative linear correlation) to $+1$ (perfect positive linear correlation). The closer Pearson's is to -1 or $+1$, the stronger the correlation is. The closer the Pearson's is to 0, the weaker the correlation is. A Pearson's of 0 implies that there is no linear correlation between two variables.

You can use the following formula to calculate the Pearson's correlation:

$$r = \frac{\Sigma XY - [(\Sigma X \, \Sigma Y)/N]}{\sqrt{[\Sigma X^2 - ((\Sigma X^2)/N)][\Sigma Y^2 - ((\Sigma Y^2)/N)]}}$$
$$= (\Sigma_{z_X z_Y})/N$$

where X is the value of one variable and Y is the value of the second variable. Z is the x-score of each variable.

Changing the measurement scales for each variable usually does not affect the Pearson's correlation. For example, the correlation between height and weight will remain the same whether height is in inches or cm or the weight is in pounds or kg.

3.5.2 Spearman's Rho

Similar to the Pearson's correlation, the *Spearman's rho* (ρ) measures the linear correlation between two variables. However, unlike Pearson's, using Spearman's rho requires ranking the values of each variable (from lowest to highest or vice versa) before calculating the correlation. For example, you can convert the following pairs of observations (50 inches and 100 pounds, 60 inches and 170 pounds, 55 inches and 110 pounds, 52 inches and 95 pounds, 51 inches and 125 pounds) into the following ranks (5 and 4, 1 and 1, 2 and 3, 3 and 5, 4 and 2). This allows you to use the Spearman's rho with nearly any type of variable, (including categorical ones such as socioeconomic class or stage of training) as long as the variable can be ranked. The following formula can calculate the Spearman's rho:

$$\rho = \frac{1 - [6\,\Sigma\,d_i^2]}{[n(n^2 - 1)]}$$

where d_i is the difference between each rank of corresponding values of x and y and n is the number of pairs of values.

3.6 HYPOTHESIS TESTING

3.6.1 The Null Hypothesis

Chance can play a role in almost everything. For example, going to your local library could by pure chance lead to you meeting a famous model and eventually getting married to him or her. If that happens, does visiting your local library tend to result in meeting and marrying a model? Similarly, if you were to give soft drink to a large number of rheumatoid arthritis patients, some patients would improve by random chance or by other unrelated reasons. Can you then safely conclude that soft drinks treat rheumatoid arthritis? It is important to distinguish whether any observed change or effect was the result of pure random chance or a specific cause. Statistics can determine the probability of random chance being the sole culprit. In general, the greater the effect and the larger the sample size, the less likely it is that random chance caused the effect.

A clinical study is essentially *hypothesis testing*. A hypothesis is a postulated theory about or suggested explanation for a phenomenon. Every formal study or experiment should consist of two rival and polar opposite hypotheses: a *null hypothesis* (H_0) and an *alternative hypothesis* (H_1). The goal of the experiment is to either accept or reject the null hypothesis. Rejecting the null hypothesis suggests that the alternative hypothesis is a viable theory or explanation. For example, the null hypothesis may be that there is no difference between two groups of patients. If the study shows a difference between the two groups that is not likely due to random chance, you may reject the null hypothesis and infer that the alternative hypothesis (i.e., there is truly a difference between the two groups) may be true.

Typically the null hypothesis is the opposite of what your study is trying to prove. So if you think your study intervention will improve a certain measure, the null hypothesis would be that the study intervention has no effect on the measure. If you think your study intervention will result in a better outcome than another intervention, the null hypothesis would be that there is no difference between the two interventions. In fact, the null hypothesis often states that there is no difference between the means of a certain measure for two populations: H_0: $\mu_1 = \mu_2$ or H_0: $\mu_1 - \mu_2 = 0$. For example, one population may receive a study intervention and the other population may receive either a placebo or a comparison intervention. Alternatively, the two populations may be the same group of patients: one population is the group of patients before and the second population is the same group after an intervention or event. Your study then aims to disprove the null hypothesis.

The null hypothesis does not always have to be that there is no difference or no change. The null hypothesis could be that a measure or the difference between two measures is equal to, greater than, or less than a certain value (e.g., H_0: $\mu = 65$ or H_0: $\mu > 65$). The null hypothesis also does not have to involve means. The null hypothesis may state that there is no difference between two or among several medians, proportions, or correlation coefficients (e.g., H_0: $\pi_1 - \pi_2 = 0$, H_0: $\mu_1 = \mu_2 = \mu_3$, or H_0: $\rho_1 - \rho_2 = 0$) (Figure 3.7).

Failure to reject the null hypothesis does not necessarily mean that the null hypothesis is true. It simply means that your study does not provide ample evidence that the null hypothesis is wrong. The null hypothesis could still indeed be wrong. An analogy helps illustrate this point. Say you were to play against your friend Byron in a game of one-on-one basketball. The null hypothesis before the game is that you are not better than Byron. You enter the game trying to reject this null hypothesis. Even though you may be better than Byron, you still may lose the game. Losing the game to Byron does not prove that you are not better than Byron. You simply failed in your attempt to reject the null hypothesis. Similarly, winning the game does not necessarily prove that you are better than Byron. It simply makes it less likely that you are not better than Byron (Figures 3.8 and 3.9).

Step 1: Specify the null hypothesis (H_0) and alternative hypothesis (H_1).
 Example 1: H_0: $m_1 = m_2$ (i.e., the mean height of Population 1 is equal to the mean height of Population 2) H_1: $m_1 \neq m_2$
 Example 2: H_0: $r = 0$ (i.e., there is no correlation between height and weight) H_1: $r \neq 0$

Step 2: Choose a significance level (usually 0.05 or 0.01).
 Examples 1 and 2: Significance level = 0.05

Step 3: Calculate the relevant measurement statistic.
 Example1: Calculate the mean height (M_1) of a sample from Population 1 and the mean height (M_2) of a sample from Population 2.
 Example2: Calculate the Pearson's correlation between height and weight.

Step 4: Use the measurement statistic to calculate a *Z*-score or *t*-score (if standard error is estimated from the sample).
 Z-score or *t*-score = (statistic − hypothesized value)/standard error of the statistic.
 Z = (statistic − hypothesized value)/(standard error of the statistic).

Step5: Use the *Z*-score or *t*-score tables to determine the probability value (*p*-value) that corresponds to the *Z*- or *t*-score. This is the probability of the statistic value (calculated in *Step 3*) occurring if null hypothesis were true.

Step 6: Compare *p*-value with significant level. If the *p*-value is:
- Less than or equal to the significance level, we say that the difference is "statistically significant." So we may reject null hypothesis.
 Example: *p*-value of 0.035.
- Greater than the significance level, the difference is "not statistically significant." We cannot reject the null hypothesis.
 Example: *p*-value of 0.10.

FIGURE 3.7 Steps in hypothesis testing.

What is the probability that rolling a pair of normal dice would result in "snake-eyes" (a pair of ones) 30 times in a row? Though possible, the probability of such an event is very low. The probability of the event is the *p*-value. The lower the *p*-value, the less likely that random chance alone caused the event. A very low *p*-value suggests that some other cause is at work (e.g., the dice are loaded, fake, or your vision is failing).
 The *p*-value tells you the likelihood of an observed event occurring if the null hypothesis indeed were true. Let us use an analogy. Say you were to watch a soccer game:

- The probability (*p*-value) of either team or neither team winning is 100%.
- Assuming that both teams are equal in strength and ability, the *p*-value of your home team winning will be around 50% or 0.50. So your home team winning would not be too shocking.
- The *p*-value of the visiting team scoring more than 10 goals is relatively low (perhaps <0.10). So a score of Visitors 15 and Home Team 2 may suggest that something is amiss (e.g., the Visitors are taking steroids or the Home Team has injuries).
- In normal circumstance, the *p*-value of every member of both teams collapsing from severe diarrhea is very low (<0.01). Such an event strongly suggests that something very unusual is occurring.

In actuality, we use *p*-values every day. Say you hear a strange noise downstairs. You ask yourself what is the probability of hearing that noise assuming that nothing unusual is happening? A high probability means no further investigation is necessary. The sound of the wind blowing or your pet barking would have a high *p*-value. A very low probability calls for further investigation. A scream or a crash would have a very low *p*-value.

FIGURE 3.8 Understanding the concept of the *p*-value.

Statistical significance does not imply practical or clinical significance. There are many reasons why statistically significant differences or findings are not necessarily relevant:
- The difference may be statistically significant but great enough to make any practical difference.
- The difference may not have any impact.

FIGURE 3.9 Statistical significance vs. practical significance.

3.6.2 Type I and II Errors

When hypothesis testing arrives at the wrong conclusions, two types of errors can result: *Type I* and *Type II errors* (Table 3.4). Incorrectly rejecting the null hypothesis is a Type I error, and incorrectly failing to reject a null hypothesis is a Type II error. In general, Type II errors are more serious than Type I errors; seeing an effect when there isn't one (e.g., believing an ineffectual drug works) is worse than missing an effect (e.g., an effective drug fails a clinical trial). But this is not always the case. One of the major decisions before conducting a clinical study is choosing a significance level. As seen in Table 3.5, changing the significance level affects the Type I error rate (α), which is the probability of a Type I error, and the Type II error rate (β), which is the probability of a Type II error, in an opposite manner. In other words, you have to decide whether you are willing to tolerate more Type I or Type II errors. Type II errors may be more tolerable when studying interventions that will meet an urgent and unmet need.

3.6.3 One-Tail and Two-Tail Tests

To understand one-tail and two-tail probability testing, let's look at an example. Imagine comparing the player heights of two football teams: the USC Trojans and the Stanford Cardinal. Your null hypothesis is that the player heights of the two teams are not different. Then your alternative hypothesis would be that the two teams' player heights are indeed different. Note that this alternative hypothesis does not specify whether the USC Trojans or the Stanford

TABLE 3.4 Hypothesis Testing Errors

	Null hypothesis true	Null hypothesis false
Reject null hypothesis	Type I error	Correct
Fail to reject null hypothesis	Correct	Type II error

TABLE 3.5 The Significance Level and Error Rates

	Type I error rate (α)	Type II error rate (β)
Higher significance level (e.g., $p < 0.05$)	↓	↑
Lower significance level (e.g., $p < 0.01$)	↑	↓

Cardinal must have the taller players. Therefore, we can reject the null hypothesis if the Stanford players are on average *significantly taller or significantly shorter* than the USC players. This is an example of *two-tail hypothesis testing*: you test whether one group's mean falls too far along the right tail *or* the left tail of the other group's expected sampling distribution of means. In other words, two-tail testing looks at both extremes, both directions along the sampling distribution.

Suppose instead that your null hypothesis is that Stanford players are not taller than USC players. Then your alternative hypothesis would be that Stanford players are indeed taller than USC players. Therefore, rejecting the null hypothesis requires Stanford players to be on average *significantly taller* than the USC players. (Being significantly shorter than the USC players will not qualify.) This is an example of *one-tail hypothesis testing:* you test whether one group's mean falls too far along the one particular side or tail (in this example, the right tail) of the other group's expected sampling distribution of means. One-tail testing only looks at one extreme or one direction along the sampling distribution.

Figure 3.10 illustrates the difference between one-tail and two-tail hypothesis testing.

If you know the direction of the effect, use a one-tail test instead of a two-tail test. Rejecting the null hypothesis is easier in a one-tailed test than a two-tailed test as long as the difference is in the same direction (Figure 3.11). At a significance level of 0.05, the *p*-value has to be less than 0.025 in a two-tailed test and less than 0.05 in a one-tailed test.

3.6.4 Confidence Interval

An *x% confidence interval* is a range which should contain the value of a variable *x%* of the time. For example, suppose a variable had a 95% confidence interval with a low boundary of 1 and a high boundary of 5. Then, 95% of the time the variable should have a value between 1 and 5. Confidence intervals may apply to sampling distributions as well. Imagine measuring the mean income in

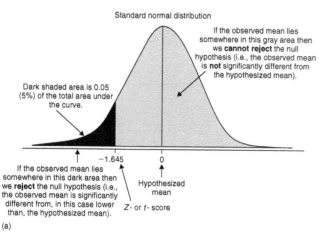

(a)

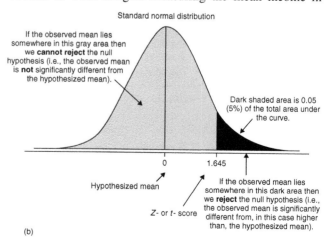

(b)

FIGURE 3.10 One-tail hypothesis testing.

an infinite number of different 10,000 person samples from a particular city. Suppose the 95% confidence interval of this sampling distribution goes from $30,000 to $60,000. Then, 95% of the sample means would be within $30,000 and $60,000.

Any variable or statistic can have a confidence interval. Table 3.6 shows how to calculate the confidence intervals for various common statistics.

You can use confidence intervals to test hypotheses. Two variables are significantly different statistically if their

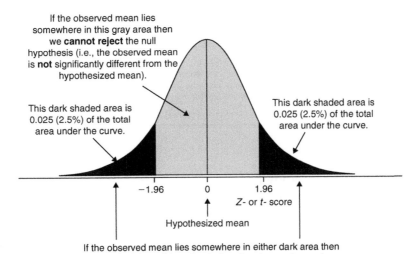

FIGURE 3.11 Two-tail hypothesis testing.

TABLE 3.6	Calculation of the confidence intervals for various common statistics		
Statistic	Lower limit	Upper limit	Components
Mean (population standard deviation known)	$M - Z\sigma_M$	$M + Z\sigma_M$	M = sample mean Z = Z-score σ_M = standard error of mean
Mean (population standard deviation not known)	$M - ts/\sqrt{N}$	$M + ts/\sqrt{N}$	M = sample mean t = t-score s = sample standard deviation N = sample size
Difference between means (Population standard deviation known)	$M_d - Z\sigma_{Md}$	$M_d + Z\sigma_{Md}$	$M_d = M_1 - M_2$ = difference between means Z = Z-score σ_{Md} = standard error of difference between means
Difference between means (Population standard deviation not known)	$M_d - ts_{Md}$	$M_d + ts_{Md}$	$M_d = M_1 - M_2$ = difference between means Z = Z-score s_{Md} = estimate of standard error of difference between means = $\sqrt{(2MSE/n)}$ MSE = mean square error = $(s_1^2 + s_2^2)/2$ s_1 = Sample 1 standard deviation s_2 = Sample 2 standard deviation
Pearson's correlation	Convert $z' - Z\sigma_{Mz}'$ to r equivalent*	Convert $z' + Z\sigma_{Mz}'$ to r equivalent*	Z' = r converted to z'* Z = Z-score $\sigma_z' = 1/\sqrt{(N-3)}$ N = sample size
Difference between correlations	Convert $z_1'-z_2' - Z(\sigma_{z1}'_{-z2}')$ to r equivalent*	Convert $z_1' - z_2' + Z(\sigma_{z1}'_{-z2}')$ to r equivalent*	Z' = r converted to z'* Z = Z-score $\sigma_{z1}'_{-z2}' = \sqrt{[(1/(N_1-3)) + (1/(N_2^{-3}))]}$ N = sample size

*using r to z' table.

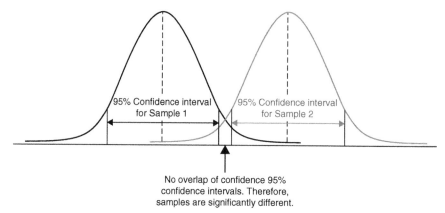

FIGURE 3.12 Using confidence intervals to test hypothesis.

confidence intervals do not overlap (Figure 3.12). Finding that the confidence interval of Sample 2 does not fall within the 95% confidence interval of Sample 1's mean rejects the null hypothesis (at a 0.05 significance level) that the two means are the same. To test at different significance levels, simply alter the percentage of the confidence interval. It is important to note however, that overlapping confidence intervals do not mean that the null hypothesis cannot be rejected.

3.7 POWER

3.7.1 Definition of Power

The *power* of a study is its ability or probability of correctly rejecting a false null hypothesis. If β is the Type II error rate then:

$$\text{Power} = 1 - \beta$$

So as power increases, the Type II error rate decreases. Low power raises the chance of an inconclusive study. While more power is always better, increasing power usually means enrolling more patients, which is time and resource consuming. So a general rule of thumb is that power below 0.25 is usually unsatisfactory and power over 0.80 is usually quite satisfactory. The power of two studies combined is greater than the power of each separate study.

Power is unaffected by whether the null hypothesis is true or false. Power only measures the chance of successfully rejecting a null hypothesis when it should be rejected.

Finding that a study has low power provides grounds for re-designing the study. You can determine a study's power before (a *priori* power analysis) or after (*post hoc* power analysis) collecting the data. *A priori power analyses* can determine the ideal sample size for a clinical study. *Post hoc power analyses* establish the power of the study after everything has been completed.

TABLE 3.7 Determinants of Power

Determinant	↑ Power	↓ Power
Sample size	Increase	Decrease
Variance (σ^2)	Decrease	Increase
Significance level (α)	Increase	Decrease
Normality	↑ Power	↓ Power
Test tails	One-tail	Two-tail
Experimental design	Within-subject	Between-subjects
Normal distribution	Yes	No
Effect size	Large	Small

3.7.2 Determinants of power

Table 3.7 lists some factors that determine power. Remember that we use the Z-score to determine if a difference or effect is statistically significant. To understand what affects power, all you have to do is to look at this formula:

$$z = \frac{M_{\text{diff}}}{\sigma / \sqrt{N}}$$

The greater the Z-score, the more likely the difference will be statistically significant. So anything that increases the Z-score increases the study's power.

Effect Size

M_{diff} is the difference between the means of two samples and reflects the *effect size*, that is, the quantitative difference between two groups. As the Z-score formula indicates, the greater the *effect size*, the greater the power of a study. When one group receives an intervention, the effect size measures the effectiveness of that intervention on the variable of interest. The effect size does not just answer "Is there a difference?" or "Does an intervention work?" It tells us "how big is the difference" and "how well does it work." You can measure the effect size as an absolute difference (e.g., 2.5% of the treatment group had heart attacks while 5% of the no-treatment group had heart attacks, making the difference 2.5%) or as a relative reduction (e.g., the treatment group had half as many heart attacks as the no-treatment group).

Study power depends on the anticipated effect size and the actual effect size seen in the study. The same study will have less power in proving a large effect size than in proving a smaller effect size. The impact of the effect size on power makes intuitive sense.

Proving something works is easier when the effect is dramatic rather than subtle (e.g., you do not have to test too many rooms to show that an air conditioner can cool a room; however, you may have to test many rooms to demonstrate that using a different kind of wall material can lower temperatures).

The effect size in a clinical study, to some degree, is under your control. The effect size depends on the biochemical and physical properties of a treatment, the physiological conditions of the patients, and the nature of the condition. In order to increase a study's power, investigators frequently will choose the right mix of treatment, patient, and disease characteristics to maximize the potential effect. For instance, they may choose a higher medication dose, a sicker patient population, and a disease state that is very treatable.

Significance Level (α)

Lowering the significance level basically raises the expectations of a study and therefore lowers the study's power. The significance level is analogous to the minimum passing test score, the qualifying time for an Olympic trial, or the minimum qualifications for a job. A more stringent cutoff makes it less likely for the treatment to "pass the test." When designing the study, you must choose a significance level that is low enough to convince others that your study is rigorous but not so low that your study has little power.

Sample Size

Larger study sample sizes mean greater study power. We see that the sample size N flips up to the numerator of the z-score calculation. Increasing N boosts the Z-score. Suppose a medication improved a person's appearance. This also makes intuitive sense. Which would be more convincing: showing an improvement in 10 people or 100 people? Increasing the sample size is costly because recruiting, retaining, treating, observing, and/or monitoring each patient can consume a lot of money and time. Therefore, investigators must balance increasing study power with expense.

Variance

Increasing the variance of the relevant outcome decreases the study power. As you can see, the standard deviation (σ), which is the square root of the variance (σ^2), appears in the denominator of the z-score calculation. The standard deviation measures the spread of different values around the mean, that is, the volatility of a variable. An analogy will help better understand this relationship. Suppose one star basketball player, John, is a very steady performer, averaging 28 points a game and rarely scoring much more or much less (i.e., he always scores between 25 and 30 points). You only need to watch a few games to see that John is better than other players. By comparison, another star player, Geoffrey, has wildly fluctuating performances: scoring as high as 50 points on some nights and as low as 2 points on other nights. However, proving that Geoff is superior to other players will require a lot more games. You have to make sure that his outstanding performances are frequent enough and his terrible games are sufficiently infrequent. Consistency and homogeneity make it easier to prove that something is better or more effective.

Therefore, making the study population as homogenous as possible will minimize the potential variance and maximize the study power. When choosing your study population, first identify the characteristics that may affect the treatment's effectiveness. Then choose study selection criteria that restrict the variability in these characteristics. For example, suppose that a patient's age influences his or her response to a medication. Restricting the trial to patients within a specific narrow age group (e.g., 40–50 years old) will then reduce variability.

The tradeoff from reducing study population heterogeneity is reduced study generalizability. *Generalizability* is how well a study's results and conclusions apply to the rest of the population (i.e., other patients in the general population with the same disease). Conclusions from a study with only 40–50 year olds are not very applicable to patients in their 20s or 70s.

Between-Subject vs. Within-Subject Designs

Within-subject studies compare the same subjects at different times (e.g., before and after a treatment or exposure to a risk factor) and *between-subject* studies compare groups of different subjects (e.g., one group received a treatment or exposure to a risk factor while another did not). An example of a within-subject design would be measuring the number of job offers a group of 10 men and 10 women receive during a 1-year period, then giving each of them plastic surgery (e.g., breast implants, nose jobs, and pectoral implants), and then measuring the number of job offers they receive the following year. Seeing their job offers increase significantly suggests that the plastic surgery increased their job marketability. An example of a between-subject design would be comparing the number of job offers in two groups: one group that receives plastic surgery and another group that does not. Seeing significantly more job offers in the plastic surgery group suggests that plastic surgery can indeed increase one's job marketability.

Within-subject designs have more power than between-subject designs. There is more variability between different subjects than within the same subject at different times. For example, the group that received plastic surgery may have better training, education, personalities, or experience than the group that did not get plastic surgery. However, time effects (i.e., changes in patient characteristics) can decrease the power of a within-subject study. For example, a disease may significantly worsen or improve regardless of whether the patient receives a treatment and, in turn, increase variability (i.e., the patients are not the same at the end of the study as when they started the study).

Two-Tails vs. One-Tail Test

Earlier in the chapter, we mentioned that it is easier to reject the null hypothesis with a one-tail test than a two-tail test. One-tail tests use a greater significance level and therefore confer greater study power than do two-tail tests.

3.8 SAMPLE SIZE

3.8.1 Determinants of Sample Size

Choosing the size of your study population (i.e., the sample size) is a critical decision. Whether you are setting up a clinical study or analyzing existing data, you need to know how many subjects to include in your study or whether you already have enough subjects. Samples that are too large waste time and resources and, in a clinical trial, may expose too many patients to potential harm. Conversely, samples that are too small confer an inadequate study power and may generate inaccurate or inconclusive results. Having patients participate in a potentially useless clinical study wastes their time and effort and, as a result, may be quite unethical.

Many factors affect the sample size. The most important factors are:

- *Power*: The most commonly used power threshold is 80%, which means that a false null hypothesis is successfully rejected 80% of the time.
- *Significance level*: The most commonly used significance levels are 5% ($p = 0.05$) and 1% ($p = 0.01$), which means that there is a 5% or 1% probability, respectively, of a chance difference mistakenly being considered a real significant difference.
- *Clinical event rate*: The relevant *clinical event* depends on what you are studying. Suppose you are studying a treatment designed to prevent heart attacks. Then the relevant clinical event is a heart attack. If you were studying a

treatment to alleviate severe diarrhea, then the clinical event is an episode of diarrhea. If you were examining the relationship between sleep and on-the-job mistakes then your clinical event is an on-the-job mistake. As you can see, the clinical event is the problem that you are trying to measure or your study treatment aims to prevent, alleviate, or cure. The *event rate* is the frequency of the relevant clinical event in your study population. A low event rate (i.e., the event rarely occurs) necessitates a large sample size, because many patients in your study population will go through study without having an event. Higher event rates (i.e., the event is common) allow you to use much smaller sample sizes: almost everyone in your study population will have the event and thus provide useful information. Predicting the event rate can be very difficult and is usually based on prior studies.

- *Expected effect size*: A study's power depends on the difference between the expected effect size and the actual observed effect size. When the study is powered to prove a certain effect size and the actual observed effect size in the study is less, the study is inconclusive (see Figure 3.13). Be realistic and perhaps a bit pessimistic when predicting effect sizes.
- *Compliance and drop-out rates*: Your sample size calculations should also take into account the number of patients that may not comply with your study protocol or withdraw from the study. So if the other factors determine that a 50-person sample size is required but half of the subjects may drop out, your study really should include a lot more than 50 people (Figure 3.14).
- *Subject allocation ratio*: Most studies assign an equal number of subjects to each study arm (called a one-to-one allocation when there are only two study arms). The allocation ratio is the ratio of the number of patients assigned to each arm. A two-to-one allocation ratio means that twice as many patients are in one study arm compared to the other study arm. Disproportionate allocations (i.e., any allocation ratio other than one-to-one) call for larger sample sizes.

Most study designs establish and fix sample sizes before the study commences. Some study designs allow you to change the sample size as the trial progresses and more

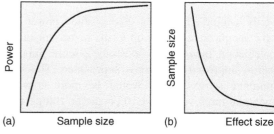

FIGURE 3.13 Important determinant of sample size: (a) Relationship between the sample size and statistical power (b) Relationship between expected effect size and sample size needed for the study.

information about factors that affect the sample size such as effect size and clinical event rate becomes available.

Sometimes studies will have multiple objectives, that is, attempt to identify or test many different things. Each of these objectives may require a different sample size. In general, use the largest sample size required by the different objectives (e.g., if one objective needs 20 patients, a second needs 70 patients, and a third needs 100 patients, you should use 100 patients). Anytime the sample size is smaller than deemed necessary for an objective, you risk not being able to draw conclusions about that objective (Figures 3.15 and 3.16).

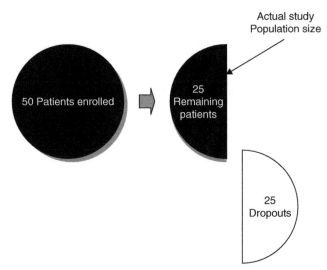

FIGURE 3.14 Sample size calculations should take into account the number of patients who may drop out of the study.

3.8.2 Calculating Sample Size

Potential strategies include using:

Most of the Population

Sometimes the entire population of patients with certain conditions or characteristics is small enough to serve as the sample. Very few patients may have the disease or condition or fulfill the selection criteria. Using the entire population (or almost the entire population) mitigates the problems of sampling error and generalizability.

The Sample Size of a Comparable Study

Imitation is not only the sincerest form of flattery but also can help identify the right sample size. Some investigators will find an equivalent study and use the same sample size. Of course, the challenge is finding a truly comparable study and not simply replicating any sample size calculation mistakes that the other study made.

Sample Size Tables and Software

There are many published tables or software programs that allow you to look up the necessary sample size based on your study characteristics. Make sure that these tables or software programs are accurate and reliable. Sometimes the tables or programs will not account for all of the characteristics important to your study.

Choosing the right sample size depends heavily on properly predicting the effect size. Overestimating an effect can cause problems:

Example: Suppose you predict that a device will reduce the risk of heart attacks by 75% and choose a sample size that will show this effect size. Conducting the study then demonstrates that the device reduces the rate of heart attacks by 25%. The study then is inconclusive and cannot reject the null hypothesis that the device makes no difference. But does this mean the device has no effect? Clearly reducing heart attacks by 25% is a good thing.

Analogy: You attend a baseball game expecting Barry Bonds to hit 3 home runs. He only hits one. Compared to your expectations, his performance was disappointing. With lower expectations, his performance would have been outstanding.

FIGURE 3.15 Effect size: Expectations must match reality.

Poor compliance affects estimated sample size in a nonlinear fashion:
Number of patients needed per arm $= N/[(c1 + c2 - 1)^2]$,
where
$N =$ Number of patients per arm from sample size calculations
$c1 =$ average compliance rate for Study Arm 1
$c2 =$ average compliance rate for Study Arm 2
Source: Adrienne Kirby, Val Gebski and Anthony C Keech (2002). eMJA, **177** (5): 256–257.

FIGURE 3.16 Adjusting sample size for compliance.

Suppose we are trying to measure the mean glucose level in a population and wanted to know the sample size that would give us 95% confidence (which corresponds to a Z-score of 1.96) in the result. If the standard deviation for glucose measurements is 15 and the we are willing to accept an error of 3, then:

$$\text{Sample Size} = Z^2\sigma^2/e^2s = [(1.96 \times 15/3)]^2 = 96.04$$

So, we would need 97 subjects.

FIGURE 3.17   Calculating sample size for a mean.

Suppose we want to determine with 95% confidence ($Z = 1.96$) the proportion of patients who will respond to a treatment. If we estimate that 70% ($p = 0.70$) will respond to the medication and are willing to accept a $+/-$ 10% ($e = 0.10$) error, then:

$$\text{Sample Size} = Z^2p(1-p)/e^2 = [(1.96)^2 \times 0.7 \times 0.3]/(0.10)^2 = 80.7$$

So, we would need 81 subjects.

FIGURE 3.18   Calculating sample size for a proportion.

Sample Size Formulae

The final method for choosing a sample is using sample size formula (Figure 3.17). The following formula calculates sample size when you are comparing the means of two groups:

$$N = \frac{Z^2\sigma^2}{e^2}$$

where Z is the Z-score, σ^2 is the population variance, and e is the margin of error (i.e., the desired precision).

The following formula calculates sample size when you are comparing the proportions of two groups:

$$N = \frac{Z^2 p(1-p)}{e^2}$$

where Z is the Z-score, p is the estimated proportion of an attribute that is present in the population, and e is the margin of error (Figure 3.18).

Chapter 4

Measures and Variables

4.1 INTRODUCTION TO MEASURES

4.1.1 The Definition of Measure

Almost anytime you want to assess something, you need to measure it. In order to measure anything, you need some *unit of measure*, such as cm, inches, pounds, color, and age. Deciding if someone is tall? Measure her height in centimeters (cm). Wondering if a car is fuel-efficient? Measure the car's miles per gallon. Trying to determine if Michael Jordan was a good basketball player? His statistics (e.g., scoring, assist, steals, championships won, and All-Star selections) seem to indicate that he was a great player. Is someone a top student? Grades and test scores separate the honors from the non-honors students. Is a television show or movie popular? The Nielsen ratings or box office sales could help answer this question.

For all these, some sort of "units" must be used to assess them. You can't measure height without using cm, feet/inches, or at least some set of categories like "short/medium/tall." How can you measure weight without using kg, pounds, or at least some categories like "light/medium/heavy"?

Similarly, in a clinical trial, you need a variety of measures to help make different assessments and answer various questions, because without measures, you cannot assess the biological phenomenon. For example, does an intervention have any biological activity? Perhaps it does if it adequately affects some biological phenomenon (e.g., hormone level, tissue growth). You need measures (such as nM, mm³/day) to assess those. Trying to determine which patients are suitable for a clinical trial? A set of measurements of biological phenomenon (e.g., age, body mass, liver function) will determine whether each patient should be included in or excluded from the trial. Evaluating the safety of an intervention? To be deemed safe, the number and severity of side effects and toxicity must fall below acceptable levels. Does the intervention have an effect? It does if it affects some measure of disease activity (e.g., mg/dL of blood

sugar levels, degree (mild/moderate/severe) of retinopathy, and mL/min of creatinine clearance to measure renal function in diabetes).

Colloquially, you would probably talk about "unit of measure" when you talk about how to measure something. In Clinical Trial Medicine, "unit of measure" is usually simply called "measure," and we will use that term in that sense. It is important to distinguish that when we talk about "measure" we are not talking about the act of measuring or the item being measured but rather what *type* of unit we should use for measuring.

A "measure" can be defined as a way of assessing a clinical event or patient characteristic by taking that characteristic and mapping it to some sort of a scale. Many things can be measured in a clinical trial such as:

- General patient characteristics (e.g., height, weight, and age)
- Different general health states (e.g., dead vs. alive, i.e., mortality, sick vs. well, i.e., morbidity)
- Physiological parameters (e.g., blood pressure and temperature)
- Anatomic parameters (e.g., organ size and tumor volume)
- Clinical events (e.g., number of myocardial infarctions or vomiting episodes)
- Presence or absence and severity of symptoms (e.g., chest pain or cough)
- Physical or mental function (e.g., ability to walk, carry out simple tasks, or solve thought problems)
- Health care resource utilization (e.g., days in the hospital, days in the ICU, or medications needed)
- Daily activities (e.g., number of times going to the bathroom, hours of sunlight exposure, number of work days)
- Attitudes, beliefs, or opinions (e.g., interest in social activities, belief in a medication's ability to treat a condition)

Measures can be very general (e.g., severe disease/mild disease) or very specific (e.g., pmol/L); absolute (e.g., pound change body weight) or relative (e.g., % change in body weight); relatively simple (e.g., presence or absence of a symptom) or complex (e.g., a score on a 36-item survey); easy (e.g., presence of skin lesions) or difficult (e.g., a positive test on a surgical biopsy tissue specimen) to obtain. For example, for complex clinical phenomenon, such as "severity of congestive heart failure," a complex measure was widely used formerly: Class I/Class II/Class III/Class IV heart failure. In those cases, measures capture some aspects of the clinical phenomenon and map those selective and hopefully representative aspects to some scale.

A given phenomenon can be measured and expressed in many different ways. As an analogy, the answer to the question, "How far is it from San Francisco to Chicago?" could come in a variety of forms, depending on the purpose of the question. In designing a railroad, you may want to know the distance in km or miles and use an odometer to measure the distance. In planning a trip, you may be more interested in the average flying time for flights from SFO to O'Hare over the past year. In shipping a package, the number of shipping zones between the two cities may be more relevant.

Similarly, there are many ways of measuring and expressing blood pressure. Interested in how a medication affects blood pressure in the long term? Check the patient's blood pressure once a day and express it in mmHg. Does a medication momentarily raise blood pressure while injected into a patient? Continuously measure the patient's blood pressure during the injection and express it as a percentage change in the patient's blood pressure. Is high blood pressure a medication's side effect? Report how many people exceeded a pre-determined cutoff for high blood pressure (e.g., 140/100) by expressing it as high blood pressure/not high blood pressure.

When choosing a measure, clearly understand the potential implications of that choice. Sometimes the method of taking and expressing a measure is not crucial. In determining whether severe diarrhea is a drug side effect, it may not be necessary to quantify the exact volume of diarrhea or report what times of day the diarrhea occurred. Just measuring and reporting whether severe diarrhea occurred may be enough. However, in many other situations, even slight changes in the measurement can profoundly affect a study's ability to answer the question, the strength of the study's conclusions, the sample size, the study design, and the resources needed.

As an analogy, several different measures can be used to assess monetary value: dollars, pounds, yen, ruble. In some cases, it will not matter which measure (currency) you use. However, imagine if everyone in the United States switched to a new currency, "megadollars" where the smallest unit of currency was a megadollar which was

equivalent to $100 in previous currency. That would be a terrible currency for the current U.S. economy. On the other hand, if the United States eliminated dollars and everyone had to use only pennies then that would be an inappropriate measure as well.

Of course, measures often are imperfect. Proper assessments may need multiple measures (e.g., can a single measure determine if someone is intelligent). Some things are very difficult to quantify or categorize. Many assessments are subjective. For instance, how do you measure attractiveness? If height alone were a measure, many movie stars like Tom Cruise would come up "short." Polling 50 people about their criteria for attractiveness could easily yield 50 different answers, especially if they are from different generations, geographic locations, cultures, or upbringings.

Clinical measures are no different, as some are more imperfect and subjective than others. Adequately capturing disease activity, physiological status, psychological effects, and behavior can be extremely difficult. Often, multiple measures are needed. For example, fully capturing a patient's cardiovascular status may involve measuring heart rate and blood pressure at rest and during exercise, exercise tolerance, and ejection fraction with echocardiograms.

4.1.2 Levels and Types of Measures/Variables

The most common way of classifying types of measures were initially proposed by Stanley Smith Stevens[1].

Quantitative Variables

Variables can be *quantitative* (numeric) or *categorical* (or nonquantitative, sometimes called qualitative). Examples of quantitative variables include: age and cardiac ejection fraction. Examples of corresponding categorical variables include: age group (adult vs. nonadult) and the New York Heart Association (NYHA) Classification for heart failure (Classes I, II, III, IV). You can mathematically manipulate (e.g., add, subtract, multiply, divide, etc.) quantitative variables but not categorical variables (e.g., adding a red head to a blonde makes no sense unless you are a hair stylist). People sometimes refer to categorical variables as qualitative variables, but "qualitative" incorrectly implies that nonquantitative variables are always subjective measures; therefore we will use "categorical" to refer to nonquantitative variables.

Since the more values a variable can have, the higher (i.e., richer) the information content, quantitative variables

[1]Stevens, S.S. (1946). On the theory of scales of measurement. *Science*, **103**, 677–680.

In a diabetic wound healing trial, the quantitative variable (e.g., % of wound surface healed) is much more informative than the categorical variable of healed/not healed. For example, if 3 out of 10 patients healed their wounds in the placebo arm vs. 5 out of 10 in the treated arm, it would be difficult to draw strong conclusions. However, presenting the same results as 25% average healing in the placebo arm vs. 90% in the treated arm would be much more informative. It would be similarly informative if there were 45% average healing in the placebo arm and 55% in the treated arm. The key point is that 3/10 vs. 5/10 could be either of these two possibilities: qualitative variables generally don't convey as much information as quantitative variables.

FIGURE 4.1 Example of quantitative variables being superior to categorical variables.

typically are richer than categorical variables (Figure 4.1). For example, the exact quantitative variable of age provides more information than the following categorical variable: adult (>18 years of age) vs. nonadult (<18 years of age). The dichotomous categorical variable (i.e., adult vs. nonadult) does not distinguish among adults who are 18–30 years of age, 31–40 years of age, 41–50 years of age, etc. To expand on this, a statement, "Adults in the study had 3% incidence of bleeding in this study and children had 1% incidence" is not nearly as informative as "Subjects who were 1–10 years old had 0% bleeding, 11–20 had 2%, 21–40 had 4.5%, and 41–80 had 10%," or "For each additional year, the risk of bleeding increased by 0.2%." This difference in information content can have a profound impact on the power, the sample size, the clinical relevance of the results, and the study's robustness to dropouts (i.e., patients who discontinue the study) and missing values. (For example, a wound healing trial using a "healed vs. non-healed" categorical variable might require hundreds of patients, whereas a trial using a continuous variable of "percentage area healed" might require one-tenth the number of patients to achieve the same degree of statistical power.)

Since they contain more information than categorical variables, quantitative variables can be converted to categorical variables (e.g., blood pressure can be categorized as "low," "normal," or "high"; tumor response can be classified as "no response," "partial response," or "complete response"). But categorical variables cannot be converted to quantitative variables (e.g., "low" blood pressure cannot be converted into a specific mmHg measure without additional information).

Quantitative variables can be continuous or discrete:

- *Continuous variables*: These variables represent real numbers (e.g., age) that can be subdivided into infinitely smaller gradations (e.g., 3.5 years, 3.75 years, 9.575 years etc.). Continuous variables always have some unit of measurement (e.g., years, degrees Celsius, and mmHg).

Continuous variables contain more information than discrete variables so they can be converted into discrete variables.

- *Discrete (count) variables*: These variables are usually integers (e.g., number of exacerbations, prior pregnancies, or hospitalizations) that cannot be subdivided (e.g., there is no such thing as half a pregnancy or 2.75 hospitalizations). Discrete variables do not have units of measurement (although they may have names – such as "number of pregnancies"). Discrete variables contain less information than continuous variables so they cannot be converted into continuous variables.

Recognize that not every numeric measure is a true quantitative variable. For example, you cannot add or divide renal tubular acidosis type I, II, III, and IV or congestive heart failure classes I, II, III, and IV, which are represented numerically but are in fact categorical variables. Similarly, although ACR20, ACR50, etc. appear on face to be quantitative variables, you should not manipulate them numerically.

Even though most biological phenomena are not strictly linear, we use continuous linear variables to approximate many clinical variables. We commonly do this with scores that are composites of many measures such as Psoriasis Area Severity Index (PASI) scores (e.g., we treat 1% of the body surface area covered with erythema as being equivalent to 1% of the surface area being covered by a plaque). It is partially because many variables used in clinical practice are only approximations of a quantitative variable that some clinicians and the FDA prefer dichotomous variables to continuous variables.

The biological significance of some continuous variables (e.g., blood pressure) may not be linear over a broad range of values. For example, even though all have a 10 mmHg difference, the difference between 75 and 85 mmHg is not the same as the differences between 115 and 125 mmHg and between 260 and 270 mmHg. Similarly, a 6-month increase in survival rate has different meaning for a patient with a 3-month life expectancy vs. someone with a 50-year life expectancy. In such cases, utilizing averages is probably not appropriate unless you use mathematical manipulations (e.g., log transformation) to transform the variable into a linear variable.

Quantitative variables can be interval or ratio variables. With *ratio variables*, absolute 0 means something (when the variable equals 0.0, there is none of that variable) and doubling, tripling, etc. the value doubles, triples, etc. the meaning of the value. With *interval variables*, the difference between two values is meaningful. For example, temperature expressed in °C is an interval variable (e.g., the difference between temperatures of 100° and 90° is the same as between 90° and 80°) and not a ratio variable (e.g., doubling the temperature does not mean that something is twice as hot and 0.0°C does not mean "no temperature"). Temperature expressed in degrees Kelvin, on the other hand, is a ratio variable (0.0°K really does mean "no temperature" and double the temperature in Kelvin does mean something is twice as hot).

Categorical Variables

Unlike quantitative variables which can assume numerical values, categorical variables can assume one of a set of categories. These categories must be:

- *Mutually exclusive*: An observation should not fall into two or more categories at the same time. For example, age categories 0–21 years, 18–30 years, and 25+ years are not mutually exclusive. A subject who is 20 years old can be in both the first and second categories.
- *Exhaustive*: There should not be any gaps in the categories. In other words, every observation should fall within one of the categories. For example, age categories 2–18 years, 19–45 years, and 46–65 years are not exhaustive. A 1-year old and a 70-year old do not fall into any categories.

Even though categorical variables typically contain less information than quantitative variables, there are many situations where categorical variables are more clinically relevant than quantitative variables:

- *Adequate quantitative variables do not yet exist.* For some phenomena, quantitative variables have not yet been developed. For example, there is no widely used influenza symptom scale. Currently, people either describe the symptoms as mild/moderate/severe or determine the presence or absence of each individual symptom (e.g., fever/no fever).
- *For some phenomena, quantitative variables do not make sense.* For example, there can only be either presence or absence of pregnancy.
- *There are clinically significant cutoffs or thresholds.* Sometimes the phenomenon being measured clearly changes past certain thresholds (e.g., fasting blood glucose >126 mg/dL suggests diabetes, age >65 years of age qualifies someone for Medicare, and therapeutic levels for Digoxin are between 0.8 and 2.0 ng/mL). Therefore, it may be more useful to use categories that reflect these changes (e.g., diabetes/glucose intolerance/no diabetes, non-Medicare/Medicare, and sub-therapeutic/therapeutic/toxic). This is especially important when patients start above a threshold and end up below a threshold (e.g., unable to walk unassisted before the treatment but able to walk after).
- *You want to count the numbers or measure the proportions of patients that exhibit some clinical phenomenon.* Say you want to count the number of patients who

have hypertension. Then you need to establish a blood pressure measurement cutoff for classifying someone as having high blood pressure. Then you can categorize each patient as having either hypertension or no hypertension.

- *Quantitative variables mask what is happening with the individual patient.* Population means and medians can be misleading. For example, measuring each patient's cardiac ejection fraction and then reporting a mean change in ejection fraction can be very misleading. Imagine two sets of patients: Set A has ejection fractions of 10%, 20%, 60%, and 70% and Set B has ejection fractions of 30%, 35%, 40%, and 45%. Both sets will have a mean cardiac ejection fraction of 40%, but are clearly not comparable. Categorizing each patient in terms of heart failure (EF < 55%) vs. no heart failure (EF > 55%) may be more useful. Set A then would have two patients in heart failure and Set B would have four patients in heart failure.
- *When measuring changes, starting and ending points are important.* Often where a value begins and ends is as important as the magnitude of change. For example, there is a 50% change when the PASI goes from 10 to 5 and from 60 to 30, two significantly different situations. In the first situation, a mild case becomes milder. In the second situation a much more severe case becomes moderate. You cannot capture this difference without using categorical variables.

Moreover, regulatory agencies often will insist on categorical variables to set a high bar. They want the clinical significance of an intervention to be clear. For example, showing that a medication can bring high blood pressure levels to normal is more impressive than showing that it can statistically significantly lower blood pressure.

Categorical variables can be ordinal, nominal, or dichotomous:

- *Ordinal (rank) variables*: These variables have an order of significance in which one category is clearly better or greater than another. For example, complete response to a therapy is better than partial response, which is better than nonresponse. NYHA Class IV is worse than Class III which is worse than Class II which is worse than Class I. Even though one category is better than another, ordinal variables are still categorical variables; you should not add or average the values.
- *Nominal variables*: These variables do not have a meaningful order (e.g., northern region, southern region, and northwestern region). Although some in New York City and California may beg to differ, no geographic regions are superior or inferior.
- *Dichotomous variables*: These variables have only two possible values (e.g., dead/alive, true/false, or responder/nonresponder) that are distinct and mutually exclusive

(e.g., regardless of what some trial lawyers may tell you, something that is true cannot be false).

4.1.3 The Difference Between Measures and Endpoints

Measures are components of an endpoint, and so it is critical to understand measures before discussing endpoints and distinguish between measures and endpoints. An "endpoint" is the clinically relevant outcome that is being measured. For example, "mmHg" is a measure, and "change in mean blood pressure after 6 weeks of therapy" is an endpoint. The measure is used to quantify the endpoint. An endpoint is expressed as a measure that is put in specific context, with specified time interval and analytical methods.

Here are some nonmedical analogies. In a sporting event, a measure could be points; an endpoint could be the final scores after all the game time has elapsed. In a college class a measure could be test and project scores; an endpoint could be the final grade after all projects and tests in that course. For a movie, a measure could be dollars; an endpoint could be box office sales from the start to the finish of that movie's run in the movie theaters.

Extending the San Francisco to Chicago analogy, you can specify the distance between San Francisco and Chicago (like clinical endpoints) in different ways. It can be from downtown to downtown, geographic center to geographic center, airport to airport, etc. It can also be specified as: driving time if one kept to the speed limit, driving time if one were transporting a manufactured home and had to drive at 55 mph, driving time with a radar detector, etc. In a clinical trial, an endpoint can be difference in blood pressure after 6 weeks, the highest recorded blood pressure at any point during 6 weeks, absolute blood pressure after 12 weeks of therapy, etc. As will be discussed in Chapter 9, specifying the endpoint is an extremely important aspect of clinical trial design. Measures can be thought of as the bricks and endpoints as houses or buildings. However, measures can also be used for other purposes – as will be seen in the next section – just as bricks can be used for other purposes, such as building roads.

4.1.4 The Definition of Variables

A variable is a quantity capable of assuming any of a set of values. These values may be numeric values, characters, or categories. Every variable has a name (i.e., the variable name) and a data type. Each variable is expressed in a specific measure. An example of a variable is "body weight in pounds," or "body weight in kg." The opposite of a variable is a constant, which is a value that never changes.

4.2 THE IMPORTANCE OF MEASURES

4.2.1 The Purposes of Measures

As we alluded to previously, measures can serve several purposes:

To Evaluate a Patient's Suitability for a Trial

Clinical trial inclusion and exclusion criteria are evaluated using measures, so patients must have measurements (e.g., blood pressure, weight, number of symptoms, or physical function level) that tells us if their characteristics fall within pre-specified ranges to be included in or excluded from the trial.

To Assign Patients to Different Study Arms/Groups

If you wanted to randomly but fairly divide a group of players among different football teams, you would want to ensure that the team rosters had a fair balance of size, ability, and experience. One team should not end up with all the tall people or all the inexperienced players. One solution would be to group (i.e., stratify) the players by size, experience, or ability and then within these subgroups randomly assign players to different teams. Similarly, in clinical trials, you must ensure that the different comparison groups and arms are reasonably similar (e.g., similar distributions of ages, weights, initial blood pressures, cholesterol levels). Therefore, before randomly assigning patients to different study arms, you must use measures to stratify patients by a variety of relevant parameters.

To Determine the Progress of the Trial

When roasting a turkey, you may make a number of informal measurements to estimate your progress (e.g., the temperature, color, and texture of the turkey). If any of these measurements suggest problems, you may make certain adjustments, such as extending the cooking time, dialing up the temperature, repositioning the turkey, or ordering fast food from the local restaurant chain.

In the same manner, measures can serve to monitor the clinical trial. You may terminate a trial when certain thresholds are reached: enough patients achieve a certain objective (e.g., regaining a certain level of physical function) or too many adverse events occur (e.g., number of heart attacks).

To Determine the Efficacy and Effectiveness of the Intervention Being Studied

As mentioned previously, measures are necessary to formulate endpoints or outcomes. Whether an intervention achieves its endpoints determines if the intervention accomplishes its aims. This will be discussed in detail in Chapter 9.

To Describe and Characterize the Study Population

To illustrate this point, let us use another analogy: deciding whether to take a job position. Someone who works in a similar position tells you that he loves his job and urges you to take the position. Should you listen to his advice? First, you will want to know more about that person and his current position. How old is he? What stage of life is he in and what is his personal life like? (For example, a 14-year old might love delivering newspapers, but you may not.) Does his current position pay the same, require the same number of hours, and involve the same amount travel as the position you are considering? The more similar these characteristics are to you and your potential position, the more likely his opinion and experience would apply to you.

Similarly, anyone interpreting trial results and deciding whether they are applicable to their patient populations will want to know the relevant characteristics of a study population. How old were the patients? How healthy were they? What kind of pre-existing medical conditions did they have? After all, results from patients who are under 20 years of age and have normal cholesterol levels may not be applicable to patients who are over 40 years of age and have high cholesterol levels. Measuring a variety of important characteristics helps characterize and profile the population.

To Determine the Safety of the Intervention Being Studied

Counting the number of side effects occurring in a trial will indicate whether the frequency of side effects is below an acceptable threshold. But not all side effects are equal. Certainly death or permanent disability is worse than nausea or mild diarrhea. Therefore, in addition to counting the number of side effects, measure the severity of each side effect. These measures are used to characterize safety endpoints.

To Determine the Relationship Between Certain Parameters and the Effects of an Intervention

A trial can not only tell you whether an intervention has any effect, it can also tell you how that effect varies by time (e.g., does the effect increase or decrease over time), patient characteristics (e.g., body weight, liver function), disease characteristics (e.g., disease stage or severity), or intervention parameters (e.g., the dose, frequency, route of administration, length of treatment). As you can see, measures can be used to classify, to rank, or to compare/establish an association between phenomena.

4.2.2 Measures Affect Clinical Trial Design and Conduct

The types of measures chosen as well as the clinical phenomena being measured can profoundly affect the design, conduct, cost, results, and interpretation of a clinical trial:

The Trial Design must Allow Adequate Time, Opportunity, and Resources to Collect Data on the Measure

Taking measurements costs money, time, effort, and potential inconvenience and discomfort to the patient. For example, if a measure is primary tumor size in mm^3 as determined by magnetic resonance imaging (MRI) 6 months after a treatment, the trial must last at least 6 months, exclude patients who have contraindications to MRI (e.g., ferromagnetic metallic objects in their bodies or claustrophobia), and include enough personnel and funding to complete the MRIs. Even though some measures (e.g., number of tumor cells) may be more accurate measures of tumor size, it may be difficult to count the actual number of cells.

The Trial must be Conducted in a Way that Allows for Accurate and Reliable Measurements

Using the same example, accurately measuring tumor size with MRI requires properly administering intravenous gadolinium (an MRI contrast agent), keeping the patient still while acquiring images, and using the correct computer sequences when acquiring the images. Failure to properly perform any of these may result in poor images and therefore inaccurate measures.

The Type of Trial Data Available Depends on the Measures Used

An MRI may show no decrease in tumor size if the measure that is used is the traditional "progression/stable disease/partial response/complete response," while there might be a clear decrease in tumor size if the measure used were "volume in mm^3." Therefore, choosing inappropriate or too few measures may lead to improper conclusions (i.e., false positives or false negatives).

The Types of Measures Used will Influence Trial Result Interpretation

Trial results may be more or less convincing depending on how adequately the measures capture disease activity and characterize the patient population. Critics may argue that the primary tumor size may be meaningless if the tumor spreads (metastasizes) to other distant locations in the body. Others may say that reducing tumor size does not necessarily prevent mortality. People may not believe or understand measures that they are not used to seeing.

4.3 CHOOSING THE RIGHT MEASURES

4.3.1 Characteristics of a Good Measure

In the previous sections, we have tried to illustrate the importance of measures and how your choice of measures can make or break a clinical study or trial. So what constitutes a good measure? How do you choose a good measure? No measure is perfect. But there are a number of characteristics that a good measure should have (Figure 4.2):

Obtaining the Measure must be Feasible

First and foremost, choose a measure that is feasible to implement from a technological, cost, personnel, resource, patient comfort, or time perspective. Measuring the total number of body cells that a drug alters would be nice but not possible … at least with current technology. Obtaining weekly surgical biopsies to characterize degree of differentiation could provide a lot of information but cause unacceptable discomfort and harm to the patient. Checking frequent serial MRIs to quantify tumor volume would provide a significant amount of data but be prohibitively expensive.

These rather extreme examples may make this point seem obvious, but in actuality investigators frequently choose measures that seem reasonable during the planning stage but in actuality are difficult or impossible to implement. Do not focus on designing the "perfect" experiment without properly accounting for cost and other "practical" issues. You may not fully recognize and appreciate the complexities and subtle implications of your choice of measures. For example, performing a functional MRI requires finding the right machine, appropriate personnel to perform the test, patients who can tolerate the procedure,

- Feasible
- Accurate
- Valid
- Precise/Reliable
- Verifiable
- Relevant
- Sensitive and Responsive
- Rich in Information
- Recognized and Accepted
- Able to Capture the Full Range of Variability
- No Significant Biological Effect
- Reasonably Objective
- Causes Minimal Harm or Discomfort

FIGURE 4.2 Characteristics of a good measure.

means of transporting patients to and from the facility, time to acquire the images, funding to pay for the test, computers to store the images, and procedures to compensate for mistakes, errors, and complications.

The Measure must be Accurate

The measurements should be as close as possible to the actual value of the physiological or disease parameter (e.g., the blood pressure reading on a machine should be close to the patient's actual blood pressure). We will discuss accuracy in greater detail in Section 4.4.

The Measure must be Valid

The measure must measure what it is supposed to measure, that is, it must be valid. We will discuss this concept in detail in Section 4.7. As an example, height is not a very valid measure of basketball playing ability. It may correlate with playing ability, but being tall does not guarantee that you are a good player and being short does not mean that you are a bad player.

The Measure Should be Precise (or Reliable)

Precision (or reliability) is repeatability or consistency, that is, a precise (reliable) measure will give identical or similar results when repeated. Section 4.4 covers this topic in greater depth.

The Measure Should be Verifiable

Once a measure is performed, you should be able to double-check and make sure (i.e., verify) that the measurement was done properly. So a measure should have clear directions and documentation on how it was obtained. Preferably, alternative methods of obtaining the same measurement should generate very similar values (e.g., since various cardiac modalities such as Doppler echocardiogram, cardiac gated radionuclide scan, and cardiac MRI should give you very similar values for cardiac ejection fraction, you can use one imaging modality to verify results from another modality).

The Measure Should be Relevant and Representative

A measure can be precise, accurate, and valid, but it should also be relevant and representative. For example, measuring the color of urine may be relevant when assessing nephrolithiasis, but not when assessing congestive heart failure (CHF). Measuring cardiac ejection fraction in percentages might be appropriate in CHF and measuring skin area affected might be appropriate in burn patients, but it is not appropriate to measure dyspnia in percentages.

The measure should be also representative. For example, height could be measured in cm, or alternatively it could be categorized as short/medium/tall. Both would be representative measures. It would not be a good measure if the categories were 5 feet/6 feet/neither 5 feet nor 6 feet.

The Act of Obtaining the Measure Should not Influence Response or have a Significant Biological Effect

Avoid using a measure that can somehow interfere with the results (e.g., a machine measuring blood pressure should not cause stress that will increase the patient's blood pressure). Of course, it is hard to find measures that have absolutely no biological effect. Just taking measurements can cause some anxiety and physiological changes in patients (e.g., Hawthorne effect, White Coat phenomenon). However, you want to either minimize these effects or know how to adjust for them.

The Measure Should Function Across and Capture Variation Along the Disease and Intervention Spectrum

Diseases can have a wide range of presentations, severity, and courses, so a measure must account for all relevant possibilities. Think about the many possible signs, symptoms, and outcomes of systemic diseases like systemic lupus erythematosus (which can affect the lungs, heart, joints, skin, kidney, brain, and/or gastrointestinal tract). So a measure of overall systemic disease severity cannot just focus on one organ system (e.g., cardiac manifestations).

The measure must remain accurate, precise, valid, etc. up and down to the potential extremes of physiological and disease parameters. For instance, a scale that is not able to capture data over 300 pounds may be a poor choice in a trial that has any patients over 300 pounds. So anticipate the range of possible values and choose a measure that functions well beyond this range.

Each time an intervention is performed, there is potential variability (e.g., different batches of the drug, particularly biologics, can have different potency or different operators of a procedure can have different skills or technical abilities), so any measure designed to characterize the intervention must capture this variability. For example, if you want to measure levels of drug toxicity, expressing toxicity per active unit (e.g., per mg of active drug) of drug may be more informative than just toxicity per drug administration.

The Measure must be Mapped so that it is Sensitive and Responsive (i.e., Rich in Information and Yield a Good Distribution of Values in a Population of Patients)

All measures map some characteristic of a phenomenon to a scale. For example, hair color might be mapped to one of the following: black, brown, blond, and red. This mapping categories must not overlap: each item being measured must map only to one value. For example, the scale for a measure cannot be made up of "red hair, black hair, long hair, curly hair." Someone could have red and curly hair, and therefore the scale overlaps. One could have three different sets of measures, such as color, length, and curliness, but one cannot have a scale that overlaps.

In addition, the mapping should not be overly specific. For example, license plate numbers can be considered to be a measure – each car is mapped to a number. However, each license plate number is unique and therefore, it is not a terribly useful way of mapping the cars to a scale for statistical. (In addition, the scale is not representative.) With a good measure, there should be an appropriate level of detail to the scale but not so fine as to make the scale useless. Multiple items and objects should map to the same categories or values.

How fine should the scale be then, and how many items should map to the same value? You should notice a change in the measurements even when relatively small changes in the phenomenon or condition occur if it is clinically significant. For example, a measure of pulmonary status should change when a patient's pulmonary status improves or deteriorates. Simply listening to the patient's lungs with a stethoscope may not yield an adequate measure. A measure base on chest X-ray and pulmonary function tests may detect differences that listening with a stethoscope cannot. Some measures are too "blunt," changing only with large alterations in physiological or disease status (e.g., presence/absence of blindness is a very blunt or crude measure of diabetic retinopathy). Such blunt measures cannot distinguish among different gradations of diseases or conditions.

If possible, avoid measures that provide very limited information, especially when alternatives are richer in information. For example, tumor volume based on a CT scan or MRI will generally provide more information than one-dimensional tumor size based on a plain film.

Ideally, the Measure Should be Widely Recognized and Accepted

Using very novel or difficult to understand measures runs the risk of regulatory agencies and the medical and scientific communities not understanding and accepting your data. Historical precedence may help choose the right measures for a clinical study. If previous trials of similar cancer drugs measured tumor volume as "progression/stable disease/partial response/complete response," your trial of a cancer drug likely should, all things being equal, include this measure rather than "no response/yes response." Using such established measures can help others compare your trial and drug with other similar trials and drugs.

Objective Measures are Preferable to Subjective Measures

All measures have some subjectivity in their collection and interpretation, but if possible strive to use ones that are more objective (e.g., calculating an ejection fraction from an echocardiogram is a more objective measure of congestive heart failure than simply relying on physical examination findings).

4.3.2 Obstacles to Obtaining Good Measurements

Obtaining correct and appropriate measurements is not easy due to many potential obstacles. Good clinical trial design, selecting good measures, blinding, randomization, and training can help overcome some obstacles. Obstacles include (but are not limited to) the following:

Cost

Although cost should not get in the way of good science, budget constraints are a fact of life and may prevent some measurements. You may need to select the least costly ways of obtaining measures that will not compromise trial conduct or results. Trial budgets should account for all the potential direct and indirect costs of measures including instrument, personnel, and consumable costs. They should anticipate that some measures may need to be repeated or done unexpectedly (e.g., safety measures when adverse events occur).

Potential Discomfort or Harm to the Patient

Not all ways of obtaining measures are benign, and some can result in substantial discomfort or harm to the patient. Measures may require invasive (e.g., surgical biopsies) or strenuous (e.g., treadmill tests) procedures; radiation (computed tomography) or other types of exposure; or time and inconvenience (e.g., travel) for the patient. Strike a balance between scientific need and potential negative consequences. Remember the diversity of your study population when trying to anticipate problems. Measures can affect different patients differently (e.g., travel can be a bigger problem for patients with limited time or living far away from the trial site; strenuous or invasive procedures can be more onerous for patients with many other medical problems).

Errors (Random and Systematic)

We will discuss errors in detail in Section 4.5.

Patient Compliance

Patients are less likely to comply with procedures that require actions that are time consuming, unsupervised, uncomfortable or harmful, or have ambiguous or difficult to understand directions. Non-compliance can manifest in varying degrees. Patients can refuse to comply at all, which is the easiest type of non-compliance to identify and remedy. They also can comply with certain aspects of the procedures and refuse others. The most challenging type of non-compliance is when patients ostensibly agree to comply but surreptitiously do not.

Inexperience and Lack of Training

Executing procedures to obtain measures can require experience and training. Even relatively simple and common procedures such as taking blood pressure can vary by training and experience (e.g., cuff placement or detecting when you hear the arterial sounds). Therefore, ensure that all measurement takers are adequately trained and experienced.

Environmental Effects

Many aspects of the environment can interfere with measurements. Poor lighting, ambient noise, extreme temperatures, and humidity are only a few of the many things that can affect subjects, observers, instruments, interventions, and even diseases. (We'll discuss more about these effects when we discuss random errors and biases.) Therefore, it is important to maintain comfortable and consistent environments and monitor and measure relevant aspects of the environment (e.g., ambient temperature and humidity).

Ethical and Legal Issues

Scientific and economic considerations may suggest using a certain measure, but ethical or legal considerations may make it difficult or impossible to perform the measure. Be careful when using measures that may potentially violate patient privacy and confidentiality. When possible, consider less personally invasive measures or employ appropriate safeguards to protect the patient. Chapter 2 covers many of the relevant ethical and legal issues.

4.4 ACCURACY AND PRECISION

4.4.1 Definitions of Accuracy and Precision

Accuracy refers to how well the measure reflects the phenomenon being measured. (For example, how well does a glucometer reading correspond to a patient's true blood sugar level?) Precision refers to how reproducible the measurement is – if we measured the blood sugar level 10 times on a patient at a given time, would the values be very similar to each other? Or will there be a lot of random variation, that is, large variability?

We can use a target analogy (Figure 4.3) to help understand the concepts of accuracy and precision. Imagine that the bull's eye in the center of a target is the actual value of a phenomenon (e.g., a patient's actual blood sugar level)

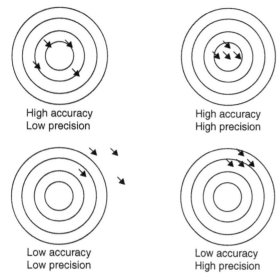

FIGURE 4.3 Target representation of accuracy and precision.

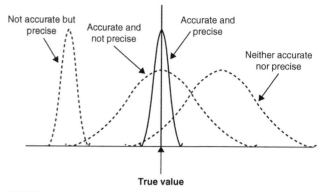

FIGURE 4.4 Accuracy and precision.

and measures (e.g., reading on a glucometer) are arrows fired at the target. Accuracy is the closeness of the arrows to the bull's eye (e.g., how close the readings are to the actual blood sugar level); the closer the arrow is to the bull's eye, the more accurate.

As Figure 4.4 shows, a measurement can be precise but not accurate, that is, repeated measurements are very close to each other but the numbers are consistently off from the true value. Using the target analogy, arrows are tightly clustered, but far from the bull's eye. An example would be using a state-of-the-art machine to measure blood pressure on a patient's arm that is too large for the machine's blood pressure cuff. The blood pressure readings will consistently be higher than the true value. Regardless of how many times you repeat the measurement, this error will persist, because it is not random but systematic.

Imprecise measures tend not to be accurate. In the target analogy, widely scattered arrows cannot all be close to the bull's eye. However, the average of many imprecise measurements can be accurate. As long as the error is random and not systematic (i.e., always in one direction), you can overcome an imprecise measure by repeating the measurement multiple times and taking the average. An example would be having many observers visually estimate a person's height. If 10 observers were to estimate a person's height, some would overshoot and some would undershoot, but whether each observer overshoots or undershoots would probably be random. Therefore, the average of 100 observers' estimates may be more accurate than the average of 10 observers' estimates. The average of 1000 observers' estimates may be even more accurate.

Characterize and document the precision of all measurements used in clinical studies. Maximizing precision is crucial, since poor precision (also called lack of reliability,

lack of repeatability, or high variability) can cause significant problems.

Imprecise Measures can Significantly Weaken the Ability to Draw Conclusions from a Study

As we mentioned, imprecise measures tend not to be accurate, and inaccurate measures can be of limited usefulness and can even be misleading.

Poor Precision can Increase the Number of Measurements or Sample Size Required to get Accurate Measures

From a scientific standpoint, avoid increasing the sample size if possible. Moreover, increasing the sample size is very costly and not always feasible. What if there are not enough eligible and available patients? What if the disease is very rare? What if your resources (e.g., medications, personnel, hospital bed capacity, or MRI time) are limited?

Imprecise Measures can Enroll Inappropriate Subjects in a Study

Imagine employing an imprecise glucometer to identify diabetics for a study of anti-hyperglycemic agents. As a result, you could accidentally enroll many nondiabetics, who then would receive medications that do not help and could even hurt them, and generate misleading results. Increasing the sample size will only enroll many more nondiabetics and not solve the problem.

Imprecise Measures Could Assign Patients to the Wrong Groups and Subgroups

Picture using an imprecise cholesterol measure to assign patients to different treatment groups or stratify patients by cholesterol level. An imprecise cholesterol measure would accidentally assign some patients with high cholesterol levels to the low cholesterol group and vice-versa. This could easily muddle the trial, analysis, and results.

4.4.2 Measuring Precision

As shown in Figures 4.4 and 4.6, precision is the spread of the curve when you plot the frequency distribution of repeated measurements, so statistics that measure this spread measure precision. The simplest measure of precision is the *standard deviation* (*SD*). The wider the spread of the curve, the larger the SD and the less precise the measurement are. Alternatively, you can use a unit-less measure, the *coefficient of variation*, to measure and compare precisions of different measures, even when they are in different units (e.g., cm vs. inches):

Coefficient of Variation = Standard Deviation/Mean

Measures with higher coefficients of variations are less precise than those with lower coefficients.

A better way of characterizing precision is to compare consistency across two or more sets of measurements:

- *Test–retest consistency (stability reliability)*: Repeating a measurement multiple times on the same set of patients can establish the *replicability* (i.e., the likelihood that the outcome of a particular study will occur again if another investigator performs the same study) of a measurement. The time between an initial test and a subsequent test is important. For some tests, repeating the test too soon will affect the second measurement (e.g., a patient asked to read letters from an eye chart may remember the letters if asked to repeat the eye test immediately). On the other hand, waiting too long could allow an actual change in the parameter being measured (e.g., vision may truly change if you wait several months between the first and second test).
- *Intra-observer consistency*: Having the same observer interpret and re-interpret the same test (e.g., an electrocardiogram or a set of photographs) at different times measures intra-observer consistency. Of course, the observer must not know his or her previous interpretation when re-interpreting the test.
- *Inter-observer consistency (inter-rater reliability)*: Having multiple observers evaluate the same set of patients or data and comparing their measurements will establish inter-observer consistency. For example, two or more investigators could use a sliding rating scale (1 being the least severe, 5 being most severe) to rate the severity of a skin disorder. If one investigator were to give a "1" rating, while another were to give a "5," the inter-observer consistency or inter-rater reliability would be inconsistent and low. Training, education, monitoring, and clear guidelines can enhance inter-observer consistency.
- *Internal consistency*: For a given test, different items that measure the same thing should generate results that agree, that is, the test should show internal consistency.

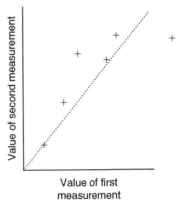

FIGURE 4.5 Measuring precision: two sets of measurements graphed against each other.

For example, if a questionnaire had two questions: "Basketball is your favorite sport" and "You dislike basketball." If the questionnaire has internal consistency, any person who agrees with Question 1 should disagree with Question 2. Similarly, blood pressure readings obtained by two different methods (e.g., noninvasively with a sphygmomanometer and invasively with an arterial line) should correlate with each other.

For each of the above tests for consistency, you could plot the resulting values on a graph (Figure 4.5). The diagonal line represents the ideal situation (i.e., perfect precision), where repeat (i.e., first and second) measurements on a given subject are equivalent. The closer the measurements are to the diagonal line, the more precise the measure is.

There are several ways to express precision statistically, but the most common ones are:

- *Correlation coefficient*: Used only for numerical measurements, the correlation coefficient indicates the statistical correlation between the first and second (repeat) measurements with 1 meaning perfect correlation and a 0 meaning no correlation at all.
- *Standard (typical) error of measurement*: The standard error of measurement or within-subject SD is the SD in each subject's measurements.
- *Coefficient of variation*: This is similar to the standard error of measurement but divided by the mean.
- *Reliability limits of agreement*: This is the 95% confidence interval for the difference between a subject's scores in two tests (e.g., a ±20 mmHg limits of agreement for a blood pressure measurement means that there is a 95% chance that the difference between a subject's two blood pressure readings will be between −20 mmHg and +20 mmHg. Also, 95% of subjects will have difference scores within −20 mmHg and +20 mmHg.
- *Change in mean*: Subtracting the mean of all the first measurements from the mean of all the second measurements gives you the change in the mean, that is, the

difference between the means for the two sets of measurements (0 being perfect precision).

- *Kappa coefficient*: The Kappa coefficient is similar to the correlation coefficient, but for nominal or categorical variables. A Kappa coefficient of 1 means perfect correlation among repeat measurements whereas a 0 means every repeat measurement was different from the other. The higher the Kappa, the better the correlation is (>0.7 is generally regarded as good statistic correlation):

$$\text{Kappa Coefficient} = [P(A) - P(E)]/[1 - P(E)]$$

where $P(A)$ is the proportion of times the model values are equal to the actual value $P(E)$ is the expected proportion of times model values are equal to the actual value by chance.

All of these methods assume that precision is the same for every subject. When the typical error varies between subjects, the data displays *heteroscedasticity*, or non-uniform error. So analysis would yield an average typical error too high for some subjects and too low for others. When measuring precision, always look for possible non-uniform error. Eliminating heteroscedasticity involves doing separate analyses on subgroups (e.g., perhaps precision is different for adults vs. children) or mathematically transforming (e.g., log transformation works when errors increase as the measure gets higher) the data so that error becomes uniform.

4.5 MEASUREMENT ERRORS

4.5.1 Random vs. Systematic (Biases) Errors

There are two general types of errors: *random* and *systematic* (also called *biases*). Random errors do not occur consistently in one direction, while biases do (Figure 4.6). As Table 4.1 indicates, random errors decrease precision; biases decrease accuracy. Repeating measurements and averaging the resulting values can reduce random errors but not biases. Once you identify and quantify biases, you can correct and adjust for biases (e.g., if a thermometer consistently gives readings 3° higher than the actual value, then you can just subtract 3° from every reading), but you cannot do the same for random errors. We will discuss biases more extensively in Section 5.5.

Three major sources of random error are subject variability, observer variability, and instrument variability. Each of these can be divided further into *intra* (within the same patient, observer, or instrument) and *inter* (among different patients, observers, or instruments) types. The distinction

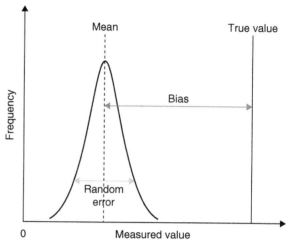

FIGURE 4.6   Graphical representation of random vs. systematic (bias) errors.

TABLE 4.1   Characteristics of Random vs. Systematic (Bias) Errors

	Random errors	Systematic errors (biases)
Consistent and repeatable	No	Yes
Mainly decreases	Precision	Accuracy
Reduced when measurement taken many times	Yes	No
Studied using	Repeated measurements statistical analysis (e.g., mean, variance, standard deviation)	Inter-comparisons, error propagation, calibration
Can be adjusted or corrected for	No	Yes

between *intra* and *inter* variability is important insofar as the tactics used to reduce the two types of variability differ (e.g., specifying that the same physician conducts the joint examination on every patient will reduce inter-observer variability but not intra-observer variability). Since these errors decrease the precision of measurements, every effort should be made to minimize them. Some of the strategies are discussed below. Remember that any of the sources of random error listed below can become sources of systematic errors (biases), when the variability occurs consistently in one manner or one direction (e.g., pollen levels change with the seasons and geography).

4.5.2 Subject Variability

A given patient is not same every hour of the day, every day of the week, and every week of the year. Sources of intra-patient variability include:

- *Physiological and disease fluctuations*: Many physiological (e.g., blood pressures, pulses, hormone levels) and disease measures fluctuate throughout the day, week, month, and year. Chronic diseases (e.g., inflammatory and psychiatric illnesses) will wax and wane, going through acute flares and periods of lower disease activity. Investigators must understand the patterns of these fluctuations and plan the timing of measures accordingly. So measuring overall disease severity for a disease that fluctuates throughout a day may require using an average or median of multiple measurements during the day.
- *Motivation, effort, and compliance*: Some measures such as treadmill tests, visual acuity charts, pulmonary function tests, and questionnaires require patients to expend focused efforts. The same patient may be more or less motivated each time he or she is tested, affecting the measurements.
- *Accidents and mistakes*: Patients may misunderstand directions or experience chance problems (e.g., marking the wrong box on a questionnaire, coughing during a pulmonary function test, injuring oneself before or during a treadmill test) that can alter measurements.
- *Subject–observer interaction*: Subjects can influence an observer's measurements. The subject may aid (e.g., help identify findings, use proper positioning) or distract the observer. An observer can influence a subject's performance by giving better directions or encouragement. An observer and subject may take more or less effort depending on their personal rapport.
- *Environmental effects*: The local environment can greatly affect different measures. Oxygen saturation varies by altitude. Disease activity can be modified by local climate conditions (e.g., sunlight may improve psoriasis, cold weather can exacerbate arthritic conditions, and allergic rhinitis can be worse in areas of high pollen counts). Room conditions such as lighting, temperature, crowdedness, size, layout, and even wall color can affect a patient's stress level, performance on tests, and behavior. Stressful situations can affect physiological and psychological parameters (e.g., increase blood pressure, heart rate, and cortisol levels) and hinder a patient's ability to understand instructions. Certain environmental extremes (e.g., high humidity and temperature or low lighting) could make patients sluggish.
- *Intervention variability*: As we mentioned previously, significant intervention variability can occur (e.g., different batches of medications can have different potencies).

Different patients can be very different from each other. All of the above-mentioned sources of intra-patient variability can also be sources of inter-patient variability. Additional sources include:

- *Socio-economic and demographic differences*: Some measures may vary by socioeconomic status, gender, culture, ethnicity, or geography. Patients who normally do not have regular access to health care may be of poorer health. The distribution of some biological parameters (e.g., body mass index or hemoglobin levels) differs between men and women. Patients of different cultures and religious affiliations may have different experiences, understanding, and compliance levels with measures.
- *Co-morbidities*: Co-morbidities are conditions and diseases other than the primary disease under study. Co-morbidities can affect test performance and measures (e.g., significant osteoarthritis or any other musculoskeletal disease can hinder a patient's ability to complete an exercise treadmill test or diabetic retinopathy can impair a patient's ability to read written directions).
- *Variation along the disease spectrum*: Diseases can have a wide range of presentations, severity, and courses. Think about the many possible signs, symptoms, and outcomes of systemic diseases like systemic lupus erythematosus (which can affect the lungs, heart, joints, skin, kidney, brain, and/or gastrointestinal tract). Measures must account for all relevant possibilities. So a measure of overall systemic disease severity cannot just focus on one organ system (e.g., cardiac manifestations).

4.5.3 Observer Variability

Observers include those preparing the patient for performing, and interpreting a measure. In general, having multiple observers to confirm each other's measurements, clear guidelines on how to perform and document findings, proper training, and appropriate quality checks can alleviate many observer errors. Sources of intra-observer variability include:

- *Time and effort*: You must also exert focused time and effort to obtain and interpret certain measurements (e.g., the more carefully a physician listens to a patient's heart the more likely he or she may detect a new murmur).
- *Training and experience effects*: Your ability to make measurements or detect certain findings changes with practice and experience. Often, it will steadily improve, which would be systematic variability (bias). However, such training and experience effects can have unpredictable consequences. If you have seen many abnormal cases or measurements, you may either look for

(i.e., "overinterpret" measures) or pass over (i.e., an abnormal finding does not "stand out" in a sea of abnormal findings) abnormalities. If you have seen many normal cases or measurements, you may be either ill-prepared (i.e., you expect normal findings and are not used to recognizing abnormal findings) or more likely (i.e., the abnormal finding stands out) to detect an abnormal finding.

- *Psychological or physical fatigue*: Fatigue can erode your ability to make precise measurements. In some situations it is clear which direction fatigue-induced errors will occur (e.g., fatigued observers tend to miss lesions on mammograms), so such errors will become biased. But in many cases, it is random whether you overshoot or undershoot with measurements.
- *Environmental effects*: The local environment also can affect your ability to administer and interpret tests. Poor lighting, ambient noise, extreme temperatures, or other distractions can hinder proper interpretation of results.
- *Subject–observer interaction*: Regardless of how objective or unbiased you believe yourself to be, your feeling about the subject may affect your effort, observations, and interpretation of results. No one is completely free of bias. Having an affinity for a patient may make you more careful and compulsive in your questioning and data gathering (e.g., you spend more time gathering measurements), tend to have a more favorable interpretation of certain types of results (e.g., if the patient rates poorly on a personality disorder scale, you may be more inclined to disregard the results and repeat the test), and be more likely to believe what a patient tells you (e.g., the patient claims that he has been compliant with taking his medications). Conversely, disliking a patient may cause you to spend less time and effort with the patient and believe the worst about the patient (e.g., that disheveled patient obviously has been noncompliant with his medications).
- *Accidents and mistakes*: Even the most experienced, well-rested, and conscientious individuals can improperly perform and misinterpret tests. For example, during an exercise treadmill test, you may inject the radiotracer at the wrong time, infiltrate the intravenous line, or fail to push the patient to his maximum exercise level. When interpreting the images, you may miss subtle defects or interpret artifacts as real defects.

Variability in how different observers interpret the same set of observations and data is common. Physicians will frequently disagree over the interpretation of imaging studies, pathology specimens, procedures (e.g., colonoscopy, bronchoscopy, electroencephalogram), or physical examination findings. Though some of these differences can be attributed to differences in skill levels and experience, uncertainty and standard error are inherent in many medical measures. In fact, the same observer may give different interpretations when viewing the same set of observations and data on different occasions (i.e., inter-observer

variability). Having multiple observers and averaging their observations can help overcome this problem. Sources of inter-observer variability include:

- *Subjective criteria and varying definitions*: Clinical medicine and many clinical measures are subjective, often involving judgment rather than hard data. This is especially true with certain diagnoses (e.g., irritable bowel syndrome, allergic reactions, psychiatric conditions, and rheumatological disorders) and disease severity scales (e.g., The Rheumatoid Arthritis Severity Scale (RASS), the TIMI scale). Ten observers may see the same data and draw widely varying conclusions.
- *Training and experience*: All "measurement takers" are not equal, which becomes more important as the subjectivity of the measure increases. The accuracy of even seemingly simple measures such as blood pressure can greatly depend on the skill and experience of the person taking the measure (e.g., taking blood pressure can be challenging when the patient's arm is large or pulse is faint). Moreover, it can be difficult to determine or test the competency of the measurer. Experience and credentials do not guarantee competency. Testing and properly training measurement takers before and even during the trial are important, especially for complicated or pivotal measures.

4.5.4 Instrument Variability

You should regularly check, test, calibrate, and maintain all instruments used in a study, including even relatively simple or peripheral instruments (e.g., blood pressure cuffs, clocks, tubing and syringes for blood draws, or buttons on a machine). Sources of intra-instrument variability include:

- *Standard test or instrument error*: No test is perfect. As discussed in Chapter 3, even fully functioning tests yield false positives and false negatives to some degree and varying results even if repeated on the same subject at the same time and place. Repeated measurements with different methods (e.g., checking the temperature with two different machines and techniques and in two different parts of the body) help alleviate this problem.
- *Instrument or measurement method defects*: Instrument defects may not be recognized. Use equipment from reputable manufacturers. Do not rely on manufacturers' assurances that an instrument is fully functioning.
- *Calibration*: Unless regularly calibrated, machines, assays, and other equipment change with time. For example, unless a scale is "zeroed" frequently, weight measurements will start drifting. If this drift is consistently in one direction, it becomes a systematic error (bias).
- *Maintenance and degradation*: All instruments steadily deteriorate in their performance over time until they

become unusable. Regular maintenance may slow this degradation, so the timing and frequency of such maintenance can affect measurements (e.g., regular cleaning and replacing parts of a machine).

- *Processing*: Many tests require some type of processing (e.g., blood cultures must be spread onto culture plates), the quality and technique of which may depend on the person performing the processing.
- *Environmental effects*: Environmental conditions such as temperature, pressure, humidity, lighting, dust, and vibration can affect an instrument's measurements.
- *Settings*: An instrument may require many settings (e.g., treadmill speed and inclination) that should be held relatively constant during measurement. Inconsistency in settings can lead to variability.

All sources of intra-instrument variability can be sources of inter-instrument variability. In addition, the following can cause variability among different instruments:

- *Differences in instrument quality*: All instruments are not the same. Even equipment of the same age and manufacturer can differ in quality, accuracy, and precision.
- *Differences among different models and manufacturers*: Just as a 1993 Honda Civic differs from a 1996 Honda Civic and a Honda Civic differs from a Geo Metro, different equipment makes and manufacturers may have different construction, calibration, or settings, even when the general design and operating principles are the same.

4.5.5 Biases

As previously mentioned, biases (systematic or nonrandom errors) decrease accuracy. In biases, the measurement is consistently off in one direction (e.g., the blood pressure measurement is always lower than the true value or an assay always determines hormone levels to be higher than they actually are). Since inaccurate measures can adversely affect the legitimacy and applicability of trial results, make every effort to minimize bias.

Any source of random errors can become biases when they consistently occur in one direction. For example, certain groups of subjects may tend to be noncompliant (e.g., non-English speakers who may not understand the directions) or have disease fluctuations or manifestations in one direction (e.g., older patients may have more severe manifestations of a disease or women may have different disease presentations than men). Certain observers may regularly have more difficulty with subjects (e.g., poor "bedside manner" or subjects may be prejudiced against an observer's appearance) or make measurements that are regularly higher (or regularly lower) than other observers. Environments may be nonrandomly different as well (e.g., the examination room is too hot on certain days or there is

a loud jackhammer sound during some of the measurements). Instruments could be miscalibrated in one direction (e.g., a scale gives readings that are 10 pounds lighter than actual weight). Also interventions can vary nonrandomly (e.g., one batch of medications has decreased potency or one interventional cardiologist performed the procedure in a different way). Therefore, it is important to measure and determine whether supposedly random errors are indeed random.

We discuss biases in greater detail in Chapter 5.

4.6 STRATEGIES TO MAXIMIZE ACCURACY AND PRECISION

4.6.1 General Strategies

General strategies to reduce errors include:

- *Trial (or test) runs*: Doing test runs of the study before actually starting the study may reveal errors that can be corrected (e.g., having study sites send in sample echocardiograms to ensure that they can perform high quality measurements).
- *Run-in phase*: For measures prone to conditioning or training (e.g., treadmill or visual acuity charts), consider using a run-in period to train the patient and observers before true measurements are obtained. A run-in period is basically akin to a warm-up period, pre-season, or Spring Training, a time during which you can get everyone used to the test and work the "kinks" out of the system (e.g., eliminate placebo responders or nonresponders).
- *Multiple measurements*: For measurements that are relatively easy to perform (e.g., blood pressure), repeat measurements, discard the highest and lowest values, and average the remaining results.

If you find some clear biases, consider doing one or more of the following:

- *Discard biased measurements.*
- *Adjustment factors*: If biases are relatively constant in quantity or magnitude, you may be able to apply an appropriate adjustment factor (e.g., for a thermometer that is consistently 10° higher, subtract 10° from every reading).
- *Group/stratify biased measurements*: When analyzing the measurements, consider grouping/stratifying the biased measurements and analyzing them separately (e.g., if the environment changed significantly in February, analyze all of the February measurements separately).
- *When analyzing the measurements, create a separate variable that measures the phenomenon that is biasing the measurement* (e.g., if environmental temperature affects pulmonary function, measure the temperature while measuring pulmonary function).

4.6.2 Subject Strategies

Subjects should be adequately prepared, informed and well rested. Specific strategies include:

- *Detailed instructions and protocols*: Instructions should be appropriate to the subjects and accommodate the potential diversity and range of patients (e.g., non-English speakers may need translated versions and visually impaired patients may require either verbal or Braille instructions). Instructions should match the reading and education levels of subjects. Minimize medical jargon, and try to keep the language simple and straightforward.
- *Compliance tools*: You can employ various tools to monitor and enhance patient compliance (e.g., electronic pill counters).
- *Diaries and home monitoring*: It may be useful to better understand what is occurring with the subjects away from the experimental setting (e.g., certain life and environmental stressors may be affecting measurements, measurements may differ significantly at home, and diseases may fluctuate in a predictable manner). So having patients keep diaries of the symptoms and relevant problems may be helpful. Also, if possible, patients may check certain simple measurements at home as well (e.g., blood pressure, pulse, or temperature).

4.6.3 Observer Strategies

As an observer, you can:

- Clearly document the process and outcomes of your decision making.
- Verify your thought processes. Sometimes in retrospect, you realize that your logic was flawed.
- When appropriate, shield yourself from outside influences.
- Identify, recognize, and understand your prior beliefs and prejudices.
- Take actions to prevent fatigue (e.g., frequent breaks).

In addition, the study can include:

- *Different and diverse observers*: Enlist multiple people from diverse backgrounds (e.g., different cultural backgrounds to prevent cultural bias and different specialities to prevent professional biases) to check and verify your findings and assessments.
- *Detailed instructions and protocols*: Instructions and protocols should be specific, clear, and detailed and account for the whole range of unanticipated situations. (e.g., the angle to hold the ultrasound probe, the number of photographs to be taken, or how long to leave the tourniquet on).
- *Site training*: Formal training programs and quality control procedures should be in place (e.g., investigator's meeting to train study site personnel and site visits to ensure that study coordinators and physicians at the sites are well trained).
- *Blinded assessors*: Where unblinding is possible, use a blinded assessor (i.e., someone separate from those who administered the intervention) to perform measures that assess the efficacy of the intervention. The blinded assessor is usually separate from the treating physician and not permitted to communicate with the treating physician regarding the study. Alternatively, use a blinded safety assessor in cases where certain unblinding information is critical to ensure patient safety. An example would be an immunosuppressive drug study in transplant patients where an unblinded safety assessor might follow hematological parameters.
- *Blind unblinding variables*: Have an unblinded investigator view all potential unblinding data, and have a separate blinded investigator perform the assessments (e.g., PTT for heparin and lymphocyte count for cellular trafficking inhibitors).
- *Discrepancy resolution procedures and adjudication of events*: There should be clearly written procedures on how to resolve discrepancies among measurements and observers. Some clinical events are so complex that they require an adjudication committee to evaluate and assess them.

4.6.4 Instrument Strategies

Ensure that instruments are well calibrated and well maintained. Measurements should be unobtrusive (i.e., not affect the outcome). Proper training, written protocols, and full documentation are important as well. Verify all instrument readings. Some specific strategies include:

- *Core laboratory or central procedure interpretation*: Having all laboratory samples go to a central core laboratory and all studies (e.g., imaging studies, ECGs, EEGs) go through a single set of interpreters can help standardize measurements.
- *Standardization*: Use identical or similar equipment and reagents for all procedures. Document and anticipate how any necessary changes (e.g., a manufacturer goes out of business or a machine is found to be inferior) may affect measurements.
- *Using high quality and up-to-date equipment*: This is not the time to skimp on equipment. The risks of using cheaper and outdated equipment far outweigh the potential savings.
- *Automating procedures*: Automating procedures can reduce or eliminate human error (e.g., using the built-in algorithms for cardiac output on MUGA scans, etc.). However, do not completely rely on automation. Monitor and verify the measurements.

4.6.5 Intervention Strategies

Interventions should be standardized as much as possible. Even seemingly minor differences can greatly affect measurements. Specific strategies include:

- *Detailed instructions, protocols, and documentation.*
- *Improving the blinding of the placebo*: There are numerous ways to make the placebo more indistinguishable from the intervention (e.g., using same color inert ingredient, same pH so that it stings the same amount as active ingredient, or covering the IV bag to mask color).
- *Sham procedures*: When it is either not feasible or ethical to administer a placebo substance, you can use sham procedures. Sham procedure is a procedure that simulates a surgery or other invasive intervention without harming the patient. An example would be sham intravitreal injections (pressing the hub of the syringe to the cornea without penetration) in age-related macular degeneration studies, where a placebo injection would be unethical due to risk of endophthalmitis.

4.7 VALIDITY

4.7.1 Definition of Validity

Validity is a test's ability to measure the phenomenon (i.e., *construct*) that it is intending to measure. A valid measure must be accurate and precise. However, an accurate and precise measure is not necessarily valid (e.g., a test that accurately and precisely measures a person's IQ is not a valid measure of a person's sense of humor). Measures are not inherently valid or invalid. A measure can be valid in some situations and populations (e.g., an IQ test for a person's ability to solve intellectual problems) but invalid in others (e.g., an IQ test for a person's golfing ability).

Although a measure can never be completely validated, you must attempt to validate all measures used for endpoints and other significant components of clinical trials. Completely unvalidated measures are unacceptable and render clinical trial results meaningless because there is no assurance that the results truly reflect the clinical phenomenon. Since there is no clear threshold at which a measure becomes valid, consider validity an argument. Validity is not binary, but continuous. You attempt to gather enough evidence to convince others that a measure is valid (or invalid). The more evidence supporting validity, the more valid the measure is.

4.7.2 Types of Validity

To illustrate the concepts of validity, let us use a fictitious experiment designed to test whether a blood test, which we will call Liver Rejectase (i.e., the *measure*), is a valid

TABLE 4.2 Types of Validity

Type of validity	Definition
Face	Does it make sense to use the measure for the construct?
Content	Does the measure sufficiently cover the phenomenon that it is intended to cover
Criterion	Does the measure (*predictor*) correctly predict an outcome (*criterion*)?
Construct	Does the measure reflect the construct and is the measure related to other variables in predicted ways?

measure of liver transplant rejection (i.e., the *construct* or the phenomenon that you are trying to measure). Table 4.2 lists the different types of validity.

Determining *face validity* (i.e., the extent to which the measure appears to assess the construct) is the simplest, weakest, and most subjective way of assessing validity. Assessing face validity means asking, "Does it make sense to use the measure for the construct?" For example, the number of professional basketball games played has face validity as a measure of a person's basketball playing ability. It makes logical sense that someone needs to have a certain amount of ability to play professional basketball. Conversely, number of visits to fine restaurants does not have face validity as a measure of basketball playing ability. What does restaurant visiting have to do with basketball playing ability? The measure (restaurant visits) and the construct (basketball playing ability) appear unrelated. Of course, it could be that star basketball players tend to visit fine restaurants, but despite this correlation, fine restaurant visits would not have face validity.

So in our fictitious experiment, determining whether Liver Rejectase levels have face validity as a liver transplant rejection measure requires a general understanding of the biology and physiology of the measure and construct. Do we expect Liver Rejectase to rise during liver rejection? The fact that Liver Rejectase is a liver related protein and is released when immune cells attack the liver supports face validity.

Content validity is the extent to which a measure represents all facets of a construct (i.e., does the measure sufficiently cover the phenomenon that it is intended to cover). Content validity is particularly important for constructs that have multiple dimensions (e.g., depression). Establishing content validity involves fully defining the construct (e.g., what is the definition of depression), defining the entire spectrum of construct indicators (e.g., what are all the possible symptoms and aspects of depression), and determining the agreement (can be expressed as a %) between the measure's indicators and the facets of the construct (>70%

is acceptable). *Content under-representation* occurs when the measure misses important aspects of the construct.

Criterion validity is the ability of a measure (*predictor*) to predict an outcome (*criterion*). Ideally the criterion should be a well-accepted "Gold Standard" measure (e.g., the "Gold Standard" for transplant rejection is histological signs of rejection on a biopsy tissue sample). If the measure (e.g., Liver Rejectase) correlates well (i.e., high specificity and sensitivity) with the "Gold Standard" (e.g., the tissue sample findings) then criterion validity has been established. When comparing the measure with the "Gold Standard," use the same statistical measures for establishing precision: correlation, errors of the estimate, and kappa coefficient. If no "Gold Standard" is available, then the criterion can be any measure or outcome that is relevant to the construct, reliable, and objective (e.g., transplant loss after 12 months).

There are three subtypes of criterion validity depending on whether the criterion variable data is collected prior to (*post-dictive validity*), at the same time as (*concurrent validity*), or after (*predictive validity*) the predictor variable data is collected (Figure 4.7). In other words, establishing post-dictive validity means comparing the measure with events that occurred in the past; establishing concurrent validity means seeing if the measure changes with the criterion; and establishing predictive validity means demonstrating that the measure predicts a future outcome.

Construct validity is the degree to which the measure reflects the construct and is related to other variables in predicted ways. Construct validity is a difficult to define term but means that the overall set of correlations among measures seem to make sense. In other words, does it measure what it is supposed to be measuring, does it change in the same way as similar measures, and does it change in different ways compared to dissimilar measures? Evaluating construct validity involves establishing the following types of validity:

- *Convergent validity*: Establishing convergent validity requires showing that measures that *should be related*

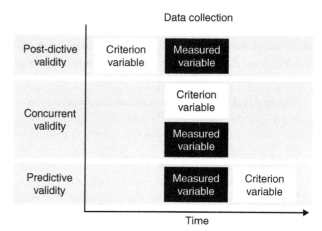

FIGURE 4.7   Timing of data collection for post-dictive, concurrent, and predictive validity.

are indeed *related*. In our example, alanine aminotransferase (ALT) and aspartate aminotransferase (AST) are markers of liver injury and should rise during liver transplant rejection (i.e., they are related to liver transplant rejection). Therefore, Liver Rejectase levels should correlate with ALT and AST levels (e.g., when Rejectase levels rise, ALT and AST levels should rise). Higher correlation means greater convergent validity.

- *Discriminant validity*: Establishing discriminant validity means demonstrating that measures that *should not be related* are indeed *not related*. In our example, body temperature and cardiac ejection fraction should not be related to liver transplant rejection. Therefore, demonstrating that Rejectase levels do not correlate with body temperature and cardiac ejection fraction supports discriminant validity. Lower correlation means greater discriminant validity.

Chapter 5

Study Groups

5.1 RATIONALE FOR CONTROL GROUPS

5.1.1 Levels of Clinical Research and Evidence

In many ways, clinical research is like an argument in a legal case or an editorial in a newspaper. The more you want to prove, the stronger your case needs to be. When addressing a specific issue or problem, there are three levels of studies that require increasing levels of evidence: descriptive study, associational study, and explanatory study (Table 5.1). To better understand these levels, let us use the analogy of instituting a dress code in your workplace. Say you notice that one woman is wearing a very short skirt and a man is wearing short pants to work. Is this a significant problem? Should there be a dress code? The first step might be to do a *descriptive study*, which would simply describe the situation. How many people are wearing short skirts and pants? How short are their skirts and pants? If only two people occasionally wear short skirts and pants, then a dress code may not be necessary. But if the descriptive study suggests that many people wear such outfits and the shorts and skirts are very short, then you might want to perform an *associational study*, which will suggest what problems may be correlated with this sartorial behavior. Associational studies are more rigorous, requiring more data and evidence. What are the potential effects of the short skirts and pants? Are people who wear these outfits less productive? Are people situated close to these short skirt and pants wearers less productive? Do others "ogle" (i.e., a technical term meaning stare or watch) these short skirt and shorts wearers? Have any clients or customers complained? How often do they complain? If the associational study suggests that there may be relationship between such revealing wardrobe and workplace productivity, you can perform an *explanatory study* to confirm that this sartorial behavior is causing problems. Institute a ban of shorts and short skirts for 1 month and see if productivity increases.

The lines between these different levels can be blurry. Pure descriptive studies are less common these days. Most studies try to show some type of association between what is being observed and potential factors. Associational studies may provide enough evidence to be explanatory. Explanatory studies may be descriptive. Some examples are:

- *Natural history study*: While largely descriptive (providing valuable information such as death rate, malignancies, and other clinical events), natural history studies can also draw correlation between patient characteristics and outcomes.
- *Epidemiological studies*: These may be descriptive and associational. In some rare cases, when the evidence is overwhelming, epidemiological studies can be explanatory (e.g., observing many skin burns after a nuclear disaster strongly suggests that the radiation caused the burns).
- *Uncontrolled clinical trial (e.g., safety study)*: A clinical trial in which all patients receive an intervention and no adequate historical controls exist is mostly descriptive.

Also, even though these different levels follow a natural order, you do not necessarily have to perform descriptive or associational studies before conducting an explanatory study. Sometimes the association between a factor and an outcome is so obvious that jumping to an explanatory study is reasonable (e.g., you do not need a descriptive study to tell you that being clubbed on the head causes pain).

Explanatory studies require the most rigorous design. Control groups are not necessary for descriptive studies but are essential for associative and explanatory studies. For a study to be explanatory:

- Patients cannot decide what intervention they receive. (Interventions are randomly assigned.)
- There is a comparator group that does not receive the intervention (e.g., half the patients receive surgery and half do not).

TABLE 5.1   Levels of Clinical Research

Level	Purpose	Uses	Controls?	Potential information provided	Examples
Descriptive	Identify the nature and magnitude of a problem or issue	Form hypotheses Target research Resource allocation	Not necessary	Incidence and prevalence of disease Morbidity and mortality of a condition Clinical event rate Medications, clinical and hospital visits, and diagnostic tests used by patients	Natural history study (often not purely descriptive) Case series Single-arm clinical trials
Associational	Identify and describe an association or correlation between factor(s) and condition	Posits a correlation between two or more factors but cannot establish a causal relationship Provide evidence to perform explanatory study	Usually necessary	Potential preventive or protective factors for a disease or condition Potential risk factors for a disease or condition	Epidemiological studies Observational studies Safety findings
Explanatory	Establish a cause-and-effect relationship	Prove that a factor is causing something Prove that an intervention is effective	Necessary	An intervention prevents or treats a disease A risk factor causes a disease or condition	Generally requires randomized prospective clinical trial, with an intervention (drug, device, surgery, etc.). In certain cases, methods other than randomization may suffice Pivotal Phase III clinical trials

- The intervention occurs earlier in time than the outcome of interest (e.g., blood pressure drops after the medication is administered).

5.1.2 Comparators and Causation

In order to make almost any kind of assessment in life, you need a *comparator* or a *comparison group*. For example, wealth is relative. If you have a job and everyone else around you is unemployed and in debt, you are by comparison wealthy. Alternatively, if your friends are all billionaires, then you will always consider yourself poor. Similarly in clinical research, determining whether an intervention has an effect requires a comparison group, one that does not get the intervention. Only with the comparison group can you tell if the intervention had any effect.

One of the toughest things to do in science (probably next to getting research grants) is to prove a cause-and-effect relationship. Life, nature, the environment, the world, and the universe are very complicated. Whenever something occurs, a host of interacting factors could be responsible. Isolating

one or two causes may be difficult or even impossible. Sometimes many factors combine to cause a situation.

Say you do not get a promotion at work. What is the reason? Was your work quality subpar? Was your boss biased against you? Did the company not have enough money to promote you? Did you not have the right credentials? Determining the exact reason could be difficult. What if they promoted another person (let's call him Jim) with almost identical credentials and work quality? Then, you may have a stronger case that your boss was biased against you. The more similar Jim is to you, the better you can isolate a specific reason why you were not promoted. If you and Jim are the same in almost every regard except for one or two characteristics, you have a strong argument that those characteristics prevented you from getting promoted. In this example, Jim serves as your *control*.

In a clinical study, a *control* or *control group* is a set of people who are very similar to the group of patients receiving the study intervention. Ideally, the only significant difference is that the control does not receive the study intervention and, as a result, serves as the comparator or comparison group. A *controlled experiment* or *trial* includes one or more treatment groups and one or more control groups. The key to running a controlled trial is to make conditions the same for both the treatment and control groups. If all conditions are truly equal in all study groups, only the intervention will be responsible for any difference in outcomes between the treatment and control groups. As you can see, controls help exclude alternative explanations for study outcomes or findings. The control group shows what may have happened to patients if they had not received the study intervention.

Usually clinical trials require a *concurrent control group* (i.e., a control group that participates in the trial at the same time and under the same conditions as the treatment group). The concurrent control group should be as similar to the treatment group as possible: drawn from the same population, undergo the same tests and treatments (except for the study intervention, of course), remain in the trial for the same length of time, and have the similar distribution of socio-demographic and other baseline characteristics. Any differences between the control and treatment groups could introduce bias. Studies that utilize concurrent control groups are often called parallel group studies.

Using a control group from outside your trial (i.e., *external controls*) from a different trial or different time (i.e., *historical controls*) raises the concern that your trial's conditions may somehow be responsible for differing outcomes. For example, what if some aspects of your trial are particularly stressful and tend to raise patients' blood pressures and heart rates? Using a control group from a less stressful trial as a comparison group would introduce (statistically) significant bias. Using historical controls may be reasonable in two situations: less rigorous clinical studies or situations where a disease or condition tends to remain very stable despite changing external conditions. A clinical study using historical controls is much less convincing than a randomized controlled trial but may serve as a prelude to a randomized controlled trial. Long-term (i.e., many years) and large-scale epidemiological studies of chronic diseases may use historical controls. The large number of patients and long time horizon may cancel out differences between the treatment and historical control groups.

5.2 PLACEBOS, SHAM DEVICES, AND SHAM PROCEDURES

5.2.1 The Placebo and Nocebo Effects

A placebo is a treatment that appears almost identical to the study intervention but does not have the pharmacological activity that the study intervention has. Sometimes referred to as a "sugar pill" or a "dummy treatment," the placebo should look, taste, and smell just like the study intervention. The patient taking the placebo should believe that he or she is taking the study medication. In fact in double-blind placebo-controlled studies, neither the investigator

nor the patients should be able to tell the difference between the study drug and the placebo.

A placebo does not have to be completely pharmacologically inert (i.e., inactive). While constructing a substance that does not have the same or similar activity as the study intervention is relatively easy, concocting a substance that has absolutely no activity is difficult. The simple act of smearing a cream on the skin (e.g., moisturizes the skin), injecting fluid intravenously (e.g., hydrates the patient), or placing something in the rectum or vagina (e.g., stretches the skin) can have therapeutic effects. The key is to make the substance characteristics as similar to the study intervention characteristics as possible, so that these therapeutic effects are present in both the treatment and placebo groups.

One of the most important reasons for using a placebo is to account for the presence of and measure the *placebo effect*. In this phenomenon, an intervention leads to improvement in the patient's condition even though the intervention should have no (or little) therapeutic benefit. In other words, the pharmacological or physical properties of the intervention are not responsible for the patient's improvement. The placebo effect appears frequently in clinical practice. Just the act of receiving treatment can be very beneficial.

Postulated explanations for the placebo effect include:

- *Subject expectancy effect*: Patients may improve because they expect to improve. In all aspects of life, initial impressions and expectations can be very powerful (e.g., if you think you will like someone before you interview the person, you will be more likely to like that person). Similarly, the simple belief that a treatment will work can lead to actual physical or physiological improvement.

- *Obedience and compliance*: Patients consciously or unconsciously may improve or at least give the impression that they are improving in order to please investigators. This phenomenon arises from the innate desire of many patients to be liked or accepted by authority figures (in this case, study investigators).

- *Classical conditioning*: Seeing a sign for a restaurant you like may make you salivate and feel hungry. Hearing a familiar song on the radio may make you feel happy or melancholic. Meeting an old girlfriend or boyfriend can cause heartache and even physical symptoms. Similarly, patients may associate receiving an intervention with improvement in health. Classic conditioning is basically training. Patients are trained to have a certain response when they see something. The response could include actual changes in physical and physiological measures.

- *Process of treatment*: Medical treatment includes many possible benefits beyond the actual intervention. Health care professionals offer many intangible things to patients: sympathy, empathy, an outlet to complain, and general care. Patients will often visit physicians just to "talk" or reassure themselves that someone is watching out for them.

- *Motivation*: The simple act of receiving an intervention to improve their health can motivate patients to improve other aspects of their lives. Perhaps they may concomitantly improve their diet and exercise, tackle sources of anxiety, become more compliant with other health care activities, and consciously change their attitudes and states of mind.
- *Hidden mechanisms*: Treatments may have undiscovered mechanisms that stimulate the release of endogenous opiates or other chemicals in the body that mediate effects. The basic acts of chewing pills or inserting things into different parts of the body may have complex physiological effects that are yet to be determined.

Placebos can also help identify a *nocebo effect*, that is, a patient's belief that a treatment is ineffective or harmful can actually worsen symptoms. The nocebo effect is a self-fulfilling prophecy; you think something is not going to work and it ends up failing as a result. Suspect the nocebo effect when patients in both the treatment and control groups experience a worsening of their conditions. Of course, you will have to distinguish the nocebo effect from a general worsening of the condition in both groups.

5.2.2 Sham Devices and Procedures

Sham devices or *procedures* can serve as placebos for interventions that are medical devices or medical procedures, respectively. A *sham* is something that is counterfeit, pretended, fake, or false. Like medications, devices and procedures can have placebo and nocebo effects. The simple act of wearing a device or going through a procedure can have powerful effects. Patients can become psychologically attached to wearing a device, consciously or unconsciously viewing it as a companion or even a lucky charm. Alternatively, devices constantly remind patients of their illness or condition, potentially leading to stress or distress. The physical properties of a medical device alone can have physical or physiological effects. A device may stretch or compress a body part, induce a local inflammatory reaction or immune response, cause pain or discomfort, or cool or warm the surrounding area. The act of placing or removing the medical device can induce comfort or distress in patients. A well known example is the relief of cardiac pain that was originally attributed to laser.

Procedures can provide several benefits to patients:

- *Make the patient the center of attention*: Procedures can make patients feel important, needed, or wanted.
- *Provide company and social support*: Performing a procedure often involves many people.
- *Provide incidental medical or personal care*: During a procedure, patients or health care providers may recognize and treat certain previously unrecognized problems or conditions (e.g., while performing a procedure on a patient's ear, the investigator may need to remove a lot of ear wax).

- *Introduce a purpose or regimentation into a patient's life*: Participating in a medical procedure may induce discipline into a patient's life. The patient may then be more attentive and diligent to other aspects of their lives and feel better about himself or herself. This is especially true if the patient is unemployed or relatively aimless.

Procedures can also be problematic by:

- *Making the patient self-conscious*: Being the center of attention is not optimal for everyone. Moreover, procedures may leave scars or other signs that may be embarrassing.
- *Disrupting a patient's schedule.*
- *Causing discomfort.*
- *Inducing side effects or complications*: No procedure is completely harmless or risk-free.

A *sham device* should closely resemble the study device but have little or no therapeutic effect. The sham device should have the same appearance, consist of the same or similar materials, make the same noises, and cause the same sensations that the study device would. Some medical devices remain on or in a patient's body for long periods of time, giving a patient ample opportunity to check if his or her device is indeed real. Therefore, the sham device should be an accurate replica that is also reasonably durable.

A *sham procedure* would proceed just as the study procedure would, except omit the few steps that are intended to confer therapeutic benefit. The sham procedure must be a very convincing act. Whoever administers the procedure should be a good actor or actress. How far you go with this masquerade depends on the procedure. For example, a sham acupuncture treatment may require inserting needles into the patient, but in a pattern that does not conform to standard acupuncture treatment.

The use of sham procedures is controversial. Decades ago, sham operations were much more prevalent. However, people have raised ethical issues about subjecting patients to invasive, uncomfortable, and potentially dangerous procedures that have no clear benefit. Every procedure, no matter how simple or noninvasive, bears a risk. Performing some sham procedures would be clearly unethical (e.g., sham heart transplant). However, where do you draw the line between ethical and unethical sham procedures? Moreover, without a sham procedure to serve as a control, can you adequately compare and interpret results from a treatment group?

5.2.3 Challenges with Placebos

Patient response to placebos can vary significantly. Some patients tend to have very strong placebo effects. Conducting a run-in period (i.e., a test period before the actual trial) in which you administer the placebo and note the effects can help identify such placebo responders. In some cases (e.g., some Phase II studies), you may exclude placebo responders from the trial. However, doing so is often not acceptable (especially in Phase III trials) because it introduces a bias into the study.

Masking the Placebo

In a clinical trial, a placebo must mirror the study intervention in nearly every way. Otherwise, patients and investigators may quickly realize who is receiving the placebo instead of the study intervention, especially when they notice any of the following:

- *Lack of expected side effects*: Some treatments have obvious side effects (e.g., nitroglycerin causes lightheadedness; some drugs cause funny metallic tastes) that will not be caused by an inert placebo. In these cases, using an active placebo (i.e., one that causes certain physiological or psychological effects) may be necessary to better masquerade the placebo. Many drugs cause a change in laboratory parameters as well that might be difficult to mask from the investigator.
- *Lack of expected benefits*: Some interventions, especially fast-acting ones, will have clearly noticeable benefits (e.g., pain relievers and blood pressure medications). Absence of these benefits may be a strong tip-off that the patient is receiving a placebo.
- *Different packaging*: This is an overlooked clue. Patient may carefully watch where their health care providers open containers and packaging out of curiosity or to make sure no mistakes are made.
- *Different administration and monitoring procedures*: If the study intervention requires a certain type of preparation or diagnostic tests, then you may need to require or perform the same procedures for the placebo group as well.

Once patients realize that they are on a placebo or an ineffective intervention, they may become noncompliant with the study. After all, many patients do not want to waste their time and effort on something that does not work, especially if the patients have debilitating diseases. Keeping control patients enrolled and engaged in a study can be quite a challenge.

As you can imagine, finding an appropriate placebo can be very difficult and in some cases impossible. Placebo design can be complicated and crucial. Sometimes multiple types of placebos may be necessary in a trial, especially if the study intervention is a regimen of different types of medications.

Ethical, Recruitment, and Retention Issues

The use of placebos also raises some ethical questions. Is it ethical to keep a patient on a treatment that is not supposed to work? Are you preventing these patients from receiving treatments that would work? Could the placebo potentially harm the patient? Can you successfully treat the patient if he or she develops complications while on placebo? The

answers are not always clear-cut and often up to the judgment of the investigator, institutional review board (IRB), and/or independent ethics committee (IEC). In general, the use of placebos is subject to much higher scrutiny in countries outside the U.S. than within U.S.

Avoid using placebos when:

- the condition is life-threatening or severely debilitating (e.g., myocardial infarction or stroke);
- patients are very unlikely to tolerate staying on placebo (e.g., severe chronic pain);
- disease prognosis could change rapidly and dramatically without warning (i.e., quickly switching the patient to real therapy is very difficult);
- no rescue treatment is available (i.e., a way of urgently treating patients should they deteriorate while on placebo).

The design of the trial can determine whether having a placebo group would be ethical. Short duration trials are less of a problem since patients do not have to be off treatment for long. Trials that do not require very sick patients also are more amenable to using placebo controls. The longer a patient has to go without proper treatment and the more severe the patients' conditions, the more ethical problems you may encounter. Moreover, groups that receive placebos are not necessarily off all treatments. In many designs, they can receive treatments other than the study intervention. In some complicated designs involving more than one study intervention, patients may never be just on placebo.

Even if administering a placebo is ethical, recruiting patients to participate in a trial with placebo groups may be difficult. Patients may be very reluctant to risk being on a placebo and receiving no treatment. Even if the patient agrees to a trial, the patient's physician, family, and/or friends may object.

Limited Placebo Period

One way of avoiding the problems of keeping patients on placebo for a long time is to use a limited placebo period. You may start the control group on placebos for a short period of time at the beginning of a trial before switching the control patients to an active treatment for the rest of trial. The short placebo period may provide enough useful information for adequate comparison with the treatment group. Of course, such a design would not inform you of the long-term effects of the placebo.

5.3 CHOOSING CONTROLS

5.3.1 General Considerations

In order to draw associations or explanatory inferences about an intervention, there must be two or more groups. Usually, there are two groups: one that receives the intervention and one that does not. The latter is the control group.

Strictly speaking, it is possible to draw associations between clinical parameters even if there is not a formal control group, so long as there is heterogeneity in both parameters. This is accomplished by modeling. For example, it could be possible to take patients who have received widely varying doses of a drug and plot a line that best fits the doses and the response.

Types of Comparisons

Control groups serve as comparison groups for the study treatment group. What you want to prove about the study treatment group affects the type of control group you choose, the sample size, and the subsequent analysis. Do you want to prove that the study intervention is as good as something else, that is, prove *noninferiority* or *equivalence*? If so, pick a control group that is already established and acceptable (e.g., a widely used treatment that is known to be effective). In other words, aim high. (Would you rather prove that you are as fast as a turtle or a hare?) Alternatively, do you want to show how much the study intervention is better than something else, that is, demonstrate *superiority*? In this case, you could choose either an established, effective comparison group (which would show the relative superiority of your study intervention) or a comparison group known to be ineffective (which would demonstrate the absolute superiority of your study intervention).

Early Escape

Providing a potential "early escape" for all trial groups, especially control groups, is important. An "early escape" is analogous to having a life raft in case a ship sinks. Patients must have potential *rescue treatment* options in case their conditions worsen significantly or do not improve to a reasonable degree. Otherwise, they may suffer significant or permanent harm. A caveat with early escape is where the primary endpoint occurs after escape is allowed. For example, if the primary endpoint in a cancer study is survival, and early escape is allowed for tumor progression, there is possibility of confounding from the recue treatment.

External vs. Internal Controls

There are two general types of controls:

- *Internal*: These subjects participate in the same clinical study during the same time as the study intervention subjects. In other words, you design and set up the clinical study to include these control groups. Since both the treatment and control groups underwent the same conditions at the same time, data from internal controls is directly comparable to those obtained from the study treatment group. In a 100-m dash analogy, internal controls would be competitors running on the same track at the same time in the same race (as in the Olympics). All internal

controls are *concurrent* (i.e., they participate in the trial at the same time).

- *External*: The data for these subjects comes from outside the study (i.e., a different, separate study or database). If the subjects were observed or treated during an earlier time, the external control is a *historical control*. In the 100-m dash analogy, historical controls would be times from previous races (e.g., world records or Olympic records). If the subjects are observed or treated at the same time as your study but in a different setting, the external control is a *concurrent external control*. In the 100-m dash analogy, concurrent external control would be times from a race conducted at the same time but in another country. If the subjects are the same subjects as the study treatment group but before they received the study intervention, the external control is a *baseline control*. External controls may be a specific group of patients (i.e., *defined*) or a general set of known parameters (i.e., *nondefined*). An example of a nondefined external control would be the average and median blood pressures in the United States.

If possible, try to include internal controls in your study. External controls alone are not as good as internal controls. There may be too many differences and interacting factors for external controls to be comparable to the study treatment subjects. However, adding external controls to a study with internal controls can be very helpful. External controls can help determine if your study results are unusual. They can show how your results may have differed under different conditions.

The weaker an external control the less it can serve as a true control. Many people consider using nondefined or baseline controls to be tantamount to not having any controls. Avoid external controls unless absolutely unavoidable.

Choosing an appropriate external control can be challenging. You have to make sure the subject and conditions are relatively similar. Sometimes finding a single external group is difficult or impossible (i.e., no single group is similar enough to your study treatment group). In such cases, utilizing multiple external control groups may be necessary. Each external control group bears some similarity to certain aspects of the study treatment group. Together the multiple groups can serve as an appropriate external control.

Externally controlled trials may be suitable when:

- *The study intervention has dramatic and well-characterized effects* (e.g., if your study intervention completely eliminates pain immediately after hip surgery, most types of controls will be able to show that this is a substantial benefit).
- *The relevant disease or condition is highly predictable.* In other words, the disease course is relatively the same regardless of differing conditions (e.g., poison ivy exposure for an otherwise healthy teenager).
- *Endpoints are objective.* A measure that is relatively clear and consistent (e.g., mortality) instead of a measure that

TABLE 5.2 Types of Controls

Control	Superiority	Noninferiority	Sample size	Efficacy	Recruitment and retention	Blinding
Placebo	Efficacy	Safety	Smaller	Absolute	May be difficult	Easier
Sham	Efficacy	Safety	Smaller	Absolute	May be difficult	Easier
No treatment	Efficacy	Safety	Smaller	Absolute	Difficult	Difficult
Dose	Efficacy and safety	Efficacy and safety	Large	Relative	Easier	Easiest
Active	Efficacy and safety	Efficacy and safety	Larger	Relative	Easiest	May be difficult

depends heavily on the subjects, the personnel performing the measurements, and the measurement scale (e.g., pain level or depression scores).

- *Detailed information is known about the external control group.* Determine if the external control is similar to the control group in a range of different characteristics (e.g., socio-demographics, co-morbid conditions, concomitant medications, baseline characteristics, etc).
- *Internal controls are contraindicated.* Internal controls may not be feasible when the condition is very serious, there is currently no satisfactory treatment, and the study intervention is very promising.

Externally controlled trials carry several potential benefits:

- *Minimal ethical problems*: In trials that have only external controls, every patient is assigned to the study intervention group and therefore gets what is supposed to be effective treatment.
- *No recruitment necessary for control group.*
- *Patient retention in the control group is not your problem.*

There are many disadvantages of externally controlled trials:

- *Selection bias*: When choosing external controls, you may have a variety of options. There is a great risk of consciously or unconsciously choosing an external control that will accentuate the efficacy of your study intervention. Therefore, if possible, choose and identify your external control as early as possible, preferably before initiating the study and certainly before doing any data analysis. Employing an independent set of reviewers to choose or assess your external control will minimize selection bias.
- *Other types of bias*: The external control group may be very different from the study intervention group and thereby introduce significant bias into the study. Since clinical trials tend to have patients better suited for the study intervention than the general population, using external controls often biases a study for the study intervention (i.e., overestimate study intervention efficacy).
- *Blinding can be very difficult.*

- *Assignment is not completely random*: The patients in the population providing the external control have already been selected. However, you could randomly choose control subjects from this population.

5.3.2 Types of Controls

Several different types of controls are available (Table 5.2). In addition to the study treatment group, a clinical study may use one or more of these types of controls. A trial may have multiple types of control groups separated or combined in a variety of ways. When possible, patients should be randomly assigned to the control and study treatment groups (we discuss patient assignment later in this chapter). Ideally, patients and investigators should also be blind to which patients are in the control or treatment groups.

Placebo Control

As we discussed in detail in Section 5.2, placebos help control for a number of different factors that may affect outcomes including those related to the natural history of the disease or condition and experimental setting. We discussed many of the advantages and challenges associated with using placebos. Unlike active and dose controls, placebo controls can help demonstrate the absolute (as opposed to relative) efficacy of the study intervention. When measuring a study intervention's effectiveness, placebo-controlled trials are superiority studies. (You want to show that the study intervention is more effective than placebo.) When evaluating safety, placebo-controlled trials are noninferiority studies. (You want to demonstrate that the study intervention is as safe as placebo. Rarely is anything safer than a completely inert substance.)

Patients in a placebo control group are not necessarily completely untreated. In some designs, placebo control patients may receive standard treatment as long as the study intervention group receives standard treatment as well. If the study intervention group does not receive standard treatment, then the placebo plus standard treatment group becomes an active control group (which we discuss later).

Using a placebo does not imply that the study is placebo-controlled. Placebos may help facilitate other types of controls. For example, placebos can aid blinding (e.g., in a *double-dummy* trial, an active control group receives an established treatment plus a placebo that makes the established treatment look like the study intervention). A trial is placebo-controlled only if the study design directly compares the study intervention to placebo.

Sham Control

A sham control is very similar to a placebo control except that patients receive a sham device or sham procedure.

No-treatment Control

A *no-treatment control* is a group that receives neither study treatment nor any type of placebo or sham treatment. Using a no-treatment control precludes complete blinding since subjects and investigators will be able to tell that they are not receiving the study intervention. Moreover, a no-treatment control will not be able to provide the information that a placebo control would (e.g., presence and nature of placebo effects). Therefore, a no-treatment control is appropriate only when a placebo control, a sham control, or blinding is not possible or advisable. Keep in mind that recruiting and retaining patients for a trial that includes a no-treatment arm may be difficult. Patients may be likely to avoid participating or leave the study when they know that they are not getting the study intervention.

Dose Control

In some trials (e.g., dose–response trials), one or more of the comparison groups receive different doses of the study intervention. Dose–response trials (which are usually double-blind) help delineate the relationship between the intervention dose, efficacy and side effects. One subtype of a dose control is a concentration control in which different groups receive doses of the drug meant to achieve different blood concentrations of the study drug. Another subtype is a regimen control in which different groups have different administration regimens (e.g., one group receives an intervention twice a day, whereas another group receives it once a day). A dose control group that has a zero dose (i.e., no active intervention or no activity) is effectively a placebo control group. Dose–response trials may also include active controls as well. Dose–response trials can demonstrate study intervention efficacy by showing increasing efficacy with increasing doses or the presence of an effect with certain doses (usually higher doses) and the absence of effect in other doses.

There are several problems with using dose controls alone to establish efficacy. The difference in response among different doses may not be great enough to demonstrate that the intervention is effective. Small inter-group differences require large sample sizes to determine if the differences are statistically significant. When all of the dose groups manifest similar efficacy, you may not be able tell whether all doses are equally effective or equally ineffective without a placebo or active control group. Moreover, if all of the dose groups have some kind of effect, you cannot quantify the absolute magnitude of the effect without a placebo or active control group. (As an analogy, if you want to appreciate the height of a professional basketball player, you do not just compare him to other professional basketball players.)

In many cases, maintaining blinding with dose controls is relatively easier than maintaining blinding with placebo and no-treatment controls. Often, administering lower doses has the same side effects and appearance as administering higher doses. However, sometimes the differences between doses can be dramatic. So maintaining blinding is not always easy and trivial.

Dose controls present some of the same ethical challenges as placebo or sham controls. Giving patients suboptimal treatments (i.e., doses are less effective) is similar to giving ineffective treatments especially if the disease is debilitating or life-threatening. What dose would be ethically too low to give? When doses are steadily increased in a dose escalation trial, how long is too long to keep a patient on a low, ineffective dose?

Active (Positive) Control

An active control group receives a known and established treatment other than the study intervention. You can use active controls to establish either *noninferiority* (the study intervention is as good as an established treatment) or *superiority* [the study intervention is better (i.e., more effective) than an established treatment].

Although many active controlled experiments are double-blinded, blinding is not always possible, since the active control treatment may be too radically different from the study intervention to hide. It may be very difficult or impossible to hide difference in dosage frequencies, routes of administration, side effects, patient preparation, and monitoring procedures.

An important bias may occur in trials that only have a study treatment group and an active control. Since patients and investigators know that every patient is receiving some type of active treatment, they may expect patients to improve and consciously or unconsciously categorize borderline cases as successes. If you expect something to work, many times you look harder for evidence that it is working.

Active controls do not raise as many ethical or recruitment problems as placebo or no-treatment controls. Active controls are receiving acceptable treatments. Patients probably are more willing to participate and stay in a group that is receiving real treatment. In fact, if the study intervention is new and relatively untested, patients may be at greater risk for not being adequately treated in the study treatment group.

As we discussed previously, a control group can consist of a limited placebo period followed by active treatment. In other words, a control group can start off as a placebo control and then soon switch over to an active control group. This design can help provide some placebo-controlled information but minimizes the length of time the control group is off any active treatment.

Active control study designs often require large sample sizes. For a superiority study, the difference between the study treatment group and the active control group effects probably would be smaller than the difference between the study treatment group and placebo group effects. Smaller differences call for larger sample sizes. By analogy, showing that U.S. professional basketball players are better than Argentinean professional basketball players requires testing a lot more basketball players than proving that U.S. professional basketball players are better than people who do not play any basketball. For a noninferiority study, you usually try to be very conservative and choose a very small maximum difference between the study treatment and active control groups. Such a small margin also calls for larger sample sizes.

5.4 STUDY GROUP ALLOCATIONS

5.4.1 Assigned vs. Unassigned

Playing any team sports (e.g., football, soccer, basketball, or team handball) requires forming teams first. How you choose teams will greatly affect which teams win and lose. Choosing teams in an unfair manner can lead to great advantages for certain teams. Some argue that team composition is the single most important determinant of a team's success. Would Phil Jackson have won any professional basketball titles if he did not have the best players in the league (i.e., Michael Jordan and Shaquille O'Neal)?

Similarly, the way you *assign* or *allocate* patients to different study groups is crucial. Haphazard or unfair subject assignment can lead to significant biases in the study. Most studies use *subject assignments* or *assigned controls*. That is, patients and treating physicians cannot decide which study group the patients enters or what treatment he or she receives. Instead, the study investigators determine which patient enters which study group. Otherwise, significant biases may occur. A treating physician may choose patients who are likely to respond to a given treatment. Patients may avoid certain study arms that may give ineffective treatments. Certain patients may want to go to certain study arms because they see other patients who are like themselves, leading to imbalances among the different study arms.

Sometimes allowing unassigned study groups or arms is reasonable. Unassigned study groups allow you to see patient preferences (e.g., which treatments will a patient choose). Unassigned study groups also allow patients to exert freedom of choice. However, most formal, rigorous clinical trials require subject assignment.

Study group allocation may be balanced or unbalanced. In *equal allocations*, every arm has the same number of patients. In *unequal or disproportionate allocations*, certain arms have more patients. Having more patients in a study intervention arm than control arms is common.

Allocation Concealment

Allocation concealment is hiding the "code" that assigns patients to different study groups. In other words, patients and investigators should not be able to predict which patients will go to which groups. Allocation concealment is distinct from blinding. The former aims to prevent *selection bias*: deliberately trying to steer subjects into particular study arms (e.g., investigators may want to steer patients with severe disease into the active treatment group rather than the placebo group). Blinding attempts to prevent *ascertainment bias*: interpreting results based on the subject's treatment group (e.g., if the patient receives an active treatment, the investigator expects to find good outcomes).

Patients and investigators can be very resourceful when trying to decipher the allocation "code": carefully examining medication labels for differences, opening, weighing, or illuminating sealed envelopes that contain subject assignments, trying to coax assignment information from central randomization personnel, and even breaking into locked files. These behaviors do not necessarily stem from malice or deviousness.

Therefore, construct an allocation concealment scheme that is as foolproof as possible. Patients and investigators should not know their study group assignment until they are fully enrolled and ready to commence the trial. Some common concealment methods include:

- *Central assignment*: A central location (e.g., central team, computer, pharmacy, etc.) should perform subject assignments so the process can be easily monitored and information leaks prevented. Email, telephone, facsimile, or any other secure communication device can then transmit patient assignments to each site.
- *Identical containers*: All containers should display only numbers or codes, not any identifying information. The containers should be equivalent in appearance, weight, color, and material.
- *Sequentially numbered, opaque, sealed envelopes (SNOSE)*: Place subject assignments in SNOSE. Pressure-sensitive (e.g., carbon paper) envelopes can detect

tampering. Internal lining (e.g., aluminum foil or cardboard) can inhibit trans-illumination.

5.4.2 Randomization

Randomization is the process of using chance or probability to assign subjects to different study arms. It is the most common method of assigning patients to study groups. Before the assignment, no one can predict which patients will end up in which study group. Each patient has a certain probability of going to each arm and until that coin flips, dice rolls, number is chosen from the hat or the equivalent, does not know in which arm he or she will be.

Randomization helps:

- *Produce groups that are balanced for both known and unknown risk factors and covariates.* The complexity of clinical status and response make it impossible to match patients exactly on each of the infinite number of variables that might affect the course of disease and likelihood of response. Randomization, if the sample size is adequate, ensures that the treatment and control groups are adequately balanced with regard to baseline characteristics.
- *Minimize selection bias.* The individual subject assignments are by chance and do not depend on the decision making of the investigator.
- *Ensure blinding.* We discuss blinding later this chapter. Patients and investigators should not know what types of treatments (e.g., study intervention vs. placebo) each patient is receiving. Otherwise, bias may ensue. For this reason, randomization should be truly random. Patients and investigators should not be able to guess the randomization order.
- *Clinical equipoise.* This ethical principle states that prior to a study there must be genuine uncertainty as to which patients will receive effective treatments. In other words, there should be no favoritism. Randomization helps guarantee that each patient has a fair chance of getting the right treatment.
- *Statistical tests.* Many statistical tests assume a random allocation of patients among different study groups.

The *ratio of randomization* is the proportional allocation of subjects to each study arm. The most common randomization ratio in clinical trials is 1:1, which maximizes statistical power for a given total sample size. A 1:1 randomization ratio means that equal numbers of patients will be randomized into each of the two study arms. However, using other ratios may be more feasible or ethical. Using a 2:1 ratio (twice as many patients in one arm as in the other) usually does not result in a significant loss in statistical power. Such a ratio may allocate more patients to receive the active study intervention than placebo, giving patients a greater chance of receiving effective treatment.

There are several different types of randomization:

Simple Randomization

This is the simplest, most straightforward method of random assignment. Each patient has fixed probabilities of ending up in each study arm. In *equal allocations*, each subject has an equal probability (=1/Number of study arms) of being assigned to each of the study arms (e.g., with two study arms, each patient has a 50% chance of being assigned to either the study treatment group or the control group). In *unequal* or *weighted allocations*, patients are more likely to end up in certain study arms than others (Probability of allocation to Study Arm n = (Total number of patients to be enrolled in Study Arm n)/(Total number of patients to be enrolled in study)). For each patient, you perform the equivalent of a coin flip (if there are only two study arms) or a dice roll. Computer programs usually do the random assignment.

Blocked Randomization

In relatively small studies, simple randomization may result in unbalanced groups. For example, if you had only 20 patients for a study and two study arms, there is reasonably high probability that one arm could have 12 patients and the other would have 8. Moreover, there may be a temporal imbalance in study group assignment. More patients early on in randomization may end up in one particular arm. To understand this problem, think about a coin flip. Even though each flip has a 50% chance of landing on heads, the first five flips could easily [$(0.5)^5$ = 3.125% chance] all be heads. The more flips you do, the greater the chance will be that 50% of the flips will be heads.

Blocked randomization overcomes these problems associated with simple randomization. Block randomization involves the following steps:

- *Step 1: Determine the number of patients that will be in a block.* The block size should be a fixed number which is a multiple of the number of arms that a study has. So a study with two arms (Study Arm A and Study Arm B) can have a block size of 2 patients, 4 patients, 6 patients, or any other multiple of 2.
- *Step 2: List the number of possible permutations of treatment assignments for each block.* The number of permutations for a block size r in an n-arm study is given by $n!/(n - r)!$ For example, a two-patient block in a two-arm study could have two possible treatment assignments: AB (the first patient is assigned to Study Arm A and the second patient is assigned to Study Arm B) or BA (the first patient is assigned to Study Arm B and the second patient is assigned to Study Arm A). A four-patient block in a two-arm study could have

six different permutations: AABB, BBAA, ABBA, ABAB, BAAB, and BABA.

- *Step 3: Randomly assign each block of patients a permutation.* So in a two-patient block randomization, the first two patients may be assigned AB (Patient 1 goes to Arm A, Patient 2 goes to Arm B), the second pair of patients may be assigned AB (Patient 3 goes to Arm A, Patient 4 goes to Arm B), the third pair BA (Patient 5 goes to Arm B, Patient 6 goes to Arm A), and so forth.

Avoid using block sizes smaller than six patients. The smaller the block size, the easier it will be for investigators (who are supposed to be blinded) to figure out the study group assignments.

Stratified Randomization

Stratified randomization is useful when certain baseline characteristics strongly influence the outcome of interest. (For example, anterior myocardial infarctions confer a worse prognosis than inferior myocardial infarctions. So, if 50% of the myocardial infarctions in Study Arm A are anterior and 20% of the myocardial infarctions in Study Arm B are anterior, Study Arm A is likely to have a higher mortality regardless of the intervention.) Using simple or block randomization may result in an imbalance in important baseline characteristics among the different study arms and, in turn, bias your study. In a very large trial, most baseline characteristics will be naturally balanced across the different study arms, but small or moderate trials run the risk that one or more characteristic will be unbalanced.

Stratified randomization involves the following steps:

- *Step 1: Identify which characteristics may affect the outcome.* These may be demographic, socio-economic, disease, physical, or physiological characteristics. Common characteristics include: the patient's enrollment site, disease severity, disease subtype, age, and concomitant medications. Clinical judgment and analysis of data from previous studies can help identify stratification variables.
- *Step 2: Divide the study population into different categories of each characteristic.* For example, if the characteristics are gender and marital status, your categories may be married males, married females, single males, and single females.
- *Step 3: Perform either simple or block randomization within each category.*

Stratified randomization helps make each of the individual subgroups more homogeneous (i.e., less variability) which will aid subsequent analysis (e.g., married males will be equally distributed among different study arms) and may increase the power of the study. However, using too many different strata could decrease the power of a study, since each stratum would have very few patients. Stratification can be logistically challenging as well. Stratification characteristics

(e.g., patient's past medical history) may be difficult to determine with accuracy. Some patients may cross several categories (e.g., ethnicity). Stratification by patient enrollment site may mean that every site would have to carry the equal amount of study intervention.

Adaptive (Dynamic) Randomization

Simple, block, and stratified randomizations involve designing and fixing the randomization scheme before the trial commences. Nothing changes in the randomization scheme once the trial begins. Although these fixed schemes aim to achieve a reasonable balance of subjects (and subject characteristics) among the different study arms, they are not always successful in doing so. If during the trial, patients are not being equally distributed among the study arms, these fixed schemes offer no solution.

Adaptive (dynamic) randomization continuously changes the assignment probabilities based on emerging information as the trial progresses. Adaptive randomization is basically a "wait and see" approach. It is analogous to a football team picking up players during the course of a football season. The team continuously assesses its needs, which may change as the season progresses (e.g., players may get injured or not perform as expected), and then acquire players who fit its needs. Similarly, the adaptive randomization scheme requires close monitoring of the clinical study and is flexible, changing to ensure that the study characteristics are balanced or that patients are getting a reasonable shot at receiving effective treatment. You should note, however, that some statisticians, including some at the FDA, look upon adaptive randomization with some skepticism because it can be difficult to implement in a rigorous manner.

Balancing (Covariate) Adaptive Randomization

Maintaining the balance of relevant characteristics among the different study arms is important. During the trial, the distribution of these characteristics becomes unequal (e.g., many more women are in Study Arm A than in Study Arm B). Covariate adaptive randomization tackles this problem by updating assignment probabilities so that the distribution is more likely to equalize (e.g., subsequent women are more likely to be allocated to Study Arm B). A randomization computer program can track the covariates distribution among the different treatment arms and change the assignment probabilities based on the characteristics of the patient being randomized.

Examples of balancing randomization techniques include (although these examples assume only two Study Arms A and B, adapting them for more than two study arms is simple):

- *Urn randomization*: Say you are trying to balance the number of patients between Study Arm A and Study Arm B. Initially, a container holds *n* balls labeled Study Arm A and *n* balls labeled Study Arm B. Random draws from this container will determine patient assignments.

If the first draw for the first patient is a "Study Arm A" ball, the first patient goes to Study Arm A and then you return the ball and add a fixed number m "Study Arm B" balls to the container. This makes it more likely to draw Study Arm B for the next patient. Every time one study group is drawn, you add m balls of the other study group to the container. This method weighs the probabilities so that Study Arms not previously selected have a higher likelihood of being selected.

- *Efron's weighted coins*: This randomization scheme uses the equivalent of a coin flip. Before each coin flip, calculate the difference between the number of patients in Study Arm A and Study Arm B. No difference means a 50–50 probability that the next patient will go to Study Arm A or B, respectively. More patients in Study Arm A means that the next coin flip is weighted ($50 - p\%$ chance that the next patient will go to Study Arm A). More patients in Study Arm A means that the next coin flip is weighted against Study Arm A (a $50 - p\%$ chance that the next patient will go to Study Arm A). Fewer patients in Study Arm A means that the next coin flip is weighted for Study Arm A (a $50 + p\%$ chance that the next patient will go to Study Arm A).

Response (Outcome) Adaptive Randomization

Prior to a trial, clinical equipoise exists, that is, investigators do not know which treatments are superior. However, as the trial progresses, increasing evidence may suggest that one study group is responding or doing much better than another. Is it then ethical to keep assigning patients equally to all study groups? Are you then denying patients effective treatment? Moreover, wouldn't assigning more patients to the effective treatment group then reduce your required sample size? Response adaptive randomization addresses these questions by continuously updating assignment probabilities based on response of the different groups to their respective treatments. This method will increase the chance of subsequent patients being assigned to effective treatment groups. To utilize response adaptive randomization, treatment responses need to be relatively rapid and easily measurable. Slow, delayed, equivocal, and subjective responses do not lend themselves well to this allocation design.

Examples of response-based randomization techniques include (although these examples assume only two Study Arms A and B, adapting them for more than two study arms is simple):

- *Play the winner*: The play the winner rule is similar to the urn randomization design, except that the previous patient's response to treatment determines what types of balls to add to the container. If the first patient is assigned to Study Arm A and has a favorable response (i.e., condition improves), then add a fixed number m "Study Arm A" balls to the container. This makes it

more likely to draw Study Arm A for the next patient. Every time a patient improves, add m balls of that study group to the container. Every time a patient fails to improve or worsen, add m balls of the other study group to the container. This method weighs the probabilities so that Study Arms that demonstrate successes have a higher likelihood of being selected.

- *Drop the loser*: This design is similar to the play the winner design, except that treatment failures lead to dropping balls from the container. In this design, the container holds three types of balls: Study Arm A, Study Arm B, and Immigration balls. If the first patient is assigned to Study Arm A and has a favorable response (i.e., condition improves), then keep the same number and distribution of balls in the container. If the patient has an unfavorable response (i.e., treatment fails), remove a Study Arm A ball from the container. If the next draw for the next patient yields an Immigration ball, add a Study Arm A ball and a Study Arm B ball to the container (Immigration balls keep the container from becoming depleted). So in general, treatment success means keep the same number of balls, and treatment failure means removing a ball of that study group.

- *Doubly adaptive biased coins*: This randomization scheme also uses the equivalent of a coin flip but weights the coin flip based on both the characteristics and responses of the different study groups.

One potential problem with adaptive randomization is potential time effects, that is, some patient characteristics and responses change over time. Characteristics (e.g., blood pressure, heart rate, co-morbid conditions) may fluctuate significantly during the course of the study. The characteristics initially may seem unbalanced but over the course of time actually be balanced or vice versa. Trying to keep them balanced may be similar to herding cats. Response to treatment can oscillate as well. Patients may respond to a treatment early on but later become unresponsive or vice versa.

5.4.3 Nonrandom Subject Assignment

Randomization is usually preferable but not always possible. Certain limitations may require that specific patients enter particular study arms:

- *Ethical considerations*: A patient may be desperate to receive the study intervention. The study intervention may be the last resort for a patient with a severely debilitating or life-threatening disease that has no other treatment option. Denying the study intervention may be unethical.
- *Patient availability*: Some patient types may be so rare that once they are identified they need to go into a specific study arm.
- *Very small studies*: A study may have so few patients that randomization is not possible.

Nonrandomized assignment, while more difficult to implement in an unbiased manner than randomized assignment, is still a legitimate method of assigning patients to study groups in some circumstances.

Older clinical trials sometimes used a *fixed pattern* to assign patients (e.g., *alternating pattern* in which the first patient would enter Study Arm A, the second Study Arm B, the third Study Arm A, the fourth Study Arm B, etc.). Unless extremely complex, fixed patterns usually are too predictable. Patients and their physicians usually can figure out the pattern fairly easily. In some cases, the fixed pattern may be *parameter-based*, which involves assigning patients to different study arms based on a set of parameters or algorithms (e.g., all patients with a glomerular filtration rate below 30 go to Study Arm A and all patients with a glomerular filtration rate above 30 go to Study Arm B).

5.5 BLINDING (MASKING)

5.5.1. Potential Biases and the Rationale for Blinding

Blinding or masking achieves two things: it reduces potential bias from investigators, and it reduces potential bias from patients.

Although many people like to think of themselves as objective, they are never completely objective. Even scientists, who pride themselves as rational thinkers, bring their own set of stereotypes, prejudices, and expectations into every experiment. Moreover, some individuals consciously or unconsciously prefer to make choices with their feelings and instincts rather than scientific objectivity. In addition, many individuals have hidden motivations and agendas. Their actions and choices may not be in line with pure scientific inquiry. Therefore, telling people to remain objective in a study is not enough.

The only way to enforce true objectivity in an experiment is blinding or masking the participants in an experiment. Blinding or masking means preventing people from knowing which patients are getting which treatments, which treatments are supposed to be effective and which are inactive, and anything else that may affect the generation and interpretation of data from the study. The goal of blinding is to minimize potential biases and prevent any behavior that may corrupt the scientific objectivity of the study.

Experimenter's Bias

As a result of your experience and knowledge of a study, you never go into an experiment or study without any expectation of the final outcome. Often, you have a strong expectation of what will happen. For example, pharmaceutical and medical device developers would not invest the time, money, and effort on a Phase III clinical trial if they did not expect their products to succeed. Having expectations is simply human nature, neither bad nor good.

When you expect something, you tend to interpret findings in ways that support your expectations. If you stereotype a certain race or ethnicity to be meek, you will interpret any period of quietness as shyness or fear rather than thoughtfulness or measured wisdom. If you stereotype a certain race or ethnicity to be aggressive, you will interpret any period of quietness as thoughtfulness or measured wisdom. Expecting someone to be rude will magnify all of their potentially impolite behaviors and obscure their considerate actions. A good first impression may lead you to overlook someone's weaknesses and negative traits.

In the same way, researchers are prone to *experimenter's bias*: interpreting data in ways that match their expectations. This is also *ascertainment bias*. Researchers will knowingly or unknowingly look for or notice any evidence that supports their expectations of the study and outcomes. Table 5.3 shows how this may work. Expectations can sway subjective interpretations (e.g., physical examination findings and equivocal responses to questionnaires), change the way you interview and examine patients, and even influence you to round up or down fractions.

In addition, the knowledge of the treatment assignment can also affect the quality of care the patient receives, or likelihood of receiving concomitant medications.

Subject Behavior

Subjects also may behave in detrimental ways if they know what treatment they are receiving. Without blinding, there are multiple potential biases that can be introduced, but one of the most important is the placebo effect. For many diseases, the response can be affected by the knowledge that the patient is receiving the drug. This is particularly true when the endpoint is subjective, such as symptoms, or dependent on effort, such as the 6-minute walk. Placebo effect is great, and the randomized blinded trials make the implicit assumption that efficacy – as opposed to effectiveness – is the goal. In real life, of course, the patients will receive the benefits of placebo effect as well as the pharmacological effect. Placebo effect can exist even in active control trials and dose-ranging trials, since patients who are on high doses or on investigative therapy might believe the drug to be superior. Blinding will not eliminate the placebo effect but will equalize them.

Knowledge of treatment can also affect the patient's willingness to stay in the study and can result in differential dropout effects:

- *Subject expectancy*: Being on an active treatment may lead patients to imagine and report more favorable outcomes.
- *Placebo effect*: In order for the placebo effect to take place in the placebo group, patients must believe that they are on the active study treatment.

TABLE 5.3   Potential Examples of Experimenter Bias

Situation	Expect treatment to work	Expect treatment to not work
Explanation for resolved symptom	Treatment eliminated symptom	Disease spontaneously improved
Explanation for worsening symptoms	Disease spontaneously worsened	Treatment failed
Find evidence of effect	No further exploration	Re-check/double-check (e.g., re-examine patient or data) for evidence
Find no evidence of effect	Look more carefully (e.g., re-examine patient or data) for evidence	No further exploration
Deciding whether to administer concomitant treatments	Less likely to administer concomitant treatments	More likely to administer concomitant treatments

- *Retention*: Patients may be more likely to stay in study treatment arms and drop out of ineffective treatment arms.
- *Personal agendas*: Patients may want to demonstrate that the study intervention is successful so that it is available on the market sooner.

5.5.2 Types of Blinds

An *open-label trial* has no blinding: everyone knows which patient is receiving which treatment. Open-label studies lack the rigor of blinded studies. Since the lack of blinding can introduce significant bias, reserve the use of open-label studies for situations in which blinding is neither feasible nor ethical or in cases where the outcome is completely objective, such as survival. Some situations include:

- *Case studies or case series*: Some studies will test a study intervention on very few subjects. These are uncontrolled, very limited studies that, in the eyes of many researchers, are not formal studies.
- *Open-label extension studies*: In these studies, which often follow a double-blind randomized placebo-controlled trial, subjects have the option of remaining on the study intervention in an open-label fashion (i.e., they know that they are on the study intervention) for an extended period of time (e.g., several years). They may be informed of this opportunity before or after the double-blind trial (or whatever study precedes the open-label extension study). Such studies can generate long-term data on the intervention's efficacy, safety, and administration.
- *Compassionate use studies*: Some serious diseases have very few effective treatments. Patients afflicted with such diseases may want or need access to certain promising experimental interventions but may not be eligible for the formal clinical trials. Such patients may enter a compassionate use study, which by definition will be open-label. Such studies can generate data on the intervention and provide patients with needed treatment.
- *Dose-ranging or pharmacokinetic studies*: In these studies, everyone receives the study intervention.

- *Other uncontrolled studies*: When there is no control, blinding is not necessary since everyone will receive the study intervention. These studies are much more limited than controlled studies.

Blinding can include almost anyone participating in a clinical study including the:

- *Patient*.
- *Investigator*.
  - *Treatment administrator*: This is the health care provider administering the treatment. Blinding this person minimizes differences in the way the treatment is administered and decreases the chance that the patient will be inadvertently unblinded.
  - *Assessor*: This is the person (usually a health care provider) assessing the results of the treatment. The treatment administrator and assessor may be the same person, but often they are different people in order to minimize bias (i.e., the person performing the intervention may not be objective enough to assess its consequences). Remember that assessors may include radiologists, pathologists, and/or anyone else interpreting test results (e.g., cardiologists reading EKGs or neurologists reading EEGs). When the treatment cannot be blinded (e.g., surgery vs. sham surgery), using a blinded assessor is an option.
  - *Site personnel*: Blinding all members of the health care team at each study site will prevent any preferential treatment or information from being inadvertently spread to patients or investigators. Sometimes, keeping certain members of the team (e.g., the pharmacist organizing and distributing the medications) unblinded is necessary.
- *Study sponsor*: Keeping a company or additional party involved in organizing or running the study blind may be important as well. In general, everyone except the safety group and monitor remains blind in a clinical trial.
- *Data analyzers*: To avoid biases in analysis, it may be useful to keep statisticians and anyone else assessing the data blind.

The terms single-blind, double-blind, and increasingly triple-blind are relatively common parlance in the clinical study world. However, their usage is not always consistent.

Single-Blind

In single-blind studies, either the patients or the researchers conducting the study (i.e., interacting with the patients) do not know which patients belong to which arm. Usually the patients are blinded and the researchers are not, but in some cases, the researchers may be the ones blinded. Maintaining single-blinds can be difficult, since the nonblinded side may consciously or unconsciously "tip off" the blinded side (e.g., nonblinded patients may ask blinded researchers questions about their intervention; nonblinded researchers may express surprise when blinded patients inform them of unexpected symptoms). Many game shows are single-blinded. The contestants do not know what is behind the door number 1, the real price of the Blender, or where the Daily Double is located.

Single-blind studies are appropriate when one side (usually the researchers) must know the treatment the patient will receive. Studies involving sham operations and sham procedures are frequently single-blind because the person performing the procedure will clearly know whether the treatment is fake (although sometimes you may have different people performing the different steps of the treatment to keep as many people blinded as possible). Moreover, researchers may have to know the treatments when they are extremely complicated or potentially dangerous. Blinding researchers may prevent them from quickly detecting something awry and remedying the situation.

Double-Blind

In a double-blind study, neither the patient nor the personnel conducting the study knows which patients belong to which study arm. This is more stringent than single-blind studies. Blinding the researchers as well as the patients helps minimize experimenter's bias. Double-blinds may differ in which study personnel are blind. Full double-blind studies blind everyone who interacts directly with the patients, including the investigator, staff members, technicians, therapists, and dispensing pharmacists. Computers often help maintain double-blinds by performing key steps that could reveal to the researchers the identity of the treatments.

Triple-Blind

Although there is some debate over what "triple-blind" means, we define it as the patient, the researchers conducting the study, and anyone analyzing the results (e.g., sponsor) do not know which subjects belong to which study arms. Triple-blinding may be useful when knowledge of study group assignment may unduly influence interpretation of the results. Some use the term total clinical study blind when everyone involved in the study is blind.

5.5.3 Blinding Techniques

Maintaining blinds can be very difficult. Many clues can jeopardize a blind including any differences in procedures or operations, labeling or packaging, test results, treatment appearance, treatment effects, side effects, and the subtle behavior of unblinded personnel. Even if patients and investigators try to stay blinded, they may inadvertently figure out the treatment groups.

Special procedures may be necessary for suppositories, eye drops, skin patches, etc. For example, for patches, the patients may need to wear a covering that prevents them from seeing which patch they are wearing. Drugs with a characteristic color may need to be administered in opaque IV lines. Drugs that have a low pH and sting on injection should be matched with a placebo that has a similar pH and also stings.

Certain drugs have a pharmacodynamic effect that can unblind the drug, such as PTT, lymphocyte count, etc. Ideally, the lab results will not be shown to the investigator, but in cases where it is important to monitor the laboratory value and adjust the treatment accordingly, a separate physician can be assigned to handle the task.

In some cases where the drug has to be prepared at the site, it is sometimes necessary to unblind the pharmacist in order to prepare the drug.

Some common techniques that you may use include the following.

Separate Steps, Separate Personnel

Dividing different steps of the study among different personnel may prevent a single person from gaining enough information about the study to figure out patient group assignment (e.g., separate physicians administer the treatment and assess outcomes). If possible, these personnel should not be allowed to communicate their findings to each other.

Dummying

A *dummy* is a fake, a mimic, or a disguise that helps conceal the identity of a treatment or study group. Dummies are necessary when the appearance of one treatment or study group is not the same as the appearance of another treatment or study arm. The formulations (e.g., intravenous vs. oral medication) or administration (e.g., one involves using a special device whereas the other does not) of two treatments may be very different. A *double-dummy* study uses dummies in two different study groups. For example, in comparing an IV drug with an oral drug, you may have to give a dummy IV drug to the oral drug group and a dummy oral drug to the IV drug group. A *triple-dummy* study uses dummies in three different study groups. A *multiple-dummy* study uses dummies in multiple arms. People may use the words dummy and placebo interchangeably.

Masking Intermediate Data

Throughout the course of the study, data from measurements may reveal treatments to patients and investigators (e.g., a steady decrease in blood pressure may suggest that the patient is on active treatment). Blinded personnel should not see this data until absolutely necessary. When such data is important for study conduct and patient safety, reveal only the amount necessary and if possible in general categories (e.g., the blood pressure was normal, the white blood cell count is significantly depressed).

Verifying and Validating the Blind

Before commencing the trial, review and check the blinding procedure, making sure that it will work under a variety of conditions. Get external reviewers to analyze each step. Run hypothetical scenarios that may challenge the blinding procedure.

Monitoring and Assessing the Blind

Your study should include ongoing assessments and checks of the blind during and after the study. Questionnaires can query patients and investigators as to whether they can guess the active treatment groups. You should document and report your blinding and blinding monitoring procedures.

5.6 BREAKING THE BLIND

5.6.1 Reasons to Break the Blind

To *break the blind* is to reveal the identity of a patient's study group to the previously blinded patient or investigator. Deliberately breaking the blind may be reasonable in the following situations:

- *Threats to patient safety*: Some severe adverse events may call for emergency treatment, which may require breaking of the blind. However, breaking the blind is not necessary for all emergent treatments.

- *Threats to investigator safety*: Investigators may suffer an accident that requires knowledge of the patient's treatment (e.g., needle stick injury or exposure to potential harmful treatments) to determine the risk and potential remedy.

- *Regulatory reporting*: Many sponsors will break the blind for serious unexpected adverse events in order to determine whether to report the event to regulatory authorities. This also allows close monitoring of the safety event pattern in the trial.

- *Disclosing assignment to Data Safety Monitoring Board (DSMB)*: For trials that have a DSMB, usually an independent third party statistician will break the blind in order to assess safety.

- *Breaking the blind for administrative reasons*: Although generally not advisable, it is possible to break the blind to trigger an independent event, such as preparation for the next clinical trial. In such a case, extreme care is necessary to preserve the blind.

To *partially unblind* is to break the blind among only certain personnel. Others remain blinded. For example, only a selected group of people may know the results after the primary endpoint but before the secondary endpoint has been attained. Such early partial unblinding may help initiate the next trial or regulatory filing. Meanwhile, the study sites and patients would remain blinded until after the secondary endpoint has been reached.

5.6.2 Consequences of Breaking the Blind

Do not break the blind until you have deemed it absolutely necessary. If possible, consult the key investigators and managers of the study before taking this drastic action. Make sure the protocol lists potential adverse effects and how to deal with them without breaking the blind. If you must break the blind, clearly document the reasoning and the potential consequences.

Breaking the blind can introduce significant biases into the study. Experimenter's or ascertainment bias may be a significant problem. While the subject may remain in some analyses (e.g., intent-to-treat), he or she should be dropped from the general protocol-compliant analysis. Breaking the blind for one patient could reveal the allocation of other patients, especially if allocation occurred in predictable patterns or blocks (e.g., if patients were randomized in two patient blocks, you could then easily guess the study arm of the other patient in the same block).

Chapter 6

Periods, Sequences, and Trial Design

6.1 BACKGROUND

6.1.1 The Importance of Time and Timing

Time and timing is critical in everything, especially clinical trials. The timing of measurements, intervention administration, patient monitoring, and other treatments can dramatically affect study results and their interpretation. There are several specific reasons why timing affects clinical trial design:

- *Timing implies causality*: When Event A precedes Event B, we often assume that A somehow caused B (e.g., if whenever a certain celebrity appears on television, we feel nauseous, we assume that the celebrity is causing the nausea). This assumption is not always correct since the timing of Events A and B can either be pure coincidence or be related to other undiscovered factors. So while A preceding B certainly is not sufficient to establish causality, it is necessary: if B preceded A, then A cannot have caused B. Clinical trials involve administering an intervention and looking to see if an effect follows. If an effect consistently follows the intervention, and does not occur in the absence of the intervention, we assume that the intervention somehow caused the effect. If the effect precedes the intervention, then we assume that it was not caused by the intervention.
- *Temporal changes can confound clinical trials*: Things change with time. Disease characteristics, clinical practice patterns, the environment (e.g., temperature, sunlight, and humidity) and patient characteristics are rarely completely static. Clinical trial design must account for these temporal changes (e.g., Asthma exacerbations occur more frequently during certain seasons. So a nonparallel trial in which half of the asthma patients receive the intervention in the winter and the other half receive placebo in the autumn might introduce a significant amount of bias.)
- *Time lag*: Many effects do not occur immediately. The delay between cause and effect is called a time lag. You have to monitor a patient long enough after an intervention is administered to see an effect. Monitoring periods that are too short may miss some effects. Monitoring periods that are too long may add unnecessary cost and delay to the trial and raise the probability that other factors may be causing the effects (e.g., if you experience nausea 3 months after seeing a celebrity, Is the celebrity really the cause?)
- *Evolution and learning effects*: Trial design can also change with time. As study results emerge, staunchly sticking to one plan may is not always prudent. Some trial designs allow you to alter the study as more information becomes available. Also, patients may improve their performance on certain measures over time (e.g., exercise tolerance, visual acuity chart is another – patients might remember the letters on a subsequent visit).
- *Timing of intervention and outcome measurements can greatly impact the trial's scientific rigor and parsimony*: All clinical development programs (i.e., sequentially moving through Phases I, II, and III or some similar sequence) alternate intervention and outcome measures. Some trial designs involve measuring outcomes during the trial before all patients have been assigned to treatment (i.e., some patients complete their course of treatment and reach their endpoints before others are randomized). For instance, iterative studies based on previous studies or flexible/adaptive designs can enhance the power of the studies and reduce sample size.

6.1.2 Definitions

A *period* is the time of observation and treatment (or in some cases no treatment). So a patient who receives a single intervention receives a single period of treatment. A patient who receives two different interventions undergoes two periods of treatment. Undergoing three different interventions in sequential order will take three periods. During a period, you may just observe the patients for a given length of time without giving any treatments. A period is analogous to a television series episode, a quarter in a football game, an act in a play, or a semester in a school calendar. During a given period a defined action occurs. *Comparator periods* are segments of time with accompanying observations that can be compared or measured against each other. Not all periods can serve as comparator periods. Some (e.g., run-in periods) occur before the experiment commences.

The *sequence* is the order in which a patient receives different interventions or treatments. If A represents Intervention A, B represents Intervention B, and C represents Intervention C, we can express sequences using the following syntax:

- *AB*: Patient receives Intervention A for one period and then switches to Intervention B for the second period.
- *BA*: Patient receives Intervention B for one period and then switches to Intervention A for the second period.
- *ABC*: Patient receives Intervention A for one period, switches to Intervention B for the second period, and then switches to Intervention C for the third period.

A *study arm* (or *study group*) is a group of patients that all receive the same interventions in the same sequence. A trial with two arms has two different groups of patients. One arm may receive Intervention A only, and another arm may receive Intervention B only. When patients in an arm are given a treatment, it is called a *treatment (or active) arm*. When

patients in an arm do not receive any treatment, it is called a *no-treatment arm*. When patients in an arm receive placebo, it is called a *placebo arm*. The no-treatment arm or placebo arm are both control arms. Once a patient is assigned to a certain arm, he or she typically should stay in that arm (i.e., study arms should be exclusive). After one or more periods, study arms may branch or arborize into additional arms (Figure 6.1).

Clinical trial designs can be traditional or flexible. *Traditional designs* involve fixing the sample size before the trial commences and performing only a single efficacy analysis after the trial has occurred. In other words, traditional designs are akin to deciding what to do at the beginning, sticking with the plan, and only really fully looking at the results at the end. Traditional designs are relatively straightforward and simple but are also rigid and not flexible. A traditional design is analogous to deciding that you want to be a neurosurgeon at an early age and adhering to this plan without any re-evaluation. By contrast, *flexible designs* entail actively monitoring efficacy during the trial (either continuously or at intervals) and altering the study based on the efficacy data. This "wait and see approach" is analogous to trying different jobs and determining whether you like the job before deciding to pursue it as a career. Flexible designs are more complicated and may necessitate more time and effort. However, they can actually save time and effort. For example, trials may be terminated early because the preliminary results suggests that the intervention

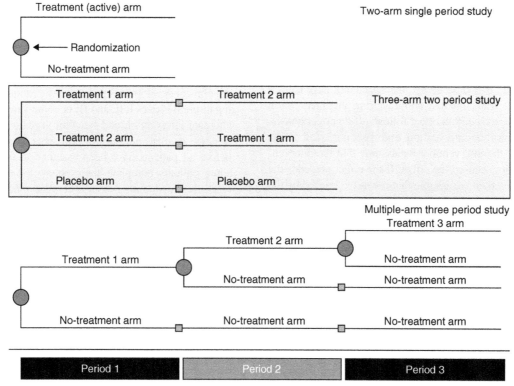

FIGURE 6.1 Study arms and periods.

is either so ineffective or so effective that continuing the trial would not provide much more additional information. Actively re-assessing the data throughout the trial can help identify trial design or safety problems. Flexible trials designs also help divert resources to get "more bang for the buck" (e.g., away from trial arms that are not providing useful data and toward trial arms that are).

Pure parallel, within-patient, and factorial designs are traditional designs. This chapter will introduce two types of flexible designs: sequential and information-based designs.

6.2 PARALLEL DESIGNS

6.2.1 Single Group (Arm)

Some clinical studies include only a single group of patients with each patient in the group receiving a single intervention. There are no placebo or comparator interventions. A single-arm design is technically not a parallel group study because there is only one track or line (i.e., there needs to be more than one line to be considered parallel). But a single-arm design can branch out into a parallel group design later in the trial if necessary (Figure 6.2).

A single-arm design is limited in its ability to compare or demonstrate efficacy of interventions. This design is analogous to timing a person when running a 100-m dash alone without any competitors (which is what football scouts do when evaluating players that they may draft for their teams). To get a sense of his or her speed, you can compare the person's time with other people's times. But without any competitors running at the same time, you are not directly comparing the person to anyone else. It is difficult to determine whether the person's speed is the result of random fluctuation, environmental conditions, athletic equipment (e.g., shoes or clothes), or other factors that are unique to that time and that run.

Usually, in single-group (or single-arm) studies, you measure the difference in certain measures before and after administering the intervention. A simple one sample *t*-test can compare the initial (pre-intervention or baseline) measurements with the post-intervention measurements.

A statistically significant difference suggests that the intervention has an effect and that the change is not just due to random fluctuation. However, a single-arm study cannot rule out bias, such as regression to the mean or natural improvement over time. Alternatively, you can tabulate the response or cure rate (i.e., the percentage of patients who had their symptoms or diseases eliminated) and determine whether this rate is statistically high enough compared to historical controls or to a previous run-in period to claim that the intervention has an effect. So using the 100-m dash analogy, to test the effects of a new pair of shoes, you could have the athlete run once while wearing her regular shoes and a second time with the new shoes. Running much faster in the second run than the first suggests that the new shoes are making a difference.

The biggest problem with single-arm designs is determining whether the difference (i.e., improvement or worsening) is due to the intervention or other factors. What if the patients would have improved (or worsened) with time regardless of whether you administered the intervention? What if other factors affecting the disease changed (e.g., the weather, patient's diet, or other medications)? In the new athletic shoes analogy mentioned above, if her time in the second run is better, are you sure that the shoes made the difference? Perhaps her performance improved after getting used to the track. Perhaps she was less ner-vous the second time. The wind could have been blowing in another direction. Depending on the length of time between the first and second runs, she could have been wearing different clothing, eaten different foods before the runs, or had different types of injuries. Distinguishing which factors were responsible is very difficult.

Additionally, without a control arm, placebo and Hawthorne effects may occur but be difficult to detect in single-arm studies. Did the patients improve because they expected to improve? Did the patients improve because they were being closely observed? A single-arm study may struggle to answer these questions.

Comparing your single-arm trial to other similar single-arm trials can help further determine if your intervention has an effect (e.g., several single-arm trials all show improvement after the intervention). Doing so is not a formal

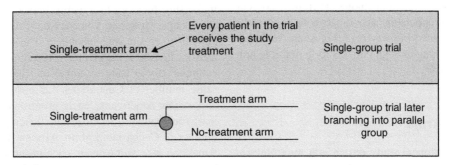

FIGURE 6.2   Single arm design.

experiment because it lacks the key ingredient of experimental design: random patient assignment. Instead it is a quasi-experiment. Quasi-experiments cannot establish cause but can suggest trends. So if a number of single-arm trials show that your intervention has a statistically significant positive effect then you can say that the patients tend to improve after receiving the intervention. This quasi-experimental design is analogous to comparing the 100-m dash time of your athlete with the 100-m dash times of other athletes from different days. If her time is better than those of other athletes, this suggests that she is faster. But until they all compete at the same time on the same track, you cannot truly establish who is faster.

Even though single group studies lack the rigor of randomized, controlled clinical trials (in many cases, they are called case series), investigators frequently employ single-arm studies because they are easier and less costly to plan and execute. Enrolling patients in single-arm studies also may be easier. Phase II and open-label Phase IV studies often are single-arm studies. Most existing studies of complementary and alternative medicines are single-arm studies.

Single-arm studies are most useful when:

- *Without the intervention, the effect is very unlikely to occur.* Very rare events are not likely to be due to random fluctuations (e.g., disappearance of a tumor is not likely to occur randomly and spontaneously). So conditions that do not improve without treatment are especially amenable to single-arm studies.
- *The anticipated effect of the intervention is large, dramatic, and obvious.* Large, dramatic, and obvious effects also are less likely to be due to random fluctuations (e.g., disappearance of severe pain or very low blood counts returning to normal levels).
- *The intervention has not been studied previously.* A randomized controlled trial (RCT) is usually not the first step in studying an intervention. You have to know if the intervention has any effect before sinking significant cost, time, and effort into more rigorous testing. Moreover, having an idea of the effects, the magnitude of the effects, and the safety of the intervention helps plan more rigorous studies like an RCT.
- *The study population is homogeneous.* Without a comparison control group, patient variability can be an even greater problem in single-arm studies. Therefore, do your best to make your population as homogeneous as possible.
- *Appropriate patients are very rare.* For some very rare conditions, recruiting enough patients for a multiple arm study is impractical.

6.2.2 Multiple Arms

The most common clinical study design is a multiple arm parallel group design (or just parallel group design, as parallel group implies more than one arm). In this design, you randomly assign patients into two or more different and exclusive groups. Each group then receives a different treatment (e.g., every patient in Group 1 receives Intervention A, every patient in Group 2 receives Intervention B, and every patient in Group 3 receives placebo). You administer treatments contemporaneously, that is, at the same time (e.g., all patients receive their assigned treatments on September 3, 2007). Each group receives only one type of treatment (e.g., patients in Group 1 do not receive Intervention B or placebo) for only one period. In other words, each patient receives treatment once and then is monitored for a specific amount of time afterwards.

Although more complex than a single-arm study, a multiple arm parallel group design is still fairly simple and straightforward way and usually has the least risk for bias. Since the treatment is given and patients are monitored at the same time, managing the trial is relatively easy (e.g., you only need to prepare a single large batch of the investigational drug once). Compared to other trial designs, the trial does not take very long to complete. Temporal bias is minimal (e.g., the weather and other environmental conditions will be the same for every patient).

A parallel group design is analogous to the 100-m dash finals at the Olympic Games. All competitors line up and race at the same time. As a result weather conditions are relatively equal for everyone. No one can complain that the wind or cold weather put him or her at a significant disadvantage. It is relatively easy to organize and monitor a 100-m dash. Reserve a track for a single day, shoot the starting gun once, and watch all the competitors at the same time. To use the 100-m race to test the effects of a new shoe, randomly assign half of the competitors to wear the new shoe and the other half to wear the old shoe. Seeing all of the new shoe-wearing runners beat the old shoe-wearing runners provides strong evidence that the new shoe makes people faster.

Unfortunately, the biggest remaining problem with parallel designs is variability. Each group may be very different from each other. For example, What if patients in Group 1 are more ill than patients in Groups 2 and 3? What if patients in Group 3 on average have a lower socioeconomic status than patients in the other groups? What if the distribution of ethnic backgrounds differs among the groups? You can do your best to measure various characteristics and make sure they are reasonably balanced among the different groups. However, you may have to include many more patients to ensure such a balance. The more relevant characteristics there are, the greater your sample size has to be. For example, if you want to make sure that each group has the same number of Caucasians, Latinos, African Americans, and Asian Americans, each group will have to have at least four patients. To ensure that each group has the same number of Caucasian, Latino, African American, and Asian American *men and women*, each group will have to have at least eight patients.

To understand these problems, let us go back to the 100-m dash analogy. The different running lanes in a 100 m dash are rarely completely equal. Their surfaces and locations relative to other runners may vary significantly. For example, runners in the outermost lanes can see the rest of the competitors without having to turn their heads both ways and do not have competitors on both sides of them. If certain running lanes were more uneven or slippery, then runners in those lanes would never get a chance to run in the smoother, better quality lanes. Their performance would be subject to the variability in lane quality. Randomly assigning competitors to different lanes does not solve this problem. Having a sample size (adequate powering) that is large enough does.

6.3 WITHIN-PATIENT DESIGNS

6.3.1 Rationale

Within-patient designs attempt to alleviate the variability problem afflicting parallel group designs. In within-patient designs, patients sequentially receive more than one type of treatment. Each patient receives one intervention, remains under observation for one period, and then receives a different intervention, followed by another period of observation. Depending on the specific design, this could continue for as many periods as necessary. For example, a patient might receive placebo for a month, followed by active drug for a month. Another patient may receive the active drug for a month first and then placebo for the second month. This design allows patients to serve as their own comparators: how a patient does on placebo can be compared with how the same patient does on the active drug. In other words, you cannot only compare different patients but the same patients as well. By comparing each patient with himself or herself you minimize the problem of variability among different patients. By reducing variability, within-patient designs also reduce the necessary sample sizes (i.e., fewer patients are needed than for parallel group designs). This is especially important when patients are in short supply (e.g., the relevant disease is rare or many other trials are competing for the same patients) or recruiting is a problem.

Within-patient designs are analogous to competitors switching shoes in the middle of a 10,000-m race (There's too little time to switch shoes in the middle of a 400-m race.) Each competitor will have the opportunity to run on the track in different shoes. For example, some runners may run the first five laps in the old shoes and then switch to the new shoes for the final five laps. Other runners may run their first five laps in the new shoes and then switch to the old shoes for the final five laps. You can see not only which runners ultimately win but also how fast each runner ran her first five laps vs. her last five laps. Seeing every runner run their laps faster while wearing the new shoes provides compelling evidence that the new shoes are helpful.

Within-patient designs are appropriate when:

- The variability among patients is greater than the variability within the same patient at different times. In other words, the difference between Patient 1 and Patient 2 during Period 1 is much more than the difference between Patient 1 in Period 1 and Patient 1 in Period 2.
- Running a parallel trial would be too expensive. Parallel trials usually require a larger sample size, which is more costly.
- There aren't enough patients available for a parallel trial.
- The treatment duration is short.

Within-patient designs may encounter several potential problems including temporal effects, carryover effects, rebound effects, time constraints, dropouts, and permanent endpoints. Often these problems are surmountable, but sometimes the problems preclude the use of within-patient designs. Carefully look at your potential study population, disease or condition of interest, intervention, environment, and budget and resource constraints to determine whether within-patient designs are feasible.

Temporal Effects

Patients, conditions, and the environment vary with time and may be different during the first intervention vs. during the second intervention. Having different patients receive interventions in different orders reduces this problem (e.g., During the first month, some patients receive placebo and others receive active drug. During the second month, those that received placebo first receive active drug and those that received active drug first receive placebo.) In the running analogy, having some runners start with the new shoes and others start with the old shoes reduces the role of variation between the first part of the race and the second part of the race.

Variation that consistently occurs in one direction is called a *period effect* (e.g., all patients' conditions are worse in the second period than in the first period). In the running analogy, runners usually run slower later in the race when they become more tired. Significant period effects preclude the use of within-patient designs. So diseases or conditions that progress in one direction (i.e., improve or worsen) with time will cause problems. Diseases that are chronic and relatively stable lend themselves best to within-patient designs. Diseases that are acute (e.g., Myocardial Infarction (MI)) or waxing and waning (e.g., multiple sclerosis) are not very suitable for within-patient designs. With such cases, there is no guarantee that the disease will be the same in different periods (e.g., the disease may be much worse in first period than the second period).

Carryover Effects

Some interventions have sustained effects that last beyond the study period, so that the order in which a patient receives different interventions matters. For example, the effects of receiving active drug during the first month may still be present during the second month when the patient is supposed to receive only placebo. In our racing analogy, wearing the new shoes may cause persistent pain or blisters that affect one's running even after switching shoes. Carryover effects occur for several different reasons: the medication may remain in the patient's body or the intervention may cause a persistent change in the disease (e.g., antibiotics eradicate bacteria) or patient's physiology (e.g., after receiving an immunosuppressant, the body's immune system needs time to regenerate immune cells) or anatomy (e.g., a surgical procedure changes the patient's anatomy).

For within-patient designs to work, the intervention's half-life must be short and effects must not have a permanent and durable effect on the disease or disease progression. The intervention must also act relatively quickly, before the switch, so that the effect can be attributed to the correct period. If the drug's effect is delayed, then the effect may be attributed to the second intervention rather than the first even if the first intervention was the active intervention.

Employing a washout period (i.e., waiting for a while before starting the second intervention) can mitigate such carryover effects. So in the racing analogy, a washout period could mean pausing the race after five laps so that all runners can recover and heal before re-starting the race for the final five laps. The washout period should be long enough for the intervention to leave the body and its effects to completely dissipate. At least three to five half-lives are generally required between the periods. Washout periods are not always possible or adequate. Some interventions permanently change a patient or condition (e.g., antibiotics will eradicate an infection). Some patients have severe conditions that must be treated at all times and cannot afford to be off therapy. In such situations, within-patient designs may not be appropriate.

Unfortunately, the required sample size to detect a significant carryover effect is usually larger than the required sample size to meet the primary endpoint. (In fact, it is usually the size needed for a parallel group study.)

Rebound Effects

Similar to carryover effects, rebound effects (which we discuss in detail in Chapter 10) can persist after stopping an intervention (e.g., after stopping some anti-hypertension medications, blood pressure may rise dramatically). Some rebound effects are so severe that treatment is necessary. Gradually tapering a patient off the intervention can prevent rebound effects. If the required taper takes a very long time then a within-patient design may be difficult to do.

Time Constraints

Within-patient designs take longer to execute. Rather than remaining on one intervention for one period, each patient has to undergo two or more interventions for a total of two or more periods. The longer trial duration may be a problem if:

- Treatment duration is very long.
- Your access to certain necessary resources will expire soon (e.g., you cannot rent time on a special Magnetic Resonance Imaging (MRI) machine for longer than 1 month).
- There is urgent need to complete the trial as soon as possible (e.g., the intervention meets an desperate need).
- The patient's conditions change rapidly (e.g., the patients will not survive for longer than a month).
- The patients are not likely to remain compliant with the trial for so long (e.g., a transient population).
- Treatment effects take a long time to appear.

Dropouts and Missing Data

Patient dropouts are a bigger problem for within-patient designs than for parallel group designs. A patient needs to be in the trial long enough to undergo the different interventions (i.e., patient cannot drop out before completing all the periods of the trial). Otherwise you will not be able to see how the patient responds to different interventions. Therefore, within-patient designs are suboptimal for relatively noncompliant patient populations.

Missing data also can play havoc with a within-patient design. Ideally data should be available for all of the patient's periods for a within-patient design to be fully effective.

Permanent Endpoints

The endpoint of interest cannot be permanent. Otherwise, once the patient experiences the permanent endpoint (e.g., death) in the first period, the patient can no longer experience the endpoint again in subsequent periods. So within-patient designs are not good for testing interventions designed to prevent death, dismemberment, or other permanent outcomes.

Converting a Within-Patient Design to a Parallel Design

When any or all of the above mentioned problems wreak havoc with a within-patient design, converting it to a parallel group design may salvage the study, even after the study has been completed. Within a given period, a within-patient design looks like a parallel group design. As long as the study was conducted appropriately, you may be able to use certain periods within the study as parallel group studies. For example, if patients drop out after the first period, the first period can serve as a parallel group study. If the disease progressively worsens during the trial according to objective measures, the first period can serve as a parallel group study at one disease stage and the second period can serve as a parallel group study at a more severe disease stage. The biggest potential problem with converting a within-patient study is inadequate sample size. Parallel group studies require larger sample sizes.

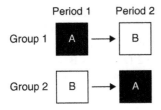

FIGURE 6.3   Two-period crossover study.

Replication

Replicate design can tease out some of the biases. This design performs the experiment more than once. For example, instead of patients receiving "placebo → drug," they might receive "placebo → drug → placebo → drug." In this way, you can determine if there is asystematic trend toward spontaneous improvement over time (e.g., by comparing placebo vs. placebo).

The next several subsections will cover some common types of within-patient designs.

6.3.2 Crossover Trial

In a crossover trial, patients start off on one arm (i.e., receive one intervention) during one period and then switch to another arm (i.e., receive another intervention) for the next period. Every time a patient switches arms, the patient "crosses over" to another arm. Depending on the study, a patient may crossover multiple times. In the racing analogy, a crossover is like switching shoes. The crossover trial is the most common within-patient design.

The simplest crossover design is the two-period crossover: during the first period, patients receive one of two treatments and during the second period patients receive the other treatment (e.g., give half the patients an AB sequence and the other half a BA sequence). Figure 6.3 shows a schematic of a two-period crossover study.

The crossover should occur only after the intervention has been completed and the effects have taken place. Crossing over prematurely runs the risk of either underestimating the intervention's effects or seeing carryover effects. Crossovers transpire immediately after the period is completed or following an intervening washout period.

Crossover designs are common in early phase studies including bioequivalence, pharmacokinetic, food interaction, dose escalation, and dose proportionality studies.

Figure 6.4 shows some examples of more complicated crossover designs. Some cases involve the same intervention being administered in multiple different periods (e.g., ABAB, ABCABC).

6.3.3 Latin Square

A Latin square design is a variation of a crossover study design. In a Latin square, each patient receives each intervention once. So, if there are *n* types of interventions or

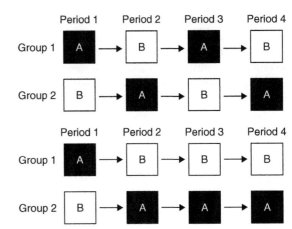

FIGURE 6.4   Examples of more complicated crossover designs.

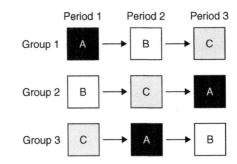

FIGURE 6.5   Latin square design.

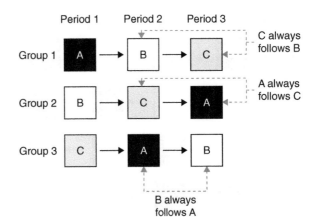

FIGURE 6.6   Circular permutation.

treatments (including placebo), the study will last *n* periods. Figure 6.5 shows a schematic representation of a three-period Latin square design. The rows represent different groups. The columns are different periods. Each group undergoes a sequence of three treatments over three periods (e.g., Group 1 receives Intervention A in Period 1, Intervention B in Period 2, and Intervention C in Period 3). As you can see, each group receives a different treatment each period. Patients in Group 2 start with Intervention B, and patients in Group 3 start with Intervention C. It is called a square because schematically the number of rows (i.e., groups) equals the number of columns (i.e., periods).

In the example in Figure 6.6, the treatment sequence is fixed. When Intervention A occurs in one period, B always occurs the next period, C the period after, and A the period after, and so forth. In other words, the sequence is never ACB, BAC, or CBA. This is an example of *circular permutation*, that is, the order of the treatments is always the same (A→B→C). In general, a circular permutation will magnify any potential carryover effects and, as a result, may introduce a systematic bias. If Intervention A has a carryover effect on Intervention B, every group will suffer since Intervention B always follows Intervention A. Noncircular permutations, that is, shuffling the order in which interventions follow (Figure 6.7), may help elucidate the presence and magnitude of this problem.

For a study with even number of treatments, you can easily modify the sequence to ensure that each treatment is followed by each other treatment (Figure 6.8a, b). This allows you to estimate the presence and magnitude of any carryover effect. As you can see, in Group 1 Intervention C follows B, Group 2 D follows B, and Group 4 A follows B. Such a design helps you compare the effects of B on A, C, and D.

Adequate sequence modifications are not possible for studies with odd numbers of groups. Instead, there are several alternatives:

- *Use two or more complementary sequences (preferred)*: The two sets in Figure 6.9 are complementary. A goes to C in the first set, and A goes to B in the second set.
- *Add an extra group to make it an even number of groups*: As Figure 6.10 demonstrates, adding an extra group allows you to have A follow B (last row).
- *Add an extra period*: In a true Latin square, each group occurs only once in each row or column. So, as Figure 6.11 shows, this is no longer a true Latin square (i.e., the BCA column appears twice).

If desired, you may repeat a treatment (e.g., in Figure 6.12, the CAB column appears twice in subsequent periods) to determine if two sequential treatment periods have a clinical effect.

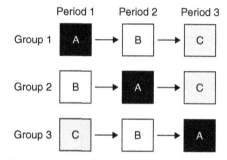

FIGURE 6.7 Latin square with non-circular permutation.

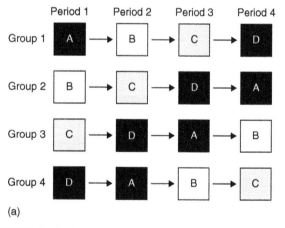

(a)

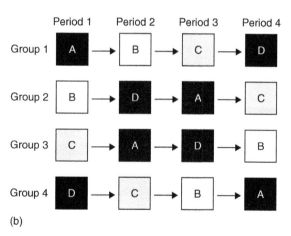

(b)

FIGURE 6.8 Study with an even number of treatments: (a) Circular permutation does not allow all treatment sequences (e.g., Treatment B never follows Treatment C) (b) Modified design ensures that each treatment is followed by each other treatment (e.g., Treatment B now follows Treatment C.)

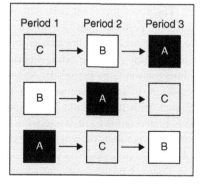
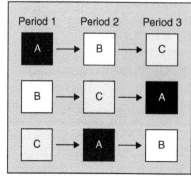

FIGURE 6.9 Complementary sequences.

If the full Latin square design is not feasible because multiple periods are not practical, you may use incomplete Latin square designs (i.e., the number of rows does not equal the number of columns) (Figures 6.13a-c). Conversely, if the availability of the patients is an issue (e.g., with orphan indications), intensive design may be used.

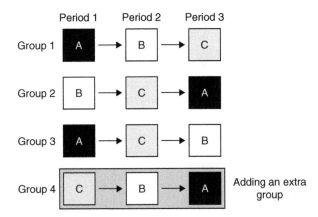

FIGURE 6.10 Adding an extra group.

6.3.4 Dose Escalation

Although often not recognized as such, dose escalation is a common within-patient design. In dose escalation studies, the same subject receives multiple, progressively increasing doses of an intervention. Then, you compare the effects of different doses given to the same patient (e.g., the effect of 1 mg vs. 5 mg vs. 10 mg of the drug). Just like any other within-patient design, dose escalation designs may be subject to temporal, carryover, or rebound effects, Time constraints, dropouts, missing data, and permanent endpoints also can wreak havoc with dose escalation studies.

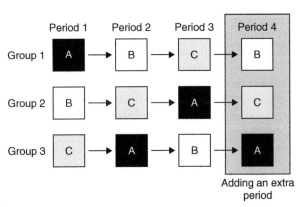

FIGURE 6.11 Adding an extra period.

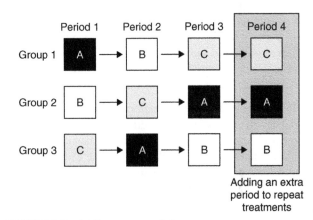

FIGURE 6.12 Adding an extra period to repeat treatment.

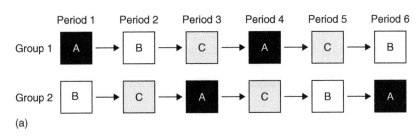

(a)

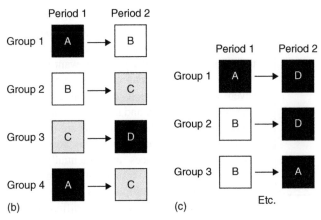

(b)

(c)

Etc.

FIGURE 6.13 Incomplete Latin squares.

6.4 FACTORIAL DESIGNS

Factorial designs involve testing two or more different interventions on the same group at the same time (i.e., in one period). In other words, different groups receive different combinations of the available interventions. By testing multiple interventions against controls simultaneously, factorial designs minimize the number of patients used.

A factorial design consists of two or more *factors* (i.e., interventions) with each intervention having two or more *levels* (i.e., degrees or quantities of the interventions). For example, two levels could be "no intervention" and "intervention." Three levels could be "0 mg of medication," "5 mg of medication," and "10 mg of medication." You can describe a factorial design by indicating the (Number of levels)$_{Factor\ 1}$ × (Number of levels)$_{Factor\ 2}$ × (Number of levels)$_{Factor\ 3}$ and so forth (e.g., a 2 × 2 design will have two factors with two levels each). To calculate the number of different possible combinations, multiply the number of levels for each factor by each other (e.g., if Intervention A has two levels and Intervention B has three levels, the total number of combinations is 2 × 3 or 6).

The most simple and common factorial design is a 2 × 2 factorial design (Figure 6.14 shows an example).

A factorial design can represent:

- *Two or more independent studies*: A so-called pure factorial design tests two (or more) different interventions, each for a different completely unrelated indication (e.g., an ophthalmologic drug for glaucoma in the eye and a dermatologic drug for dermatitis in the hand, in patients who have both diseases). If performed with appropriate rigor and relatively devoid of drug–drug interactions, such a study is fairly equivalent to two or more independent, separate studies (e.g., a study testing the drug for glaucoma and a study testing the drug for dermatitis).

- *A single study looking at interventions alone and in combination*: More often, factorial studies test two or more interventions for the same or similar indications (e.g., the HOPE trial examined the effect of ramipril and of vitamin E on cardiac events; the Phase IIb Rituximab trial examined different steroid doses and Rituximab doses on rheumatoid arthritis).

Interactions as a Drawback

The main drawback to factorial design is the potential for *interaction* among different interventions. When given simultaneously, interventions can affect each other in many different ways. One intervention can affect the absorption, distribution, or elimination of other interventions (e.g., giving two drugs that are metabolized by the liver will slow the metabolism of both). One intervention can either potentiate (e.g., Bactrim can increase the anti-coagulation effects of Coumadin) or inhibit (e.g., an immunosuppressant opposes the effects of an immunostimulant) the action of another intervention. Interaction refers to this synergy or dys-synergy between two or more interventions. With interactions, factorial designs do not demonstrate the true effects of giving an intervention alone. For example, giving cyclosporine plus azathioprine is not the same as adding the effects of giving cyclosporine alone with the effects of giving azathioprine alone. In other words, combining the medications may have more than an additive effect (2 + 2 = 5). Alternatively, giving Cetuximab with other chemotherapy agents may be less effective than giving Cetuximab alone (2 + 2 = 1). Interactions can cause safety problems as well. Combining certain interventions can result in excessive medication levels, unusual adverse events, or severe effects.

Studying Interactions

Factorial designs can help to investigate intervention–intervention interactions. For instance, you may need to know what interventions to avoid when a patient is on a certain treatment. Alternatively, you may want to find combinations of interventions that can enhance treatment efficacy. Many severe medical conditions call for intervention combinations (e.g., cancer, complex and severe infectious diseases, or organ failure) since individual treatments are frequently inadequate. Factorial designs can help define dose–response surfaces. Dose–response surfaces are essentially multi-dimensional dose–response curves. Instead of having a single *X*-axis for the dose, you have multiple axes for the doses of each intervention. Varying the doses of the different interventions and

---

Example: Simple 2 by 2 factorial design

Group 1
Placebo/Placebo

Group 2
Placebo/Glaucoma drug

Group 3
Dermatitis drug/Pacebo

Group 4
Dermatitis drug/Glaucoma drug

---

3 by 3 Rituximab rheumatoid arthritis

Phase IIb design

A1	B2	C3
B3	C1	A2
C2	A3	B1

A – no steroid   1 – no Rituximab

B – low dose steroid   2 – 1 gram Rituximab

C – high dose steroid   3 – 2 gram Rituximab

FIGURE 6.14 Examples of factorial designs.

plotting the resulting response results in a multi-dimensional surface instead of a two-dimensional curve.

Reduced Sample Size and Increased Power

Factorial designs can address more than one question in one study in an elegant manner and significantly reduce the required sample size. In general, an *n*-factor study decreases the required sample size by a factor of *n*. So a two-factor study (e.g., 2×2, 3×3, or 4×4) requires half the number of patients that running two separate studies would need. A three-factor study (e.g., $2 \times 2 \times 2$) needs a third of the patients that three independent studies would require (Figure 6.15).

When used to answer two independent questions and interactions are minimal, factorial designs can significantly increase the power of a study. For example, Figure 6.16 shows that a 3×3 design with 50 patients in each group would yield 150 patients per arm to answer each question.

Having a smaller sample size brings potential problems as well, such as imbalance in groups and potential for bias. Combining the groups when analyzing results can ameliorate some but not all of these problems.

A factorial design is *incomplete* if it does not include every possible combination. Logistical issues, such as cost, resource or recruitment limitations, can prevent complete factorial designs. Incomplete factorial designs can still provide useful information in a parsimonious manner but do not provide as powerful results.

In the past, factorial designs often had logistical problems that prevented their implementation. Without computers, arranging and operationalizing complex randomization schemes and assembling and tracking numerous types of drug kits was unwieldy. However, modern computer systems have alleviated much of this logistic complexity.

Greco-Latin Square

A Greco-Latin square is a factorial design within a Latin square. Although rarely used in clinical trials, Greco-Latin squares can help evaluate two sets of factors. All of the problems and caveats of Latin square designs and factorial designs apply. The example illustrated in Figure 6.17 evaluates

---

Impact on sample size, 3 by 3 factorial design:

Sample size is reduced 2-fold

A1	B2	C3		50	50	50	= 150
B3	C1	A2		50	50	50	= 150
C2	A3	B1		50	50	50	= 150
				150	150	150	

With 50 patients per group

A *vs.* B *vs.* C compares 150 pts *vs.* 150 pts *vs.* 150 pts

and

1 *vs.* 2 *vs.* 3 compares 150 pts *vs.* 150 pts *vs.* 150 pts

If the studies were conducted independently, the sample sizes for each of the studies would have been 450 each, for a total of 900 patients in the two studies.

FIGURE 6.16 Impact on sample size.

---

3 by 3 by 3 factorial design:

Sample size is reduced 3-fold

A1X	B2X	C3X
B3Y	C1Y	A2Y
C2Z	A3Z	B1Z

A – placebo drug 1   1 – placebo drug 2   X – placebo drug 3

B – low dose drug 1   2 – low dose drug 2   Y – low dose drug 3

C – high dose drug 2 3 – high dose drug 2 Z – high dose drug 3

---

2 by 2 by 2 factorial design:

Sample size is reduced 3-fold

A1X	B2X	B1X	A2X
B2Y	A1Y	A2Y	B1Y

A – placebo drug 1   1 – placebo drug 2   X – placebo drug 3
B – drug 1   2 – drug 2   Y – drug 3

FIGURE 6.15 Three factor study reducing sample size.

A1 → B2 → C3

B3 → C1 → A2

C2 → A3 → B1

A – placebo

B – 1 mg/kg of drug

C – 5 mg/kg of drug

1 – traditional counseling

2 – psychotherapy

3 – no counseling

FIGURE 6.17 Greco-Latin square.

a psychoactive medication that has different doses and psychiatric counseling that has different levels (traditional, psychotherapy, and none).

6.5 CLUSTER AND NESTED DESIGNS

Cluster designs randomizes patients at a group level, as shown in 6.18a. Nested designs have one or more factors imbedded within one or more other factors as shown in 6.18b (e.g., randomly select hospitals to do testing and then within each selected hospital, randomly select patients to be tested). In the first five hospitals, randomly selected myocardial infarction (MI) patients receive aspirin, and in the second five hospitals, randomly selected MI patients receive Clopidogrel. Of the patients in the first five hospitals, a randomly selected

half receive thrombolysis and the other half percutaneous transluminal coronary angioplasty (PTCA). The patients in the second five hospitals may be randomized in a similar way to receive thrombolysis vs. PTCA, or they might be allowed to receive therapies at the physician's discretion. A nested design is different from a factorial design in that the randomization occurs hierarchically, and the first randomization can influence the second randomization (which can influence the third randomization, etc).

Nested designs are also known as *hierarchical designs*, because factors are randomized in a clear hierarchy (i.e., order). A nested design has multiple *levels*. Figure 6.19 is an example of a 3-level design (e.g., hospitals, patients, and anti-platelet therapy). At each level, a nested design appears to be a simpler design (e.g., at one level, you are randomizing only hospitals; at another level, you are randomizing

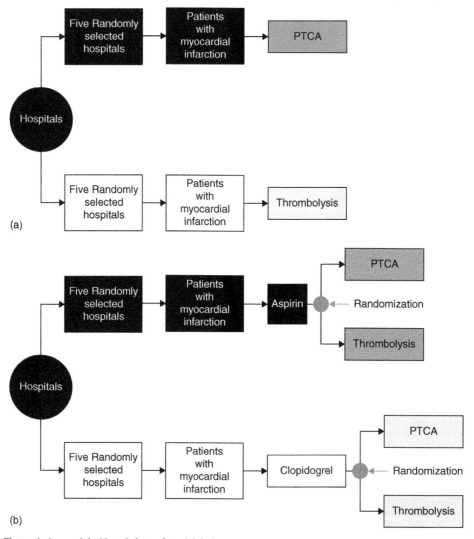

FIGURE 6.18   (a) Cluster design; and (b) Nested cluster factorial design.

only oral medications). A nested design allows testing for difference across multiple levels (e.g., at the hospital level and at the patient level).

Nesting is different from stratifying. Figure 6.20 illustrates this difference. When stratifying, you randomize patients within each strata. When nesting, you randomize by groups, and then again by patients.

Let us use an analogy to further shed light on the differences between nested and stratified designs. Pretend that you have a mall or avenue of stores and shops (e.g., Fifth Avenue in New York City, Newberry Street in Boston, or the Great American Mall in Minnesota). In a nested design, you would select some of the stores and then enter the selected stores to shop and buy items. You never even enter the stores that are not selected. Your final collection will have shopping bags from only some of the stores. A stratified design is similar to entering, shopping in, and buying items from every store in the mall or on the avenue. Ultimately your collection will have items and shopping bags from every single store.

At each level, selections or treatment assignments can occur either randomly or nonrandomly. So for example, you may randomly select hospitals or choose hospitals with the largest number of patients. You may have every patient in Hospital 1 receive Clopidogrel or randomly select some to

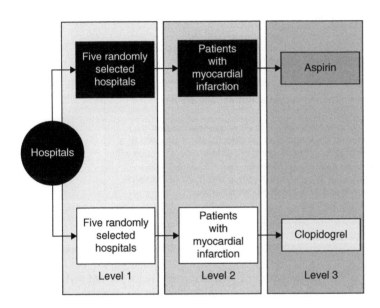

FIGURE 6.19 Heirarchical or nested three-level design.

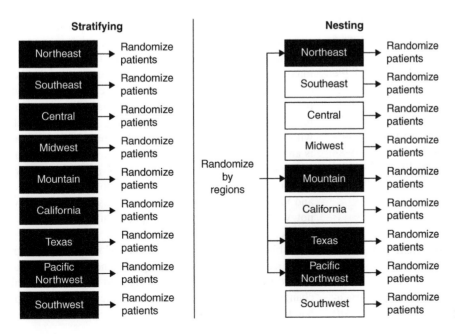

FIGURE 6.20 Stratifying vs. nesting.

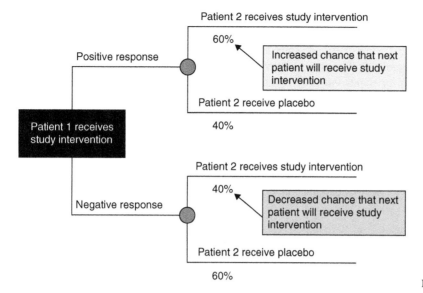

FIGURE 6.21   Sequential design.

Pharmacokinetic studies appear sequential but usually are not

At first glance, Phase I pharmacokinetic studies appear to be sequential studies. You administer a dose, check for effects, and, depending on the effects, either proceed to a higher dose or stop. However, such studies primarily compare different dose groups with each other and do not compare doses vs controls. So rather than sequential studies, Phase I pharmacokinetic studies are actually non-parallel group design or (if the same patient is dosed repeated with different doses of the drug) within-group crossover/modified Latin square design studies.

FIGURE 6.22   Phase I pharmacokinetic studies are not sequential studies.

receive Clopidogrel and others to receive aspirin. Selection or assignments at each level significantly influence selections or assignments at subsequent levels. So if everyone in Hospital 1 is assigned to receive only Clopidogrel, it will be impossible for any patient, regardless of his or her race, age, or co-morbid conditions, in Hospital 1 to be given Clopidogrel in your study. If Hospital 1 serves a pre-dominantly African American community, then many more African American patients will end up receiving Clopidogrel in your study. So your study's nesting structure and selection methods are very important. Inattention to these aspects may introduce significant bias to your study. Blinding relevant study personnel to the nesting structure and selection methods can avoid important biases (e.g., physician might deliberately send patients to one hospital in order to ensure that they receive a particular treatment).

6.6 SEQUENTIAL DESIGNS

6.6.1 Individual and Group Sequential Design

In a sequential design study, you administer the intervention or control to a single patient (*individual sequential*)

or a group of patients (may be a pre-defined number as in a *group sequential* design), analyze the results, and then based on the analysis modify the study for the next patient or group of patients (Figures 6.21 and 6.22). For example, when comparing several different candidate drugs, every time a patient responds to a particular drug, you may increase the probability of the next patient being randomized to receive that particular drug. This helps to maximize the number of patients who receive the beneficial drugs and minimize the number of patients who receive the no-effect drugs. In turn, this will substantially reduce the necessary sample size. You can do all of this without breaking the blind. An individual sequential study is analogous to approaching a salad bar or buffet table and trying small samples of each food. For subsequent trips to the bar or table, you continue to eat those foods you liked and ignore those foods you disliked. As a result, you will not waste time and stomach space eating food that you dislike.

Table 6.1 lists the requirements of sequential designs. The success of a sequential design depends on readily available results, quick decision making, and the ability to make changes in an agile manner. Bureaucratic and administrative hassles and barrier can impair such a design.

TABLE 6.1   Requirements of Sequential Designs

Requirement	Examples in which sequential designs are …	
	Possible	Not possible
Intervention's effects occur rapidly	Pain relief medication	Multiple sclerosis medication (outcomes may takeover a year to occur)
Measurement and analysis of effects is relatively easy and straightforward	Blood test	Specialized surgical procedure required to check change in tumor size
Altering trial is feasible	Can easily reallocate resources	Facilities and resources need to be reserved 1 year in advance

6.6.2 Group Sequential Design: Drop the Loser

Here is an analogy to illustrate the "Drop the Loser" design. Say you are exploring careers. While you shadow a dentist, seeing some blood makes you faint. This episode compels you to drop any health care related field (e.g., physician, emergency medicine technician, nurse, etc.) from your list of possible career choices.

Similarly, a "Drop the Loser" design involves performing an interim analysis during the course of the study and dropping one or more of the arms that are showing negative or undesirable results (e.g., If preliminary results show that a 2 mg dose of a medication has no effect, why continue any patients in that study arm?). "Dropping the Loser" can occur unexpectedly or as planned. Interim analysis may show an unexpectedly and unacceptably high adverse event rate in one arm. So dropping the arm may be in the interest of patient safety (e.g., recommendation of the Data Safety Monitoring Boards). Also, cost overruns can compel investigators to eliminate the study arms that are showing no effect. Alternatively, dropping one or more arms is part of the overall plan. For example, Phase II data may not strongly suggest a single ideal dose. So a Phase III study may start off giving different doses to different study arms with plans to drop those arms that show little or no effect.

6.6.3 Group Sequential Design: Play the Winner

Modifying the previous analogy demonstrates the "Play the Winner" design. While you follow the dentist, a patient expresses significant gratitude for relieving her chronic tooth pain. Seeing this convinces you to keep any career that directly helps people on your list of possible career choices (e.g., physician, nurse, EMT, immigration lawyer).

The "Play the Winner" design is the opposite of "Drop the Loser" design. Instead of eliminating arms that show no or undesirable effects, the "Play the Winner" design entails enrolling additional patients into arms that appear the most promising (and, in turn, away from arms that are not promising). For example, a dose escalation Phase I study might proceed with four patients per study arm until detecting some drug effects, at which time an additional 10 patients are enrolled into the more promising arms. This allows you to collect more data on the targeted dose, to make a better estimate of efficacy and safety.

Various randomized play-the-winner (RPW) rules can assign patients to study arms after preliminary results are available. Here are the basic steps for RPW designs:

- Analyze preliminary results.
- Determine which study arms are showing promising results (and by how much).
- Weight probabilities so that patients are more likely to be randomized into promising arms.

Figure 6.23 shows an example of a simple RPW rule. In this case, there are only two study arms and a dichotomous outcome (i.e., only two possible outcomes: yes effect or no effect). As you can imagine, RPW rules become more complex when the number of study arms or possible outcomes increases.

6.6.4 Group Sequential Design: Modify Dose

Group sequential designs frequently are used for intervention dosing decisions. The goal is to minimize the number of patients exposed to futile or toxic doses. After administering a dose of an intervention to a patient group, assess the response and determine whether you should change the dose. Toxicity means you should lower the dose. A relative lack of effects may prompt you to raise the dose. Such a design is common in oncology trials (see Figure 6.24). As with the other sequential designs, sequential dosing designs require intervention response to be relatively rapid. Otherwise, many patients would be subjected to unwarranted doses before the decision is made, unless

Simple randomized play-the-winner (RPW) rule

Example:
1. Preliminary results:
    Study Arm A (Intervention): 14 of 20 patients showed an effect.
    Study Arm B (Placebo): 7 of 20 patients showed an effect.

2. Twice as many patients showed an effect in Study Arm A vs. Study Arm B.

3. *Alter randomization probabilities*: 66% (Instead of 50%) chance of being assigned to Study Arm A and 33% (instead of 50%) chance of being assigned to Study Arm B.

General Rule:
Preliminary Results: δ = Number of Arm A patients showing effect/(Number of Arm A patients showing effect + Number of Arm B patients showing effect)

Probability of being assigned to Study Arm A = δ
Probability of being assigned to Study Arm B = $1 - \delta$

FIGURE 6.23 Simple randomized play-the-winner (RPW) rule.

Sequential design in oncology trials

Oncology trials often use group sequential trials. Many oncology studies are single arm studies. So an oncology trial often has a series of prespecified efficacy bars with a different bar in each stage of the sequential trial.

Example: For instance, there might be 18 patients in the first stage with the minimal cutoff being 5 responses by Response Evaluation Criteria in Solid Tumors criteria, with many more patients to be enrolled in the second stage of the study if the cutoff criteria is met.

FIGURE 6.24 Sequential design in oncology trials.

you halt enrollment and treatment until the clinical effects are manifested and assessed.

6.7 PERIODS PRECEDING THE STUDY PERIODS

6.7.1 Run-In Periods

A run-in period occurs before randomization and gives patients an opportunity to wean off other medications or get started on the study drug. A run-in period is analogous to pre-season games before a football regular season or dress rehearsal before a Broadway musical. The run-in period allows subjects and study personnel to get ready for the real experimental periods. Results from the run-in period are not official study results.

A run-in period can help:

- *Exclude patients who do not tolerate the intervention*: A run-in period is a good opportunity to determine who will suffer adverse effects and exclude them from the trial before randomization. Without a run-in period, such patients would have to drop out of the trial, raising the trial dropout rate.

- *Wean off current therapy*: Patients may not be able to abruptly stop their regular treatments. A run-in period allows them to slowly reduce their doses and be monitored for a time after discontinuing their treatments.

- *Washout current therapy*: Current treatments may have carryover effects (i.e., treatment effects may take a while to dissipate). Run-in periods help ensure that these effects are gone by the time the trial begins. In some patients, effects may persist despite the run-in period (which serves as a washout period). Run-in periods can help identify and exclude such patients. Unfortunately, disease may flare during the washout period. So washout periods are not always feasible.

- *Standardize other treatments*: Many patients will be using other treatments during the clinical trial. Standardizing these treatments (e.g., in a trial for a congestive heart failure drug, making sure that everyone who is taking a medication for angina is taking the same type and dose of medication) can reduce variability among the patient population. For example, if asthma patients are all taking different brands of inhaled corticosteroids, and the protocol calls for steady reduction in their steroid dose, it may be necessary to have a run-in period to switch the patients to the same type of corticosteroid.

- *Establish baselines*: Sometimes observing patients over a period of time will help you better understand the severity and natural history of their conditions. (e.g., for multiple sclerosis patients, performing MRI over 6 months of run-in period in order to establish a baseline). Seeing a patient at a single point in time does not tell you whether the patient's disease waxes and wanes or is getting progressively worse or better. A run-in period helps you appreciate the full spectrum of the patient's symptoms and treatment requirements. A patient's past medical records and tests do not always provide enough reliable information. In diseases in which the endpoint has high patient-to-patient variability but good intra-patient reproducibility, establishing a baseline is necessary to conduct a reasonably sized study. Run-in periods also help establish a baseline frequency of relevant clinical events (e.g., number of anginal episodes or headaches per month).

  A run-in phase may be necessary to ensure that a patient's disease is of a certain severity (e.g., at least two asthma exacerbations within 6 months).

- *Screen out ineligible and noncompliant patients*: A run-in period can be equivalent to a test run of the trial, like an exhibition season for baseball or football. The "test-run" may demonstrate that certain patients are unsuitable for the trial (e.g., disruptive, noncompliant, or do not meet the inclusion criteria).

- *Screen for placebo response*: Placebos may have significant effects on patients. A run-in period can help exclude patients with significant placebo effects or determine whether the placebo should be replaced by another type of placebo.

- *Screen for intervention response*: Sometimes identifying those patients most likely to respond to the intervention is necessary. For example, knowing the response can affect study arm assignment (e.g., you may want a balance of different responses in different study arms). However, beware of introducing any biases when using patient response for study arm assignment.

- *Establish dosing and other intervention parameters*: During a run-in period, you can tinker with and adjust different intervention parameters (e.g., dose size, dose frequency, medical device setting, or medical device positioning) so that they are optimized for the actual trial.

- *Adjust clinical trial operations*: Having a test or practice run can help personnel get familiar with the workings of the trial and make any necessary adjustments.

- *Improve clinical realism*: Sometimes having a run-in period makes the trial more similar to real clinical practice. For example, physicians often will slowly wean a patient off old medications before starting a new medication or try test doses of the new treatment before beginning the full treatment. All of the above mentioned reasons can apply in real world clinical practice. Making the trial more clinically realistic can enhance the applicability of the study results.

Employing run-in periods can introduce some problems:

- *Changing eligibility*: During a run-in period, patients' characteristics (e.g., disease severity, weight, or lab values) may change so that they are no longer eligible for the trial.
- *Disease exacerbations*: Patients may suffer disease progression or flares while off their usual medications.
- *Increased cost and resource use*: Run-in periods require time, effort, and resources that may otherwise be used for the study periods.
- *Introduce biases*: Excluding nonresponders, placebo-responders, or noncompliant patients may not be appropriate. For study results to apply to the real world population, the study population should mirror the real world population.
- *Fatigue*: Including a run-in period extends the length of the trial. Subjects and study personnel may be more likely to withdraw or quit the longer the trial continues.

Randomization should occur after the run-in period

In general, perform randomization after the run-in period. Otherwise, you risk in introducing significant bias into the study.

6.7.2 Induction Period

An *induction period* is very similar to and sometimes considered a subtype of the run-in period. The purpose of an induction period is to prepare the patients for the study intervention. Many interventions do not need an induction period. Patients are already ready to receive treatment and the trial and data collection can commence immediately.

However, some interventions need time to take effect. Medication levels may build up slowly to therapeutic levels (e.g., certain anti-arrythmics take several days to achieve the right blood levels). The body and mind may have to get acclimated to the intervention (e.g., adjust to having a foreign body like an implanted medical device; become used to certain diet or routine). Physiological or psychological response to an intervention may be very gradual. Sometimes no response is evident before a time threshold has been crossed (e.g., physical therapy or psychotherapy). Patients may need time to learn certain methods. Sometimes establishing a trusting relationship between subjects and study personnel is essential, especially in psychiatric and chronic treatments.

In some cases, certain procedures or conditions must precede your intervention to prepare the patient. Without such preparation, your intervention may be less effective or your trial results may be invalid. Sometimes you will need to adjust patients so that they all exhibit the same symptom or physiological state (e.g., a trial of an atrial fibrillation drug that is designed to maintain sinus rhythm may require that all patients be cardioverted into normal sinus rhythm before the beginning of a study; a trial of a drug designed to maintain lupus remission may require another intervention to put patients into remission first).

Such conditions do not always imply that an induction period is necessary. Preparing the patients for the intervention or building up the intervention's effects can be part of the actual trial. However, an induction period can help:

- *Guarantee that patients and their conditions start the trial at the same level*: An induction period can weed out patients that cannot be adequately prepared.
- *Save time and cost*: Using trial time to prepare patients consumes valuable trial time and resources.
- *Make necessary adjustments*: Sometimes patient preparation requires more time, effort, and procedures than expected.

6.7.3 Screening Period

A screening *period* is also similar to the run-in period but often is considered a specialized type of period. It is the time necessary to conduct screening tests and for the laboratory to determine eligibility criteria. It is due solely to logistics of performing the tests (e.g., if an oncology trial requires histological confirmation of the tumor type as part of the inclusion criteria, then the time spent waiting for the central laboratory to read and prepare the report are part of the screening period).

6.8 TREATMENT AND FOLLOW-UP

6.8.1 Treatment Administration and Follow-Up

A period may consist of several components:

- *Patient preparation*: Depending on the trial patients, patient preparation may be part of the run-in or induction period or part of the study period.
- *Baseline measurements.*
- *Treatment administration and follow-up.*
- *Post-study follow-up.*

Treatment administration and follow-up starts with randomization and ends with the last patient visit or last patient contact/data point. Typically, the last patient visit takes place during or shortly after the primary endpoint measurement (e.g., in a psoriasis trial, and the primary endpoint is a Psoriasis Area and Severity Index (PASI) score at 12 weeks, the last patient visit is typically at week 14 or 16; similarly, a rheumatoid arthritis study with primary endpoint at 12 months might have the last patient visit at

13 months). In most cases, treatment continues throughout most of the duration. However, sometimes treatment is very brief, followed by lengthy "treatment follow-up." (e.g., a vaccine trial follows patients for a year after a single vaccine administration).

There are two main ways of determining treatment administration and follow-up:

In *event-driven* studies, follow patients until each experiences a pre-specified event. (e.g., death in a cancer trial, a relapse of multiple sclerosis, or progression of the disease). Since some patients may not experience certain events within a finite period of time and following patients forever is impossible, follow-up usually terminates when a pre-specified number of events have transpired. (e.g., 160 of the 200 patients have experienced a relapse). You can then classify each patient as having had or not having had the event and use survival analysis (discussed in Chapter 10) to analyze the results.

Alternatively, you can select an arbitrary length of follow-up time. While event-driven studies require the outcome to be binary (dichotomous), outcomes in this method can be either dichotomous (e.g., deaths) or for nondichotomous (e.g., PASI scores). Length of follow-up depends heavily on what you are trying to measure (i.e., the hypothesis of the study). Are you trying to measure an intervention's maximal effect, average effect over a period of time, or peak and trough activities? Does the intervention prevent (which typically need longer follow-ups) or treat diseases? Is this a dose selection or exploration, safety, or efficacy study?

Important considerations include:

- *Duration of treatment*: Interventions may be episodic (i.e., last a finite length of time) or chronic (i.e., continuing). In most trials of episodic interventions, follow-up should be at least as long as the duration of treatment. Usually follow-up extends beyond treatment completion. For chronic treatments, other factors determine follow-up length.
- *Pharmokinetics and pharmacodynamics of the intervention*: Interventions that stay in the body longer typically have longer effects and, as a result, follow-up. Follow-up should be long enough for the intervention to take effect. An intervention may not exhibit effects until it reaches a steady state, which in some cases may not occur until many weeks have elapsed (e.g., amiodarone). Follow-up also should be long enough to determine whether the intervention exhibits tachyphlaxis, enhanced efficacy, or continued efficacy over time. Ideally follow-up duration should allow you to address as many safety questions as possible, including cumulative and patterns of toxicity. However, keep in mind that you may need more than one study to address all safety questions.
- *Natural history (timing and duration) of disease*: Follow-up must be long enough for the disease course to be altered by the intervention. The follow-up duration must give diseases an opportunity to progress or

wax and wane (e.g., if on average one flare of a disease occurs every 6 months, follow-up should be at least 6 months long). A rapidly progressive disease will be more amenable to shorter follow-up.

- *The intended effect/indication*: Follow-up duration can be short for interventions that provide only immediate or temporary symptom relief. (e.g., it takes only a few days to see if oral analgesics have any effect). Follow-up duration should be longer for interventions designed to provide chronic symptom relief (e.g., corticosteroid injections for arthritis pain relief). Studying interventions designed to prevent the progression of disease (e.g., Alzheimer's disease or age related macular degeneration) may take many years.

- *Statistical powering*: Variables that affect statistical analysis (e.g., the rate of disease progression or incidence of relevant clinical events) may drive length of follow-up. More clinical events or greater disease progression enhance statistical power (e.g., in an HIV vaccine study, more cases of infections; in a human growth hormone study, enough body growth to see a difference between groups).

For some diseases, already established standards may guide length of follow-up. Be aware of any relevant standards and guidelines. However, such standards and guidelines should only serve as starting points and not immutable rules when designing a study.

Determining the optimal length of follow-up is complicated. Shorter follow-up durations may lead to insufficient results. Longer follow-up durations provide more data but also cost more and may delay analyzing and releasing study results (and, in turn, delay drug or device approvals). Studies that are too long will be prone to dropouts and other biases. Longer follow-ups mean more dropouts. In planning the follow-up duration, consider the expected dropout rate and the effects dropouts will have on your sample size and study analysis (e.g., in a study of etidronate, longer follow-up resulted in decreased effect size because of dropouts. The study showed an effect at 1 year but no effect at 2 years).

6.8.2 Safety Post-Study Follow-Up

Even after completing the main study period, you may need a follow-up period to monitor for adverse events. A patient can be on an intervention for a long time before any adverse events appear. Therefore, just because a patient did not have adverse events during the study period does not mean the patients will not experience adverse events in the future. Typically, at least 6 to 12 months of follow-up may be necessary for new interventions. Follow-up may be shorter (at least 1 month) for interventions with already well-characterized safety profiles.

6.8.3 Open-Label Follow-Up Period

After a study has concluded, patients can continue into an *open-label follow-up study*. Such a study consists of observing patients on the study intervention for an extended period of time after the main formal study is concluded. This can provide:

- *Long-term efficacy data*: Over time, tolerance to the intervention may develop.
- *Long-term safety data.* Some adverse events only occur after the patient has been receiving the intervention for an extended period of time.
- *Efficacy and safety as the disease evolves*: Diseases or conditions evolve over time. A follow-up period can offer better insight about how the intervention performs when the disease or condition changes.
- Additional data to support intervention claims or approval.
- *Continuing treatment for patients*: Patients with chronic diseases who respond to the study intervention may benefit from continued treatment.

6.9 ADDITIONAL MULTI-PERIOD DESIGNS

6.9.1 Symptomatic vs. Disease Modifying Interventions

Interventions may have either temporary (i.e., symptomatic) or permanent (i.e., disease modifying) effects or both. Disease modifying interventions actually change the natural course of the disease, altering either the anatomy or pathophysiology of the disease. Symptomatic interventions do not affect the natural course of the disease in any way and instead decrease or mask symptoms. A lipid lowering agent is an example of a disease modifying intervention for coronary artery disease. By lowering cholesterol levels, the drug prevents coronary artery plaque formation. Nitroglycerin is an example of a symptomatic intervention for coronary artery disease. Nitroglycerin will relieve a patient's chest pain but does not alter the progression of coronary artery obstruction in any way. Once you take a patient off a symptomatic intervention, the patient is the same as if he or she had never been on the intervention.

Many clinical trial designs have difficulty distinguishing between temporary and permanent effects. You need a period of time after an intervention is discontinued to tell if the effects persist or dissipate. Traditional crossover designs offer one solution but are not always optimal. As we discussed earlier, crossover designs face problems when the disease progresses (either worsens or improves naturally). In this section, we discuss several multi-period designs that can help separate temporary from permanent effects even in progressive diseases.

6.9.2 Withdrawal Design

Withdrawal designs involve randomizing patients to either study intervention or placebo during the first period and then switching all patients to placebo for the second period (Figure 6.26). The first period should be long enough for the intervention to take full effect. The second period is typically longer than the first period and should be long enough for all intervention effects to dissipate ("washout"). If the intervention is disease modifying, then the effectiveness curves for the two groups should remain separate (i.e., the intervention caused permanent change in the disease). If the intervention is symptomatic, the curves should converge (Figure 6.27). This design is particularly useful in distinguishing symptomatic from disease modifying interventions in diseases that cause a progressive

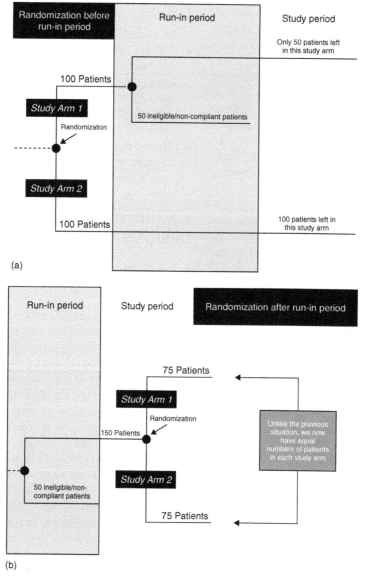

(a)

(b)

FIGURE 6.25   Randomization should occur after the run-in period.

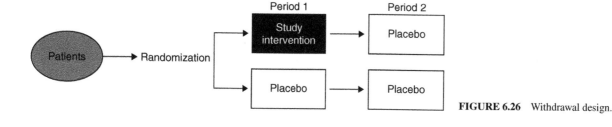

FIGURE 6.26   Withdrawal design.

decline in function (e.g., Alzheimer's disease). Crossover designs are suboptimal for such progressive diseases. The biggest problem with withdrawal designs is that patients have to remain on placebo for a fair amount of time, which can be a problem if the disease is debilitating or fatal.

6.9.3 Randomized Withdrawal Design

Randomized withdrawal designs (Figure 6.28) involve initially treating some or all patients with the study intervention in the first period, and then randomizing responder patients to either placebo or continued study intervention treatment for the second period.[a] Patients remain on the study intervention or placebo until the treatment fails (e.g., symptoms return). If the study intervention has long-term efficacy, the responder and the non-responder efficacy curves should remain separate with time if the study intervention has long-term efficacy (Figure 6.29). If the study intervention has only short-term efficacy (e.g., tolerance develops) then the two curves will converge.

Randomized withdrawal design is an option when you desire long-term efficacy data but long-term placebo-controlled design is not practical or ethical. Like withdrawal designs, randomized withdrawal designs are superior to crossover designs in evaluating progressive diseases. It is also appropriate if long term place to treatment is not possible. Compared to withdrawal designs, this design minimizes the amount of time a patient is on placebo and the amount of time a patient receives an intervention that does not work.

However:

- *Carryover effects may be a problem.*
- *Taking patients off treatments abruptly can be dangerous.* Randomized withdrawal designs work best in trials of healthy volunteers (e.g., Phase I and II trials) who can

tolerate being off treatments. When you must take patients who need treatment off treatments in such designs, use caution, make sure you obtain informed consent, and provide adequate care during the withdrawal period.

- *Changes in the natural course of the disease can confound results.*

6.9.4 Active Extension Design

Active extension designs are similar to withdrawal designs in that patients are randomized to either study intervention or placebo during the first period. The difference is that for the second period, all patients are switched to the study intervention (Figure 6.30). Both periods should be long enough for the intervention to take full effect. The group that started on the study intervention during the first period will have a head start (i.e., have been on the study

---

[a] Katz, R. FDA, Evidentiary standards for drug, development and approval. *NeuroRx*, **1**:307–316, 2006.

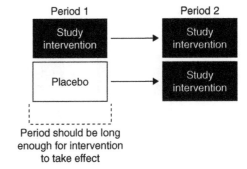

FIGURE 6.29 Randomized withdrawal design efficacy curves.

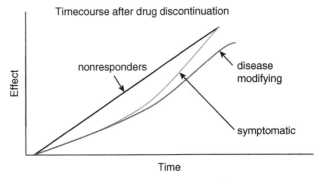

FIGURE 6.30 Active extension design.

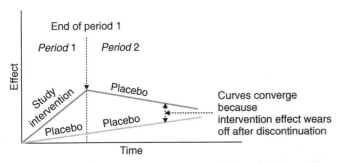

FIGURE 6.27 Efficacy curves in withdrawal design when intervention is symptomatic.

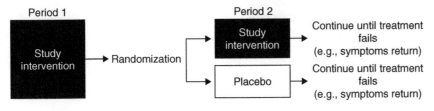

FIGURE 6.28 Randomized withdrawal design.

intervention for a longer period of time). If the intervention is disease modifying, then the effectiveness curve for this group should remain ahead of the curve for the other (placebo first then study intervention) group. If the intervention is symptomatic, the effectiveness curve for the placebo first group should "catch-up" (i.e., converge) with the study intervention first group (Figure 6.31).

6.9.5 Randomized (Staggered) Start Design

Staggered start designs switch different groups of patients from placebo to study interventions at different times (e.g., one group might start at time 0 and another group after 6 months). Randomized start designs do this in a randomized fashion. Figure 6.32 illustrates an example. If measurements of the treatment effectiveness in the different groups converge over time, the intervention probably has a symptomatic rather than a disease modifying effect. Conversely, if the effectiveness curves separate over time, the intervention either just works better over time or actually modifies (i.e., changes) the nature of the disease.

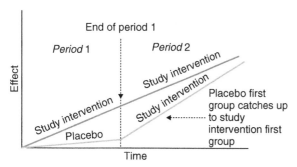

FIGURE 6.31   Active extension design effectiveness curves.

6.10 DESIGNS TO MINIMIZE EXPOSURE TO INEFFECTIVE TREATMENTS

6.10.1 Placebo and Ineffective Treatments

Unfortunately, as we discuss in Chapter 2, many clinical trial designs subject patients to placebo or ineffective treatment for an extended period of time. By definition, placebos have no biological effect, and study interventions have undetermined effects (which is why you are doing the study). Some diseases require continuous effective treatment. Otherwise, patients will suffer debilitating or even fatal effects. Examples of such diseases include nearly any type of organ failure (e.g., congestive heart failure), moderate-to-severe diabetes, infectious diseases, and cancer. In many cases, early and consistent treatment is essential to curing or limiting the damage of the disease (e.g., diagnosing and treating cancer in its early stages offers the best chance at cure). Even if the disease is not life threatening or does not cause permanent damage, withholding standard established treatments can induce a lot of suffering in the patients (e.g., not giving pain-relief medications for severe back pain). Two different ways of approaching this problem are continuing patients on effective treatments while conducting the trial (add-on design) or minimizing the amount of time patients are off known effective treatments (early-escape design).

6.10.2 Early-Escape Design

The early-escape design involves removing participants from the study when their diseases attain a certain pre-defined severity level or do not respond to a pre-defined extent. Figure 6.33 illustrates an example of this design. The failure rate and time to withdrawal can serve as efficacy measures. This design requires close, continuous monitoring. As soon as patients pass or do not pass the pre-defined

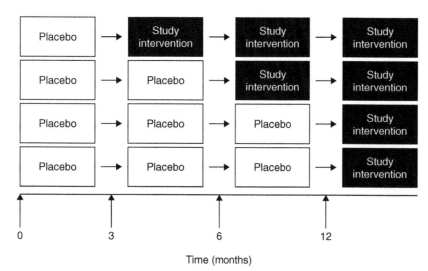

Time (months)

FIGURE 6.32   Staggered start design.

thresholds, you must quickly withdraw them from the study and place them on their regular treatments.

This early-escape design is analogous to watching closely a turkey cooking in the oven. You have to be very careful that the turkey is cooking evenly and not getting overcooked and burned. The key is setting and sticking to specific thresholds before putting the turkey in the oven (e.g., stop cooking if the turkey changes to a certain color; do not continue at the same cooking temperature if the turkey temperature is not high enough or the color has not changed after a certain amount of time).

The early-escape design is more suitable for slowly progressive diseases than for wildly waxing and waning diseases. In a waxing and waning disease, distinguishing between a temporary worsening or permanent worsening of the disease can be very difficult. Rapidly progressing diseases may not afford enough time to make proper assessments and treatment decisions.

Here are some potential challenges:

- *Close monitoring must be possible.* Patients must be accessible and compliant. They must be able to return frequently for monitoring measurements.
- *Close monitoring is very time, labor, and resource intensive.* You may not have the necessary personnel and resources to do such close monitoring.
- *Measures of disease progression must be convenient, reliable, and accurate.* Some diseases are easy to monitor (e.g., checking symptoms and physical exam findings and measuring ejection fraction for congestive heart failure). Others are much more difficult to monitor. Some measurements (e.g., checking an MRI for tumor growth) are too expensive or invasive to perform frequently.
- *Time lag of intervention response.* This design works better for interventions that have relatively rapid measurable effects. If an intervention's effects take 3 months to manifest, then you will have to wait at least that long before deciding whether to keep the patient in the trial.
- *Time lag of measurements.* A disease may progress significantly before measurements change. Once measurements have changed, treatment may be too late.

6.10.3 Add-On Design

In an add-on design, a placebo-controlled trial of a study intervention takes place while patients stay on established effective treatments (Figure 6.34). In other words, the trial occurs "on top" of patients receiving regular treatment. Patients on placebo are also on established effective treatments. Patients on the study intervention also remain on established effective treatments. This design confers several advantages:

- *No one ever goes completely untreated.* Placebo patients basically are on established effective treatments. Unless the study intervention counteracts the effects of the established treatment, patients on the study intervention will be on multiple treatments that could treat the condition.
- *Allows you to study intervention interactions.* Like factorial designs, add-on designs offer the chance to see how multiple interactions interact with each other.

The add-on design does have some potential problems:

- *Treatment interactions may occur.* Being on simultaneous treatments can be dangerous. The study intervention may counteract or potential the side effects of the established treatment. For these reasons, this design works best when the study intervention has a different mechanism from the established treatment.
- *Ascribing effects can be difficult.* If a patient improves, Is it due to the study intervention or the established effective treatment? The "placebo" arm may help but does not always fully answer this question.

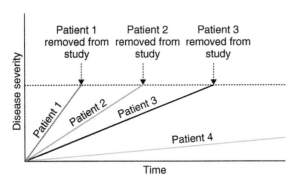

FIGURE 6.33 Early escape design.

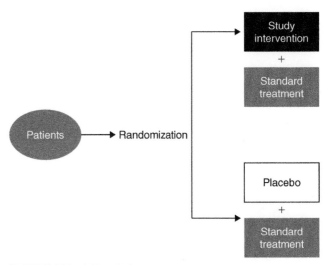

FIGURE 6.34 Add-on design.

Chapter 7

Endpoints

7.1 CHOOSING THE RIGHT ENDPOINTS

7.1.1 Characteristics of a Good Endpoint

As discussed in Chapter 4, an endpoint is defined as an overall outcome that a clinical trial aims to measure. This outcome can be a disease characteristic, health state, symptom, sign, or test (e.g., laboratory, radiological) results. Using the same analogies from Chapter 4, endpoints are like final scores in sports, final grades in college courses, and final box office receipts for a movie. Whether an intervention (e.g., drug, device or procedure) achieves an endpoint determines if it is a success or a failure. Regulatory agencies such as the Food and Drug Administration (FDA) base drug and device approval decisions on clinical trial endpoints. Early in the development and evaluation of an intervention, endpoints are used to determine the safety and biological activity of an intervention. Later on, endpoints help decide whether a drug provides a clinical benefit. These results are then extrapolated to entire populations of patients based on similarities to the patients in the clinical trials.

The terms "endpoint" and "measure" are terms that are sometimes used loosely in clinical trials. For example, "endpoint" and "measure" are sometimes used to refer to any one of the following:

1. General clinical phenomenon being measured: the general disease or disease characteristic
   - Blood pressure
   - Congestive heart failure
2. Specific clinical phenomenon being measured: an aspect, usually the most significant aspect of a disease
   - Systolic blood pressure
   - Mean blood pressure
   - Exacerbations of congestive heart failure
3. Specific clinical parameter at a specified interval: the aspect of the disease, with a specification regarding duration of observation or follow-up
   - Systolic blood pressure at 12 weeks
   - Congestive heart failure exacerbations over 6 months

4. Specific measure at a specified interval: same as #3, but with specification of the scale used for the measurement
   - Systolic blood pressure at 12 weeks measured in mmHg
   - Number of congestive heart failure exacerbations over 6 months
5. Specific measure at a specified interval, with measurement methods: same as #4, but with detailed method of obtaining the measurement
   - Systolic blood pressure at 12 weeks measured in mmHg, measured after sitting for 5 minutes, repeated 3 times and averaged
   - Number of congestive heart failure exacerbations over 6 months, as defined as need for hospitalization or ER visit
6. Specific measure at a specified interval, with analytic methods: same as #5, but with specification about how the data will be manipulated to draw inferences and conclusions
   - Mean change in systolic blood pressure at 12 weeks compared to baseline measured in mmHg
   - Percentage of patients who had at least 5 mmHg decrease in systolic blood pressure at 12 weeks compared to baseline
   - Frequency of congestive heart failure exacerbations over 6 months, as defined as need for hospitalization or ER visit
7. Specific measure at a specified interval, with analytic methods and comparator group: similar to #6 but specifies a comparator group
   - Mean change in systolic blood pressure at 12 weeks compared to baseline measured in mmHg, compared to placebo
   - Frequency of congestive heart failure exacerbations over 6 months, as defined as need for hospitalization or ER visit, compared to frequency during the previous 6 months

Often, the details of the measure and endpoint are not well described, because sometimes the clinical phenomenon can be measured or characterized in different ways with similar results (for example, many drugs have collinear effects on mean blood pressure and systolic blood pressure so measurement of either yields similar results) or because the researcher chooses to use endpoints that have been used previously by previous researchers. In many cases, this is acceptable.

However, in many other situations, even slight changes in the measurement, the time interval, comparator group, etc. can have a profound effect on the ability of a study to answer the question, the strength of the conclusions that can be drawn, the sample size, and so on. It is therefore imperative that the endpoint and measure be chosen with clear understanding of the implications of the choice.

It is important to distinguish between measure and endpoint. We define "measure" as a numeric, mathematical, or other way of assessing a clinical event or characteristic. A measure maps some aspect of the item or phenomenon onto a scale. Some common measures include mmHg, mortality rate, and number of days in the intensive care unit.

We define "endpoint" as the clinically relevant property that is being measured. For example, "mmHg" is a measure, and "change in mean blood pressure after 6 weeks of therapy" is an endpoint. The measure is used to quantify the endpoint. An endpoint is expressed as a measure that is put in context, with specified time interval and analytical methods.

The endpoints chosen can dramatically affect results and interpretation of a clinical trial. In sports and college courses, the scoring system and grading criteria can dramatically affect the final scores (and hence the winners and losers) and final grades (and hence the honor students and those who flunk), respectively. For example, using a racket to hit a ball past your opponent will result in points in tennis, but not in basketball. Similarly, writing a nice essay may help your grade in a history class, but not in a mathematics class. Similarly, if inappropriate endpoints are used, then a clinical trial may mistakenly show that the intervention has or does not have a benefit or that the intervention is safe or not safe.

As discussed in Chapter 4, there are many different ways to measure the same phenomenon. We mentioned that even a simple question like "how far is it from San Francisco to Chicago?" can have a myriad of different answers. Therefore, it is crucial to specify the criteria being used. Measuring the air, driving, or postal distance from downtown to downtown,

SFO to O'Hare, or city limit to city limit can give very different answers. Therefore, in clinical trials, it is essential to be very specific when choosing and defining endpoints.

Figure 7.1 lists the characteristics of a good endpoint. We will discuss *clinical relevance* and *responsiveness* in detail in the following sections but there are several other key characteristics of a good clinical endpoint.

First, the endpoint must closely and comprehensively reflect the overall disease being treated. Using our previous analogies, counting only the number of field goals made would not be an appropriate way to score a football game, and considering only class participation may not be the best way to grade a freshman history class. Field goals only represent one part of a football game, and class participation may reflect only one aspect of a student's abilities and knowledge. Similarly, an endpoint that only captures one aspect or component of a disease may not suffice. For example, if the disease being treated were systemic lupus erythematosus (SLE), an endpoint focusing just on skin manifestations may miss the cardiac, pulmonary, and renal manifestations of lupus. If the intent of the therapy were to improve the overall status of a patient with SLE, a skin manifestations measure would be an inappropriate endpoint. On the other hand, if the drug is only intended to improve skin manifestations, this endpoint may be acceptable.

Second, the endpoint should capture enough appropriate information for you to analyze and draw appropriate conclusions. In general, knowing more useful information is better. For example, knowing the actual cardiac ejection fraction by percentage is usually better than just knowing whether the ejection fraction was normal or reduced. Checking for disease remission at 12 and 48 weeks provides more information about when remission actually occurs than just checking at 48 weeks.

Third, the endpoint should be reliable. Reliability is the "consistency" or "repeatability" of the endpoint. Double-checking (or triple-checking) the measurements for an endpoint should produce similar values, that is, the endpoint should be reproducible and verifiable. The measurement should not vary significantly depending on who measures it. In the same way, a written test for a college course should not yield wildly changing scores every time the same person takes the test. Ideally, you should record and archive endpoint measurements as well as the settings and

- Clinically relevant
- Closely and comprehensively reflects overall disease being treated
- Rich in information
- Responsive (sensitive, discriminating, and has good distribution)
- Reliable (precise, low variability, and is reproducible) even across studies
- Robust to dropouts and missing data
- Does not influence treatment response or have biological effect in and of itself
- Practical (implementable at different sites, measurable in all patients, economical, and noninvasive)

FIGURE 7.1 Characteristics of a good endpoint.

techniques used to obtain them, so that people can review them at a later date.

Fourth, the endpoint should be robust to dropouts and missing data. Patients will drop out of trials. Data will be lost. So you will have to predict what measurements would have been for those instances. For example, all-cause mortality is relatively robust to a few dropouts because you may treat dropouts as deaths. However, the frequency of flare is not robust because you cannot predict how many flares the patients who dropped out would have had during the study.

Finally, two characteristics that were mentioned in our Chapter 4 discussion about measures are particularly important for endpoints. The endpoint should not influence treatment response or have a biological effect on the patient; and the endpoint should be practical from an implementation, economic, and patient comfort standpoint.

7.2 CLINICAL RELEVANCE

7.2.1 Overview

One of the most important aspects of selecting and defining an endpoint is its *clinical relevance*. The most sensitive and reliable measure is of little use if the results do not have clinical meaning or cannot be extrapolated to an endpoint that has clinical meaning. Clinical relevance is dependent on several factors, including importance of the endpoint being measured, the magnitude of the change, and functional outcome. Ultimately, though, what is clinically relevant is what matters to the patient.

As the *Pyramid of Clinical Relevance* in Figure 7.2 depicts, emotive feelings from symptoms are most important to patients (and therefore, most clinically relevant) followed by symptoms, signs, and then medical test results. Patients care about symptoms and any threats to their functional status and survival. They only care about laboratory values, radiology findings, or other test results if they impact their symptoms, functional status, or survival. The emotional reaction to the symptoms determines which symptoms are worse: the worse the feelings, the more the patient will want to avoid or eliminate the symptoms. For example, pain would not be relevant if it caused absolutely no distress. It is important to distinguish between symptoms and the emotive response to the symptoms, because different patients may have different emotive reactions to the same set of symptoms (e.g., a stoic person may not have the same reaction to a given level of pain as a more emotional person). As patients often have emotive feelings attached to common diagnoses, the diagnosis associated with a disease can sometimes become a highly clinically relevant endpoint (e.g., telling a patient that he or she had a myocardial infarction can be very distressing).

Treatments can target different points in the Pyramid of clinical relevance. An intervention may affect the emotive response to the symptoms without affecting the symptom itself [e.g., ziconotide can significantly decrease the negative emotive component of pain but only have a moderate effect on traditional pain scales such as visual analog scale of pain intensity (VASPI)]. By contrast, there are drugs directed solely toward the symptoms themselves (e.g., diazepam reduces the symptoms of atrial fibrillation without affecting the atrial fibrillation itself).

Unfortunately, the Pyramid of Clinical Relevance in Figure 7.2 also shows that the more clinically relevant an endpoint is, the more it is subjective and difficult to measure. It is very challenging to quantify symptoms and their emotive responses. Evaluating signs can be subjective too, as it requires a fair amount of judgment from the physician. Even some laboratory measurements are subjective, as discussed in Chapter 4.

Ultimately, you have to decide the balance between clinical relevance and objectivity when choosing endpoints for your study. It is most common to use signs as endpoints, since they fall in the middle of the Pyramid of Clinical Relevance. Moreover, many endpoints rely on a

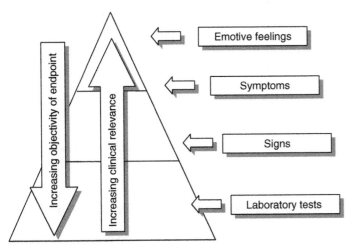

Emotive feelings. How patients feel about their symptoms and disease. Captured as quality of life or patient reported outcome measures.

Symptoms. What patients feel, such as pain, dizziness, shortness of breath. Sometimes captured as quality of life, sometimes as clinical endpoint.

Signs. Observations by physician or other personnel, such as cough, skin rash, or heart murmur. This is the most common level of clinical endpoint measurements.

Laboratory test. Surrogate measurements such as radiograph, ECG, or blood count. Generally, this is the most objective measurement, but least clinically relevant.

FIGURE 7.2 Pyramid of Clinical Relevance.

Example: Psoriasis area and severity index (PASI)

The PASI is a widely-used gold standard for assessing extensive psoriasis. To calculate the PASI, the observer grades the average redness, thickness, and scaliness of the lesions on a 0–4 scale and weights the scores by the area of skin affected. As a result, the PASI also is very subjective (e.g., in estimating these areas of skin involvement, the observer must judge where on the body a patient's arms and legs begin) that does not capture all clinical relevant aspects of psoriasis, such as degree of itching.

FIGURE 7.3 Example of the challenges of a clinical endpoint.

mixture of measures from different locations on the pyramid. For instance, an endpoint may consist of symptom measurements and laboratory test results.

The measured magnitude of effect also helps determine clinical relevance. Even though a study shows a statistically significant difference between control and treatment groups, the difference may be too small to be clinically relevant (e.g., showing that drug reduces the average length of hospitalization by 2-hours is not clinically relevant). Therefore, the endpoint should be a measure that the treatment can change significantly enough to matter to the patient (e.g., reducing hospital length of stay by 2 days will be important to the patient).

The occurrence of disease cure or remission often is most clinically relevant, simple to measure, and therefore most suitable for an endpoint. After all, ultimately a patient wants to be free of a disease and all its accompanying symptoms and emotive effects. Such endpoints have clear magnitudes of effect (i.e., the difference between having and not having active disease is significant). Frequently, presence or absence of disease is an objective measure (e.g., all of the signs and symptoms are absent and the laboratory tests are normal).

However, the presence of disease remission or cure is not always the best endpoint because they can be difficult to define. It is not always clear if and when active disease is occurring. For example, how does one delineate remission for a pleomorphic (i.e., able to assume different forms) disease, such as SLE? Any disease activity endpoint must capture all of the possible presentations and manifestations of the disease. As shown in Figure 7.3, even well-established measures of disease activity can be highly subjective and omit important aspects of the disease.

7.2.2 Example of the Challenges in Choosing Appropriate Endpoints: Mean Value

A clinical trial endpoint must be able to capture all different possible clinical scenarios. Even endpoints that appear adequate may yield misleading conclusions in some situations. The mean value (or the average value) commonly used as an endpoint, is a good example. Often in comparing the pre- and post-treatment means of a measurement (e.g., blood pressure), we assume that the shape of the

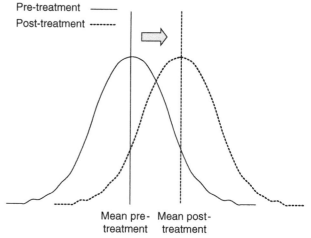

Pre-treatment ——
Post-treatment ------

Mean pre-   Mean post-
treatment   treatment

FIGURE 7.4 Treatment response in entire population with overall mean improving.

distribution curve does not change. Figure 7.4 depicts this situation with the solid line representing the pre-treatment blood pressure distribution and dashed line representing the post-treatment blood pressure distribution.

However, the curve does not necessarily remain the same. In fact, many drugs only show a response in a subgroup of patients. So as shown in Figure 7.5, just looking at the change in means is misleading.

In another scenario (Figure 7.6), the mean can actually improve with some patients doing much worse.

Or as shown in Figure 7.7, the mean might not change significantly but a subgroup might do better.

As can be seen, if a specific definable subgroup behaves differently from the overall group of patients, using just the mean as an endpoint will not adequately portray the effects of the intervention. Understanding the intervention and the population will help investigators choose more clinically relevant endpoints such as changes in means of different subgroups or numbers of patients who cross certain thresholds (e.g., how many patients went from a blood pressure of <140 mmHg to a blood pressure of >140 mmHg).

7.2.3 Determinants of Clinical Relevance

The choice of clinically relevant endpoints depends on the type of disease. What is relevant to one disease may not be

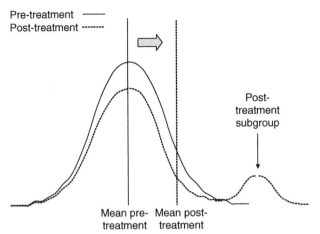

FIGURE 7.5 Positive treatment response in subgroup with overall mean improving.

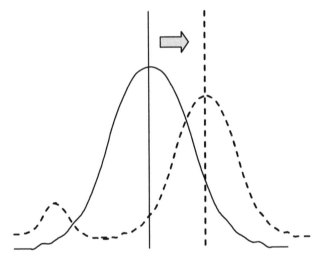

FIGURE 7.6 Negative treatment response in subgroup with overall mean improving.

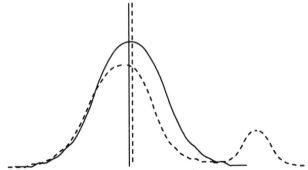

FIGURE 7.7 Positive treatment response in subgroup with no change in overall mean.

relevant to another disease. Reduction in symptoms would be a better endpoint than mortality for acute self-limited, nonfatal diseases like seasonal allergies or colds. But mortality would be a more appropriate endpoint for potentially rapidly fatal diseases like aneurysm ruptures or myocardial infarctions. For chronic debilitating diseases like arthritis,

- Sensitivity of the measure (driven by type of variable: continuous, dichotomous, etc.)
- Type of analysis (mean change, survival, etc.)
- Susceptibility to treatment
- Length of follow-up
- Robustness to drop-outs

FIGURE 7.8 What determines an endpoint's responsiveness?

endpoints such as degree of physical impairment, physical functioning, quality of life, and/or pain may be most useful. For diseases with waxing and waning courses, endpoints that have time components, such as times between flares or frequencies of flares, may be most clinically relevant.

The type of intervention also influences the clinical relevance of potential endpoints. Mortality alone would not be a correct endpoint for a drug that is designed only to ameliorate symptoms. A study of any preventive measure, such as a vaccine, may use incidence of disease as an appropriate endpoint.

The disease durations and the intervention's effects are important as well. An endpoint should extend far enough in time to include all the possible clinically relevant disease manifestations and intervention responses. For example, using tumor size at 3 months as the only endpoint for a medication that is administered over a 6-month period will underestimate response to the medication.

7.3 RESPONSIVENESS AND ANALYSIS

7.3.1 Background

Responsiveness (i.e., sensitivity of the measure to actual changes in a phenomenon) is a critical characteristic of a good endpoint, that is, when there is a change in the phenomenon, the value of the endpoint should change as well. Figure 7.8 lists the characteristics that determine an endpoint's responsiveness. Endpoints with good responsiveness (i.e., large changes in the endpoints when the phenomenon changes) allow smaller sample sizes and permit a better estimate of the clinical benefit. Of course, when the endpoint is too sensitive, it may detect too many small clinically insignificant changes, such as a 3% decrease in tumor size or a 6-hours increase in the median survival. The key is balancing responsiveness and clinical significance. In situations where investigators simply want to characterize the effects of an intervention (e.g., Phase I or II studies), a highly sensitive endpoint that detects almost any change may be desirable. When investigators want to prove the clinical benefit of an intervention (e.g., Phase III trials), a less sensitive and more clinically relevant may be indicated.

Choosing the appropriate type of analysis to perform on the endpoints is also very important. You specify the endpoints and analysis plan during the design phase (i.e., before study initiation), because they will determine the power of the study and ensure that the research question is specific. While possible and sometimes necessary, changing the endpoints and analysis plan during the trial is considered poor form and might raise suspicions of faulty blinding.

7.3.2 Landmark Analysis

A *landmark analysis* is like a photograph or snapshot in time. You choose a time point in the trial and take measurements. These measurements can be quantitative or qualitative. Examples include: how many subjects are alive 30 days after a myocardial infarction; how many patients are in remission 12 weeks after starting a therapy for Crohn's disease; what proportion of patients have healed wounds at 8 weeks; and what is the average percentage of healed area at 8 weeks.. Like a snapshot or photograph, if you have enough neighboring information, it may be easy to fill in missing information or values. (By analogy, seeing eyes, a mouth, and ears on a photograph will make it easy to draw in a nose.)

Like a snapshot or photograph, a landmark analysis cannot answer questions about what happened before or after that time point. For instance, among the patients whose diseases resolved, how long did their symptoms last and how severe were their symptoms? Figure 7.9 illustrates this problem. In evaluating a drug designed to reduce the duration of varicella symptoms, a landmark analysis would mistakenly show no difference between study groups. Landmark analyses also require larger (often significantly larger) sample size than some other types of analyses.

Landmark analyses come in two general flavors: *unpaired analyses* and *paired/change analyses*. An *unpaired landmark analysis* is akin to taking a single snapshot at the end of a trial. A *paired or change analysis* is akin to taking at least two snapshots during the trial and comparing them. An unpaired analysis is adequate if all the patients in each study group begin with relatively similar values of a measurement. Take as an example a trial evaluating the effects of growth hormone treatment on patient heights over 1 year. If all patients in the intervention and control groups start at similar heights, you may only have to do a snapshot of the patients' heights at 1 year. But if the starting heights are not similar, then taking snapshots at the beginning of the trial and at 1 year will be necessary. You would then have to calculate the change in the measure (i.e., a *change score*) for each patient (e.g., a patient who goes from 100 to 103 cm would have a change score of 3 cm or 3%). Then you could calculate the mean or median change scores for each study group (e.g., the group that received growth hormone had a mean change score of 7 cm or 7% vs. the control group which had a mean change score of 2 cm or 2%). A change or paired analysis, which offers and requires more information, is usually more sensitive and powerful than an unpaired analysis but not always necessary.

For change scores, you can calculate either absolute changes (subtracting the starting value from the ending value, e.g., 3 cm growth change) or relative differences (subtracting the starting value from the ending value and dividing this by the starting value, e.g., 5% growth change). As seen in Figure 7.10, absolute and relative change scores can look quite different. For many biological parameters (e.g., height, heart rate, blood pressure), relative changes are more appropriate because these are independent of the starting value. An absolute 5 cm change in a patient starting at 100 cm and an absolute 10 cm change in a patient starting at 200 cm would both represent 5% relative changes. It may be reasonable to use absolute changes for other measures (e.g., body temperature).

7.3.3 Frequency Analysis

Landmark analyses will not tell you how often certain events (e.g., disease flares, adverse events) occurred during the course of trial. Therefore, *frequency analyses* (i.e., counting and comparing the number of events per

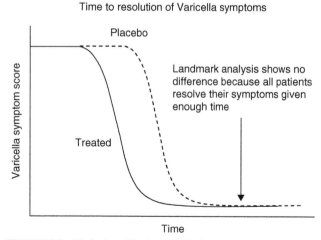

FIGURE 7.9   Limitation of landmark analysis.

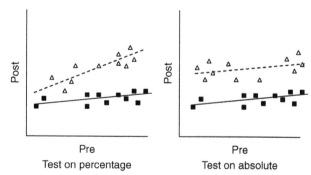

FIGURE 7.10   Change analysis – absolute vs. relative difference.

time period) may be more appropriate when studying diseases that have multiple events or recurrences such as SLE flares and asthma attacks. However, in order to use frequency analyses, the events should ideally be independent of each other; that is, the occurrence of an event should not affect the probability of a future event. When past events increase the likelihood of future events, this accentuates the difference between patients who have had an event and patients who have never had an event. For example, to see whether watching a fitness show stimulates a person to go jogging, counting the frequency of jogs would not be the best way of analyzing the results. Someone who jogs tends to do so regularly, much more often than someone who never jogs. A better measure might be to divide people into categories such as those who never jog, those who jog less than once a week, and those who jog more than once a week.

It also can be challenging to do frequency analyses when many people drop out of the trial. Predicting how many events someone would have had can be very difficult. The fact that dropouts are often the sickest patients (i.e., more likely to have many events or flares) compounds this problem. Ignoring or excluding these dropouts may dramatically bias the results.

7.3.4 Repeated Measures Analysis/Slope Analysis

Some studies involve taking measurements on each patient multiple times over the course of the study (e.g., patient blood pressure at week 1, week 2, week 3, etc.), especially when the disease or drug effects change over time. Investigators frequently will not use all of these measurements and will simply calculate the differences between the first and last measurements because dealing with repeated measurements can be difficult. Having to take so many measurements could result in many missing values, requiring investigators to predict what those missing values would have been. Also, measurements that follow complicated nonlinear patterns are challenging to analyze.

However, when an intervention is designed to change the progression of a disease, analyzing the full sets of measurements can be very useful and important. Looking at only the starting and ending points of a measurement may not be enough. This would be similar to knowing the origin and destination of a trip without knowing what occurs during the trip. *Repeated measure analysis* involves analyzing the full set of measurements and can be straightforward when the studied phenomenon (e.g., loss of glomerular filtration rate in polycystic kidney disease) follows a linear progression. Graphing the measurements as a function of time would yield a straight line. You can

then calculate the *slope of change* (i.e., the change in measurement divided by the time period over which the change occurred) for each patient and study group. Calculating the slope of change makes it easy to estimate (impute) any missing values by extrapolating or extending the line to predict what the missing value would have been. Even if the change in the endpoint is nonlinear, a repeated measure analysis is possible if the change in measurements follows a distinct predictable shape (e.g., a smooth curve). You can plot the curves and calculate and compare the areas under the curves using a variety of statistical techniques.

Repeated measure analyses can be very useful in diseases that wax and wane; but they may not be very powerful in diseases that progressively worsen. When diseases progressively worsen over time, the differences in measurements between the treatment group and control group should become greater over time (i.e., if a drug aims to slow the progression of heart failure, there should be a greater difference in cardiac function between treatment and control patients later in the trial). Therefore, using only the first and last measurements may be more sensitive in detecting differences between the treatment and control groups. Using a sports analogy, if one athlete were to start regularly lifting weights while another athlete did not, there might not be any difference in their game performance during the first year. However, after four years, the differences might be readily apparent.

A variation of repeated measure analysis is looking for a *sustained response analysis* (i.e., does the intervention have the same response at multiple time points). An intervention showing positive effects at weeks 5 and 10 is more convincing than one having effects just at 5 weeks. This is especially helpful when there is a high placebo rate. For instance, a Crohn's disease drug may induce disease remission at weeks 10 and 12 while a placebo may demonstrate remission only at week 10. Defining endpoints as disease remission at both weeks 10 and 12 therefore decreases the rate of false remission in the placebo group.

7.3.5 Time-to-Event (Survival) Analysis

Imagine that you were evaluating an intervention designed to shorten the duration of a disease, delay the onset of a disease, prevent the occurrence of an event, or extend a patient's life. You would be interested in how long it takes each patient to reach certain outcomes (e.g., disease remission, symptom resolution, disease onset, death), rather than just whether these outcomes occurred. This is especially true when the outcomes are inevitable (like death … and taxes), and the only thing you can do is delay or expedite the onset of the outcomes. You could calculate and compare the average or median time it takes for patients to reach the outcome of interest. However, some patients will have only partial information, including those who did not experience the outcome by the study completion time and those with whom you lost contact (e.g., patients move away or do not return phone calls or return to clinic). Excluding these patients from the study could introduce significant bias because you cannot predict when these patients would have experienced the outcome of interest, especially if this outcome is inevitable. Observations that contain only partial information are called *censored* observations. A *time-to-event (or survival or hazard) analysis* can handle censored observations.

An example can show why using a survival analysis is preferable to just calculating the mean or median time to events. Imagine a trial of a drug that promotes wound healing. In the placebo group of 10 patients, 2 patients healed after 2 weeks and none of the remaining 8 patients healed by the end of the trial. In the treatment group of 10 patients, 2 patients healed at 2 weeks and 8 more healed at 6 weeks. Calculating average time for healing erroneously makes the placebo group (average healing time of 2 weeks) look better than the treatment group (average healing time of 5.2 weeks).

In a time-to-event analysis each patient is followed until the trial ends. The investigator measures how long (e.g., minutes, hours, days, etc.) it takes each patient to experience the outcome of interest. If the outcome can occur more than once (e.g., myocardial infarction, syncope, hospitalization) then the investigator may do a *time-to-first event analysis* and measure the time until the patient experiences the outcome for the first time. Patients do not have to enter the study at the same time. Each patient's "stopwatch" begins when he or she starts the trial (i.e., the intervention is administered) and ends when the outcome is achieved, the trial ends, or the patient is lost to follow-up (whichever comes first).

Computing a *life table* is the simplest way to describe and analyze data in a survival analysis. The entire time course of the trial can be divided into a certain number of intervals. For each time interval, you can then compute the number and proportion of patients who remained "alive" (i.e., have not experienced the outcome of interest yet), "failed" (i.e., experienced the outcome of interest), and were censored (i.e., were lost) in that interval. Using these numbers and proportions, you can calculate the following:

$$\text{Number of cases at risk}_{\text{interval}} = \frac{\text{Number of cases that entered the interval alive}} - \frac{[(\text{Number of cases lost or censored in that interval})/2]}$$

$$\text{Proportion failing}_{\text{interval}} = \frac{(\text{Number of failures}_{\text{interval}})}{(\text{Number of cases at risk}_{\text{interval}})}$$

$$\text{Proportion surviving} = 1 - \text{proportion failing}_{\text{interval}}$$

$$\begin{aligned}\text{Cumulative proportion surviving (survival function or survivorship)}_{\text{Interval } i} &= \text{Cumulative proportion of cases surviving up to the Interval } i \\ &= (\text{Proportion surviving})_{\text{interval 1}} \\ &\quad \times (\text{Proportion surviving})_{\text{interval 2}} \\ &\quad \times \dots (\text{Proportion surviving})_{\text{interval } i-1}\end{aligned}$$

$$\begin{aligned}\text{Probability density}_{\text{interval}} &= \text{Estimated probability of failure in a specific interval per unit of time} \\ &= F_i = (P_i - P_i + 1)/h_i\end{aligned}$$

where F_i is the probability density in the ith interval, P_i is the estimated cumulative proportion surviving at the beginning of the ith interval, $P_i + 1$ is the cumulative proportion surviving at the end of the ith interval, and h_i is the width of the interval.

$$\begin{aligned}\text{Hazard rate}_{\text{interval}} &= \text{Probability per time unit that an alive case will fail in that interval} \\ &= \frac{(\text{Number of failures per time unit})_{\text{interval}}}{(\text{Average number of surviving cases})_{\text{mid point of interval}}}\end{aligned}$$

$$\text{Median survival time} = \text{Time at which the cumulative proportion surviving equals } 0.5.$$

(Note: the 50th percentile (median) for the cumulative survival function usually is not the same as the point in time up to which 50% of the sample survived unless no censored observations occurred prior to this time).

You can then compare these measurements among study groups using various statistical techniques that are beyond the scope of our current discussion.

Survival analysis allows full use of all data from patients even if they had different lengths of follow-up. This is particularly helpful when it is difficult to enroll patients (e.g., the disease is rare or the study requires a lot of time and effort from the patient). Figure 7.11 outlines an example of a multiple sclerosis study. Each bar represents

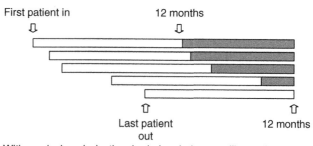

With survival analysis, the shaded periods can still contribute data, whereas in landmark analysis, only the white part can.

FIGURE 7.11   Survival analysis vs. landmark analysis.

a patient. The white portion of the bar represents the patient being "alive" (i.e., did not have an event yet) and the gray portion represents after the event when the patient becomes a "failure." If the study enrolls patients for 1 year and requires a minimum 1 year of follow-up, then the first enrolled patient will have had 2 years of follow-up by the time the last enrolled patient completed the 1 year follow-up. Unlike a survival analysis, a landmark analysis would not include information from the first patient's second year.

There is another advantage to a time-to-event analysis. If the event rate is not known prior to the study, it may be difficult to determine the length of time to run the study (e.g., if you do not know how many asthma exacerbations occur each month, how would you know how many months to run the study to see enough exacerbations?) In a time-to-event analysis, you can run the study until a certain number of events have occurred.

Survival analyses usually assume that the hazard ratio remains constant over time. However, in some clinical situations (Figure 7.12) hazard ratios cross. For example, during an initial time period the survival for a first group may be better than the survival for a second group, and after that time period the situation reverses, and survival for the second group may be better. A classic example was the prospective (though nonrandomized) study of transplantation vs. chemotherapy after induction of remission in acute myelogenous leukemia. In that study, the transplantation group fared worse in the first 6 months, but at 5 years, 49% of the patients in the group survived, compared to 20% of the control group.

7.3.6 Susceptibility to Treatment

Another important factor in responsiveness is susceptibility of the endpoint to the treatment or intervention. The chosen endpoint should be related to the potential effect of the intervention. Even though an endpoint is intimately related to the organ affected by the disease, it may not be affected by the intervention. For example, although an anti-IgE antibody should, by its mechanism of action, decrease asthma exacerbations, it would not alter a patient's forced expiratory volume (FEV_1), a measure of pulmonary function. Therefore, FEV_1 would not be a good endpoint. Figure 7.13 details another example.

7.4 PRIMARY AND SECONDARY ENDPOINTS

7.4.1 Primary Endpoint

The primary endpoint is analogous to the final score, grade, or box office receipts of a clinical trial. It is the main measurement that determines whether an intervention has worked. A positive result on the primary endpoint may be enough to establish a causal relationship between the intervention and outcome. Regardless of how many other endpoints are used in a trial, a negative

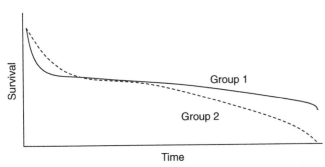

FIGURE 7.12   Crossing hazard ratios.

Case Study: Pexelizumab in coronary artery bypass surgery

Pexelizumab was studied in a double-blind, randomized, placebo-controlled Phase II trial. Investigators enrolled a total of 914 patients and stratified them into two groups: those undergoing only coronary artery bypass surgery or those undergoing coronary artery bypass surgery with concomitant valve surgery. Patients were treated with placebo, pexelizumab 2 mg/kg bolus, or with pexelizumab 2 mg/kg bolus followed by a 24-hour infusion of pexelizumab at 0.05 mg/kg/h

The primary endpoint was 30 day composite of one or more of the following:

- Non-Q-wave myocardial infarction (NQWMI) defined as CK-MB elevation (mild, moderate, or severe)
- Neurological deficits
- Left ventricular dysfunction

Investigators obviously designed the primary endpoint to maximize the event rate to reduce the required sample size. They probably expected that NQWMI was going to drive the events.

The study missed the primary endpoint. This was not surprising. Multiple prior studies had shown that surgical procedures themselves caused small clinically insignificant CK-MB leaks which could not be prevented by the medication.

If the investigators had narrowed the primary endpoint to include just moderate/severe NQWMI (CK-MB > 100 ng/ml) and death, the study would have shown a significantly positive effect. They should have heeded the prior clinical study results and understood the effects of surgery. Trying to increase the event rate by including a broad range of possible outcomes led to a negative study.

FIGURE 7.13   Case study.

result on the primary endpoint, on the other hand, means that the intervention has not achieved its purported effect. Phase III or pivotal studies generally have only one prespecified primary endpoint (usually an efficacy endpoint) with an alpha of 0.05. (Alphas and p-values are discussed in detail in Chapter 3. Although arbitrary, a p-value of 0.05 has been widely accepted as the threshold for a positive study. A p-value less than 0.05 can establish causality or an effect, while greater than 0.05 rejects the possibility of an effect. A p-value of <0.05 means that there is less than a 5% probability that the study results occurred by pure random chance. In other words, if the same trial were performed an infinite number of times and the intervention had absolutely no efficacy, the same study results or better would be seen only about once every 20 repetitions of the trial. Also, as discussed in Chapter 15, p-values are not as informative as confidence intervals, which are becoming a more common standard in study result interpretation.) (Figure 7.14)

7.4.2 Co-primary Endpoints

Some diseases and interventions can affect multiple measures. Improving one measure may not be enough to demonstrate true success in treatment, making it difficult to find one single endpoint that can demonstrate the success of an intervention. Also, sometimes demonstrating improvement at different points in time may be necessary. As a result, regulatory agencies recently have required more than one primary endpoint (or co-primary endpoints) for some trials.

Using our college education analogy, a single high grade in one course may not be enough to demonstrate ability in mathematics. The student may have to garner high grades in more than one course and potentially over different time periods (e.g., sophomore, junior year) to truly confirm his

or her ability. The multiple grades are like co-primary or multiple primary endpoints.

Splitting the Alpha

When you have multiple primary endpoints, you can "split the alpha." What does this mean? As stated previously, with one primary endpoint, the standard alpha is 0.05. With two primary endpoints, then the required alpha for each could be 0.025 or half of 0.05. If either endpoint meets a p-value of less than or equal to 0.025 then you can infer a causal relationship. Any combination of primary endpoints with p-value of 0.05 (e.g., 0.04 + 0.01, 0.01 + 0.01 + 0.01 + 0.01 + 0.01) would be acceptable.

Hierarchical Testing

Some trials have a series of related objectives, hurdles, or primary endpoints that an intervention must pass (i.e., there is a hierarchy of endpoints). For instance, an intervention may first have to prove that it can reduce the acute symptoms of a disease (the most important primary endpoint) and then prove that it can prevent disease progression (the second most important primary endpoint). An intervention may have to show a mortality benefit first (the most important primary endpoint) and then demonstrate prevention of other serious but nonfatal conditions (subsequent primary endpoints).

Using our college analogy again, in order to graduate with honors in mathematics, a student has to pass the introductory course first and then progress through a series of increasingly more advanced courses. When multiple primary endpoints fall on a distinct hierarchy, you can test whether each endpoint was fulfilled in its order of importance (i.e., *hierarchical testing*). For example, you can first determine if an intervention prevented mortality (using a p-value of <0.05). If this test is passed then you can test whether it pre-

---

Regulatory Point: Reproducibility of Studies and p Value

In general, the FDA requires two studies with a p value <0.05 (two sided). There are multiple reasons for this requirement, but the main reason is to increase confidence in the validity of the study results. They want reproducibility–to ensure it was not a fluke, due to some special aspect of the study (certain sites, the batch of drug, etc.), or fraud. Also, they want to improve the validity of the study by ensuring that in a slightly different population or slightly different endpoint that the drug works as well. In this way, they add to the confidence in convergent validity.

This requirement was put into place by CDER a while ago when the studies were not as robust. Now that the studies in general are well-designed, double-blind, placebo-controlled studies, there is an argument that there is less need for this. Furthermore, the FDA has stated that a single study can be acceptable for approval if it is robust. By this, they mean:

- $p < 0.00125$ (0.05 $\times$ 0.05 divided by 2)
- Internal consistency across subgroups
- Internal consistency across endpoints

It should be noted that in very large trials (e.g., 17,000-patient thrombolytic trial), trials with very clear results (mortality endpoint and low p value), trials that would be unethical to repeat, or for CBER products, the FDA has not been as strict with the requirement for the two trials.

FIGURE 7.14   Regulatory point: reproducibility of studies and p-value.

vented disability (again using a p-value of <0.05). You do not need to split the alpha.

Hierarchical testing works for subgroups as well. For example, if a drug meets a p-value of <0.05 for the overall group, then you can test a subgroup using a p-value of <0.05 to see if there is a significant effect. Similarly, if a study shows that Intervention 1 is noninferior to Intervention 2 (i.e., Intervention 1 is not worse than Intervention 2), then you may determine if Intervention 1 is indeed superior to Intervention 2 using a p-value of <0.05. In each of these cases, the second test is a sub-question of the primary question. You cannot perform the second test if the first test is negative. This is intuitive for the noninferiority/superiority question: an intervention cannot be superior if it is inferior. However, it is less intuitive for subgroup questions: an intervention can benefit a subgroup without benefiting the group as a whole (e.g., Herceptin works only for breast cancer patients with HER2 over expression and not for all breast cancer patients). Therefore, you carefully sequence such multiple comparisons when they can lead to spurious results. If you know that a drug will work only for a subgroup, do not do hierarchical testing in which you try to test the overall group and then the subgroup. Instead, test the subgroup then the overall group.

7.4.3 Secondary Endpoints

As we have emphasized, the success of a clinical trial depends on meeting the primary endpoint (or endpoints). However, during the trial, you may measure many other outcomes in addition to the primary endpoint. These other outcomes, otherwise known as *secondary endpoints*, provide additional, potentially valuable, information from the trial. Although secondary endpoints should be specified during the planning of the trial, interpret secondary outcomes with caution. Well-chosen secondary endpoints can enhance information provided by the primary endpoint. Achieving the primary endpoint may simply show whether an intervention has a positive effect on a disease but not fully characterize and quantify the magnitude of this effect. Prespecified secondary endpoints can examine pharmacokinetics and pharmacodynamics, important safety parameters, nonclinical endpoints, alternate ways of evaluating the primary endpoint, pharmacoeconomic results, resource utilization, quality of care outcomes, time to response, relapse/durability of response, rebound effects, and tachyphylaxis.

In general, minimize the number of secondary endpoints used in a clinical trial. Increasing the number of secondary endpoints increases the likelihood of both Type I and Type II errors and, in turn, may lead to spurious negative results. Therefore, you should ensure that each secondary endpoint addresses a clinically meaningful question and does not duplicate information already being collected.

7.5 COMPOSITE ENDPOINTS

7.5.1 Background

As we mentioned in our discussion of co-primary endpoints, often a single endpoint cannot adequately capture the potential effects of an intervention on a disease. A cardiovascular drug, for example, may cause small reductions in a variety of different potential endpoints such as mortality, incidence of myocardial infarction and stroke, and the need for cardiac catheterization and surgery. Using any one of these endpoints as a primary endpoint could require a very large sample size, since the intervention's potential impact on each endpoint may be relatively small. Also, excluding any of these endpoints may overlook potentially important drug effects. Having multiple primary endpoints would require a substantial and probably impractical increase in the sample size needed. Therefore, in these situations, using *composite endpoints* (i.e., combinations of multiple clinically relevant endpoints) may be the best way to fully characterize a disease and properly assess a treatment's effects. Extending one of our previous analogies, college course grades frequently are composite endpoints, combinations of many different components such as test scores, paper assignment, oral reports, and class participation.

Choosing and using an appropriate composite endpoint is a much more complex task than choosing and using a simple primary endpoint. The composite endpoint, of course, must be clinically relevant and consist of measures that are combined in a logical and appropriate manner. Some diseases have fairly well-established composite endpoints. But in many cases, there can be a fair amount of subjectivity in how the component measures are chosen and combined. Moreover, any combination of multiple measures rarely follows a simple linear pattern (e.g., an intervention may have a positive effect on one component measure and a negative effect on another component measure), making it difficult to analyze statistically. Therefore, in most situations, simple primary endpoints are preferable to composite endpoints.

However, there are a number of specific situations in which composite endpoints are extremely useful and potentially necessary. These include the following.

Composite Endpoints can Increase a Low Event Rate and, In turn, Sensitivity

When the outcome of interest occurs too infrequently, having a single primary endpoint may require a sample size that is too large (e.g., when mortality, which is currently ~5%, is a single primary endpoint, thrombolytic trials require over 20,000 patients). However, you must be careful when designing composite endpoints to increase the event rate. Unless each individual component endpoint is sensitive to the treatment effect, using a composite endpoint will dilute the positive effects of the drug. In our college course grade analogy, including measures that have nothing to do with a student's performance (e.g., the clothes they wear or their socioeconomic status) will decrease the ability of the final grade to truly differentiate between honors and nonhonors students. Also, the various component measures of a composite endpoint should not be competing risks. In Figure 7.15, Scenario A shows mortality as a single primary endpoint and Scenario B shows a composite endpoint that includes mortality and the incidence of congestive heart failure. Scenario B underestimates the positive effects of a cardiovascular drug, since many of the prevented deaths ended up with congestive heart failure instead.

Composite Endpoints Can Help Better Diagnose the Disease/Condition and, In turn, Increase Specificity

One measure may not be enough to diagnose a disease or condition. Sometimes multiple measures are needed. For example, determining the presence of a multiple sclerosis exacerbation may require magnetic resonance imaging (MRI) findings in addition to symptoms. So a primary endpoint of MRI findings would not be enough in evaluating a drug designed to prevent multiple sclerosis exacerbations. You would need a composite endpoint to decide which patients actually suffered exacerbations.

Composite Endpoints can Fully Capture the Heterogeneity of a Disease

Some diseases can be extremely varied in their signs, symptoms, and sequelae. Diseases (e.g., lupus, rheumatoid arthritis) can affect many different organ systems, change and evolve over time (e.g., multiple sclerosis patients may

be able to walk certain distances early in their disease, but not later), and differ in the ways they affect various subpopulations (e.g., hepatitis B in alcoholics may progress much more rapidly). Single primary endpoints may not capture all of these variations (e.g., walking distance will not be an appropriate measure of disease severity for a patient already unable to walk).

Composite Endpoints can Include Dropouts, Crossovers, and Rescue Medications as a Component

You may anticipate that many patients will drop out, crossover to other study groups, or require rescue medications because the disease symptoms, drug side effects, or testing procedures are difficult to tolerate or the study population is historically noncompliant. These occurrences in and of themselves may be important outcome measures. For example, dropouts may be a sign that a drug has too many side effects or is not adequately reducing disease symptoms.

Composite Endpoints can Help Avoid Survivor Bias When There Is Competing Risk

Sometimes you need to use a composite endpoint that includes more severe potential outcomes even if the expected primary outcomes are less severe. Figure 7.16 portrays an example of this situation: a trial of a drug expected to have little effect on mortality and significant effects on congestive heart failure hospitalization. Using hospitalization alone as a primary endpoint may underestimate the number of events, because many of the patients who would have been hospitalized may have died instead.

Composite Endpoints Can Capture Both Efficacy and Safety

Sometimes, the study's main question is whether an intervention's benefits outweigh its potentially serious side effects

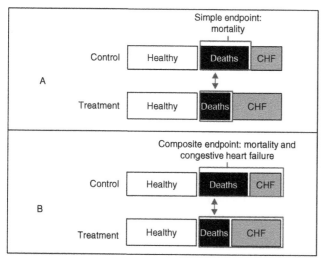

FIGURE 7.15 Example of how a simple endpoint can better capture the positive effects of a treatment: (a) Simple endpoint (b) Composite endpoint.

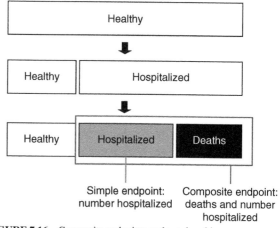

FIGURE 7.16 Composite endpoints and survivor bias.

(e.g., thrombolytic therapy can abort a potential myocardial infarction but also can cause serious intracranial hemorrhage), or whether a new intervention has similar efficacy but fewer side effects when compared to an older intervention. Both of these situations call for composite endpoints that calculate the net clinical benefit (i.e., positive effects minus negative effects) of the interventions. Simple primary endpoints that do not include either efficacy or safety measures would be inadequate.

7.5.2 Types of Composite Endpoints

Composite endpoints can be *rating scales* that yield a total score or index (e.g., the Hamilton Depression Rating Scale for depression and the ACR20/ACR70 for rheumatoid arthritis), *event rates* with an event being any one of a given set of clinically relevant occurences (e.g., in a study of organ transplant patients, the composite endpoint can be the "failure" rate 6 months after treatment, with "failure" being defined as acute rejection, graft loss, or death), or *times to the first event,* with an event again being any one of a given set of occurences (e.g., time to acute rejection, graft loss, or death).

There are several different ways to construct a composite endpoint.

Unweighted Composite Endpoints with Alternate/ Exclusive/Independent Events

Some composite endpoints treat different possible events as equivalent. Achieving a certain endpoint means having any one of a list of events. For example, glycoprotein IIb/IIIa trials have used composite endpoints that determine whether each patient experienced any one of the following: death, myocardial infarction, or refractory ischemia. A patient did not achieve the endpoint if he or she did not have any of those three events. There are two major problems with using such an endpoint. It asserts that a death is similar in clinical significance to an episode of recurrent ischemia and suggests that the three types of events are biologically related. The composite endpoint above is dichotomous or binary. There are two alternatives: "yes" the patient had one of those events or "no" the patient had none of those events. However, if each event is exclusive, composite endpoints can be non-dichotomous. Each event can be treated as a point, so that a composite endpoint with 3 $$ assume a value between 0 and 3.

Weighted Composite Endpoints with Exclusive Events

Weighting each of the events can account for the differing clinical significance of possible events in a composite endpoint. For example, you may give death a score of 5, myocardial infarction a score of 3, and recurrent ischemia a score of 2. Figure 7.17 shows some more examples of weighted composite endpoints. Ideally, the events should be exclusive and independent of one other. Otherwise the scoring becomes very complicated. For example, someone who dies cannot have further events, so death is not independent of any other event. In such a case, rather that adding the scores, the single highest score may need to be used.

You may arithmetically manipulate (e.g., add, subtract, etc.) the components of weighted endpoints only if the different components are identical or very similar in clinical significance. Adding, subtracting, dividing, or multiplying two very different components (e.g., the presence of cerebritis and the presence of urinary casts) would be like combining apples and oranges and may not make any sense.

Reaching consensus on how to weight each component of a composite endpoint can be difficult. Using novel weighting schemes that have not been well established brings the risk of having your results called into question. Moreover, the weights may have to change depending on the situation. For certain types of patients or disease presentations, a given measure may be more or less important (e.g., a measure may be a stronger indicator of a disease in African Americans).

Nonweighted Composite Ordinal Endpoints

Some composite endpoints consist of two or more different categories with a set of criteria to qualify for each category. For example, if Measure 1 is above Threshold 1, Measure 2 is above Threshold 2, and Measure 3 is above Threshold 3 then the endpoint has a value of 3. If Measure 1 is above Threshold 1, Measure 2 is below Threshold 2, and Measure 3 is above Threshold 3 then the endpoint has a value of 2. Although the endpoint looks like a quantitative measure, it is actually an ordinal measure (i.e., different categories that have a rank order), so mathematically manipulating their values would not make sense.

ACR scores are good examples of such endpoints. ACR20 (Figure 7.18) is not a 20% improvement in rheumatoid arthritis. It is a complex composite endpoint, requiring at least 20% improvement on several parameters, which must include both tender joint count and swollen joint count, and 3 out of 5 other parameters. Similarly, ACR50 requires 50% improvement on multiple parameters, and ACR70 requires 70% improvement on multiple parameters, and so forth.

One of the goals for ACR20 is to have high specificity for improvement, which requires multiple separate improvement outcomes. ACR20 is specific and sensitive in determining improvement in individual patients, but is not a continuous measure (i.e., ACR 70% is not 20% better than ACR50, and ACR50 is not 2.5 times better than ACR20). In order to achieve ACR50, the patient must have 50% improvement in multiple parameters, which is usually much more difficult than achieving an overall 50% mean improvement. Even if a patient has a dramatic improvement in one or two parameters, sub par improvement in the other

Systemic lupus erythematous

disease activity index (SLEDAI) score endpoint

Each sign or symptom is given a weighted score, and the sum of the scores is the SEDAI score.

Score		Definition
8	Seizure	Recent onset. Exclude metabolic, infectious, drug causes.
8	Psychosis	Altered ability to function in normal activity due to severe disturbance in the perception of reality. Include hallucinations, incoherence, marked loose associations, impoverished thought content, marked illogical thinking, bizarre, disorganized, or catatonic behavior. Exclude uremia and drug causes.
8	Organic brain syndrome	Altered mental function with impaired orientation, memory, or other intellectual function, with rapid onset and fluctuating clinical features. Include clouding of consciousness with reduced capacity to focus, and inability to sustain attention to environment, plus at least 2 of the following: perceptual disturbance, incoherent speech, insomnia or daytime drowsiness, or increased or decreased psychomotor activity. Exclude metabolic, infectious, or drug causes.
8	Visual disturbance	Retinal changes of SLE. Include cytoid bodies, retinal hemorrhages, serous exudate or hemorrhages in the choroid, or optic neuritis. Exclude hypertension, infection, or drug causes.
8	Cranial nerve disorder	New onset of sensory or motor neuropathy involving cranial nerves.
8	Lupus headache severe, persistent headache; may be migrainous, but must be nonresponsive to narcotic analgesia.	
8	CVA	New onset of cerebrovascular accident(s). Exclude arteriosclerosis.
8	Vasculitis	Ulceration, gangrene, tender finger nodules, periungual infarction, splinter hemorrhages, or biopsy or angiogram proof of vasculitis.
4	Arthritis	More than 2 joints with pain and signs of inflammation (i.e., tenderness, swelling, or effusion).
4	Myositis	Proximal muscle aching/weakness, associated with elevated creatine phosphokinase/aldolase or electromyogram changes or a biopsy showing myositis.
4	Urinary casts	Heme-granular or red blood cell casts.
4	Hematuria	>5 red blood cells/high power field. Exclude stone, infection, or other cause.
4	Proteinuria	>0.5 gm/24 hrs. New onset or recent increase of more than 0.5 gm/24-hours.
4	Pyuria	>5 white blood cells/high power field. Exclude infection.
2	New rash	New onset or recurrence of inflammatory type rash.
2	Alopecia	New onset or recurrence of abnormal, patchy or diffuse loss of hair.
2	Mucosal ulcers	New onset or recurrence of oral or nasal ulcerations.
2	Pleurisy	Pleuritic chest pain with pleural rub or effusion, and pleural thickening.
2	Pericarditis	Pericardial pain with at least 1 of the following: rub, effusion, or electrocardiogram or echocardiogram confirmation.
2	Low complement	Decrease in CH50, C3, or C4 below the lower limit of normal for testing laboratory.
2	Increased DNA binding	>25% binding by Farr assay or above normal range for testing laboratory.
1	Fever	>38°C. Exclude infectious cause.
1	Thrombocytopenia	<100,000 platelets/mm^3.
1	Leukopenia	<3,000 white blood cells/mm^3. Exclude drug causes.

Crohn's disease activity index (CDAI)

CDAI = 2 × 1 + 5 × 2 + 7 × 3 + 20 × 4 + 30 × 5 + 10 × 6 + 6 × 7 + (weight factor)

Crohn's disease activity index was originally designed for comparing the status of patients across two timepoints. It is still useful for pairwise comparisons. However, it is now often used for a cross-sectional assessment of patients as well.

1. Total number of liquid or very soft stools in a week
2. Sum of seven daily abdominal pain ratings:
   (0=none; 1=mild; 2=moderate; 3=severe)
3. Sum of seven daily ratings of general well-being:
   (0=well; 1=slightly below par; 2=poor; 3=very poor; 4=terrible)

FIGURE 7.17   Examples of weighted composite endpoints.

4. Symptoms or findings presumed related to Crohn's disease
   Add 1 for each set that corresponding to patient's symptoms:
   set 1: arthritis or arthralgia
   set 2: iritis or uveitis
   set 3: erythema nodosum, pyoderma gangrenosum, apthhous stomatitis
   set 4: anal fissure, fistula or perirectal abscess
   set 5: other bowel-related fistula
   set 6: febrile (fever) episode over 100° during past week.
5. Taking Lomotil or opiates for diarrhea
   0=no; 1=yes
6. Abnormal mass
   0=none; 0.4=questionable; 1 = present
7. Hematocrit [typical − current] × 6]

Weight factor: 100 × [(standard weight-actual body weight)/standard weight]

Best WR, *et al.* (1976). Development of a Crohn's disease activity index. *Gastroenterology* **70**, 439–444.

FIGURE 7.17   (Continued).

Both of the below criteria must be met	Three out of the following five criteria must be improved by ≥20%
1. ≥20% improvement in tender joint count	1. Patient pain assessment
	2. Patient global assessment
	3. Physician global assessment
2. ≥20% improvement in swollen joint count	4. Patient self-assessed disability
	5. Acute-phase reactant (ESR or CRP)

FIGURE 7.18   ACR 20 definition of improvement in rheumatoid arthritis.

Characteristics of safety endpoints

- Detrimental to the patient
- Not always pre-specified
- Not always validated
- Not always randomized or stratified in advance
- Do not necessarily have to be statistically significant

FIGURE 7.19   Characteristics of safety endpoints.

parameters will keep the score low. Back to our college course analogy, it is much more difficult to do well on all components of a college course (i.e., tests, oral presentations, class participation) than exceptionally well on just one component (i.e., perfect on the test scores).

Although, in general, a patient with ACR70 will have had a better clinical response than a patient with ACR20 or ACR50 response, this is not always the case. A patient with a 90% improvement in 6 out of 7 parameters and a 20% improvement in tender joint count have ACR20 response, while a patient with a 50% improvement in 5 out of 7 parameters could have ACR50 response. So in fact, ACR score is actually a nominal endpoint (i.e., the categories do not necessarily follow a rank order), but most people in practice treat ACR scores as an ordinal endpoint since it is a close approximation of one.

7.6 SAFETY ENDPOINTS

7.6.1 Characteristics of Safety Endpoints

Just as efficacy endpoints determine if an intervention works, safety endpoints determine if an intervention is safe. All endpoints can be safety or efficacy endpoints, depending on the context. An efficacy endpoint in one circumstance can be a safety endpoint in another, and vice versa. Efficacy endpoints are endpoints that change for the better; safety endpoints change for the worse. For example, if a drug decreases mortality, death is a survival benefit or an efficacy endpoint. If a drug increases mortality, death is a fatality, a serious adverse event, or a safety endpoint. Figure 7.19 lists the characteristics of safety endpoints.

You should specify primary and secondary efficacy endpoints before conducting a study. But you do not necessarily have to identify all safety endpoints prior to the trial, unless, of course, it is a safety study, (i.e., designed specifically to evaluate the safety of an intervention.) Unexpected efficacy events (i.e., the intervention has a surprise positive event) are usually not "valid" clinical events, because the study was not designed to evaluate them, although such events may form the basis for future studies. For example, in a trial looking at a drug's effects on heart disease, even though a patient's rheumatologic condition is cured after receiving the drug, investigators cannot claim the drug treats rheumatologic disease because the condition was not a pre-specified primary endpoint. On the other hand, even an unexpected safety endpoint is a valid clinical event. If only one patient receiving the drug had a severe allergic reaction, investigators would still have to consider a possible negative effect of the drug.

Any clinically relevant, detrimental event that is not specified as an efficacy event qualifies as a safety endpoint. For example, if the primary efficacy endpoint is reduction in asthma, asthma exacerbations, hospitalizations, or mortality can be safety endpoints.

Efficacy endpoints require a minimum number of events before they are statistically significant. In other words, until a certain number of positive efficacy events occur, you cannot claim that an intervention has an effect. For example, even if an intervention completely cured a single patient of a disease, you cannot claim that the intervention is a cure, until enough other examples occur. On the other hand, there is no minimum number of safety events that need to occur for the safety endpoint to be considered important. For example, a single case of eosinophilia myalgia syndrome or a single case of a highly unusual course of a common disease can be very meaningful.

Limitations of Safety Endpoints in Clinical Trials

Investigators use efficacy endpoints, and not safety endpoints, to determine sample size. Since safety events tend to be rarer, studies usually are not large enough to have sufficient power to statistically evaluate adverse events, unless they occur relatively frequently. It is almost impossible to make a trial large enough to detect very rare adverse events with any reliability. (e.g., even a trial with 30,000 patients cannot detect a very rare severe adverse event that occurred in 1 in 100,000 patients.) Therefore, although all safety events should be described and reported, you may not have enough cases to statistically definitively say that the intervention caused the safety events. So, if you anticipate certain safety events before a trial, prepare a prospective safety analysis plan specifying the anticipated safety events so that you may draw much stronger conclusions. Such a plan makes it less likely that a safety event could be hidden by re-categorizing events or analyzing the data in an inappropriate fashion.

Safety Endpoint Characteristics

You must understand the nature of different safety endpoints while planning and conducting a trial. Proper knowledge will help better in the design, data collection, and analysis of the trial. Here are some important concepts to remember.

Know the Population's Baseline Risks

Some safety events will occur in patients regardless of whether they receive a treatment. Even completely healthy patients have a baseline risk for many different adverse events including hospitalization and death. Patients with many pre-existing conditions will have increased risk. Therefore, to properly interpret safety data, you should know these baseline risks and choose patients in a way that minimizes these risks (e.g., healthy patients).

Be Aware of Harbinger or Sentinel Events

Harbinger or sentinel events (e.g., amaurosus fugax for stroke, nuisance gum bleeding for intracranial bleeding) warn investigators that certain safety events are occurring or will occur, allowing easier early detection and intervention.

Avoid Irreversible Safety Events and Prepare for Reversible Events

The reversibility and treatability of potential safety events affects the design and conduct of a trial. Certain safety events (e.g., asthma exacerbations) are reversible or treatable, while others (e.g., stroke) are not. You should try to avoid irreversible safety events and build in safeguards to help reverse reversible events (e.g., have antidotes available).

Understand the Timing and Time Course of Safety Events

Some safety events develop and progress slowly, allowing time for appropriate action even if they are completely unanticipated (e.g., thrombocytopenia that develops over several weeks). Others arise abruptly and progress rapidly (e.g., agranulocytosis) and can be devastating if safeguards are not already in place.

7.6.2 Clinical Trial Design Aspects

Anticipated Safety Events

You may be able to anticipate certain safety events. Data from pre-clinical studies, previous clinical studies, and studies of related compounds can provide important clues. A new drug may have the same side effects as other drugs in the same class (e.g., most beta-blockers can exacerbate asthma). A drug that caused certain problems in animals may be expected to do so in humans as well. Drugs of certain chemical structures always affect certain receptors or types of cells. The biological action of a drug can also help predict what may happen in humans. For example, any drug designed to dissolve blood clots should have bleeding as a potential side effect. Any drug that suppresses the immune system could promote infections. Any drug metabolized and excreted by the liver may lead to liver problems.

You should prospectively collect information on all anticipated safety events during the trial. Rather than passively wait for such events, actively look for them. This means performing relevant lab, radiologic, and other diagnostic tests and asking patients if they are experiencing such events.

Harbinger Safety Events

Some safety events are not in and of themselves causes for alarm but may be harbingers of more rare and serious events.

Examples include nuisance bleeding that might progress to more serious bleeding, mild thrombocytopenia that might evolve into severe thrombocytopenia, and liver function test abnormalities that may develop into liver failure. These so-called harbinger safety events should be recorded.

Unanticipated Safety Events

It is very difficult to anticipate all possible safety events, especially when the studied intervention is completely novel. Even if you have reams of data from animal studies or even prior human studies, you never know what may happen whenever you apply an intervention to humans. Even the safest interventions can have unexpected negative effects. Therefore, investigators must routinely monitor the study population and build enough flexibility into the data collection process to capture these unanticipated events.

In addition, you should always look for and collect information on certain types of unanticipated safety events. First of all, some classes of interventions are associated with specific sets of unanticipated events. For example, small molecule drugs are associated with QTc prolongation, liver toxicity, nephrotoxicity, bone marrow toxicity, and drug–drug interactions; and biologics tend to manifest immunogenicity and infusion reactions. Secondly, severe, catastrophic safety events, such as death, malignancies, and hospitalization can almost always occur. Most of these are collected by the serious adverse event reporting system. Thirdly, any drug can manifest rebound effects and tachyphylaxis. In drug rebound, when a medication wears off or is withdrawn after being used over a period of time to treat specific symptoms, the lack medicine itself can trigger the same symptoms. In tachyphylaxis, patients rapidly develop tolerance to the effects of a drug.

7.6.3 Safety Endpoint Collection and Classification

Safety endpoint collection techniques can affect the number of safety events collected. Patients are more likely to remember experiencing certain events if you ask them more frequently or inquire specifically about those events (e.g., a patient is more likely to recall having a headache if you asked him if he had a headache). Keep in mind that distinguishing an adverse event from disease progression can sometimes be difficult (e.g., is a patient death the result of the disease or the intervention?)

You can classify safety events in a number of different ways. The severity is often graded *mild*, *moderate*, or *severe*. Safety events can also be graded by regulatory definitions. The FDA defines an adverse event as any undesirable experience associated with the use of a medical product in a patient. They classify events as *serious* or *nonserious*, and as *expected* or *unexpected*. An adverse event is *serious* and should be reported when the patient outcome is death (i.e., as a direct outcome of the adverse event); a life-threatening event (i.e., the patient was at substantial risk of dying or continuing the treatment would have resulted in the patient's death); hospitalization (i.e., due to the adverse event); disability (i.e., significant, persistent, or permanent change, impairment, damage, or disruption in the patient's body function/structure, physical activities or quality of life); or a congenital anomaly (i.e., as a result of exposure prior to conception or during pregnancy). An adverse event is also serious if it requires some intervention to prevent permanent impairment or damage.

With *mild* adverse events, the signs or symptoms are transient, easily tolerated and at most irritating. They do not cause loss of time from normal activities or require medical treatment or evaluation. *Moderate* adverse events are persistent, cause discomfort severe enough to interfere with usual activities, or require treatment.

Unexpected adverse events are any events not listed in the investigator brochure. Even if an event is listed, if the severity is greater than described (e.g., severe pain occurs when only minor pain is listed), it qualifies as an unexpected event. By contrast, expected adverse events have already been listed and characterized in the trial documentation.

7.6.4 Special Circumstances and Interactions with Other Factors

Some safety events are not initially apparent. They may remain hidden until the affected organ or immune system is sufficiently damaged. They may only appear when a patient suffers psychological or physiologic stress. Some events become active only with the presence of certain concurrent conditions or situations (e.g., antiarrhythmic drug side effects occurring when there is hypokalemia, tumor necrosis factor inhibitor reactivating latent tuberculosis).

The risk of experiencing a safety event may vary among different types or subgroups of patients. Medication adverse events may occur more commonly or even exclusively in certain age groups, ethnicities, genotypes, or phenotypes (e.g., body types). Certain preexisting conditions (e.g., diabetes, heart disease, cancer), habits (e.g., smoking, alcohol consumption) or environmental factors (e.g., climate, sunlight, diesel exhaust) may also influence the risk. Long-term and short-term diet (e.g., taking medications on a full or empty stomach can influence absorption, green vegetables containing vitamin K may counteract the effects of coumadin, and grape juice can interfere with calcium channel blocker metabolism by impairing cytochrome P450-dependent metabolism), metabolism, and concomitant medications can all affect the risk and severity of adverse events.

When designing a trial, account for these potential factors and design the trial and data collection appropriately.

For example, if you anticipate that a platelet inhibitor will be used frequently in conjunction with anticoagulants, you might design the trial so that the different groups are taking different anticoagulants. This would help draw conclusions about the interaction between the platelet inhibitor and the anticoagulants. At a minimum, collect information on which patients used what anticoagulants. It is also important to identify in advance which populations may be at risk for adverse events. You may be able to modify the clinical trial design to minimize the number and impact of such events. For instance, if the onset of toxicity is gradual, you may aggressively monitor the at-risk patients and quickly discontinue the medication as soon as signs of toxicity appear.

7.7 SURROGATE ENDPOINTS

7.7.1 Definition

Surrogate endpoints are measures that correlate with and can replace measuring clinically important outcomes in a trial. Using our sports analogy, the presence of a victory celebration may be a surrogate measure for the final score of a game. If one team is celebrating, you may assume that they had a higher final score than the other team. The number of yards a football team gains may be a surrogate measure for the final score of a game, although it is a weaker surrogate measure because the team that gains more yards does not always win.

Figure 7.20 lists examples of surrogate endpoints. One of the examples is hypertension, which in and of itself is not clinically meaningful. Hypertension correlates with clinical outcomes such as the risk of stroke. If a drug could eliminate all the negative outcomes associated with hypertension, then hypertension alone would not be a cause for alarm. This also would be the case for cardiac ejection fraction, another surrogate endpoint. Contrast these examples with nonsurrogate endpoints such myocardial infarction, prolonged hospitalization, and pneumonia that are in and of themselves clinically meaningful.

7.7.2 Need for Surrogate Endpoints

We employ surrogate endpoints whenever using real clinical outcome endpoints is not practical or feasible. It may take too much time (when the outcome occurs in the distant future) or too many patients (when the outcome is relatively uncommon) to see a real clinical outcome endpoint. Also, it may be too costly or cause too much discomfort to measure a real clinical outcome.

Since surrogate endpoints commonly guide treatment decisions in clinical practice (e.g., a 95% stenosis in a coronary artery may lead to a percutaneous coronary intervention (PCI), high glucosylated hemoglobin levels might lead to increase in the insulin dose, and active urine sediment might precipitate aggressive immunosuppression in a lupus patient), many clinical trials use surrogate endpoints, and their results often can drive clinical practice.

However, a surrogate endpoint is never as informative as the clinical endpoint, and in many instances, surrogate endpoints have turned out not to be predictive of clinical response at all. For example, antiarrhythmics that prevent premature ventricular contractions (PVCs) have actually increased mortality (Figure 7.21). Some drugs that lower

---

- Pharmacokinetic/pharmacodynamic measures
- *In-vivo* biomarkers (e.g., CD4 count, viral load, glucose level, cholesterol level)
- Clinical surrogates (e.g., Blood pressure)
- *Ex-vivo* measures
- Minimal inhibitory concentration (MIC) of an anti-bacterial agent
- ADP-induced platelet aggregation inhibition
- Non-clinical measures (e.g., FEV1, radiographic findings)

FIGURE 7.20   Examples of surrogate endpoints.

Example: Cardiac arrhythmia suppression trial (CAST) study

High rates of PVCs are predictive of sudden death after myocardial infarction. Several drugs were developed with suppression of PVCs as the goal, with the ultimate goal of reducing death after myocardial infarction. The CAST study was initiated in 1987 with fl ecainide, moricizine, and encainide, which had been shown to be highly effective at reducing PVCs. At initiation of the trial, there was debate over whether it was ethical to randomize patients to placebo when the drugs had been demonstrated to reduce PVCs. In all, 2,309 patients were randomized.

The Data Safety Monitoring Board (DSMB) stopped the study early because the patients receiving antiarrhythmic therapy had an unacceptably high mortality. The relative risk (RR) of death and nonfatal events at 10 months was 4.6 in favor of placebo.

As an aside, the rate of mortality seen in the antiarrhythmic group was lower than historical controls. If it had been deemed unethical to conduct a placebo-controlled trial, then we may still be using these drugs in post-myocardial infarction patients.

FIGURE 7.21   An example of a failed surrogate endpoint.

blood pressure do not lower the risk of cardiovascular problems. Moreover, a surrogate endpoint that works for one drug may not for another drug with a different mechanism of action. As a result, regulatory authorities and many clinicians insist on clinical rather than surrogate endpoints.

Surrogate endpoints are highly useful in the following situations:

- *Studies with small sample sizes and short study durations.* Phase II trials typically fit this description. When you are not able to observe enough patients for a long enough time to experience real clinical outcomes (e.g., diabetic complications), you still may be able to see changes in surrogate endpoints (e.g., high blood sugar level which eventually will lead to diabetic complications).
- *Dose response determination studies that have multiple study arms with each arm being too small to be powered adequately for clinical endpoints.* Similar to the first scenario, if the study arm population is too small to expect enough real clinical outcomes, a surrogate endpoint may suffice.
- *Diseases with slow progression.* Using a true clinical outcome endpoint would make the trial time frame too long (e.g., it would take too long to wait for osteoporosis patients to suffer bone fractures, so you can use bone density as a surrogate endpoint instead).
- *Diseases with low event rates.* Using a true clinical outcome endpoint would require a very large study population. (e.g., hypertension, a surrogate endpoint of stroke, is a lot more common than stroke itself).
- *Subgroup analysis when the subgroup is underpowered for the nonsurrogate endpoint.* This is another example where the event rate may be too low.

7.7.3 Characteristics of a High Quality Surrogate Endpoint

A surrogate endpoint should be:

- Predictive of the clinical endpoint
- Sensitive to treatment effect in the same manner as the clinical outcome

Also compared to the clinical endpoint, it should be one of the following:

- More sensitive (e.g., ejection fraction instead of mortality)
- Occur sooner (e.g., you can detect decreased bone mineral density before hip fractures occur)
- More convenient to obtain (e.g., it is easier to see resolution of ST segment changes on electrocardiograms than open coronary arteries on angiography)

Surrogate endpoints also may precede an irreversible outcome (e.g., signs of organ rejection on biopsy precede actual organ rejection), so that a surrogate endpoint can warn you to intervene before the irreversible outcome occurs. The ideal surrogate endpoint is in the causal pathway (Figure 7.22). Choosing a surrogate that is not in the right location in the pathway can lead to spurious results. A surrogate endpoint may correlate with disease activity and be predictive of outcomes without being sensitive to treatment effect. For example, the presence of H. pylori antibody may be predictive of duodenal ulcers. But antibiotic treatment that eradicates the infection will not reverse a patient's antibody-positive status.

7.7.4 Validating a Surrogate Endpoint

Validating a surrogate endpoint (i.e., proving that it can serve as a true surrogate) is very difficult. It should have good positive predictive value (e.g., drugs that affect the surrogate also affect the clinical endpoint) and good negative predictive value (e.g., drugs that did not affect the

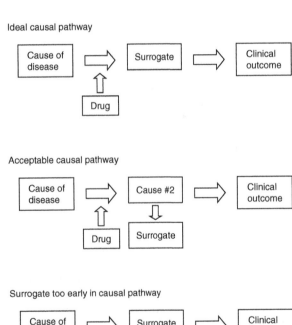

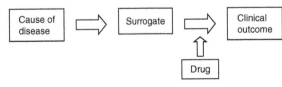

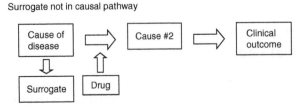

FIGURE 7.22   Surrogate endpoints and the causal pathway.

surrogate failed to show clinical effect). You should also understand its role in the causal chain relative to the drug (Figure 7.22). Also, ideally you should validate the surrogate using a drug similar to the new drug that you want to study. It is very difficult (and frequently impossible) to fulfill all of these conditions, so often investigators use surrogates that have not been fully validated. Even many surrogates commonly used in clinical practice (e.g., cardiac ejection fraction) have not been validated.

7.8 DIFFERENT TYPES OF ENDPOINTS

As we mentioned earlier in this chapter, primary, secondary, and safety endpoints can be simple or composite endpoints and actual clinical outcome or surrogate endpoints. They can also come in many different forms and dimensions, some of which we will discuss in this section.

7.8.1 Individual vs. Aggregate Endpoints

The best endpoint (i.e., the highest sensitivity and specificity) for evaluating an individual patient (*individual endpoint*) is not necessarily the best endpoint for evaluating the efficacy of a medication in a whole population (*aggregate endpoint*). Patients are interested in their symptoms and general functional status. A treatment may improve certain measures of disease activity that a patient does not immediately appreciate. For example, a patient will not say that a treatment really improved his joint count, cardiac ejection fraction, or diabetic retinopathy. However, he will be interested if a treatment alleviates his pain, breathing difficulties, or eyesight.

For example, ACR20 is better than joint count in discriminating clinical response on an individual patient basis. Having a 2–3 joint improvement may not be clinically significant if the patient is otherwise doing no better. It is partly because joint count alone tends to overestimate response that the ACR chose ACR20. However, if joint count is responsive to therapy and a more sensitive measure of drug activity, it might be a good endpoint for a clinical trial assessing the presence of drug activity or comparing responses to different doses of the drug (e.g., Phase II trials). In other words, even though improvement in joint count in the absence of other improvements may not be significant to a patient, it can serve as a useful surrogate endpoint for drug development.

7.8.2 Clinical Practice vs. Clinical Trial Endpoints

A practicing physician uses many signs, symptoms, and test measurements – all of which can be considered endpoints. However, endpoints well suited for clinical practice may not

be the best for clinical trials, and vice versa. Practicing physicians choose clinical endpoints that are easy, quick, and relatively inexpensive to use. Clinical practice endpoints should be able to discriminate findings to guide therapy and discriminate findings to render prognosis. Finally, they should be rich in descriptive data, even if they cannot be well quantified. By contrast, a clinical trial endpoint is chosen based on its ability to be standardized across sites (even if it requires training), to document results, and to reproduce results and methods at different sites, countries, and times.

So, for example, listening to a patient's breath sounds with a stethoscope may help practicing physicians guide therapy. But breath sounds is a poor clinical trial endpoint. It is not easy to quantify or record (e.g., they may not sound the same on a tape recorder) breath sounds. There is tremendous variability in how they are evaluated and interpreted.

7.8.3 Objective vs. Subjective Endpoints

Objective endpoints (e.g., walk distance, joint count, or viral load) are measured quantitatively or with an instrument. Softer *subjective endpoints* (e.g., pain, dyspnea scale, quality of life) require much judgment by patients or investigators and are therefore more difficult to standardize and reproduce. Subjective endpoints are also less amenable to aggregate data collection, analysis, and interpretation. As a result, objective endpoints are generally preferred. But the distinction between objective and subjective endpoints can be blurry. Well-designed and standardized subjective endpoints are acceptable and sometimes the only viable option.

7.8.4 Clinical vs. Nonclinical Endpoints

Nonclinical endpoints are often considered to be surrogate endpoints. In some instances, the addition of clinical judgment can transform a nonclinical endpoint into a clinical endpoint. For example (Figure 7.23), a chest X-ray alone is not a clinical endpoint, but a clinical diagnosis of pneumonia, which may be based on chest X-ray findings, can be a *clinical endpoint*.

Not a clinical endpoint in itself:	Clinical endpoint:
Infiltrate on chest x-ray Low pO$_2$	Clinical diagnosis of pneumonia, based on both of the following: 1) Clinical judgment of pneumonia *and* 2) Either infiltrate on CXR and/or low pO$_2$

FIGURE 7.23   Example of clinical and nonclinical endpoints.

7.8.5 Static vs. Dynamic/Change vs. Cumulative Change

Static endpoints (e.g., ejection fraction, blood pressure) measure absolute numbers. *Dynamic endpoints* (e.g., ACR20, change in blood pressure) measure changes. Using a financial analogy, a static endpoint would be similar to a stock price (e.g., Yahoo is currently $30 per share), and a dynamic endpoint would be similar to a stock price change (e.g., Yahoo went up by 2.5% yesterday). It is possible to derive a dynamic endpoint (e.g., change in blood pressure) from a static endpoint (e.g., absolute blood pressure), but not vice versa. Some endpoints measure disease severity at one time point (e.g., joint pain) while others are *cumulative endpoints* that measure changes that have occurred over a period of time (e.g., the amount of joint erosion).

7.8.6 Remission vs. Response

Traditionally, *response* means that the disease is nearly or completely gone, but the patient remains on the treatment. *Remission* suggests that the disease was modified to the point that the patient no longer needs the treatment. Both of these may be very relevant clinical endpoints, but, as we mentioned previously, determining remission and response is not always easy. In some cases, finding objective, accurate, and valid criteria can be difficult. For example, how long should you observe a patient to conclude that he or she has experienced a response or remission? What if 8 out of 10 patients with a given set of symptoms no longer require treatment? Are those two patients still requiring treatment truly not in remission? As you can see, definitions can be so subjective or complicated that surrogate measures are needed.

7.8.7 Need-for-Intervention and Drug Sparing as Endpoints

Some treatments can help patients reduce the amount or number of other medications that they have to take (i.e., *drug sparing*) or avoid certain other treatments or interventions (i.e., reduce the *need-for-intervention*).

A Treatment May Prevent Patients from Having to Undergo Certain Treatments or Procedures that Are Part of the Diagnosis and Treatment of a Certain Disease

For example, a cardiovascular medicine may save patients from having to under coronary catheterization or bypass surgery. Using such endpoints is controversial, however. Some researchers argue that needing interventions is not an appropriate proxy for disease progression, since there is considerable controversy over whether and when patients should get many types of treatments and procedures.

A Treatment May Reduce the Need for Rescue Medications

Some diseases have flares and exacerbations that require intense short-term or rescue medications. Asthma is an example. A severe asthmatic exacerbation requires oral or intravenous corticosteroids. A primary benefit of a chronic asthma medication may be to reduce the frequency and severity of such exacerbations and, in turn, the need for rescue medications.

A Treatment May Reduce the Required Dose of Another Medication

Some patients are chronically on medications that can have serious short- or long-term side effects. These patients can benefit from treatments that help reduce the doses and need for these chronic medications. In some cases, a treatment may be able to completely wean the patient off another medication. As a classic example, many patients with severe rheumatologic conditions require chronic systemic corticosteroids. Systemic steroids have recognized detrimental side effects on many organs, creating a need for rheumatologic medications that can lower the requirement for steroids.

Unless designed carefully, medication weaning or drug sparing studies could lead to confounding. For example, imagine that one group has a higher number of patients able to wean off chronic medications but at the same time has a greater number of disease exacerbations. How will you be able to tell if the treatment is having a positive effect? Are the patients who are able to wean off medications having exacerbations because they are no longer taking their chronic medications or do they have more severe disease? In the former situation, the treatment is not effective, and in the latter, the treatment is effective.

When using drug sparing as an endpoint, you have to demonstrate that your treatment (which we will call Treatment 1) is actually lowering the required dosage and in turn the toxicity of another drug (which we will call Drug A). This effect must be maintained (i.e., not temporary or transient) and should not be the result of other factors such as natural disease progression or poor patient compliance (i.e., make sure that the same patients who can reduce their medication use also have improvements in their disease conditions). You have to know the relationship between Drug A dose reduction and toxicity. This relationship may not be linear (e.g., reducing the average dose of Drug A by 50% may only lead to a 10% reduction in safety problems), so not all dosage reductions are necessarily meaningful. Of course, if Drug A has a better safety or efficacy ratio than Treatment 1, then reducing the dose of Drug A is not beneficial. For example, although several acute coronary syndrome trials have used reducing need for PTCA as an endpoint, it is not clear that reducing the need for PTCA is clinically meaningful. So when using dose reduction of another drug as an endpoint, you implicitly are comparing the two drugs, asserting that one drug is better.

7.8.8 Pharmacoeconomics

Pharmacoeconomic endpoints are becoming increasingly popular. They are very relevant in many situations. Insurance companies, health care facilities, employers, and government agencies are concerned if they can pay for certain treatments, especially in this age of limited resources. In some cases, pharmacoeconomic measures may be superior to clinical measures in approximating disease severity (e.g., allergies, depression). A treatment may help reduce different measures of health care resource utilization (e.g., emergency room visits, hospitalizations, days in the intensive care unit, or number of procedures needed) or worker productivity (e.g., days of work missed or worker output), all potential surrogates for disease severity. Some trials are designed to measure the cost–benefit or cost-effectiveness of a treatment or intervention. This is especially true when two interventions with equivalent clinical efficacy but different costs are being compared. In such a study, cost and other such economic measures can be endpoints. Similar rules that apply to clinical endpoints, apply for pharmacoeconomic endpoints. The pharmacoeconomic endpoint should be relevant, responsive, rich in information, etc. In addition, the endpoint should be relevant to the perspective, which should be specified prior to the trial (perspective is discussed in Chapter 8: Pharmacoeconomics).

7.8.9 Disease Symptom vs. General Symptom Endpoints

You should be able to distinguish between *general symptom* and specific *disease symptom endpoints*. In some cases, a symptom can be very specific (pathognomic) to a disease. In other words, only patients with that disease will have that symptom. However, most symptoms (e.g., pain, diarrhea, and breathing difficulties) can be the product of many different causes, including a variety of disease conditions, normal aging (e.g., joint pain), and the environment (e.g., rhinitis from seasonal allergies). You can define some symptoms as generally (e.g., pain) or as specifically (e.g., knee joint pain) as you choose. Remember that very general symptom endpoints bring the risk of confounding (e.g., a general pain score can reflect pain from any part of the body). Conversely, very specific symptom endpoints may reduce the likelihood of seeing an effect (e.g., an anti-inflammatory may reduce pain everywhere else besides the joint you specify). Even relatively specific symptom endpoints can have confounders (e.g., does the knee pain come from arthritis, other medications that the patient is taking such as statins,

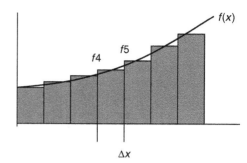

FIGURE 7.24 The area under the curve.

exercise, or traums?) Directly linking the symptom to the disease of interest often is not easy.

7.8.10 Area under the Curve

As we mentioned in the section on repeated measures analysis, you can measure and compare the *areas under a curve*, which can be a continuous endpoint. Figure 7.24 shows an example of calculating the area under a curve. The curve is a function $f(x)$. The area under the curve is approximated by a series of rectangles. Integration, making the rectangles increasingly narrow and calculating their areas, is a mathematical method of computing the area under the curve. Using such a continuous variable can increase the power of the study, just as with the repeated measures method. The area under the curve is an attractive endpoint intuitively, because the course of the disease over time is an important clinical endpoint in many chronic diseases.

7.8.11 Quality of Life

Quality of Life is considered one of the more subjective endpoints. It is also called patient reported symptoms. It is a valuable endpoint for many diseases, but prone to methodological weaknesses. We will discuss this in detail in Chapter 8.

7.8.12 Durability and Maintenance of Response

Sometimes it is not enough just to demonstrate that a treatment has an effect. You may also want to know how long this effect will persist while the treatment is being given (i.e., *maintenance of response*) and after the treatment is stopped (i.e., the *durability of response*). These endpoints are especially important for waxing and waning diseases (e.g., psoriasis) and chronic diseases (e.g., rheumatoid arthritis). Some treatments improve over time (e.g., reducing the disease activity makes the disease even more susceptible to treatment). Some worsen over time (e.g.,

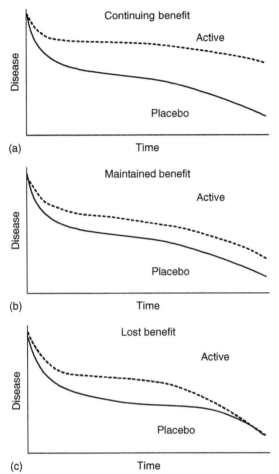

(a)

(b)

(c)

FIGURE 7.25 Disease activity curves in three different treatment scenarios: (a) treatment has continuing benefits (b) treatment has a maintained benefit (c) treatment has lost benefit.

patients become habituated to the effects of the medication). Treatments that actually modify some aspect of the disease process and medications that have long pharmacodynamic half-lives (e.g., alefacept) tend to have long durabilities of response. Figure 7.25 shows three different scenarios, one where the treatment has continuing benefit (i.e., the treatment continues to improve the condition), a second where the treatment has maintained benefit (i.e., the benefit and the condition stays the same), and a third where the benefit has been lost. In each, the dotted line represents the disease activity in the treatment group and the solid line represents the disease activity in the placebo group.

7.8.13 Cure vs. Treatment

Some drugs *cure* a disease (e.g., antibiotics,infections), fundamentally changing the pathophysiological process so that the disease no longer exists, while others *treat* a disease (e.g., enbrel, rheumatois arthritis), reducing or eliminating the disease's symptoms and effects while the underlying cause of the disease remains. Distinguishing between a cure and treatment requires in-depth knowledge of the disease pathophysiology. Determining when and if a cure has resulted is not always easy. Many diseases may remain dormant or smoldering, only to return or reactivate years later. Demonstrating a cure requires significantly more rigor and evidence than demonstrating a treatment.

7.8.14 Symptom vs. Disease Modification

Treatments and, in turn, endpoints can address the symptoms (e.g., pain), the biological effects of a disease (e.g., long-term progression of joint erosion), or both (e.g., composite endpoints can incorporate both of these parameters). You should not confuse *symptom modification* with *disease modification*. Treatments that do just the former do not alter the natural course or history of the disease. However, symptom modification can be an indication that disease modification is occurring (e.g., decreasing coronary artery occlusion may decrease chest pain). Moreover, disease modification does not always imply symptom modification (i.e., some disease activity can decrease without an improvement in symptoms.)

7.8.15 Induction of Remission vs. Maintenance

There are endpoints that account for the fact that some drugs induce remission of a disease during active flares (*induction of remission*), while others prevent or reduce the recurrence of flares (*maintenance*). You can measure the frequency and severity of flares as well as the time intervals between flares. Measuring the severity of a flare requires an acute disease activity measure as opposed to a chronic disease activity measure. Acute disease activity can be tricky to determine, since signs, symptoms, and test results can rapidly change and oscillate. Also there may be significant natural variation from flare to flare and from patient to patient. You must be very specific about when and how you will measure flare severity.

7.8.16 Improvement vs. Prevention of Progression

Some treatments improve a disease condition (e.g., restore vision), while others prevent or inhibit progression (e.g., prevent vision from worsening). This is an important distinction. Timing of the intervention may be particularly important for treatments that prevent disease progression, since delay may result in missed opportunities. Trials should be structured with this in mind (e.g., a drug that prevents further damage in stroke might need to be given as early as possible, but a drug that enhances re-growth of nerve tissue might be given long after the stroke).

7.8.17 Speed of Onset of Effect

Trials may measure the speed and patterns of onset of an intervention's effect. Two treatments may have the same effect, but one may act sooner because of mechanism of action or bioavailability. This is important when dealing with life-threatening or disabling conditions or severe symptoms that need to be addressed as soon as possible. The most effective medication for treating heart attacks, bleeding, or severe diarrhea will not be useful if it requires a week to take effect. Potential endpoints may be time to peak effect, slope of effect, or percentage of effect at various time points. Survival analyses could be useful in these situations with the outcome event being maximal effect of the treatment or resolution of the clinical problem.

7.8.18 Tachyphylaxis

Various aspects of *tachyphylaxis* (i.e., a drug losing part or its entire efficacy over time as the body becomes tolerant or counterregulatory processes occur) can serve as endpoints. For example, since nitroglycerine demonstrates tachyphylaxis, you should wait for some time (i.e., drug-free intervals) between doses to allow patients to remain sensitive to the drug effects. Studying tachyphylaxis is important in establishing proper dosing. Potential endpoints are presence or absence of tachyphylaxis, speed of onset of tachyphylaxis, and drug-free intervals needed between doses to avoid tachyphylaxis. One challenge is distinguishing between declining efficacy because of tachyphylaxis and declining efficacy because of worsening disease.

7.8.19 Efficacy upon Re-treatment

Since some drugs (e.g., streptokinase, murine antibodies) work well only a limited number of times before losing their effects, measuring *efficacy on re-treatment* can be a useful endpoint. Drug effects can dramatically decline between administrations; and once the effects disappear they may not return, even after a drug-free interval. This may be acceptable for diseases such as acute myocardial infarction, where few patients have more than one or two episodes, but unacceptable for diseases that require repeated treatments. Do not confuse this with tachyphylaxis, where the effects may decline gradually and return after the drug has been discontinued for a while.

7.8.20 Oncology Endpoints

In oncology clinical trials, a set of endpoints that are somewhat unique has been developed. The definitive endpoint is overall survival, but in addition, disease–free progression, progression–free survival, and RECIST response rates have been frequently used. Disease–free survival (DFS) is length of time until either disease recurs or the patient dies. Progression–free survival (PFS) is the time until the tumor grows or until the patient dies whichever comes first.

Disease–free survival and progression–free survival are problematic in many ways. They are difficult to measure, since they require careful imaging studies that are read in a standardized manner. Depending on when and how frequently the scans are performed, DFS and PFS can be biased. For example, if the scans for the control arm patients happen to be scheduled later than placebo arm patients, then there can be a false signal because the earlier visits can translate into earlier detection of progression. It is controversial as to whether either correlates with survival very well. However, some would argue that the period of time without disease is of value in and of itself, particularly if the disease causes discomfort or symptoms.

One disadvantage of DFS or PFS is that in many oncology studies, the patients are crossed over to the active arm as soon as there is recurrence or progression. This can confound overall survival, especially if the drug is very active. This occurred, for example, with the phase 2 study of renal cell carcinoma with bevacizumab. An advantage is that DFS and PFS allows a shorter study than a survival study since it takes shorter time to reach those endpoints.

RECIST criteria is based on changes in the size of target tumor lesions. There are four response categories:

- CR (complete response) = disappearance of all target lesions
- PR (partial response) = 30% decrease in the sum of the longest diameter of target lesions
- PD (progressive disease) = 20% increase in the sum of the longest diameter of target lesions
- SD (stable disease) = small changes that do not meet above criteria

There are some important assumptions behind RECIST, such as assumption that linear measures are an adequate substitute for 2-D or 3-D measures, and assumption that size of tumors is correlated with survival. RECIST was sometimes helpful in the early days of oncologic drug development, because most agents were non-targeted, general cytotoxic agents, and their anti-tumor activity corresponded to their ability to shrink tumors in some instances. With newer, targeted agents, however, RECIST criteria may not be as helpful.

Chapter 8

Economics and Patient Reported Outcomes

8.1 HEALTH ECONOMICS AND PHARMACOECONOMICS

8.1.1 Importance of Economics

Money changes everything.

Cyndi Lauper, singer and philosopher

Show me the money!

Cuba Gooding, Jr. in the movie Jerry McGuire

Do you want to own a premium sports car like a Porsche? Are you willing to pay for one? How much is the performance, luxury, and/or style of a Porsche worth to you? Wouldn't a car like a Honda Civic, which offers reasonable performance at a much lower price, suffice? How badly do you need the Porsche? What are you willing to sacrifice for less cost?

These are the types of questions you ask whenever making any kind of purchase. You want to know the relative worth and cost of your options. Some items may be essential to you (e.g., a reliable air bag system, ability to function in the snow, or adequate trunk space) and others may be optional or luxuries (e.g., a surround-sound stereo system, temperature controlled seats, or a pair of fuzzy dice to hang on the rear-view mirror). The relative costs and benefits of a given item can vary significantly from person-to-person. A car like a Porsche then becomes essential. For people who live in a very large city with convenient public transportation, a car could even be a burden.

You have to make such assessments and decisions, especially when your resources are limited. There is a finite amount of money in your bank account that could go toward buying other things like food, clothing, and this book. Buying one thing means less money for other things. On the other hand, with unlimited resources, you could easily get any car. You could choose the fastest, longest-lasting, and best-looking car available.

This is in essence *economics*, the study of resource allocation when resources are limited. Economics looks at where money is coming from, where it can and is being spent, and what people are getting in return for spending money. Economists aim to provide rational and objective decision–making in the face of financial realities.

Many argue that health care is different from other industries and that economics should not play a significant role in decision making. Isn't health care a right to which everyone should have access rather than a commodity that can be bought and sold? Does the harsh objectivity of economics lack the compassion and sympathy needed in health care? Is the most economically sound decision necessarily the morally and ethically right decision? Can things such as saving lives, easing pain, and reducing suffering be adequately captured and quantified in economic studies?

Although moral or ethical principles are important in any industry, disregarding economic realities in health care is foolhardy and dangerous. Realistically, health care resources are limited. Drug and medical device development is very costly. Delivering health care is an enormous and expensive enterprise. Many people want the best possible health care for themselves and their families, but many fewer are willing to pay for it. Healthy individuals do not want to subsidize other people's health care until they themselves are ill. Then they welcome or even expect others to subsidize their care. Ignoring economic considerations will lead to some terrible consequences such as patients not being able to afford desperately needed treatments, patients facing financial ruin, and health care providers, organizations, and companies no longer being able to deliver essential services.

Moreover, health care is not the only industry with moral, ethical, and legal concerns although these issues do play a more important role in health care. The automobile industry cannot just focus on making money without paying attention to the quality and safety of their cars. The U.S. Postal Service cannot arbitrarily decide not to service certain cities because they are not profitable enough. The food industry has to worry about meeting nutritional and safety standards. Even the entertainment industry cannot be entirely obsessed with financial gain. Otherwise there may be even more sex and violence in movies. In reality, every industry affects the health and welfare of the general public. An investment firm that collects and pockets billions of dollars may take away available resources from industries such as health care and eventually hurt patients. On the other hand, the investment firm may stimulate the growth of some biotechnology companies that in turn can develop the medications that eventually save thousands of lives.

Every day, economic considerations are becoming more and more important in clinical research and health care. As the costs of health care and medical interventions continue to increase, proving that an intervention is safe, effective, and easy to use is often not enough. You frequently have to prove that an intervention will be worth its cost. This is especially true when the intervention being developed or researched is not significantly superior in efficacy or safety to existing interventions. In fact, the crisis of rising health care costs has been a real impetus for researchers to develop less expensive alternatives to existing interventions.

All of these issues help make *health care economics*, the study of the allocation of health care resources, a very complicated but important part of clinical research. (*Pharmacoeconomics* is health care economics applied specifically to medications.) One part of health economics is *technology assessment*, studying the economic value of different medical interventions.

8.1.2 Audience and Arenas

Economic studies come in a wide variety of shapes and forms. They range from very simple, "back-of-the-envelope" calculations to sophisticated models that require substantial computer power. So who is interested in health economics and pharmacoeconomic studies? Almost, everyone involved in health care, including:

- *Local, state, federal, and international organizations*: Decision makers in many organizations often must choose among different alternatives. Should we institute a mass immunization program? Which vaccine should we use for a mass immunization program? Should we commit funds to develop this medication? Which will have a greater effect, building a bridge or providing medications?
- *Patients*: Is the intervention worth the cost? Is there a lower cost alternative?
- *Health care providers*: To whom should we provide this intervention? Will this intervention cost the patient and society too much? What are the various alternatives?

- *Health care organizations*: Should we include this intervention on our formulary? A *formulary* is the list of approved interventions that a health care organization allows its providers to use. Using interventions not listed on the formulary may require special approval. The health care organization's *formulary* or *pharmacy and therapeutics (P&T) committee* will periodically review studies on different interventions and decide whether to approve their use.
- *Payors (e.g., insurance companies)*: Should we provide insurance coverage (i.e., be willing to provide payment) for that intervention? How will covering that intervention affect our business? Payors are third parties (e.g., insurance companies, Medicare, or Medicaid) that help defray patients' health care bills.
- *Employers*: How will that intervention affect worker productivity? Should we encourage insurance companies to cover that intervention?
- *Regulatory bodies*: The manufacturers are claiming that their intervention reduces costs and improves productivity. Can they make such a claim? Is it reasonable for them to include those claims on product labels or advertising?
- *Medical product developers and manufacturers*: Should we continue to develop and manufacture this intervention? Will it be worth the time, effort, and cost? How does our intervention compare against competing interventions? What can we claim about our intervention vs. other interventions? How much should we charge for the intervention? How much will payors cover the intervention?
- *Investors and research funders*: Is it worth investing in this medical intervention? What will our rewards be for investing our resources?

So when is it appropriate to perform an economic analysis? Anytime. For example, you can perform an economic analysis:

- *Before an intervention even exists*: Economic studies can be important planning tools, helping determine if an intervention is even worth developing, what resources will be required, and which directions research and development should take.
- *During the development of a medical intervention*: An economic analysis can be part of a clinical study. You can either have the primary or secondary endpoints be economic endpoints or add an economic analysis to a clinical study (i.e., a *piggyback study*). Doing so will delineate the potential of the intervention and what claims can or cannot be made about the intervention. Near the end of clinical development, economic studies can help set the price of the intervention and serve as justifications for insurance coverage.

- *When the intervention is on the market*: Economic studies can demonstrate the relative advantages and disadvantages of your intervention compared with other interventions.

8.1.3 Perspective

Let us go back to our car buying scenario. The benefits and costs of a car purchase depend on who you are and what is your point-of-view. A car buyer who is single with no family to support only has to worry about himself or herself. (For example, what will the car cost? How much enjoyment will this car provide? Will this car attract the right women or men?) The casual girlfriend or boyfriend of the car buyer may not have to worry about the costs of the car and may focus only on the conferred benefits. (For example, will my friends envy me if my boyfriend or girlfriend has this car? How much enjoyment will I gain from riding in it?) If the car buyer is married, the car buyer's spouse may be very upset about money being spent on a car rather than on household items, a vacation, or the children. A car salesman may not care about the actual benefits of the car and just wants the car buyer to spend as much money as possible.

This example illustrates the importance of the *perspective* or point-of-view of an economic study. Decisions, available choices, costs, and benefits depend on whom you are. For example, the economic concerns and motivations of a *payor* are very different from those of a *patient* or *health care provider*. Therefore, every economic study should clearly identify what perspective it is taking. Common perspectives are those of an individual, a health care provider, a hospital, an insurance company, a managed care company, a pharmaceutical or medical device company, a government body, or society in general. In all cases, the economic study assumes selfish or self-centered behavior. For example, a study taking an individual's perspective will assume that the individual is only interested in himself or herself and does not care about what happens to others. (In reality, an individual may show concern for strangers, organizations, or society.) Similarly, a study taking a payor's perspective will assume that the insurance company is only interested in maximizing its profits. Changing the perspective of a study can drastically alter the study's results. The correct choice for one individual or organization may not be right for another individual or organization. Therefore, the perspective of the economic study should match that of the decision maker.

8.2 TIME

8.2.1 Period of Analysis

As with clinical studies, economic analyses can be *retrospective* (looking at events that have already occurred),

prospective (looking at events as they occur), or *predictive* (looking at theoretical events that could occur in the future). Different approaches are appropriate in different situations. Each approach has its relative advantages, disadvantages, and applicability. Retrospective analyses are useful since the past often repeats itself or may help predict the future. However, the past may be quite different from current and future situations. Moreover, collecting accurate and comprehensive data on past events can be difficult. Prospective analyses, which involve collecting data while a clinical study occurs, give you much more control over the information collected. You can design a clinical study to directly compare the costs and rewards of different treatments. However, results from such a prospective analyses may only represent specific situations. Will the results apply to situations unlike the clinical study's conditions? Predictive analyses (i.e., building mathematical models or computer simulations of hypothetical situations) offer the most flexibility. You can create a predictive model to mirror nearly any scenario. However, since such predictive models represent hypothetical situations, they incorporate a number of assumptions and speculations. Often, a combination of retrospective, prospective, and predictive analyses can help answer a question.

8.2.2 Time Frame

Good economic decisions in the short term are not always good economic decisions in the long term. Suppose you were choosing between getting that Porsche and investing in your child's education. Over the next year that Porsche may give you a lot more pleasure than putting money away for your child. Your child's education will not allow you to blaze down the streets and make heads turn. No one will say, "cool investment in your child's education." However, in the long run (perhaps 20 years from now), your child's education may bring greater benefits to you (e.g., your child's happiness and success, family harmony, and invaluable memories).

Therefore, the *time frame*, *time horizon*, or *period of analysis* of an economic study is important. The time frame should be long enough to capture all relevant rewards and costs but not so long that collecting or estimating all rewards and costs is unrealistic. For example, suppose you are trying to measure the costs of having a major stroke. Let us look at the effects of using different time frames:

- *Measuring costs up to 1 month after the stroke.* This may significantly underestimate costs, since a major stroke may cause substantial long-lasting disability (e.g., long-term rehabilitation and medical care costs).
- *Measuring costs for 200 years after the stroke.* This may be unnecessary. The patient's lifespan is far less than 200 years. Either collecting or estimating costs for the next 200 years is clearly impractical.

- *Measuring costs over the remaining lifetime of the patient.* This may be more accurate and reasonable than the two previous options. However, if the life expectancies of patients vary significantly, you may see a wide distribution of costs.
- *Measuring costs for the first 5 years after the stroke.* This may result in less variability in costs than the previous option. However, it may underestimate the costs for patients with substantially longer-life expectancies.

8.2.3 Time and Value

Time also affects the worth or value of things. The value of some things *appreciate* (i.e., increase) over time, while the value of many other things *depreciate* (i.e., decrease) over time. The value of property, gold, and a good company stock may increase with passing years. By contrast, is the car that you bought 7 years ago worth the same today as it was brand new? The car has suffered wear and tear. The car's technology and style may be outdated. The car like all other functioning items has a limited lifetime, that is, at some point the item no longer functions. Accounting for this *depreciation*, that is, decrease in value with age, may be important in an economic study. For example, a medical device has a specific lifetime. The value of the device goes from its maximum when the device is first manufactured to its *residual value* at the end of its lifetime (which is usually zero unless the device has some re-sale value or some other use). The value of the device slowly decreases from the maximum to the residual with use and time at a certain *depreciation rate*. When this rate is expressed as change in value over a unit of time (e.g., value of the device decreases by $100 every year):

$$\text{Current value} = \text{Initial value} - (\text{Depreciation rate} \times \text{Time})$$

When the depreciation rate is expressed as change in value over a unit of use (e.g., value of the device decreases by $10 every time it is used):

$$\text{Current value} = \text{Initial value} - (\text{Depreciation rate} \times \text{Use})$$

Sometimes using a depreciation rate can account for both time and use (e.g., the value will decrease by $10 with each use and $100 with each passing year) is more accurate. For example, a car that sits in your driveway without being used is not retaining the same value that the car had when it was brand new. At the same time, a 7-year old car that has been driven continuously will have less value than a 7-year old car that has been largely idle.

Discounting and Net Present Value

Having something today is not equivalent to having the same thing years from now. Which one would you rather have: $10,000 today or $10,000 in 10 years? If you receive $10,000 today, you can invest or spend it on something that will help you for the future. Moreover, inflation slowly and continuously devalues the worth of $10,000. Similarly, would you rather have a skin blemish removed today or 10 years from now? Waiting for 10 years may sacrifice lots of dates and job interviews. You will lose 10 years of being skin blemish-free.

Opportunity costs are the value of missed alternatives due to taking a certain course of action. Anytime you choose a course of action when several options are available, you forfeit the potential rewards of other options. For example, choosing one job means that you miss out on the benefits of the jobs you declined. When you spend an extra hour at work, it is one less hour that you have to spend with your family or friends. A 6-month break to travel the world may result in 6 months of lost income. The value of your chosen option may exceed the opportunity costs of not choosing other options. However, the net value of a choice is always the value of that choice minus the opportunity costs of missing the other options. Delays in receiving something of value cause opportunity costs. For example, losing 10 years of skin blemish-free existence is opportunity cost.

As a result of inflation and opportunity costs, a dollar (or any other cost or reward) in the future is worthless than a dollar today. So in an economic study, you must adjust all future values to present day values (i.e., the *net present value*). The net present value is today's value of the future good or service. *Discount rates* can adjust future costs and rewards to their net present values:

$$C_0 = C_n/(1 + r)^n$$

C_0 = current or net present value of C_n
C_n = cost n years from now
r = discount rate (most often between 3% and 5%)

Example: Using a 3% discount rate, an intervention that earns $100 ten years from now will be worth $100/(1 + 0.03)10 = $74.41 in today's dollars.

The discount rate that you should use depends on the situation and study. Frequently, people use the inflation rate or the consumer price index. Conventionally, health economic studies use 3–5% discount rates. The correct rate to use is the subject of many health economist debates. Alluding to the discount rate is a great way to stir up trouble in a room full of health economists.

8.3 VALUATION

8.3.1 Tangible Costs and Rewards

Every action or decision has its *costs* and *rewards*. The costs of buying a Porsche may include the price that you have to pay for the car, its accessories, any potential increase in car insurance, and its maintenance. The rewards may be the satisfaction, image enhancement, and confidence that the car brings. Some costs and rewards are relatively straightforward and easy to estimate, while others are complicated and difficult to obtain. For example, the sale price of the Porsche should be clearly listed. The costs of keeping the Porsche clean may be a little more difficult to estimate. Buying the Porsche may infuriate your spouse, which may result in many unexpected and difficult to predict costs. Similarly, some of the rewards are easier to quantify than others. Owning a Porsche may get you into a coveted social club and facilitate the beginning of a social or business relationship. Some of these rewards are more tangible, whereas others are intangible.

Valuation is the process of quantifying the costs and rewards of an item or event. In some cases, valuation is relatively straightforward. Many items have frequently updated and publicly available prices. For example, the current prices of precious metals (e.g., gold and silver) and commonly used natural resources (e.g., oil and natural gas) are readily available. The prices of some health care resources such as medications and surgical equipment are also readily available. Calculating the costs from these prices can be fairly simple. From the perspective of someone purchasing these items, the cost of each item is simply the price. From the perspective of someone selling these items, the reward is the net profit earned (i.e., Profit = Price − Cost). However, in many cases, determining the true value of something is complicated. An item or event can have both tangible and intangible costs and rewards. Tangible costs and rewards are ones that are easily touched and counted (e.g., costs of medications and surgical supplies). Intangible costs and rewards are not easily touched or counted (e.g., cost of pain, suffering, and loss of life).

Costs and rewards can be either *fixed* (remain constant) or *variable* (vary by frequency of use). Monthly apartment rent is an example of a fixed cost. The rent for a given month does not depend on how many hours each day and how many days each week you stay inside your apartment. On the other hand, electricity is a variable cost, increasing with increased electricity use. Therefore, calculating a variable cost requires knowing the total use of the resource.

Both costs and rewards can be very subtle and hidden. Realize that even seemingly small actions or events can have far-reaching consequences. For example, a major stroke can result in not only many *direct costs* (e.g., hospitalization, medication, and physical therapy costs) but also many less obvious *indirect costs* (e.g., lost income from not being able to work and costs of reconfiguring the house to make it more accessible for the disabled patient). The total indirect costs may even outweigh the more obvious direct costs.

Some of the most common methods of gathering or estimating medical costs include:

- *Charges*: Hospital, clinic, or any other health care provider charges (found on bills) may be reasonable proxies for costs. Since health care providers rarely receive full reimbursement from insurance companies for their charges (e.g., a physician who charges $500 for a procedure may receive only $200), established *cost-to-charge ratios* or other conversion factors can convert charges to costs. Moreover, bills may not offer the level of detail needed. For example, an emergency room visit charge may aggregate many components (e.g., placing an intravenous line and transporting the patient to different locations) of the visit and not identify what fraction of the charge is associated with each component. Finally, bills and charges often do not accurately reflect all of the resources consumed or services provided.

- *Micro-costing*: Micro-costing is the process of identifying every resource consumed, assigning a cost to each resource, and totaling up the costs. As you can imagine, this process is more accurate than using charges but potentially very tedious and labor intensive. *Time-and-motion studies* can provide the information needed for micro-costing. In a time-and-motion study, you follow a patient during the relevant time period and count every item used (e.g., medications, catheters, saline, gauze, and radiology film) and every service performed (e.g., 30 minutes of a nurse's time and 10 minutes of a patient transporter's time).

- *Resource unit use*: In this approach, you choose a resource that can be easily measured (e.g., number of hospitalizations, length of hospital stay, and number of radiology procedures), determine the cost of a single unit of that resource (e.g., cost per hospitalization, cost per hospital day, cost per radiology procedure), and then tabulate how many units of that resource are used. So, for example, if a patient with a stroke must stay in the hospital for 7 days, the cost of hospitalization equals the cost of a hospital day multiplied by seven. This method tends to provide gross estimates that do not account for significant variability (e.g., fluctuation in cost of a day in the hospital). Moreover, the resource unit may not represent every cost incurred.

Cost values can come from a variety of sources, including the medical literature, insurance reports, and other publications. Before using any value, ascertain whether the source is credible and the source's circumstances are comparable. For example, the cost of physical therapy for a patient with a minor stroke is not the same as the cost for a major stroke. When cost values vary significantly among different sources, consider using either a simple or a weighted average of the costs.

One component of many interventions is personnel costs. An intervention may require different health care personnel to deliver the intervention. Personnel costs can be quite high when the intervention is a procedure or involves professionals interpreting diagnostic tests. For example, a major surgery could involve one or two surgeons, an anesthesiologist, several nurses, a pathologist to interpret the tissue samples, a radiologist to read any X-rays, and physical therapists after the surgery. Either professional charges or each person's time and salary can serve as estimates of personnel costs. Here's an example:

$$\text{Cost of nurse} = (\text{Hours spent assisting procedure}) \times (\text{Hourly wage})$$

8.3.2 Intangible Costs and Rewards

Intangible costs and rewards may have significant value, but quantifying their value can be difficult. What is the value of entertainment, peace-of-mind, good health, and happiness? What is the cost of suffering, unhappiness, making enemies, or poor physical or mental health? Economic studies that ignore these intangibles can sorely under or overestimate the economic impact of something. However, you cannot count or measure intangible costs and rewards unless they are expressed in quantitative terms. Therefore, converting intangible effects into quantitative (e.g., monetary) terms is often necessary.

Revealed preferences can help quantify the value of intangible costs and rewards. This method involves identifying measurable costs that are closely associated with what you are trying to quantify. For example, a vacation to Hawaii entails paying for an airplane ticket and hotel room. Presumably, people are willing to pay these costs because the value of the vacation (e.g., happiness, relaxation, and experience) either equals or exceeds the cost of the airplane ticket and hotel room. Using a health care example, to quantify the value of having larger breasts, you may need to look at what people have been spending on breast implant surgery.

Revealed preferences have several drawbacks. Spending often does not reflect the real value that someone places on an item. We frequently purchase things on impulse or due to the influence of friends, co-workers, and/or advertisements. Moreover, perfect information is rarely available when we purchase an item or service. We do not know what the item and service will actually provide or what our needs will be. If we had perfect information, we would never have to throw away or re-sell anything sooner than anticipated.

Additionally, the price of an item or service does not necessarily reflect its true value. Items and services may be underpriced or (more frequently) overpriced. While price eventually may reflect demand, such is not always the case. Markets can be very inefficient, that is, there can be a tremendous lag time between changes in price to reflect demand. For example, a manufacturer may charge $1,000 for a handbag. It may take a year or two before the manufacturer realizes that not enough people are buying the handbag and then lowers the price accordingly. Moreover, many items, services, or events do not have obvious price tags. What is the cost and reward of a nurse making extra effort to ensure a patient feels more comfortable? What is

the cost and reward of being able to play in a recreational baseball league? What is the reward of eliminating those blemishes from your face?

An alternative to determining revealed preferences is using surveys or experiments (i.e., *stated preference or contingent valuation techniques*) to ascertain the value that subjects place on intangible costs and rewards. Contingent valuation techniques aim to determine a subject's *willingness to pay (WTP)* for something. The WTP is the maximum amount of money a subject would agree to expend. The WTP value usually differs among different people. One person may be willing to pay $100,000 for a car while another may only be willing to spend $50,000. What is extremely valuable to one person may be worthless to another. Breast implants may be very valuable to a fashion model but be much less valuable to a carpenter. The answers to two questions determine a WTP value:

- *What is the item or service worth to you?* An essential item will have more value (e.g., a cool drink in a desert) than a luxury item. Limiting the supply of an item may increase its value (e.g., diamonds would not be so valuable if they were abundantly available). An item with longer-lasting or more permanent effects (e.g., house) may be more valuable than an item with transient effects (e.g., hotel room).
- *What is your disposable income?* Bill Gates may be willing to pay more money for a car with a built in sauna and wide screen television because he probably has a little more disposable income than you.

A common contingent valuation technique is the *bidding game*, which proceeds as follows:

- *Step 1 – Describe situation*: Show the subject the situation that you are trying to quantify (e.g., removal of a skin blemish).
- *Step 2 – Initial bid*: Ask the subject if they would pay $X to achieve that situation. (For example, would you pay $10 to remove the skin blemish?)
- *Step 3 – Raise or lower the bid*: If the subject accepts this bid then offer a higher price. (For example, would you pay $12 to remove the skin blemish?) If the subject rejects this bid then offer a lower price. (For example, would you pay $8 to remove the skin blemish?)
- *Step 4 – Find the maximum bid*: Repeat *Step 3* until you find the maximum price that the subject will pay (e.g., the subject will pay no more than $11 to remove the skin blemish).

A variation of the bidding game is the *discrete choice* approach, that is, asking subjects to choose between two or more different alternatives at a time. For example, you may ask a subject if he or she would rather have $50 or remove the skin blemish. Like the bidding game, the discrete choice approach may continue for any number of iterations until arriving at a final value. In addition, the *paired rating* approach is a variation of the discrete choice approach in which you ask subjects not only to choose among alternatives but also to rate them (e.g., strongly, moderately, or slightly). So a subject may prefer $50 but only slightly over removing the skin blemish. A paired rating approach may help you arrive at the final value faster.

Another contingent valuation technique is *contingent ranking*, that is, asking subjects to rank different situations or alternatives from most to least desirable. Contingent ranking will help establish the relative value of different possibilities. Including tangible possibilities can in turn help estimate the intangible possibilities in the list. For example, a subject ranking the removal of a skin blemish under buying a $30 DVD but above going to a $10 movie suggests that getting rid of that skin blemish is worth somewhere between $30 and $10.

Stated preferences or contingent valuation techniques overcome many of the drawbacks of revealed preferences. Stated preference techniques offer you complete control over the situations or alternatives that you pose to subjects. Carefully constructing the situation and questions can eliminate other possible factors that may influence the price that a subject is willing to pay.

However, a vulnerability of stated preference techniques is that the subjects' responses may not accurately reflect their true behavior. As we discuss later in this chapter, surveys, questionnaires, and any patient reported information are subject to a wide variety of biases and inaccuracies. People's words and statements frequently do not match their true beliefs or actions.

8.3.3 Productivity Losses

Patients may have to miss work due to illness, debilitation, health care visits, or hospitalization, resulting in *productivity losses*. Studies from the societal or employer's perspective should include productivity losses. For many economic studies, the following formula can estimate productivity losses:

$$\text{Productivity loss} = \text{Hours missing work} \times \text{Hourly wage}$$

When considering the general population, you may use the average workday length (8 hours) and the mean or median hourly wage to estimate productivity losses from missing a day of work.

Studies that measure all costs and rewards in monetary terms must also express death in monetary terms. In many such cases, the cost of a death is the lost productivity of removing that person from the labor force for the rest of that person's potential working life. The following formula can calculate this loss:

$$\text{Cost-of-death} = (\text{Retirement age} - \text{Age at death}) \times \text{Annual income}$$

For example, a 20-year old who dies will cost society 45 years of lost income.

Even though the productivity formulas above are used for many economic studies, they are only rough estimates that do not accurately measure all productivity losses. For some conditions (e.g., sleep disorders, allergies, depression, anxiety, or injuries), productivity losses comprise a significant proportion of the overall costs. Therefore, a blunt, inaccurate measure of productivity may grossly under or overestimate productivity losses. For example, an employee afflicted with such conditions may not only miss days of work but also may be less productive while at work. Such conditions may lead to reduced or poor-quality output (e.g., more mistakes). Patients may have to take frequent breaks or, in some cases, exhibit behavior that inhibits the productivity of others (e.g., reduce the overall performance of the team or assembly line). Therefore, using more detailed measures of productivity losses may be necessary. For example, you could follow patients with and without the condition in a time-and-motion study and calculate the work output of each patient.

8.3.4 Externalities

Any event can have effects that reach beyond the people and things directly associated with the event. Such effects are termed externalities: *positive externalities* when the effects are beneficial and *negative externalities* when the effects are detrimental. For example, instituting an exercise program at work may motivate employees to be more concerned about their health in general (which in turn may improve their diets) and create a positive image of the company (which may help the company gain more business).

Since the impact of an event and interactions among different people and the environment are very complex, capturing all of the possible externalities in an economic study is impossible. You have to decide for each study how extensive you want the study to be. The more distant or remote the externality is from the event, the more you have to convince others that the effect is indeed related to the event. In general, do not ignore sizable and easily quantifiable externalities (e.g., knee surgery on a professional basketball superstar could have substantial economic externalities such as attendance at basketball games and sales of items that the player endorses). Identifying an effect as an externality requires assumptions, which should be clearly stated in an economic study (e.g., you assume that the superstar not playing will affect attendance).

8.3.5 Measuring Rewards

You can measure rewards in a variety of different units such as money, lives saved, quality-of-life improvements, productivity increases, suffering prevented, or adverse events avoided. Different rewards are relevant to different situations. For example, an acne cream is not going to save lives but may improve quality of life (or the number of dates).

Different reward measures have emerged over the years:

- *Money*: The earliest economic studies expressed all rewards in purely monetary terms, converting all potential benefits of an intervention into dollars, pounds, yen, francs, etc.
- *Life years saved*: Not all rewards can be easily expressed in monetary terms. Saving a life does not necessarily save money (e.g., a patient who dies may actually save the health care system money by not consuming any more hospital resources). Therefore, "life years saved" may be more appropriate as a reward for some interventions.
- *Quality-adjusted life years (QALYs)*: Some interventions do not save lives but instead improve a patient's life by reducing symptoms or suffering (e.g., pain medications, walking devices, and physical therapy). One QALY represents a year of perfect health, and less than one QALY represents a year of impaired health (the smaller the fraction of the QALY, the worse the health status).
- *Others*: Many reward measures are specific to particular interventions or diseases (e.g., the number of bypass operations prevented for cardiac medications).

TABLE 8.1 Common Health Economic Analyses

	Question	Costs	Rewards
Cost-of-illness (COI) analysis	Economic impact of disease	Monetary units	None
Cost-of-treatment analysis	Economic cost of intervention	Monetary units	None
Cost-minimization analysis (CMA)	Choose best alternative when effects are equal	Monetary units	None
Cost-benefit analysis (CBA)	Choose best alternative when rewards can be expressed in monetary units	Monetary units	Monetary units
Cost-effectiveness analysis (CEA)	Choose best alternative when rewards expressed in simple clinical units	Monetary units	Clinical units (e.g., life years saved and hospitalizations averted)
Cost-utility analysis (CUA)	Choose best alternative when rewards expressed in health status units	Monetary units	Health status units (e.g., QALYs)

8.4 TYPES OF ECONOMIC ANALYSES

8.4.1 Choosing the Right Analysis

Choosing the right economic analytic method entails defining the question first. Do you want to know whether a disease or condition is worth addressing? Do you want to choose among different alternatives? Are you unsure about how much money to invest in developing a treatment? What should the price or reimbursement for your intervention be? In many cases, one analytic method will not suffice, and a progression of different methods will answer a question. Table 8.1 lists some common health economic analyses.

A *cost-of-illness (COI) study* can help quantify a disease's total monetary effect, including all the resulting medical and nonmedical costs (e.g., loss of productivity). A well-performed COI study will show not only the total cost (e.g., disease A costs society $750 million annually), but also different strata and categories of cost, such as the amount spent on medications, hospitalizations, emergency care, and days off from work (e.g., $100 million from hospital visits, $200 million from clinic visits, $250 million from lost productivity, and $200 million from medications), allowing you to target the areas of greatest economic burden. Often, the first step in tackling a new and unfamiliar disease is a COI study to map out the problem.

A COI study can serve multiple purposes, such as:

- *Determine whether a problem is worth tackling*. A COI study can identify which diseases and conditions should be addressed. For example, acne and hangnails are two very common conditions. However, acne probably has more economic cost than hangnails. People purchase a variety of facial washes, creams, and medications to prevent or conceal acne. Therefore, an economic study could show that pursuing an acne treatment may be more worthwhile than pursuing a hangnail treatment.
- *Demonstrate the size and importance of the problem*. A COI study can convince others that a disease or condition should receive more attention. Sometimes the full impact of a disease or condition is very subtle but far-reaching. An example is sleep disorders. While failing to get regular sleep may not have consequences as dramatic as a heart attack, over time, insomnia can result in substantial loss in productivity and increased health care expenditures from developing depression, suffering fatigue and getting sick more often. A COI study could delineate the economic impact of these effects.
- *Find unexpected costs*. Often people will not realize the effects of a disease or condition. For example, if an

employer learns that a disease affects an employee's productivity, the employer may be willing to subsidize treatment for the disease.

There are different types of COI studies. Prevalence COI studies tabulate the total cost of a disease per year. Incidence studies calculate the total cost of a disease throughout a patient's lifetime. A COI study may sum the costs of a single patient, a specific group of patients, or all patients with the disease. Establishing the costs-of-illness for a "typical" patient can be challenging, since patients may vary substantially. Therefore, it may be more useful to identify a median, mean, and standard deviation of disease-related costs.

After profiling a problem, a cost-of-intervention or cost-of-treatment analysis can profile all the monetary costs associated with administering an intervention. While some interventions are relatively simple to administer (e.g., simply taking a pill), others involve a range of different steps and materials (e.g., surgery). Cost-of-intervention studies should include and clearly identify every important fixed and variable cost. Running multiple scenarios may show how variable costs change with different situations.

Cost-of-intervention studies can serve several purposes:

- *Outline which interventions are economically feasible.* No matter how effective, an intervention may be prohibitively expensive to use. Moreover, you may want to reserve relatively expensive interventions for unusual, very-difficult-to-treat situations.
- *Identify targets for cost reduction.* Cost-of-intervention studies may help determine which steps or materials in an intervention are particularly expensive and find less expensive alternatives. Sometimes the *cost-driver* (i.e., the item or step that contributes the most to the overall cost of the intervention) of the intervention is unexpected.
- *Choosing the best intervention among equally effective, safe, and convenient interventions.* When two or more interventions are no different in efficacy, safety or ease of use, the primary factor in choosing an intervention is cost. Insurance companies and health care organizations will often use cost-of-treatment studies to determine the cost savings from switching to a generic version of a medication or an alternative "equivalent" treatment.

After you profile possible treatments, a *cost-minimization analysis (CMA), cost-benefit analysis (CBA), cost-effective analysis (CEA),* or *cost-utility analysis (CUA)* can help choose among multiple alternative treatments. The type of problem guides the choice of analysis. If all treatments have equivalent effects, a CMA, which focuses only on costs, can help choose the least expensive treatments. For example, if Medication A and Medication B have the same success rate in treating a disease, a CMA might find that Medication A should be used because it costs $200 less. If the potential effects are different but easily translate to monetary

terms (e.g., dollars, yen, pounds), a CBA is suitable. A CBA converts all rewards and costs of each option into comparable monetary terms. A *benefit* is a reward expressed in monetary terms. All costs and rewards must be in equivalent monetary terms (e.g., you cannot have some rewards in dollars and others in yen) and present day values (i.e., net present value). So, for instance, a CMA may find that Medication A that costs $300 but potentially could save $1000 from preventing lung disease (a net benefit of $700 = $1000 − $300) to be favorable to Medication B that costs $100 but could save only $400 (a net benefit of $300). However, if all the potential rewards do not translate easily into pure monetary terms, a CEA (which measures rewards in simple clinical units such as life years saved, deaths avoided, or operations avoided) or a CUA (which measures rewards in health status measures like QALYs or utilities) is more useful. A CEA and CUA will measure the costs and rewards of each alternative separately and compare the alternatives using incremental cost-effectiveness (or cost-utility) ratios.

Any CBA, CEA, or CUA should not include *sunk costs*, that is, costs that already incurred before the time frame of the study and thus are not recoupable. Such costs would be part of any possible option and therefore will not help decide among different options. For example, in deciding what medication to give a patient after heart surgery, do not include the cost of the heart surgery. The sunk costs of heart surgery should not affect the choice of medication.

A common mistake in CBA's, CEA's, and CUA's is *double-counting* of costs and rewards. An intervention may result in seemingly two separate rewards that are in fact different variations of the same reward. For example, an asthma medication may help a person breathe better and improve her productivity at work. If you were to use days present at work as a measure of productivity, do not also use the number of projects completed. Counting and summing both will result in double-counting. Someone who is at work more often most likely will complete more projects.

Some costs and rewards may be *contingencies*, that is, there is a chance that they may occur. For example, after knee surgery, some (but not all) patients may need very strong pain medications. In some cases, a repeat operation may be necessary. The value of a contingency is equal to its cost or reward multiplied by the probability of the contingency occurring.

8.4.2 Marginal and Incremental Analyses

Incremental analyses quantify the resulting differences in choosing one alternative over others. In CBA, the incremental cost indicates the change in cost when moving from one alternative to another. For example, if C_A and C_B are the net costs and rewards of Treatments A and B, respectively, then the incremental cost of using Treatment B instead of A is $C_B - C_A$. A negative incremental cost suggests that B is favorable or dominant to A, while a positive one favors A.

Similarly in cost-effectiveness analyses, an incremental cost-effectiveness ratio (ICER) is the change in cost per change in effectiveness when shifting from one alternative treatment to another, and in cost-utility analyses, an incremental cost-utility ratio is the change in cost per change in health status when shifting from one alternative treatment to another. For example, if C_A and C_B are the costs of Treatments A and B, respectively and E_A and E_B are the resulting effectiveness of A and B, respectively, then an ICER is $(C_B - C_A)/(E_B - E_A)$. Interpreting this ratio is somewhat more complicated than interpreting an incremental cost. If the ICER is negative, then Treatment B is favorable or dominant to Treatment A. If the ICER is positive, then the magnitude of the ICER matters. If for instance, the ICER is $10/life year saved, then choosing Treatment B requires only $10 more for each life year saved. Most, except for the most penurious, would view this as a worthwhile investment and choose B. However, if the ICER is $100,000/life year saved, then you would have to question whether this reward is worth the investment.

Marginal cost and marginal cost-effectiveness can help see the implications of changing a certain parameter (e.g., number of medications given, dollars invested, items used, and people employed) by a single unit. For example, in CBA, to measure the added cost of giving every patient an extra day of a medication, if C_N represents the net monetary value of giving a medication for N days and C_{N+1} the net monetary value for giving it $N+1$ days, then the marginal cost would be $C_{N+1} - C_N$. In a CEA, if C_N and E_N represents the cost and effectiveness, respectively, of giving a medication N days and C_{N+1} and E_{N+1} represents the cost and effectiveness, respectively, of giving the medication $N+1$ days, the marginal cost-effectiveness of an additional day of medication is $(C_{N+1} - C_N)/(E_{N+1} - E_N)$. A similar calculation would yield a marginal cost-utility in a CUA.

8.4.3 Assumptions and Sensitivity Analyses

Collecting perfect data is impossible. So you frequently have to rely on a series of assumptions based on findings from prior studies, expert opinion, educated guesses from personal experience, or, in some cases, truly random guesses. Is the available data truly representative? Are your estimates about unavailable data accurate? People will ask such questions when interpreting your economic study. An economic study is only as strong as its assumptions. Clearly stating your assumptions is very important. Some assumptions may be minor and have little bearing on study results, but others may be very controversial and dramatically influence study conclusions. *Sensitivity analyses* can help ascertain the impact of these assumptions.

As even the best executed and most comprehensive economic studies incorporate many uncertainties and potentially variable data, properly performed sensitivity analyses are important and, in some cases, the most important part of the study. Performing sensitivity analyses involves changing important variables along a range of different values and measuring the consequent effects on the results. For example, What would happen to the results if the discount rate varies from 2% to 6%, the cost of a specific medication ranges from $100 to $500, the percentage of people receiving a certain test changes from 40% to 60%, or the study excluded certain costs that were previously included? Running these different scenarios will not only identify the variables that have an important impact on the results, but also demonstrate the credibility of the economic study. When an economic study's results do not change significantly during sensitivity analyses, the study is "*robust*," that is, its results are considered definitive. However, just because the results fluctuate significantly during sensitivity analyses does not mean the study is useless. Sensitivity analyses can help target the items and issues that are most responsible for the costs and rewards of a situation. If, for example, finding that results depend heavily on the wait time for a procedure suggests that extra efforts should be made to reduce the wait time.

8.5 PATIENT REPORTED OUTCOMES (PRO)

8.5.1 Roles and Uses

Nowadays medical technology allows you to measure an array of physiological, psychological, economic, and physical phenomena. Imaging devices, laboratory tests, tissue samplers, and monitoring devices can quantify the size and function of organs, the levels of different chemicals in various body fluids, and the movement of certain molecules throughout the human body. Many of these measurements do not even require talking to the patient. All the patients have to do is be present and obey instructions.

However, technology will never be able to measure everything. Technology alone cannot tell you:

- *Whether a patient is experiencing certain symptoms.* Many symptoms are not obvious to observers (e.g., headache, abdominal pain, back pain, dizziness, chest discomfort, nausea, or fatigue). Some symptoms are psychological or psychiatrical (e.g., depression or anxiety). Some occur only when research personnel are not present (e.g., sexual side effects or sleep disturbances).
- *The frequency of certain symptoms.* (e.g., does the headache occur once a day, once a week, or once a month?)
- *The severity of certain symptoms* (e.g., is the headache mild, moderate, or severe?)
- *The severity and nature of a patient's disability.* (e.g., when and how long does the chest pain occur? Does

the chest pain occur during exercise? How severe is the chest pain?)

- *The impact of a disease or condition on a patient's daily life.* (e.g., does the disease interfere with certain activities such as exercise, work, or sex?)
- *The patient's perceptions and feelings about a disease, condition, or intervention.* (e.g., is the patient satisfied with the treatment? Is it very frustrating to have recurring headaches?)

As they often say in clinical medicine, nothing replaces listening to the patient. The patient can tell you many things that technology and physical examinations cannot measure. Quite often, patient opinions, thoughts, and complaints become lost in the sea of diagnostic tests and physician interpretation. Disregarding patient comments and statements can overlook valuable information. In fact, for some diseases, conditions, and interventions, the patient is the only possible source of data.

A *patient reported outcome (PRO)* is any measurement that comes directly from the patient. A true PRO is not altered or filtered in any way by the clinician or researcher. You can use different *instruments* to collect PROs such as a questionnaire or a formal interview session. When a clinician or researcher filters or interprets a patient's statements before recording them, they become observer reported outcomes (ORO) instead. For example, a patient's revelation in a written questionnaire that she is experiencing severe hot flashes is a PRO. A physician asking a patient to describe the nature and frequency of her hot flashes and then determining that the hot flashes are severe is an ORO.

A PRO can serve a variety of functions:

- *Determine patient eligibility for a clinical study*: Many selection criteria for study enrollment depend on PROs (e.g., an inclusion criterion is having chronic pain for at least a year).
- *Confirm or validate other measures*: PROs can help confirm other measures (e.g., a patient with a very low cardiac ejection fraction and jugular venous distention most likely will have symptoms of congestive heart failure, such trouble breathing when lying flat or walking up stairs). Discrepancies between the PROs and other measurements may suggest that either your measurement devices are faulty or the patient is not being forthcoming about his or her symptoms or experiences.
- *Help interpret other measures*: Some measurements can have many different possible explanations or interpretations. A PRO can eliminate some possibilities (e.g., enlarged lymph nodes associated with upper respiratory symptoms are more likely due to infection; enlarged lymph nodes without upper respiratory symptoms may be due to cancer).
- *Characterize patient compliance*: Frequently, there is no way for most of us to know if a patient is taking a treatment without asking the patient. Moreover,

understanding the reason for noncompliance is important. (For example, is the treatment too inconvenient to take? Does the treatment cause too many side effects?)
- *Serve as study endpoints*: In many cases, PROs can serve as a primary or secondary efficacy (e.g., pain level for a pain medication) or safety (e.g., nausea or diarrhea) endpoint.
- *Provide feedback to investigators*: Patient comments can help you improve your intervention, study design, and operations (e.g., the patient may relate factors that are making the study or treatment inconvenient).

8.5.2 Collecting PROs

There are many different ways of collecting PROs. Your choice of *instrument* depends on the nature of the PROs, potential biases, the use of the PROs, budgetary constraints, and the frequency at which you want to collect PROs. Live interviews and questionnaires are two general ways of obtaining PROs.

Live interviews can occur in person or via a communications medium such as the telephone or Internet. Live interviews have several advantages:

- *Provide guidance for the respondent*: The interviewer can help clarify questions that the patient does not understand.
- *Cues from the respondent*: The interviewer may detect audio cues (e.g., pauses or voice inflections) or visual cues (e.g., signs of nervousness or anxiety such as tapping, hand wringing, or eye movements) that can provide additional information.
- *Additional probing*: The interviewer can elicit additional information from the patient, especially if the patient offers vague or unusual answers.
- *Increased response rate*: It may harder to ignore or turn down a person wanting an interview than a mailed written questionnaire.
- *Confirming the identity of the respondent*: The live interviewer can ensure that the person answering the questions is indeed the patient.

However, live interviews have several disadvantages as well:

- *Costly and time consuming*: Hiring personnel to perform interviews can be costly.
- *Variability in questions*: Unless you precisely script the interview (i.e., provide a written transcript for the interviewer to strictly follow), the interviewer consciously or unconsciously may change the questions. Even subtle differences in wording, tone, or inflection can change the meaning of a question. For example, a patient may answer, "Have you had pain?" differently from "Have you *ever* had pain?".

- *Interviewer interpretation*: An interviewer may consciously or unconsciously filter or alter a patient's responses. The interviewer may miss, misunderstand, or make assumptions about a patient's answer.
- *Intrusiveness*: A live interview can seem more intrusive. Patients may be less willing to reveal sensitive or embarrassing details to a live person.
- *Time pressure*: Patients have to provide answers within a limited time frame. As a result, they may offer hasty and poorly thought-out answers.

Questionnaires can come in multiple forms: paper questionnaires that are either handed out or mailed to subjects, electronic questionnaires located on a computer or on the internet, or audio questionnaires administered through the telephone or other devices. Questionnaires have several advantages:

- *Cost-effectiveness*: Preparing and administering questionnaires is usually less expensive than hiring personnel.
- *Standardized questions*: Questions on a questionnaire are fixed and unalterable.
- *Unfiltered answers*: Questionnaires allow you to see the subjects original answers, not subject to an interviewers interpretation.
- *Reduced time pressure*: Patients can take their time to consider and answer the questions.

Questionnaires can have the following disadvantages:

- *No interviewer to provide guidance, probe for more answers, or pick cues from the respondent.*
- *Lower response rate.* Patients may fail to answer questions within the questionnaire.
- *Inability to confirm the identity of the respondent.* Unless you supervise or watch the subject, you cannot be sure who helped answer the questionnaire.

Focus groups are similar to interviews but with multiple interviewees at a time. The focus group can have any number of interviewees but 6 to 12 is typical. There can also be more than one interviewer or moderator. The session can be as structured or unstructured as needed. The interviewer or moderator can control the conversation or be more of an observer or bystander. When there is more than one moderator, each moderator can assume a different role. For example, one moderator can ask the questions while the other moderator ensures that all topics are covered. Focus groups can be superior to one-on-one interviews when different interviewees help each other recall information and think of ideas that they would not have come up with alone. However, the biggest problem with focus groups is that certain interviewees may influence other interviewees. Domineering interviewees could overpower others. *Groupthink* (i.e., members of the group going along with the crowd) could occur.

8.6 INSTRUMENTS

8.6.1 Developing an Instrument

Developing the right instrument for your study can be a complicated and time consuming process. If the instrument is an interview, you may have to *script* (i.e., write out what to say) the interview in advance. You also have to decide where and how the interview will take place. If the instrument is a questionnaire, you will have to design the questions and the physical layout of the questionnaire.

Using Existing Instruments

Developing your own instrument may not be necessary if an appropriate validated and published instrument already exists. Using an existing instrument can save considerable time, effort, and resources. Keep in mind that instruments can lose their validity if they are used in different ways and populations. So carefully compare your study population with the ones for which the existing instrument was developed.

Ordering of Questions

The order in which you ask questions is very important. Earlier questions can influence the responses to subsequent questions. A question can serve as a memory trigger for the next question. For example:

> *Question 1*: When were you last hospitalized?
> *Question 2*: During your last hospitalization, did you receive physical therapy?

Putting *Question 1* first helps the patient recall his last hospitalization so that he may better answer *Question 2*.

Response contamination occurs when earlier questions unduly influence responses to later questions. Make sure that the initial questions do not contain information that will change the way respondents will answer later questions. For example, if the first 10 questions suggest that certain activities are deviant or abnormal, the respondent may not be willing to admit that he or she practices those activities.

Respondents often consciously or unconsciously look for patterns in the questions. They subsequently may provide answers that match the pattern. A respondent may accidentally answer one question in the same way as the previous question. For example, if a respondent answers "yes" to the first 9 questions, he may automatically answer "yes" to Question 10 without reading the question carefully.

The ordering of questions can affect different people in different ways. Earlier questions can train the respondent, getting him or her used to answering the questions. As a result, the respondent may be more facile at answering later questions. However, fatigue and boredom may make respondents less likely to answer later questions.

Transitions between questions should be relatively smooth. Jumping from topic to topic may disorient and frustrate respondents. Grouping similar questions (e.g., all questions about the patient's urinary habits) together can help patients recall information. Placing appropriate headlines or section titles in front of each group can assist recall as well as help the patient move to and from different sections in case they want to skip some questions to answer later.

Instrument Appearance

Appearance matters when designing an instrument. Friendly appearing and visually appealing questionnaires can elicit higher response rates. The words and pictures should be large enough for patients to read with ease. Remember that many elderly patients may be visually impaired. The physical layout of the questionnaire can help respondents find and better understand each of the questions (e.g., a picture of a heart next to heart-related questions can be a good visual cue). Color and changes in font-types can emphasize important instructions, words, or statements (e.g., which of the following would you *NOT* take).

Similarly, the appearance or sound of an interviewer during an interview can affect responses. The interviewer should not be intimidating, rude, or unprofessional. Remember that many patients are hearing impaired. The interviewer should speak slowly and clearly, pausing between sentences. The interviewer should make transitions between questions obvious and frequently ask if the patient understands the instructions and questions.

Validating the Instrument and Testing Its Reliability

We discussed *validity* and *reliability* when we discussed measures in Chapter 4. An instrument is valid if it measures what it claims to measure. To establish an instrument's validity, the instrument should appear like the right kind of measure (*face validity*) and produce comparable results as other similar measures. An instrument is reliable if it consistently reproduces the same results from repeated samples and by different researchers. Therefore, you must test the instrument repeatedly to make sure the results remain relatively consistent.

Respondent Diversity

Remember that respondents may come from a variety of cultural, racial, ethnic, geographic, socioeconomic, language, and educational backgrounds. All respondents must be able to fully understand the instructions, questions, and answers. If the diversity of your study population is too great for one instrument, multiple versions of the instrument may be necessary (e.g., Spanish, Chinese, and English versions).

Pilot-Testing

Pilot-testing before administering a questionnaire or interview can identify potential weaknesses and circumvent problems. Pilot-testing is analogous to a practice or trial run. Identify a small group of people, who can complete and provide feedback on the questionnaire or interview. Information from this test run can help you revise and refine the instrument and procedure. Make sure the diversity of the pilot group matches that of your study population (e.g., if the study population has many people of Korean descent, then your pilot group should have some people of Korean descent). Otherwise, the pilot-test will not identify all potential problems.

8.6.2 Administering an Instrument

Pre-notification

Prior to distributing a questionnaire or contacting the patient for an interview, a *pre-notification message* (e.g., a letter, email, or phone call) may be helpful. The pre-notification message warns the subject to be on the lookout for the questionnaire or interview. With such a warning, patients may be less likely to miss the interview or misplace the questionnaire. Such a message also can help confirm the legitimacy of the questionnaire or interview. In turn, pre-notification messages can increase the response rate. A pre-notification message should describe the purpose of the questionnaire or interview, identify the sponsors of the study, and explain the general purposes of the study. Do not assume that the patient knows or remembers this information. Even if the patient is already aware of this information, re-iterating and re-emphasizing it can be useful.

Questionnaire Cover Letters

Having a well-composed cover letter can significantly improve the response rate to your questionnaire by providing valuable guidance and making the questionnaire seem more official. Write the cover letter in a clear, concise and friendly manner. The cover letter should describe the purpose of the study and questionnaire, identify the study sponsors, list contact information in case the respondent has any questions. Include a statement about patient confidentiality and privacy. The cover letter also can instruct the patient on when and how to return the completed questionnaire.

Interview Environment

The environment in which you administer an interview can dramatically affect responses and compliance. The environment should be quiet and comfortable with minimal distractions. Stressful environments may keep patients from opening up and revealing information. Sometimes certain settings, objects, images, and sounds can serve as memory triggers, helping the patient recall information. Bringing patients back to where certain events occurred may aid recall, as long as those places are conducive to interviews.

Respect patient privacy and dignity during interviews. Do not interview patients while they are in the middle of a procedure, eating, showering, or using the bathroom. Give them adequate warning before conducting an interview. Patients should have the option of deciding who can remain in the room during the interview. If possible, patients should have the opportunity of changing into more comfortable or respectable clothes.

8.7 QUESTIONNAIRE AND INTERVIEW QUESTIONS

8.7.1 Characteristics of Good Questions

Asking the right questions is more difficult than it seems. The way you ask a question can dramatically change the answers evoked. For example, here are five similar questions that may have very different answers:

- *Do you have a Porsche (or similar car)?*
- *Do you not have a car like a Porsche?* This question implies that you are unusual or different if you do not own a Porsche. The respondent may want to fit in and answer "no."
- *Do you have an overpriced car like a Porsche?* This suggests that having a Porsche is somewhat foolish. The respondent may be embarrassed to admit that he or she has a Porsche.
- *Do you have a luxury sports car like a Porsche?* This suggests that having a Porsche is good thing. The respondent may be more likely to answer "yes."
- *Do you own a Porsche?* The respondent may lease a Porsche but not own it.

As you can see, similar questions with slightly different wording can elicit very different responses. When designing questions keep in mind the following:

Questions Should be Single-Dimensional

Questions should ask about one characteristic or issue (i.e., dimension) at a time. Beware of asking "double-barreled" questions such as "do you like that person's looks and personality?" Such questions actually consist of more than one

question and you have no idea which part of the question a respondent is answering. When a subject answers "no," does the answer apply to the person's "looks," "personality," or both? Try to minimize the use of the words "and" or "or" in your question.

Questions Should be Clear and Unambiguous

Respondents should be able to readily understand what the question is asking. The question should not have different possible interpretations. Remember that some words or phrases may have multiple meanings to different people. For example, the following question would be too vague and ambiguous:

Is he nice?

A. Yes   B. No

What is the meaning of "nice"? Does it refer to his looks, actions, or demeanor? Under what circumstances are we evaluating the person? No one is "nice" to all people or in all situations. A clearer question would be:

Does he behave courteously to his elders?

A. Yes   B. No

Such a question is better but still not completely clear. Who is an "elder"? What does courteous behavior entail?

Does he help his grandmother lift heavy items?

A. Yes   B. No

This question is even better. Now we know the specific behavior and recipient of the behavior. There is still some ambiguity. What is a "heavy item" and what does "help" mean? But, as you can see, the question is a lot more specific than our previous two questions.

Questions Should Use Plain, Lay Language

Remember that the educational and experience levels of respondents may vary significantly. Every possible respondent should be able to fully understand your questions. Avoid using technical terms and jargon that lay persons will not understand. Keep sentences plain and simple. Refrain from employing abbreviations unless they are very commonplace.

Keep Questions Short and Simple

Patients' have short attention spans and low tolerance for tedious and long questions. Remember that answering questions may be keeping them from other important activities such as work, time with family and friends, or hobbies. Keep questions relatively short. The longer the question, the less likely a respondent will thoroughly read the question. Also, the longer the questionnaire, the less likely a respondent will complete the questionnaire.

Questions Should be Assumption-Free

The question should make no assumptions about the respondent. For example, the following question assumes that the respondent is working:

Does your condition affect you at work?

A. Yes   B. No

The question should include either a third response option ("C. Not currently working") or a statement that allows the respondent to skip the question (e.g., "Answer only if you are working").

Questions Should Clarify and Explain Important Concepts and Terms

Do not assume that the respondents will completely understand all issues, concepts, and terms. For example, the following question presupposes that the respondent knows about a certain piece of legislation:

Do you agree with the Medicare Act of 2001?

A. Yes   B. No

The question should include either an overview of the Medicare Act of 2001 or a third response option ("C. Not familiar with Medicare Act of 2001").

Questions Should Not "Lead" Respondents

A question's wording may suggest that a certain answer is correct or more desirable. Avoid such *leading questions* that "push" respondents to choose a particular answer. Questions that begin with phrases such as "don't you think ...," "wouldn't you like ...," "isn't it better ...," or "have you not ..." tend to be leading.

Minimize Branching Questions

A *branching question* directs the respondent along different pathways depending on which answer the respondent selects. An example of a branching question is:

1. Have you been hospitalized in the past year?

A. Yes   B. No (if no, go to Question 3).

2. Did you receive intravenous medications in the hospital?

A. Yes   B. No

Branching questions can confuse respondents. Respondents may not follow directions or fail to answer

questions out of frustration. Combining the two questions will eliminate the branching question and may be clearer for the respondent:

1. Have you received intravenous medications in the hospital over the past year?

A. Yes   B. No   C. Have not been hospitalized

Avoid Emotionally Loaded or Controversial Questions

Questions should appear as objective and emotionally detached as possible. When possible, ask about facts and not assessments. For example, avoid questions such as the following:

Are you a mean person?

A. Yes   B. No

Very few people would answer "Yes" to this kind of question. Most people either do not believe or will not admit that they are "mean." Better questions would be:

Have you thrown rocks at someone over the past year?

A. Yes   B. No

Have you kicked any animals over the past year?

A. Yes   B. No

These are more "objective" and "factual" questions and involve less value judgment. They do not specify whether someone is right or wrong in throwing rocks or kicking an animal. They are also easier to determine. Regardless of the reason or intent, those who threw rocks and kicked animals would have to answer "yes." (Of course, some may argue about the definition of "throwing rocks" and "kick.")

Avoid Offensive or Judgmental Questions

Insulting or offending respondents will only decrease their willingness to cooperate and complete your questionnaire or interview. What may not seem offensive to you could be highly offensive to someone else. Never include racial or ethnic slurs, sexist remarks, or inappropriate comments unless there is a real scientific need to do so. (One exception would be if you were studying the effects of such comments or remarks: for example, have you ever been called one of the following slurs?)

Remember that everyone is different and has had a different path in life. Without knowing the full story, making uneducated judgments and assessments about why a person takes certain actions and holds certain beliefs is unfair and unreasonable. As they say, "unless you've walked in someone's shoes you cannot fully appreciate his or her experiences and perspectives."

Therefore, your questions should not make any value judgments. Doing so can be difficult. We all bring unconscious biases into all our activities. If we are opposed to certain actions or people, we are more likely to portray them in a negative light. Examples would be:

How often do you engage in fun activities such as wine tasting?

How often do you indulge in gambling?

These questions suggest that wine tasting is fun and gambling is bad and indulgent. Not everyone will agree with such assessments. Better questions would be:

How often do you go wine tasting?

How often do you gamble?

As you can see, these questions do not include such significant judgments about wine tasting and gambling. They are more factual and "objective" questions.

Questions Should Not Have "Right" and "Wrong" Answers

Unless your questionnaire or interview is an aptitude test, do not design questions to have correct and incorrect answers. Respondents often worry about choosing the right answer and not appearing stupid, strange, or deviant. They will avoid answers that appear socially or intellectually "incorrect." Look at the following example:

Is your intelligence above average?

A. Yes   B. No

How many people will answer "B. No"? By definition (assuming a normal distribution of intelligence in the general population), 50% of all people should be below average and answer "B. No". But the wording of the question makes answering "no" seem like a wrong or incorrect answer. In actuality, intelligence is only one aspect of a person's abilities. Moreover, there are many different measures of intelligence.

8.7.2 Open-Ended vs. Close-Ended Questions

A question can be open-ended or close-ended. An *open-ended question* allows and encourages a subject to respond in practically any manner. Here are some examples:

- *What do you think about her?* You could answer "I like her," "she has beautiful long hair and a fantastic personality," or "she is a very talented writer and a good leader."

- *How does your symptom make you feel?* You could answer "okay," "very badly," or "like a slow, worthless individual."

- *Tell me about your condition.* You could answer "it's a very rare condition," "it causes a lot of problems," or "it is very severe."

As you can see, potential answers to open-ended questions can vary significantly in length, focus, and content. Open-ended questions are useful when you cannot anticipate the subject's answers or want to encourage the subject to raise unexpected issues. However, the potential wide variability of answers may make analysis difficult. Subjects may provide vague, unusual, or uninterpretable answers. Subjects may fail to address the exact issues that you want them to address (e.g., when you ask, "what do you think about her," a subject may focus on her looks and not her personality or abilities). Subjects may not understand the meaning or implications of an open-ended question, which can be rather vague.

By contrast, a *closed-ended question* restricts subjects to a limited number of different short answers. Examples include:

- *Do you like her?* Your answer can only be "yes," "no," or "I don't know."
- *Rate the severity of your symptom on a scale of 1 to 5.* Your answer can only be "1," "2," "3," "4," or "5."
- *Is your condition mild, moderate, or severe?*

Potential answers are predictable and finite. Answers to closed-ended questions are usually easier to tabulate and analyze. By forcing subjects to provide specific answers, closed-ended questions usually result in fewer uninterpretable or vague answers. However, closed-ended questions can be inappropriately limiting. For example, a subject may like a woman but only under certain conditions (e.g., when the woman is trying to be friendly). A closed-ended question may not allow the subject to qualify his answer or provide additional important details. As a result, open-ended questions often can elicit more information than closed-ended questions.

8.8 RESPONSE OPTIONS

8.8.1 Characteristics of Response Options

Once you have designed a question for an instrument, you must offer a way for the respondent to answer (i.e., *response options*). The respondent may have to choose one of several different possible answers, place a mark on a scale, rank different possibilities, assign a score to some items, or provide a written or verbal answer. The type of response option can substantially affect the respondent's ability and willingness to answer the question, the accuracy and validity of the instrument, and the analysis and interpretation of the result. So take time and effort to design and choose appropriate response options.

When designing a question's response options, try to maximize the questions' *discriminability*. Discriminability is how well the question can show true differences among different respondents. In other words, will the question be able to separate respondents that are truly different? Both the wording of the question and the available response options determine the question's discriminability. For example, the following question has poor discriminability:

Are you human?

A. Yes   B. No

Presumably all respondents will answer "A. Yes," (unless you have some panda bears and dolphins participating in your study). This question will not separate respondent into different groups. Consider the following question:

What is your favorite color?

A. Red   B. Something else

This question has some discriminability. It separates the red-lovers from everyone else. But it clumps everyone else into one category. The following question has better discriminability:

What is your favorite color?

A. Red   B. Green   C. Blue   D. Something else

This question has even more discriminability. Now the green-lovers, blue-lovers, and red-lovers are separated.

It may appear that the more answers, the better. But such is not always the case. Too many answers that are too similar may not separate respondents sufficiently. For example:

What is your favorite color?

A. Greenish-Blue   B. Green   C. Reddish-Green …

In this situation, the answers may be too close to each other. Respondents may float between different categories becoming indistinct.

Many questions have an option for respondents who cannot answer the question (e.g., "Don't Know," "Undecided," or "Neutral"). This "*neutral point*" option is for respondents who cannot provide a definitive answer or do not believe the question applies to them. The decision whether to include a neutral point as an option can be very important. Not including such an option may force some respondents to guess or even randomly select one of the available answers. Including a neutral point may allow some respondents to avoid selecting a definitive answer. Some questions should not have a neutral point answer (e.g., how many hours do you work a week, how often do you have pain, or how old are you?)

8.8.2 Multiple Choice Response Options

Multiple choice questions ask respondents to choose among a number of different response options. The question should clearly specify whether respondents must choose only one answer or may select more than one answer at a time. Otherwise, you may end up with uninterpretable data. Also, the positioning of the different choices may be important. The first and last response option may be more noticeable than options located in the middle. The biggest advantage of multiple choice questions is the ease of tabulating and analyzing the results.

Multiple choice questions should include all possible answers to a question. In other words, every possible respondent should be able to select an answer. For example, the following answer options are inadequate:

What medications are you taking?

A. Aspirin   B. Amoxicillin

Obviously, aspirin and amoxicillin are not the only medications that a patient may be taking. There are no options to select if a patient is taking a cholesterol-lowering or blood pressure medication. Which answer should a patient select if she is not taking any medications? What if the patient is taking both aspirin and amoxicillin?

Instead, any of following options may work better:

Option 1: *Do you take aspirin?*

A. Yes   B. No

Do you take amoxicillin?

A. Yes   B. No

Option 2: *Which of the following medications are you taking?*

(*Select only one answer*) A. Aspirin B. Amoxicillin C. Both aspirin and amoxicillin D. Neither aspirin nor amoxicillin

Make sure the different response options are mutually exclusive. One option should not be a subset of another option. Otherwise, a respondent may be confused as to which option to select. For example, the following question can cause problems:

Which is your favorite food?

A. Fish   B. Sushi   C. Salmon   D. Broccoli   E. Steak

Does a respondent who likes salmon sushi pick A, B, or C? Salmon sushi is a salmon, sushi, and fish.

Construct the answer options so that different people will be likely to select different answers. The question and option should be able to separate people into different categories. In other words, if almost everyone will select one option, then your question will not be useful. For example, the following question is relatively useless:

Do you feel unhappy sometimes?

A. Yes   B. No

Everyone has felt unhappy at some point and should answer "A. Yes." With a 100% answering "A," this question offers no important information. By contrast, the following question will provide more information:

Do you feel unhappy about your marriage?

A. Yes   B. No

Although this question is far from perfect, some will answer A, and others will answer B.

8.8.3 Rank Order

Some questions require a respondent to *rank* a series of items in some type of order (e.g., best to worst, worst to best, least to greatest, greatest to least, least important to most important, or most preferred to least preferred). While such questions may be necessary in some situations, they can be very problematic. The more items that need to be ranked, the less reliable the question becomes. For example, look at following two examples:

Example 1: *Rank the following cities in terms of desirability*: Chicago, San Diego, San Francisco

Example 2: *Rank the following city in terms of desirability*: Boston, New York City, Philadelphia, Chicago, Atlanta, Houston, Dallas, Miami, Los Angeles, San Diego, San Francisco, Seattle, Washington, D.C., Portland, Pittsburgh, Cleveland, Denver, Minneapolis, St. Louis

For example 2, ranking the top three or bottom three cities may be easy. But distinguishing among the middle pack is difficult. When there are too many items to rank, respondents lose concentration and have difficulty making comparisons. It is much easier to compare an item with one, two, or perhaps three items. But comparing more than five items with each other is challenging and confusing. So, in general, if you must use such ranking questions, try to keep the number of items to at most five.

A problem with simple rank order is that you do not know how far apart the different items on the list are from each other. Number 1 and Number 2 may be very close in desirability. But Number 2 may be much more desirable than Number 3. One way of circumventing this problem is to have the respondent assign a score to each item on the list. In this way, the respondent assigns a relative value to each of the listed options. For example:

Score each of the following cities in terms of desirability (0 for least desirable, 100 for most desirable):

Chicago _____

San Diego _____

San Francisco _____

Suppose the respondent assigns the following scores: San Diego 97, San Francisco 95, and Chicago 50. We then know that the respondent much prefers San Diego and San Francisco to Chicago. The higher the score, the higher the city is ranked. This type of response option really combines rank order with response scales (which we discuss in the following section).

8.8.4 Response Scales

A response scale is a set of answer choices that fall into a sequence or order (e.g., lowest to highest or least to most). A scale can have a finite number of discrete choices or an infinite continuum of choices. (We will discuss continuous response scales later in this section.) A scale can consist of numbers, categories, or pictures. A graphic rating scale is a set of pictures or diagrams on which the respondent can place a mark or circle. The graphic rating scale may have words, numbers, both, or neither. Figure 8.1 depicts some common examples.

Continuous Response Scales

Some variables have values that are continuous and do not fall into clear discrete categories. In fact, many symptoms (e.g., pain, weakness, depression, or fatigue) and attitudes (e.g., political, sociological, or sexual beliefs) have gradations of differences. For example, how important is sex in a relationship? Few would say that it is completely unimportant. Few would say that it is everything in a relationship. Most believe that sex has at least some importance. Forcing people to choose one of several specific choices may limit the amount of information you can collect. If you had only three choices, such as unimportant, important, and most important, the vast majority would answer "important." For the vast majority, they still would not know how important sex is. Is it mildly important, moderately important, or very important? Even expanding the choices to five categories (not important, mildly important, moderately important, very important, and most important) would not alleviate some potential problems. What is the difference between moderate and mild? Are all cases of moderately important the same? Should you classify mild-to-moderate as mild or moderate?

Therefore, a continuous set of response options may be more appropriate for a continuous variable. A continuous set of response options allows a subject to select a point along a continuum rather than a specific category. In other words, the subject has an "infinite" number of response

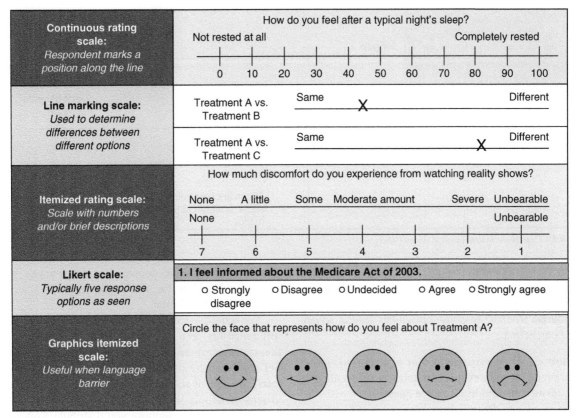

FIGURE 8.1   Examples of graphic rating scales.

options along a continuum. A *visual analog scale (VAS)* provides a set of continuous response options. A VAS is usually is a straight line with one end being the minimum value of the variable (e.g., no pain) and the other end being the maximum value of the variable (worst imaginable pain). A subject then marks a point along that line (e.g., if the subject's pain is severe, the subject would place a mark close to the maximum end; if the pain is mild, subject's mark would be close to the minimum end). The line can have any number of landmarks along the line to guide the patient (*Anchored or Categorized VAS*). Figure 8.2 shows example of VAS.

However, the biggest problem with a VAS is that different people with the same symptoms or attitudes may place their marks at different locations. The VAS is relatively imprecise. Are marks 2 mm or 3 mm apart significantly different? How far apart should marks be to be considered different? For example, one patient with relatively severe pain may put a mark 2 mm left of the maximum while another patient with equally severe pain may place a mark 4 mm left of the maximum. Therefore, a VAS is limited in its ability to compare small differences among various people or groups. A VAS is most useful in measuring change over time in the same individual. For example, one person may put a mark 2 mm left of the maximum and then after a pain medication treatment place a mark 5 mm to the left of maximum. This suggests that the patient's pain improved.

Scale anchors help alleviate some of the variability in where respondents place their marks. Scale anchors are landmarks along the scale that help guide respondents. Almost all scales have anchors at the two ends of the scale (i.e., the minimum and maximum values). Additional anchors may identify ratings between the minimum and maximum. For example, if the minimum and maximum values are "never" and "always," you may have anchors for "sometimes" and "frequently." More anchors provide more landmarks and may help reduce the variability in mark placement among different respondents. However, too many anchors can clutter the scale, making it difficult to read. The wording, number, and placement of scale anchors can dramatically affect where respondents place their marks. Anchors are usually equally distributed along the scale. In other words, if the scale is 10 cm long and has five anchors, the minimum anchor should be at 0 cm and the rest of the anchors should be at 2.5 cm, 5 cm, 7.5 cm, and 10 cm. Using unequally distributed anchors can confuse the patient.

8.8.5 Free Text

Some questions give respondents opportunities to make comments in addition to or rather than choosing among different pre-specified options. In other words, respondents

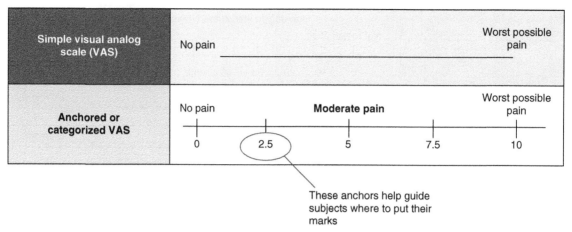

FIGURE 8.2 Examples of visual analog scales (VAS).

can say or enter *free text* in response to a question. Free text response options are common for open-ended questions but may also be used for closed-ended questions.

Including a free text response option has several advantages and can help:

- *Capture response possibilities that were not previously considered*: Sometimes it is difficult to include all possible answers in a multiple choice question.
- *Clarify answers*: Respondents may want the opportunity to qualify or explain their answers.
- *Raise important issues and concerns:* Even comments not directly related to the question may provide valuable insights about the patient, the patient's condition, the intervention, or the study.
- *Give the respondent an opportunity to voice opinions*: Respondents may be more likely to complete the instrument if they feel that their concerns and opinions are being heard.

Analyzing free text can be very challenging. Usually you have to classify the free text responses into different categories before applying statistical methods. Determining these categories and then deciding which responses fit into each category can be difficult because responses may vary significantly in type, style, and complexity. Some free text answers may cross several categories. For example, a person may say that he likes the medication when it works, is neutral about the medication when it works but produces side effects, and dislikes it when it does not work. Does this mean that the person likes or dislikes the medication?

8.9 RESPONSE RATE

8.9.1 Nonresponse Bias

An instrument is only as strong as its *response rate*, that is, the percentage of the study population completed the

instrument (e.g., questionnaire or interview). When the response rate is low, the results may not be indicative of the overall study population.

Nonresponse bias occurs when there is a fundamental difference between responders (i.e., people who complete the instrument) and nonresponders (i.e., people who do not complete the instrument) that affects the analysis and interpretation of results. In other words, specific types or groups of people were less likely to complete the instrument. For example, suppose you distribute a questionnaire to assess people's exercise habits. Respondents have to return the completed questionnaires to drop boxes that are only located in women's bathrooms. This arrangement will result in a clear nonresponse bias: few men will enter women's bathrooms to return the questionnaire (and those that do may be quite unusual). As a result, your sample will be predominantly women, which may not be representative of the whole study population.

Minimizing response bias can be very difficult, since responders will frequently be different from nonresponders in many ways. Patients may not respond if they are:

- Very busy or occupied with more urgent matters.
- Dissatisfied with or opposed to the study.
- Physically or psychologically inhibited from responding.
- Unable to read or comprehend the instructions.
- Forgetful.

You can evaluate the presence of nonresponse bias by analyzing and comparing the available characteristics of responders and nonresponders. For example, you can compare the distributions of age, gender, ethnicity, socioeconomic status, and disease severity among the responders with those of the nonresponders. Any statistically significant difference raises the possibility of nonresponse bias. For example, finding that certain groups (e.g., women, elderly, African Americans, or people with more severe disease) tended not to respond would raise questions about the validity of your results. The responders may not be representative of the overall study population.

8.9.2 Strategies to Increase Response Rate

The design of the instrument can dramatically affect whether a patient complies. Clear, concise, and friendly instruments are superior to vague, long-winded, and uninviting instruments. Remember that patients are not obligated to comply. You must convince them that donating their time and efforts is worthwhile.

In addition to the instrument design, you can increase response rate by:

- *Reducing the work or time commitment involved.* Make the questionnaire or interview session as short as possible.
- *Emphasizing the importance of the study and how the instrument is essential to the study.* People may comply if they feel that something is useful and important.
- *Making it convenient for respondents or interviewees.* Provide stamped addressed envelopes to return mailed questionnaires. Conduct interviews in close-by locations. Choose convenient times for the study subjects.
- *Offering incentives.* A small prize or reward for returning a questionnaire or completing an interview can go a long way. Even something simple like a letter or document of appreciation can have significant effects.
- *Establishing a bond with study participants.* Study subjects are more likely to comply when they like you.
- *Sending follow-up reminders.* Sending reminder postcards or email messages and making follow-up phone calls can nudge subjects into complying.
- *Offering assistance and guidance.* Some subjects who do not know how to complete the questionnaire or interview will abandon it.
- Treating the patients with respect.

Chapter 9

Patient Selection and Sampling

9.1 DEFINING THE STUDY POPULATION

9.1.1 Defining the Disease or Condition

Before selecting patients or sites, clearly determine and define the study population (i.e., the type of subject that you want for your study). While this may seem obvious, doing so is not necessarily as easy as it seems. Although some conditions and diseases are relatively easy to define (e.g., significant fractures, ligament tears, other types of anatomic damage, pregnancy, infections, and heart attacks), many conditions and diseases have more vague and complicated definitions and criteria. For example, evaluating an antidepressant requires recruiting patients who have depression. But how do you determine if a patient is depressed? The Diagnostic and Statistical Manual of Mental Disorders specifies a number of criteria. But each of these criteria can be ambiguous and have alternative explanations:

- *Depressed mood (feeling sad or low)*: What constitutes feeling low? Many of us feel sad and low at some point during the week.
- *Loss of interest or pleasure (in activities you normally enjoy)*: Many things, including being engrossed in reading this book, may make you lose interest in other activities.
- *Significant appetite or weight loss or gain*: If significant weight gain was not a problem, diet companies would be out of business.
- *Insomnia or hypersomnia (sleeping too little or too much)*: Stress, weather, and noisy neighbors can interfere with sleeping.
- *Psychomotor agitation or retardation (being restless and jittery, or alternatively, slower than usual)*: Concerns about where to recruit patients can make you jittery and restless.
- *Fatigue or loss of energy*: Many corporate lawyers, surgeons, and investment bankers feel fatigue on a regular basis. Are they depressed?

- *Feelings of worthlessness or excessive guilt*: Where is the boundary between normal guilt and excessive guilt?
- *Impaired thinking or concentration, indecisiveness*: Indecisiveness may or may not be a symptom of depression... possibly.
- *Suicidal thoughts/thoughts of death*: Not everyone who has thought of death is suicidal.

In addition, some diseases overlap considerably, making it difficult to draw the line between one disease and another (e.g., systemic lupus erythematosus and mixed connective tissue disease, rheumatoid arthritis and psoriatic arthritis, polymyositis, and dermatomyositis all have similar features).

Remember disease definitions are arbitrary. They are intellectual constructs that change over time. They are based on a number of possible criteria including:

- *Histological changes* (e.g., Crohn's disease and ulcerative colitis alter the intestinal lining in different manners).
- *Pathophysiologic mechanisms* (e.g., lack of insulin secretion results in Type I Diabetes while lack of response to insulin results in Type II Diabetes).
- *Causative agent* (e.g., hepatitis A is caused by the hepatitis A virus, asbestosis is caused by asbestos).
- *Physical manifestations* (e.g., rheumatologic conditions are defined by the joints they affect and how they affect them).
- *Symptoms and signs* (e.g., stable angina is the presence of chest pain during exertion and unstable angina is the presence of chest pain at rest).
- *Body part, organ, or organ system affected* (e.g., iritis is inflammation of the iris and uveitis is inflammation of the uvea).
- *Pre-disposing, preceding, or concurrent conditions* (e.g., concussions occur after head trauma, frostbite occurs with extreme cold).
- *Prognosis and natural history* (e.g., cancerous masses can spread to distant locations while benign masses do not).

- *Measurement thresholds* (e.g., hypertension is defined as a systolic blood pressure above 140 and a diastolic pressure above 90).
- *Response to treatment*: Two very similar conditions may have different treatments (e.g., the distinction between an ST-elevation myocardial infarction and a non-ST elevation myocardial infarction emerged only after it was found that thrombolytics were effective in one and not in the other). Sometimes several conditions with very different mechanisms and clinical manifestations will be defined as a single disease if their treatments are the same.

Of the above, the most common way to classify disease is by response to therapy. In fact, you may classify several distinct conditions with very different pathophysiology and clinical manifestations as the same disease if the treatment is the same – or more commonly, if no good treatments exist for any of the conditions. For example, schizophrenia has very different possible manifestations that range from catatonic to paranoid schizophrenia; these conditions all fall under the umbrella of one disease partly because they respond, or fail to respond, to similar therapy. Classifying diseases based on the available treatment options is often more pragmatic. (e.g., distinguishing between ST elevation myocardial infarction and non-ST elevation myocardial infarction was not necessary before thrombolytics were shown to be effective in one but not the other; since that discovery, one disease has become two).

So, think carefully about the "disease" that a clinical trial is targeting. You may have to expand the trial beyond the normal confines of a disease – such as lumping all patients with arterial atherosclerosis together, including patients requiring coronary artery bypass surgery, percutaneous coronary interventions, and stroke interventions – or limit the trial to a subgroup of patients such as classic or occult age-related macular degeneration. There are many different ways to lump conditions together. For example, you can lump conditions that have:

- The same symptoms (e.g., patients with joint pain).
- Any combination of signs or symptoms from a list of criteria (e.g., different lupus patients have different symptoms; but all must have a minimal number of symptoms from an established list).
- The same pathophysiological criteria (e.g., a positive blood culture for an organism).
- The same cause (e.g., patients with tuberculosis may have pulmonary or gastrointestinal manifestations).

Using cause to lump conditions can be problematic. Although assigning a single cause to diseases is common, very few diseases have just one cause. Most are the result of interaction among the environment, genes, and other factors. Here are three examples:

- *Helicobacter pylori*: H. pylori is present in many people. Although H. pylori causes peptic ulcers, many infected patients do not have ulcers. Other factors must be present for ulcers to result.
- *Phenylketonuria (PKU)*: Many consider PKU a genetic disease. But if the normal human diet had very low levels of phenylalanine, even people who were homozygous for the recessive PKU gene would not demonstrate any signs of PKU. Only people with abnormally high levels of phenylalanine in their diet would exhibit PKU. In that case, many may say that an abnormal diet causes PKU.
- *AIDS*: Mutant versions of CCR5 can keep HIV in chronic dormant state. If 99% of the population had these mutations then most would never develop AIDS despite being infected by HIV. Only those without the mutation would be susceptible. In such a scenario, you could call AIDS a genetic disease.

So for the purposes of defining diseases for clinical trials, think of disease causes as disease risk factors instead. Moreover, consider defining a disease by treatment response or clinical manifestations rather than by causes or risk factors (unless, of course, the trial tests an intervention designed to prevent or treat the causes or risk factors). Using such definitions will preclude questions such as "Does someone who has an infection without manifesting it have the disease?"

Also, when choosing a study population, keep in mind that disease definitions may change over time as scientists gain a better understanding of the biological processes. Medical knowledge changes at a rapid rate. Conditions that were not considered diseases 20 years ago are defined as diseases today (e.g., the normal ranges for blood pressure and cholesterol continue to change). Continuing research may reveal that diseases and conditions currently considered separate may indeed be one unified disease process (e.g., a patient with hypertension, diabetes, and coronary artery disease may have the same disease: metabolic syndrome) and certain individual diseases may actually be conglomerates of multiple conditions.

9.1.2 Additional and Alternative Study Population Characteristics

Using traditional disease definitions is not always the best way to define your study population. Many situations call for either expanding the study population beyond the normal confines of disease definitions (e.g., lumping coronary artery disease, cerebral vascular, and peripheral vascular disease patients together) or limiting the population to a subpopulation with a disease (e.g., patients with uncontrolled diabetes). In general, the study population should mirror the population that the intervention targets. Interventions do not necessarily target specific diseases (e.g., ibuprofen can be used for a number of different conditions) although they usually do. So the study population may consist of patients who exhibit or have certain:

- *Symptoms*: Some interventions alleviate particular symptoms (e.g., pain) rather than treat a disease. In such situations, defining your study population as patients who have that symptom (e.g., joint pain, which would include patients with osteoarthritis, rheumatoid arthritis, and traumatic injury) may be a better alternative.
- *Phenotypes or signs*: Interventions may be for certain body characteristics.
- *Genotypes*: Sometimes interventions may be for patients with specific genetic sequences or types (e.g., BRCA mutation, Tay Sach's disease, or Down's syndrome).
- *Past medical history*: When studying interventions designed to prevent diseases (i.e., prophylactic studies), you may use the patient's past medical history (e.g., history of transient ischemic attacks).
- *Diseases caused by certain agents*: If the intervention (e.g., antibiotic) targets a particular causative agent (e.g., streptococcus bacteria), your study population may be patients with that causative agent (e.g., patients with streptococcal infections).
- *Values of a measure*: For interventions that alter specific measures (e.g., blood pressure), choosing patients with certain values of that measure (e.g., blood pressure above 140/90).
- *Behaviors, habits, or activities*: Interventions may benefit individuals who exhibit certain behaviors (e.g., medical devices for those who snore), have certain habits (e.g., nicotine patches for smokers), or participate in specific activities (e.g., orthopedic braces for athletes playing sports).
- *Demographic characteristics*: Interventions can target certain age groups (e.g., vaccinations for newborns), genders (e.g., hot flash prophylaxis for women), ethnicities (e.g., sickle cell screening tests for African Americans), socioeconomic groups (e.g., special programs for patients who cannot pay for medications), or occupations (e.g., ventilators for miners).

Some parameters are easier to define than others. For instance, genetic tests can identify the presence or absence of a genotype, but symptoms (e.g., how many headaches a week is abnormal?), demographic characteristics (e.g., mixed race patients do not fall neatly into one demographic category), and phenotypes may be more vague or ill-defined. In many cases, defining the study population requires a combination of the parameters listed above. For example, you may specify that the subject must have a certain causative agent (e.g., *H. pylori*) and symptoms (e.g., epigastric pain) or a certain set of demographics (e.g., women in their teens), phenotypes (e.g., thin), and symptoms (e.g., amenorrhea).

You can group different patients together only if you can measure their response to your intervention with the same common endpoint (e.g., you can study patients with previous history of stroke along with patients with high blood pressure if the endpoint is prevention of strokes; on the other hand, since patients with cerebral lupus and discoid lupus have different measures of diseases severity, you should study them separately).

9.1.3 Considerations When Choosing a Study Population

Choosing the appropriate study population takes significant clinical and scientific judgment. There are several important elements that you should consider.

Targeted Clinical Event

The targeted clinical event is the symptom, condition, or disease episode that the intervention is intended to prevent or treat. An intervention that alters some psychological or physiological process potentially could prevent or treat many different things (e.g., lowering blood pressure may reduce the risk of heart attacks, strokes, or renal disease; a drug that alters lymphocyte activity may affect many different autoimmune diseases or prevent rejection of organ transplants). Choosing the appropriate clinical event depends on the intervention's mechanism (e.g., a medication inhibits a molecule involved in the blood clotting), the mechanism's potential clinical consequences (e.g., blood clotting is involved in strokes, heart attacks, and pulmonary embolism), and pre-clinical study results (including *in vitro* and animal studies). Every disease or condition has multiple potential targeted clinical events (e.g., potential clinical events for coronary artery disease include angina, myocardial infarction, occlusion of an artery as determined by angiography, hospitalization, and death). The targeted clinical event should be clinically important (e.g., laughing, in general, is not a clinically important event) and preventable or reversible.

Prevalence, Incidence, or Likelihood of Targeted Clinical Event

The targeted clinical event must occur frequently enough in the study population to allow demonstration of a difference between the control and treatment groups. If the targeted clinical event is too rare in the chosen study population (e.g., 20–30 year old healthy women probably will not have enough heart attacks to test an intervention designed to prevent heart attacks) then there will not be enough events for the intervention to prevent or treat (Figure 9.1). A study population that will have more events (e.g., diabetic 50–60 year old male smokers with family histories of heart disease) would be a better study population.

Ceiling and Floor Effects

Demonstrating that an intervention can improve a condition requires enough room for improvement. In other words, the condition has to be severe enough to allow for a statistically significant change. Figure 9.2 demonstrates ceiling and floor effects. The measures cannot assume a value higher than some "ceiling" or lower than some "floor." If you only include patients who are already close to the ceiling or floor (e.g., including only patients with mild headaches in a trial testing a headache medication), then the majority of values are at or near the maximum or minimum possible for the test (e.g., at the end of the trial, every patient will either have a mild headache or no headache). This prevents you from seeing the full potential effect of the intervention (e.g., the medication may adequately treat a mild headache but would it treat a severe headache?). Also, most statistical tests assume that values are variable and evenly distributed (most frequently the normal or bell curve distribution). Strong ceiling or floor effects distort distributions and significantly reduce variability, violating statistical assumptions, and limiting the possibility of finding effects. Therefore, make sure you include patients with conditions severe enough that a benefit can be demonstrated (e.g., patients with moderate and severe headaches).

Likelihood of Therapy Response

Your study population should have a chance of responding to your intervention. While you should not bias your study for your intervention, give your intervention a fair chance of proving its worth. This is analogous to competing in a basketball game. Having baskets that are too high above regulation height will prevent you from scoring and proving that you can beat the other team. When evaluating the likelihood of a patient responding to your intervention, keep in mind several things:

- *Diseases are usually easier to treat in their early stages than their later stages.* Some diseases eventually cause irreversible damage (e.g., macular degeneration causing retina scarring; myocardial infarction causing irreversible loss of myocardium) or weaken the body so that other diseases may occur (e.g., patients with immune system disorders may eventually develop infections and

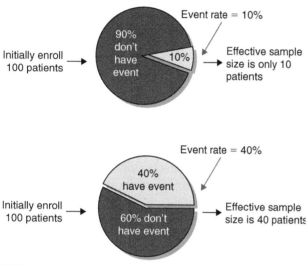

FIGURE 9.1   The importance of the frequency of the targeted clinical event in the chosen study population.

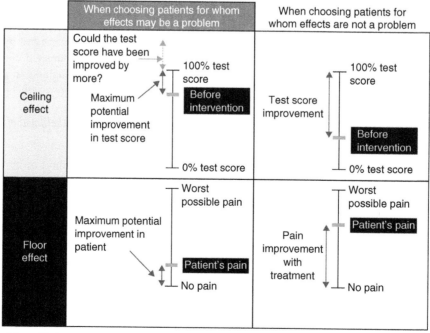

FIGURE 9.2   Ceiling and floor effects.

cancers; severe artery disease may ultimately lead to heart and kidney problems).

- *Prior treatment may either increase or decrease a patient's likelihood of responding to your intervention.* In some situations, prior treatments may have already extracted all the possible benefits or altered the anatomy or physiology of the patient (e.g., a patient who has received many coronary bypass surgeries may be less likely to benefit from one more). Also, patients who have not been cured by prior treatments may be "tougher cases," that is, have conditions that are more refractory to treatment (e.g., a tumor that has survived several rounds of radiation and chemotherapy). On the other hand, prior treatment may have weakened or reduced the disease so that it is more easily treatable (e.g., prior radiation and chemotherapy may reduce the size of the tumor).
- *Concomitant diseases or conditions may affect response to therapy.* Beware of other drugs or conditions that may inhibit response to your intervention (e.g., gastrointestinal disease, congestive heart failure, and liver failure may affect the absorption, distribution, and elimination of your drug).

Greatest Unmet Need

An important consideration is the unmet medical need. Some patient populations are desperate to find a treatment for a disease. The disease is debilitating or deadly, and there is a current lack of viable alternatives (e.g., AIDS in the 1980s). So if a drug may be used for different possible populations, choosing the population that most desperately wants the drug developed and approved may be the best option, from an ethical as well as a regulatory viewpoint.

Recruitability

If you cannot get the patients, you cannot do the trial. Therefore, choose a population that you are able to recruit. While narrowing your study population (e.g., elderly patients who are not taking any other medications) helps decrease heterogeneity and the chance of other factors interfering with or confounding your results (e.g., no other medications will interfere with your intervention), it also makes it more difficult to recruit patients (e.g., many elderly patients are taking at least one type of medications such as aspirin or ibuprofen). Therefore, factor in recruitability when defining your study population.

Feasibility

Even when a study population is recruitable, conducting a trial on that population may not be feasible. Members of the study population must be able to consent to (e.g., they should be sufficiently conscious, aware, and communicative to understand and agree to the study) and participate

in (e.g., they must reliably come in for scheduled visits and perform the necessary procedures) the study. Unfortunately, this feasibility requirement may be biased against certain populations (e.g., indigent patients' financial constraints, busy professionals' time constraints, and disabled patients' physical constraints may prevent them from traveling to appointments to participate).

Identifiability/Diagnosability

Choose a study population that is relatively easy and straightforward to identify. Avoid vague or nonspecific parameters. If possible, define study populations in ways that do not require extensive testing to identify (e.g., instead of specifying that a study population must have completely normal livers, which may require liver biopsies, specify that the population must have normal liver function tests, a simple set of blood tests). Opt for more objective measures over highly subjective measures and parameters (e.g., instead of 100% compliant patients specify that patients must have made over 80% of their physician appointments).

Matching with Endpoints

The patient population and endpoint are intimately linked. Choose each while considering the other. Some examples are as follows:

- *Remission induction endpoint*: If the endpoint is the induction of disease remission, the patient must be having active disease which is not likely to resolve without treatment (e.g., an active, recalcitrant case of ulcerative colitis instead of a mild case that shows few symptoms).
- *Prophylactic endpoint*: If the endpoint is prevention of disease, then the study population should be patients who do not yet have the disease, but are at reasonable risk of acquiring it. If the risk is too low, then you may have to enroll an impractically large number of patients for any to develop the disease (e.g., for a trial studying a drug to prevent heart attacks, 50 year old men with high cholesterol is a better study population than 20 year-old healthy men). Therefore, understanding the risk factors for the disease is important (e.g., high cholesterol and age for heart attacks).

9.2 SELECTION (INCLUSION AND EXCLUSION) CRITERIA

9.2.1 Definitions

Selection criteria are the characteristics and qualities that a patient should or should not have in order to participate in your clinical study. Selection criteria include *inclusion criteria* (the characteristics and qualities a patient must have to be included in or participate in the trial) and *exclusion criteria* (characteristics or qualities that prevent a patient from participating in the trial). Most inclusion criteria can be worded as exclusion criteria and vice versa (e.g., "patient is female" as an inclusion criterion is equivalent to patient is male as an exclusion criterion).

Selection criteria must be well defined, precise, unambiguous, and clearly established before patient recruitment begins. Vague selection criteria can lead to the wrong patients being selected and cause a number of significant problems. Patients may be subject to inappropriate treatments that may cause harm (e.g., a patient with heart failure may receive a drug that worsens heart failure). Choosing the wrong study patients may invalidate results (e.g., if some study patients do not actually have a disease, you may not be able to claim that your drug improves the disease).

Selection criteria are analogous to dating criteria. In dating, your criteria should match what you ultimately want. Irrelevant dating criteria (e.g., if you are mainly interested in finding a nice person who is supportive, the type of car that he or she drives should not matter) may preclude you from finding the right person. Being too lax about your dating criteria (e.g., anyone who is older than 21 and is alive) may result in too many bad or unproductive dates. Being too strict or specific about whom you will or will not date (e.g., the person must be of a certain age and have a specific appearance, job, and set of interests) may make finding people to date very difficult. In fact, being too strict about your dating criteria can preclude you from ever finding the right person. In the end, choosing dating criteria should factor in needs, time and effort available, and probability of success.

Similarly, keep in mind the repercussions of choosing different selection criteria. The more stringent your selection criteria, the narrower and more homogenous your study population will be. Greater homogeneity means less variability in the study population. Less variability allows for more precise and accurate comparisons and results. Greater homogeneity also limits the generalizability of results (e.g., results from a study population consisting of only white men in their 40s cannot necessarily be applied to women, Asian Americans, or people in their 60s). Additionally, more stringent selection criteria make it more difficult and costly to find appropriate patients (e.g., it is much easier to find men between the ages of 20–65 than men who are between the ages of 20–65, 150–200 pounds in weight, and Samoan). Selection criteria may be so stringent that you cannot find enough patients to conduct your trial (e.g., how many 20–25 year old, 150–160 pound Samoan men do you expect to find if you are recruiting patients in Iowa).

The type of inclusion and exclusion criteria you use will depend on the condition, intervention, study population, and trial. Table 9.1 lists some of the types you should consider. Patient characteristics (e.g., age, weight, geographic location,

or cardiac function) and in turn patient trial eligibility may change during the course of recruitment and the clinical trial. So specifying the exact date at which these criteria apply (e.g., on the date of randomization, the patient must be less than 45 years old) may be important. For many criteria, specifying the duration, frequency, and degree may be relevant. The impact of diseases, medications, habits, and environmental risk factors can vary by how long, how often, and how much the patients have been exposed.

Changing Selection Criteria

If recruitment does not go as planned you may have to change your selection criteria. Relaxing the selection criteria may allow you to recruit more patients (e.g., excluding patients over 65 years of age instead of over 55 years of age will make patients between 55 and 65 years old available). However, changing the selection criteria (especially the major criteria) should be the last resort, because the enrolled patients before the change may be different from those after the change. Any efficacy and safety differences between the pre- and post-change subjects can wreak havoc on the analysis and the generalizability of the results. Do not loosen criteria to the point where you may jeopardize the integrity or safety of the clinical trial.

Employing a Run-In Period

Sometimes you may observe your study patients for a period of time (run-in period) before starting the study (Chapter 6 covers run-in periods in greater detail). The run-in period helps weed out ineligible or noncompliant patients. Run-in periods can help decrease your study population's heterogeneity in many ways. During the run-in period, you can confirm the severity, stage, and stability of the disease. You can test whether the patient can tolerate your intervention. You can also standardize each patient's background therapy (e.g., patients receiving several different types of beta-blockers may be switched on to a single uniform beta-blocker before the study is initiated). A run-in period becomes a *wash-out period* when it allows patients to stop their regular treatments and the regular treatments' effects to dissipate (e.g., a patient has to be off blood thinners for at least several days before their blood coagulation returns to normal).

9.2.2 Patients to Include

Patients with Specific Objective Measurements

Selection criteria should be as objective as possible. Vague subjective measures that are open to interpretation will increase the heterogeneity (perhaps to point of being unacceptable) of your study population. Avoid using terms such as normal, abnormal, large, small, or unusual. Terms like

TABLE 9.1 Possible Selection Criteria Categories

Category	Examples	Comments
Demographics	Sex, age, race, ethnicity, marital status, geographic location, nationality	Should match the population that the intervention will target. Certain conditions or interventions may be specific to certain demographic groups (e.g., prostate disease, vaginal problems, menopause, Sickle Cell Anemia)
Disease or Condition of Interest	Formal diagnosis, Diagnostic tests, staging, severity, previous or current treatment (and outcome)	Beware of ceiling effects and significant heterogeneity. There needs to be strict criteria for the disease diagnosis, which can include more subjective clinical findings and/or more objective test results
Allergies	Allergies to Intervention as well as other Medications and Substances	Consider all materials and equipment used in the trial (e.g., latex, radiographic contrast material, rescue medications)
Screening Test Results	Laboratory, imaging, electrocardiogram results	Specify acceptable/unacceptable ranges
Ability to Consent	Reading ability, level of consciousness, alertness, education level,	In some conditions (e.g., Alzheimer's) that may affect cognition, you may need to document ability to consent with a cognitive test
Ability to Comply	History of complying with medical visits and treatments, physical condition, travel ability, schedule flexibility, ability perform the required tests, ability to receive the drug language	Some conditions (e.g., poor venous access) may prevent patients from receiving certain interventions (e.g., IV medications). Some situations (e.g., lack of transportation, no telephone, or language barrier) or conditions (e.g., cannot walk) may inhibit a patient's ability to make required visits, communicate with study personnel, or understand directions. In some cases, the patients must have a caregiver who can administer the drug or perform the required assessments
Other Diseases	Current and previous	Other diseases may confound results or threaten the safety of patients. (e.g., , a history of heart disease may exclude a patient from receiving a drug with potential cardiotoxicity; a brain metastasis may exclude a patient from receiving a drug that can cause bleeding
Psychological and Emotional History	Psychological or emotional problems	Patients must have emotional and psychological fortitude to complete trial
Physical Exam Findings	Presence/absence as well as severity	Indicate the details and thoroughness of the physical examination required. Use objective measures when possible (e.g., 20/20 vision instead of normal vision)
Pregnancy, Presence of Lack of Fertility	Birth control, post-menopausal	Typically, two or more simultaneous forms of birth control are required

normal are relative. What is normal to one person's eyes may be abnormal to others eyes. So employing the term normal in inclusion criteria is fraught with problems. For example, what does stating that the subject must have normal mental status mean? The boundaries of normal may vary from laboratory to laboratory. Changes in altitude can change hematocrit. When possible, use objective measures and specific ranges (e.g., hematocrit should be between 36% and 45%; the Mental Status Exam should be above 29%) rather than the term normal.

Patients with Stable Measurements

Many patients characteristics will fluctuate minute to minute, hour to hour, day to day, month to month, or year to year. Physiologic parameters (e.g., blood pressure, heart rate, temperature, and respiration rate), laboratory values (e.g., hematocrit and liver function tests), sociodemographic characteristics (e.g., place of residence, income, education level, or marital status), and psychological states (e.g., mood or mental status) can vary from measurement to measurement. Therefore, specifying when, how often, or how long the patient needs to fulfill the measurement is important. For example, you may indicate that you will take five blood pressure measurements during five consecutive days and all of the measurements must be under 120/80. Or you may specify that three of the five measurements or the mean of all the readings must be under 120/80. You can also specify that the measurements cannot fluctuate beyond a certain range. Your choice depends on how strict you will need to be (e.g., if your intervention will cause problems with even only momentary blood pressure elevations, then specifying that all measurements should be under 120/80 is the better choice).

Remember that recruitment and enrollment can occur over a long period of time, during which patient characteristics can change (or drift) drastically. The course and severity of a patient's condition can change from when he or she is first recruited to the conclusion of the study. Patients' conditions may naturally wax or wane, improve, or deteriorate. Avoid problems with regression to the mean. In other words, a patient's condition that waxes during recruitment is likely to wane during the trial and vice versa. Observing a patient over a period of time before enrolling him or her will help you assess the true nature of the patient's condition.

Patients with Particular Physical Exam Findings

Physical exam findings can be extremely subjective. Different examiners can interpret the same finding differently. Specifying the experience of the examiner and the extent of the exam can be important. In some cases, multiple examiners may have to confirm a given finding (e.g., rebound tenderness as determined by three separate examiners). Also, some physical exam findings may be fleeting or fluctuate. Indicating how long a finding should be present (e.g., abdominal tenderness for more than 10 days) may be necessary. Ideally, each patient should be examined by the same examiner on every visit.

Patients of Particular Races and Ethnicities

There are three major reasons why race and ethnicity may be important in inclusion criteria. First of all, some conditions or interventions are more common or behave differently in different races (e.g., keloid formation after surgery and sickle-cell disease are more common in African Americans). Secondly, some trials specifically aim to answer questions about race or ethnicity (e.g., what (not what) is the effect of a hypertension medication on Latino patients?). Third, not including different races limits your ability to apply your study results to the entire population (e.g., if (not if) you do not include patients of Chinese decent in your trial, how do you know how they would respond to your intervention?).

There are several challenges to using race or ethnicity as inclusion criteria:

- *Determining whether a patient qualifies as a certain race*: Identifying a patient's race can be tricky. How do you categorize a mixed race person? Does someone 20% Black, 40% Hispanic, and 20% non-Hispanic white qualify as Black, White, or Hispanic? At what point does one "become" Black, White, Hispanic, or Asian? Aside from superficial appearance, it is difficult to "verify" a patient's race.
- *Knowing how specific to make the criteria*: Great diversity exists within racial categories. For example, Asian Americans include patients of Korean, Japanese, Phillipino, and Vietnamese descent. The differences among these subpopulations of Asian Americans are in many ways greater than the differences between broader categories such as African Americans and Caucasians. Even if you use racial "subpopulations," you will encounter tremendous diversity (e.g., Chinese descent includes Taiwanese, Cantonese, etc.).
- *Offending and excluding people*: Anything involving race can be very controversial and sensitive. People may feel that you are unnecessarily limiting trial participation (e.g., why is this trial being limited to Caucasian and African American patients) or bringing stigma upon certain races (e.g., advertising a depression trial for Latinos may imply that Latinos tend to be depressed). Be sensitive about the potential repercussions of any selection criteria involving race and ethnicity. Make sure your criteria are reasonable from a scientific perspective.
- *Obscuring relevant variables*: Race and ethnicity in many ways are artificial constructs. Evidence suggests that some biological differences are present but that many perceived differences may actually be attributable to socioeconomic, environmental, and cultural differences.

Patients on Other Therapies

When standard existing therapy is clearly effective or the disease consequences are devastating, conducting a placebo-controlled trial may be unethical. In such cases, new drugs become add-on (to be used along with the standard existing therapy) rather than alternative therapies. Therefore, one of the inclusion criteria may be that the patient is already on the standard existing therapy. Specifying the duration and dose of the standard therapy may be important. Combination treatments may become toxic or negate each others effects (e.g., a cancer drug that prevents proliferation of tumor cells and one that depends on proliferation for its effects) at certain doses or after certain durations.

Patients Refractory to Other Therapy

Sometimes the new intervention can never serve as add-on therapy (e.g., due to toxicity or conflicting mechanisms) but starting a patient on the new intervention without trying existing therapies is unethical. In such cases, you may choose a population shown to be refractory to existing therapies. Using such a strategy may help expedite drug or medical device approval because patients who are refractory to other therapies are desperate for a treatment alternative (i.e., they have the greatest unmet medical need). On the other hand, such patients may be too sick to reap much benefit from the intervention (e.g., patients with longstanding disease might have lost most function already or cancers that have been resistant to all standard therapies may be the least likely to respond to the new drug). If you use patients refractory to other therapies, specify in your inclusion criteria what it means to be refractory to other therapies (e.g., patient tried Standard Drug X for 10 months with no improvement in the patient's liver function).

9.2.3 Patients to Exclude

Excluding more patients from your study will generate a more homogenous study population and reduce bias and confounding but will also limit the generalizability of your study results. Choosing whether exclude a certain set of patients is a balance between these two considerations. Some commonly excluded populations include the following.

High-Risk Patients

Consider excluding patients that have either a high probability of suffering side effects or a possibility of experiencing catastrophic side effects (e.g., death, permanent disability, or disfigurement). Of course, the probability of a catastrophic event is never zero (e.g., even a completely healthy patient could in theory die from ingesting aspirin). But do your best to minimize risk to patients. So, for example, avoid administering interventions that may cause bleeding (e.g., anticoagulants) to patients who are at increased risk for falling (and hitting their head which may cause intracranial hemorrhages) or gastrointestinal bleeding (e.g., peptic ulcers). Unless necessary, do not give interventions that may suppress immune systems to patients at high risk for serious infections (e.g., positive PPD). Beware of any conditions that the intervention may exacerbate (e.g., congestive heart failure in patients getting drugs that increase stress on the heart; patients with weak immune systems getting immunosuppressants).

Patients Unable to Give Consent

For ethical and legal reasons, avoid including patients who cannot consent to studies out of their own free will unless the trial is specifically for those patients. These include children who must get parental (or guardian) permission, patients with impaired thought processes or consciousness

(from psychiatric illness, substance use, medications, or other conditions), and patients who may be under duress to participate (e.g., prisoners). When trials require these populations (e.g., interventions designed for the infants or patients with psychiatric illness), identify people who can serve as the patients' legal guardians.

Pregnant Patients

Including patients who are either pregnant or planning to conceive runs the risk of fetal harm or birth defects. Moreover, pregnancy-induced alterations in the mother's physiology may influence the intervention's effects. Therefore, most trials exclude any patients who are or may become pregnant. In fact, many trials (e.g., most Phase I trials) exclude any women of child-bearing age.

Children

Clinical trials often exclude children since many interventions may affect development, obtaining consent is more difficult, many adult diseases are not common in children, and interventions often act differently in children (e.g., different dosing and pharmacokinetics). Unless the intervention will be used in children, excluding children is reasonable.

Elderly

The elderly are potentially a high risk, vulnerable population. Many have other medical conditions and are taking other medications that may confound your results. Moreover, many feel the duty to respect and protect the elderly. On the hand, many medical conditions are most common in the elderly. It is sometimes prudent to exclude the very elderly unless necessary or the disease is common in the elderly.

Patients with Extreme Body Sizes

Since the effects of many interventions (e.g., drug pharmacokinetics, pharmacodynamics, and side effects may vary significantly) depend on patient body size, excluding patients with extreme body size measurements (e.g., significantly under or over weight) compared to the general study population may be necessary. Extreme body sizes also may cause logistic problems as well. Patients may exceed (e.g., CT tables may collapse or the patient may not be able to fit into a machine) or fall short of the height or weight limits of trial equipment. Body size may impair (e.g., body fat can distort images such as ultrasound and make it difficult to find anatomical structures such as veins to insert catheters) or prevent (e.g., fasting in underweight patients may be dangerous) certain procedures.

Confounding Diseases or Conditions

Beware of diseases, conditions, or medications that may cause or alter the effects that you are trying to measure. For example, if you are trying to measure an intervention's effects on cancer mortality, consider excluding patients who are at high risk of dying from other causes (e.g., severe heart failure patients). However, keep in mind that many patients in real clinical practice will have multiple medical conditions and be on multiple medications. So aggressively excluding patients with any other diseases or medications may limit the generalizability of your results (e.g., it may be unrealistic to exclude patients who have been on any other breast cancer medications from a breast cancer drug trial or exclude diabetics for a trial involving peripheral vascular disease).

Other Medications/Interventions

Ideally, patients should stop taking their other medications during the course of the trial, since other medications may interact and interfere with your intervention. The patient should not start the trial until after a *washout* or medicine-free period has elapsed to ensure that the medications and their effects are completely eliminated from the patient's body. Stopping other medications abruptly is not always feasible or prudent and may cause withdrawal or rebound effects. Slowly tapering (i.e., decreasing the dose each day until the patient is completely off the medications) the medications may be necessary.

Sometimes stopping medications will have unacceptable consequences (e.g., leading to flare ups of symptoms or even death). In such cases, there are several possible options:

- *Perform separate studies on the other medications to determine their effects on your intervention.*
- *Switch the patient to alternative medications that do not interact with your intervention.* Switching should be gradual and done well in advance of the study start to ensure that the patient tolerates the change.
- *Require patients to adhere to pre-determined regimens (i.e., specific doses and schedules) when taking other medications.* Fluctuating doses and regimens throughout the trial make it difficult to determine their effects on results.

Previous Treatment

Including patients who have received previous treatment (for the disease or condition that you are studying) can bias the results in several possible ways. The previous treatment may have weakened or attenuated the disease or condition, so that your intervention appears more successful. Conversely, patients who have received treatment may represent treatment failures (i.e., cases that are more difficult to treat), so that your intervention appears less success-

ful. Previous treatment can alter the patient's physiology (e.g., chemotherapy can weaken a patient's immune system) and anatomy (e.g., artery bypass surgery changes the blood circulation in that area) or the disease process. Again, excluding such patients may not be possible if your intervention is intended for patients who have had previous treatment or most patients in real clinical practice have received previous treatment. If the patient has received previous treatments, there should be an adequate *washout period* (i.e., time between the last treatment and applying your intervention) to prevent *carryover effect* (i.e., effects that are really the result of the previous treatment and not attributable to your intervention).

Participation in Another Study

Since clinical trials can provide money, medical care, attention, and other potential perquisites, some patients try to enroll in multiple studies, which can cause problems with your study. The other studies may administer interventions that treat the same disease as your study or interact with your interventions. Other study protocols may interfere with your study operations (e.g., both studies may require patient visits on the same day; studies may require different diets; retained barium from an upper GI exam in one study could interfere with a CT scan in another). Since establishing whether another study will interfere with your study is difficult, excluding all patients who are participating in any other clinical study may be a safer route. Establishing a wash-out period after a patient has participated in another study can minimize carry-over effects.

Noncompliant and Difficult Patients

Avoid enrolling patients that may cause problems for your study. These include patients that are noncompliant with your study protocol (e.g., fail to take the study medication or show up for required visits), threaten legal action (i.e., lawsuits) if their study outcomes are not favorable, or abuse study personnel. Identifying such patients can be difficult. You may look for warning signs such as histories of missing physician visits, lawsuits, or criminal behavior. Obviously, do not stereotype or profile patients (e.g., assume that certain race, ethnic, or socioeconomic groups will be more problematic).

9.3 SAMPLING

9.3.1 Sampling Process

Since it is usually impossible to test an intervention on every single patient with a certain disease or condition, the study population of a clinical study is by definition a sample (i.e., a subset of the overall population). Ideally, this sample should be representative of the population and not biased, that is, the proportions of different characteristics in the sample should be the same as the proportions of different characteristics in the population (e.g., the age distribution and male-to-female ratio of the sample should be the same as that of the overall population). In a biased sample, certain members are underrepresented or overrepresented relative to others in the population. In extreme cases, certain types of subjects are completely excluded. For example, a study population from Beverly Hills may be biased and not include any patients from lower socioeconomic groups or certain ethnicities.

Sampling biases may not be obvious at first. For example, imagine going to the mall to select a sample of patients to test a drug that prevents angina (i.e., chest pain from coronary artery disease). Such a sample could be biased in many ways. Patients have to be healthy and wealthy enough to go to the mall. Depending on the mall location, your sample may have very few members of certain ethnic groups. Going to the mall at 10 a.m. on Tuesday will select for people who do not work.

The sampling process consists of several stages.

Define the Theoretical and Accessible Study Populations

Section 9.1 broached the subject of defining your study population. It is important to distinguish between the *theoretical* and *accessible study populations* (Figure 9.3). The *theoretical study population* is the group of people to whom you would like to generalize your study results (e.g., men above 50 years old with coronary artery disease). To truly determine whether an intervention works, you must take a sample from this theoretical population. However, doing so may be impractical or impossible (e.g., there is no accurate list of every man over 50 years old with coronary artery disease). Not every member of the theoretical study population is "accessible" (i.e., available to be sampled). The *accessible study population* is the population that can realistically be sampled (e.g., men over 50 years old listed in a coronary disease registry; men over 50 years old found to have coronary artery disease in any of 20 hospitals over the past 5 years). In other words, the accessible population is a pool of people from which you can randomly or nonrandomly choose. Ideally, the accessible study population should be as similar as possible in composition and characteristics as the theoretical study population.

Using an analogy from the dating world, the theoretical dating population would be every woman or man (depending on your preference) in the world, including celebrities, models, top athletes, and people from different countries and social strata. But not all of these people are accessible. The accessible dating population is anyone you would actually have a chance of meeting (e.g., people in your city, listed on internet dating sights, or friends of friends). Depending who or where you are, this accessible dating population may be very similar or very different from the theoretical dating population.

Specify the Sampling Frame

After identifying the theoretical and accessible populations, the next step is assembling a list of (or a way of reaching or contacting) the members of the accessible population (i.e., the *sampling frame*). You then will draw your sample from this sampling frame. (In the dating analogy, the sampling frame could be dating service listings or members of a particular club.) Your choice of sampling frame is extremely important. Choosing the wrong sampling frame can introduce significant biases (e.g., a sampling frame of all women listed in a phone book will miss women who do not have listed land lines or have moved into the area after the phone book was printed). Examples of sampling frames include specific patient populations (e.g., all patients who visited the University of Pittsburgh Medical Center emergency room with chest pain from 2000 to 2005; this is the list of the accessible population from which you will draw your sample), lists or directories (e.g., the telephone book can serve as a sampling frame for phone surveys; doing so has significant limitations as significant portions of the population either do not have a phone or have moved in or out of the area since the last phone book was printed), and specific sampling procedures (e.g., randomly digit dialing, which is randomly dialing telephone numbers).

Unfortunately, many investigators do not specify the sampling frame when designing clinical studies. In fact, specifying the sampling frame is usually an afterthought, delegated to the clinical operations people, who frequently select study sites purely on the basis of patient recruitability.

Example: Psoriasis area and severity index (PASI)

The PASI is a widely used gold standard for assessing extensive psoriasis. To calculate the PASI, the observer grades the average redness, thickness, and scaliness of the lesions on a 0–4 scale and weights the scores by the area of skin affected. As a result, the PASI is also very subjective (e.g., in estimating these areas of skin involvement, the observer must judge where on the body a patient's arms and legs begin) that does not capture all clinical relevant aspects of psoriasis, such as degree of itching.

FIGURE 9.3 Example of the challenges of a clinical endpoint.

Therefore, relying completely on clinical operations people to select study sites is a serious flaw in how clinical trials currently are conducted.

Determine the Sampling Method

Once you identify the sampling frame, you must decide how you will pick or choose patients from the sampling frame. Random (otherwise known as probability) sampling is the best way of avoiding bias. (Unfortunately, clinical trials often do not use pure random sampling, since site selection, patient consent, and a number of other factors significantly influence sampling.) A sample is random if each member of the population has an equal chance of being selected for the sample (in contrast to a nonrandom or nonprobability sample in which certain members are more likely to be selected). In *simple random sampling*, all members of the sampling frame have an equal chance of being selected. You do not divide the frame in any way. It is analogous to putting all members of the sampling frame in a big bucket and then blindly pulling names out of the bucket.

There are different methods of random sampling:

- *Stratified random sampling*: For this method, first, divide the population into different logical categories or strata (e.g., different socioeconomic groups, disease severity levels, or ethnic groups) and then take random samples within each category or stratum. It is analogous to first dividing all of the members of the sampling frame into different buckets based on their characteristics and then blindly pulling names out of each bucket. The sample size in each category or stratum is usually proportional to the relative size of the stratum (e.g., if Asian Americans consists of 40% of the population and white Americans 60% and you want a study group of 100 people, you can take a random sample of 40 Asian Americans and 60 Whites). However, when the variances differ significantly across strata, sample sizes should be proportional to the stratum standard deviation.
- *Proportionate sampling*: This variation of stratified random sampling is useful when the strata vary dramatically in size (e.g., a study of people on the Wellesley College campus will have significantly more women than men). The number of patients you randomly select from each stratum is proportional to the stratum size relative to the whole population size (e.g., if the population is 90% women and you need to select 100 patients, you select 90 from the female stratum and 10 from the male stratum).
- *Systematic sampling*: In this method, you select every *n*th patient (e.g., every 5th patient) in the sampling frame or list. If the list is in random order then this is a random sampling method. Otherwise it is nonrandom. This method is relatively easy and efficient to implement. However, if every *n*th patient is somehow consistently different from the others (e.g., every 5th patient on the list is related), then there will be significant bias.
- *Cluster sampling*: Sometimes identifying everyone in a sampling frame is impossible or impractical (e.g., assembling a list of every hospitalized diabetic patient in Philadelphia is feasible but extremely difficult). In cluster sampling, you group the patients into naturally appropriate clusters or groups (e.g., by hospitals, geographic locations, or physician), randomly select clusters (e.g., 5% of the hospitals, zip codes, or physicians), and then use every patient within each selected cluster. So, for example, if there are 100 hospitals in Philadelphia, randomly select 5 hospitals then use every diabetic patient hospitalized in those 5 hospitals. Cluster sampling may save administrative and travel expenses (e.g., you only have to get records from 5 different hospitals). However, cluster sampling is only viable if you select clusters that are reasonably representative of the total population (e.g., clustering by zip code and only selecting clusters in the wealthiest neighborhoods will introduce bias). Moreover, depending on the type and size of the clusters, finding and using every patient in each selected cluster can be difficult and prohibitively expensive.
- *Multistage sampling*: This method is similar to cluster sampling (i.e., like cluster sampling, you first group the population into clusters and then randomly choose a certain number of clusters), except that you randomly select patients (rather than use all of the patients) in each selected cluster.

A sample that is not random is called a nonrandom sample or a nonprobability sample. Examples include:

- *Quota sampling*: This method is similar to stratified sampling, except that the patient selection is nonrandom. First, divide the population into different strata and then pick a pre-determined number of patients from each stratum (e.g., must get 20 women between the ages of 25 and 30, 10 men between the ages of 30 and 40, etc.) Stop when you have filled the quotas (i.e., pre-determined numbers) for each stratum. Quota sampling is relatively quick and inexpensive to perform but does not yield as representative a sample as other sampling methods.
- *Judgment sampling*: In this method, you look at the population and use your expertise or "judgment" to select patients from the population. This method is completely nonrandom and may be useful when the desired patients are rare or hard to find.
- *Convenience (grab or opportunity) sampling*: In this method, you arbitrarily choose patients from the sampling frame without any structure or rigor (e.g., patients you encounter in the park; patients that happen to come by your recruitment table).
- *Snowball sampling*: In this method, existing study subjects help recruit more subjects into the sample (e.g., their friends, family members, or co-workers).

Unfortunately, clinical trials almost always rely on convenience sampling. Since a patient's likelihood of consenting to a study is not purely random, the consent process further confounds and biases the sample (i.e., certain patients characteristics may influence whether a patient participates in a study).

Determine the Sample Size

Sample size calculations are discussed in Chapter 3.

Implement the Sampling Plan

The sample is the patients whom you select to be in your study. The key word here is *select*. Not every patient you select will ultimately participate in your study. Some may be unreachable. Some will not meet your inclusion criteria. Some will refuse to participate or drop out of the study. Your study population actually ends up being a sub-sample of the sample.

9.3.2 Clinical Trial Sample Characteristics

Nonrepresentative Samples

A nonrepresentative sample is one that does not reflect the overall patient population (e.g., a sample including only Latino men is not representative of the New York City population). Using a nonrepresentative sample can limit the generalizability of the study results. Unfortunately, as stated above, in clinical trials, random sampling is usually impossible. The patient population is almost never truly representative of the patient population at large, which is probably the greatest weakness of randomized prospective clinical trials.

Sampling Biases

Significant biases are unavoidable when patients are recruited into clinical trials. Patients who enroll in studies tend to be more motivated and younger. Usually they will be more compliant with treatment regimens and respond better to interventions than the "real world" population. Academic centers usually attract patients with more severe and complicated conditions. Different socioeconomic classes may be more or less likely to enroll (e.g., patients who cannot afford treatments may be more likely to enroll to receive free treatments or patients who cannot afford transportation to and from the study site may be excluded from the trial).

Biased samples can significantly influence results. Patients in a biased sample may have a different natural history of disease (e.g., a more severe course than the population at large, which would tend to overinflate the study intervention's benefits) or a different efficacy or safety response to the intervention.

Changing Sample Characteristics

Your sample will not be static. Patient characteristics may change over the course of the study, particularly in studies with a long enrollment periods. Many factors such as environmental changes, news stories, and scientific breakthroughs can affect the types of patients you are able to enroll in your trial. Results from similar trials can influence who enrolls in your trial (e.g., good results can encourage and bad results can discourage patients from enrolling in your trial). As enrollment progresses, finding the most appropriate patients becomes more and more difficult. Moreover, diseases and patient conditions change (e.g., diseases progressively worsen or improve, wax or wane). Also, the same patients that you initially screened may be very different when they are enrolled, when the trial starts, and when the trial concludes. Remember that no matter how tight you make the inclusion and exclusion criteria, population drift (i.e., a shift in patient characteristics) will occur.

Limited or Restricted Samples

Selecting a homogenous patient sample usually reduces variability and therefore the required sample size. This is because different subpopulations may have different natural histories and different responses to the drug – for both efficacy and safety. Selecting a homogeneous patient sample for a trial is often important in reducing the study size and increasing the likelihood of a positive trial. However, one of the most common methods for decreasing heterogeneity is to limit enrollment to a subset of the patients with a disease or a condition which unfortunately also limits the generalizability of the study's results (e.g., if only patients with lupus nephritis were enrolled in a trial, then the probability of showing a benefit may be significantly higher than if patients with lupus of any severity were enrolled; however, such a trial would address whether the drug would work in lupus patients who do not have nephritis). In addition, it may be more difficult to find and recruit a select group of patients. Another important way of decreasing heterogeneity is to institute strict criteria for confirming or establishing diagnosis and severity of disease (e.g., requiring a retinal angiogram to confirm the diagnosis of classic age-related macular degeneration; documentation of prior chemotherapy to ensure that the patient has refractory cancer; using a run-in period to confirm that the patient does have at least one exacerbation of asthma in 6 months).

Multi-center and Multi-geography Samples

With multi-center (and multi-national) studies becoming more prevalent, understanding their effects on the study sample is important. While multi-center trials bring multiple significant advantages (including speed, generalizability, and replication), they do add, increased variability and statistical

TABLE 9.2	Probability of Treatment Reversal by Random Chance							
Probability of At Least One Center Showing Treatment Reversal								
Number of Centers	1	2	3	4	5	6	7	8
Probability of Treatment Reversal	0.003	0.05	0.15	0.29	0.43	0.56	0.67	0.75

interactions. Having multiple centers decreases the likelihood of having a spurious result due to a systematic bias at one center, or due to practice pattern peculiar to one institution or region (e.g., some sites may or may not use IV nitroglycerin in acute myocardial infarction or coumadin post-myocardial infarction). Having multiple sites across the country reduces the likelihood that the results would depend on presence or absence of a concomitant medication or a particular practice pattern. Inconsistencies are very likely in a multi-center clinical trial. Practice patterns and patient populations vary across regions and countries. Patients in different countries frequently respond differently to the same intervention (e.g., European or Japanese patients vs. U.S. patients).

Moreover, by pure random chance, some sites may have results that are completely opposite to those of the rest of the sites (i.e., treatment reversal). So even if most sites show a treatment to improve mortality, by random chance, one or more sites may actually show the treatment to worsen mortality. The probability of at least one center demonstrating this kind of treatment reversal increases with the number of sites. Table 9.2 shows these probabilities when the alpha is 5% and the power is 80%.

A basketball analogy may help demonstrate this idea of chance treatment reversal. Michael Jordan is widely acknowledged as perhaps the best basketball player of all time. Throughout his career, he made many fantastic plays. However, since his career lasted so long and he played so many games, he also made some very foolish and embarrassing plays. These poor plays do not detract from his greatness and are the result of chance. There is no way anyone can play so many games and not have such "talent reversals." Similarly, famed cellist Yo-yo Ma cannot avoid playing some concerts poorly and well-known investor Warren Buffet will make some very bad investments.

Chapter 10

Dosing and Intervention

10.1 BACKGROUND

10.1.1 Definition of Intervention

Most clinical studies involve an intervention, that is a drug, a medical device, a technique (e.g., psychotherapy, an exercise, a muscle or spinal manipulation), or a behavior modification (e.g., change in diet or habits) designed to affect a clinical phenomenon. The goal of many clinical studies is to assess the effectiveness and safety of an intervention. This intervention can be:

- *invasive* (i.e., an intervention, such as an angioplasty stent or a needle, that somehow enters or penetrates the body) or *noninvasive* (i.e., an intervention such as psychotherapy, a bandage, a heating device, or a compression device that does not enter or penetrate the body);
- *preventive* (i.e., prevents the occurrence of an event, such as a vaccine) or *therapeutic* (i.e., treats symptoms or a disease, such as a drug);
- *acute* (i.e., administered over a short period of time) or *chronic* (i.e., administered regularly over a long period of time).

Not all interventions are amenable to clinical studies. For an intervention to be adequately studied in a clinical study, the intervention must be:

- *Reproducible*: For results of clinical study to be generalizable, the intervention must be reproducible, that is, practicing clinicians should be able to perform the intervention in the same manner in real-world settings. An intervention that can be performed by only one person in the world, requires very scarce resources or environments (e.g., a ritual that requires a solar eclipse), or lacks clearly defined protocols and instructions (e.g., magical healers that cannot explain their techniques) is not reproducible.

- *Standardized*: Standardization is essential. Different batches of the same drug should have equivalent quantities of active ingredients, bioavailability, and routes of administration. A medical device should have the same specifications (e.g., size, weight, and materials) and be built, assembled, and placed in or on patients in the same manner. Standardization is especially important with nondrug interventions such as surgery or behavioral techniques. Performing the intervention differently each time (e.g., using different techniques, doses, or timing) will make it impossible to draw any consistent conclusions about the intervention.
- *Clearly defined*: Know and define what the intervention is and when it begins and ends. Minimize the number of interventions occurring at one time so that you can establish which intervention is having the effect. You cannot adequately characterize the effects of an intervention until you know how long the intervention took place and when the intervention was completed. For acute and short-term interventions, the start and stop times may be easy to define. For chronic interventions, you may have to arbitrarily set start and stop times.

In addition, you must know the intervention's *operator dependency*. Any intervention must be administered. Intervention administration ranges from the simple and straightforward (e.g., giving a patient a pill to swallow) to the complex and difficult (e.g., surgical procedure). Understand how much the operator (i.e., the person or persons administering the intervention) affects the characteristics and impact of the intervention. For example, surgical procedures are highly operator dependent (i.e., a skilled surgeon will perform the intervention much more effectively than an unskilled surgeon), but giving a patient an oral medication is not very operator dependent (i.e., most people can put a pill in a patient's mouth). If an intervention is highly operator dependent, then your study will have to account for the operator's skill and experience levels, and you will need training and other standardization processes.

10.1.2 Definition of Dosing

A dose is the amount of an intervention administered. Every intervention can be administered in varying amounts and degrees. Giving a patient a metric ton of acetaminophen is not the same as giving her a microgram. Placing 18 cardiac stents probably will be a lot riskier than placing 1 stent. A patient may emerge from 2,000 hours of psychotherapy in a different state of mind than if he had only 3 hours. Therefore, simply saying whether an intervention does or does not work is not enough. Clinical studies help determine at what doses an intervention begins to work, at what doses an intervention becomes dangerous, and how changing the dose affects both efficacy and safety.

The units used for doses can vary by intervention, convention, and geography. You can administer drugs in an almost infinite variety of gradations (e.g., from microgram quantities to gram quantities or kilogram quantities). By contrast, you cannot administer fractions of surgical interventions (e.g., $2\frac{1}{4}$-vessel bypass surgery) or medical devices (e.g., half a pacemaker). Establishing dosing units for complicated procedures, noninvasive techniques, or behavioral interventions can be difficult. There is tremendous potential variability in one session of acupuncture or psychotherapy. "Increasing exercise" can mean one of a number of different interventions.

The doses of most medications, especially oral medications, are set during the manufacturing process. Each unit of medication (e.g., pill, suppository, or patch) may contain a specific amount of:

1. *Active drug*: Active ingredients are the part that does what the medication is designed to do or provides "pharmacological activity." This is usually fixed and consistent from batch to batch (e.g., 500 mg tablets of Tylenol will contain the same amount of acetaminophen). However, standardization of content and potency is not always trivial, especially for biologics. Biologics derived or purified from nonrecombinant sources, and in many cases even from recombinant sources, can have significantly different chemical structures (e.g., glycosylation patterns and *N*-terminal modifications) that can affect pharmacokinetics, pharmacodynamics, clinical efficacy, or clinical safety.
2. *Adjuvant*: Adjuvants are compounds that modify the effects of the active medication (acting like chemical catalysts) but have minimal direct effects when given by themselves. Therefore, the presence and quantity of adjuvant can affect the dosing of the medication. You can combine adjuvants with the active medication (e.g., vaccines suspended in aluminum slats designed to stimulate the immune system) or give them prior to (*neoadjuvants*) or concurrent with the administration of the active ingredients.
3. *Inactive ingredients (or excipients)*: Inactive ingredients do not have any direct pharmacological effects and include preservatives, stabilizers, buffers, absorption modifiers, distribution modifiers, fillers, and dilutions. They often are included to modify the stability, shape, appearance, and taste of the medication and can affect the absorption (and in turn the bioavailability) of the medication.

The doses of many medical devices are set during manufacturing as well. Characteristics of medical devices include:

1. *Physical dimensions*
2. *Delivery/release rate*: Some devices will deliver or release an active medication at a certain rate.

However, not all doses are set during manufacturing. A number of intervention administration techniques and factors can affect dosing. Therefore, documenting and standardizing the following administration parameters may be very important aspects of dosing:

1. *Dosing interval*: Dosing interval is the period of time between doses. For a once–a–day medication, the interval is 1 day or 24 hours. If you hold the individual dose quantity constant, decreasing the dosing interval increases the dose.
2. *Rate and duration of administration*: For interventions that are administered over a period of time, the rate and duration of administration can be very important. Infusing 500 mg of a medication over 10 minutes (which may result in higher levels of medication in the blood at a given time) can be very different from infusing 500 mg over 1 hour (which may result in lower levels over a longer period of time). Delivering three rounds of radiation therapy over 3 weeks is different from delivering three rounds over 6 months. Increasing the length and flow rate of hemodialysis can have significant implications.
3. *Patient positioning*: The patient's body positioning can affect the success of a surgical technique (e.g., changing body position can change accessibility of different organs, blood flow, and blood loss), receptability to an invasive or noninvasive technique (e.g., having a patient stand vs. sit vs. lie down could influence a patient's psychotherapy experience), and test results (e.g., cortisol levels and imaging tests).
4. *Route, location, and positioning of administration*: For some interventions, the positioning (e.g., the orientation and location of pacemakers, vascular or urological stents, or drug infusion pumps) or route of administration (e.g., the target and depth of injections) can vary significantly and greatly affect their efficacy and safety.

Remember that dosing goes far beyond just the size of pill you give to a patient. Therefore reporting that a patient was given 500 mg of a medication may not be enough. You may have to specify that the 500 mg was delivered over 60 seconds via an injection into the bicep while the patient was recumbent. Changing any of these parameters may change the dosing. The key is to identify what parameters might have the greatest impact and standardize those parameters as much as possible.

10.2 OVERVIEW OF DOSE SELECTION

10.2.1 Definitions and Objectives

Dose selection, exploration, and characterization are essential components of clinical trials. To better understand these terms, we can use the analogy of shopping for pants … not just for yourself but for a whole group of people. *Dose selection* is deciding which doses to test on a group of patients, which would be analogous to choosing which pants to take to the fitting room. *Dose exploration* involves testing the different doses and observing their effects and safety, similar to trying on the pants in the fitting room and seeing how they fit. *Dose characterization* is discovering and defining the relationships between the dose and different clinical and nonclinical effects (e.g., characterizing the safety margin, drug interactions, and dose–response relationship and determining the optimal starting dose and maximal dose), which would be akin to determining and understanding what aspects and features of the pants (e.g., their inseam, waist size, crotch length, thickness, and material) influence their fit and appeal.

The overall goal of dose selection, exploration, and characterization is not just to identify doses that are safe and effective but also to paint a comprehensive picture of the:

- relationships between dose and different efficacy, safety, and convenience parameters;
- parameters that affect these relationships;
- dosing regimens that appropriately balance efficacy and safety.

You will want a full understanding how different doses behave in a wide variety of situations, that is the distribution of efficacy and toxicity in the population and whether the patients experiencing the adverse events are the ones exhibiting response. Being able to predict (if possible) which patients will respond and which will suffer toxicity would allow clinicians to select the right doses and appropriate measures to avoid or alleviate adverse effects.

Using the pants shopping analogy, the goal is not just to find a single pair of pants to wear but to understand how all sizes and kinds of pants fit and look. Remember you are shopping not only for yourself but also for a larger group of people. Knowing and understanding the factors that affect the fit and appearance of pants will help you choose pants for all kinds of situations and people in the future.

Designing appropriate dosing regimens requires close collaboration with the pharmacokineticists, toxicologists, and preclinical scientists. Data from preclinical experiments such as animal, modeling, and pharmacokinetic data help determine the dosing interval and the initial doses in the early clinical development. Later in clinical development, the clinical efficacy and safety profiles from early phase studies play a much larger role in guiding dose selection, but understanding pharmacokinetics, toxicology, and pre-clinical information is still important.

In the "real world," clinicians often do not use the optimal doses recommended by clinical trials. In fact, they frequently use medications and other interventions "off label," that is for conditions and situations not indicated on the medication label or, in other words, not approved by relevant regulatory agencies such as the FDA. Using their clinical judgment and experience, clinicians will decide whether to administer an intervention and how to adjust the dose based on the specific situation. There are many reasons clinicians will use doses different from those deemed optimal by clinical trials. The patient may be of a different height, weight, ethnicity, age, or gender from those studied in the clinical trial. The patient's co-morbid conditions (i.e., other diseases), concomitant medications, and relevant physiological parameters (e.g., heart, lung, liver, or kidney function) also may be unlike those in the clinical trial population. The same toxicity effects may be more or less problematic to different patients (e.g., losing sensation in the fingers may be more significant for a surgeon than an accountant). Furthermore, the situation may be unusual. For example, a patient may not be able to pay for a full dose. The patient may have a terminal disease and have no other option, prompting the clinician to try higher and riskier doses.

Clinical practice and decision making is part science, part judgment, and part experience. A clinician does not and should not base every decision on pure scientific evidence. Often scientific evidence can be lacking or, even worse, misleading. Moreover, recommendations based on scientific evidence frequently change from year to year, and many times experts cannot come to any consensus.

Therefore, when it comes to dosing, a clinical trial should not just provide a "right-or-wrong" answer. Instead of determining the right dose, the trial should fully characterize the range of possible effects from different doses. The trial should provide information not make decisions for the clinician. This way clinicians will have a better picture of what may happen if they change doses or try any less orthodox strategies.

Of course, fully characterizing the effects of every potential dose is not always practical. Collecting and analyzing additional information consumes valuable time and resources. Balancing between adequate dose characterization and practical considerations can be challenging. When

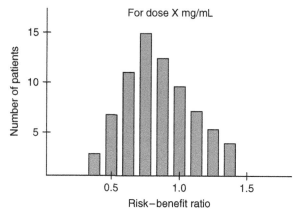

FIGURE 10.1   A histogram of risk-benefit ratio for specific tested dose of a drug.

there is a dire unmet need for a medication, generating scant dose–response curves may be adequate, so that the drug can be approved and reach patients as quickly as possible.

10.2.2 Challenges

Two of biggest challenges in dose selection are *risk–benefit ratio optimization* and *heterogeneity management*. The two are intimately related. Risk–benefit ratio optimization means finding doses that maximize the benefits of the intervention while minimizing the dangers. All drugs and doses have at least some toxicity, so completely eliminating risk is impossible. Rarely does the most efficacious dose have the least toxicity. Similarly, the least toxic dose usually is not the most effective dose. In fact higher doses tend to be more effective and more toxic. So, the challenge is finding the right "middle ground," the appropriate balance between benefits and risks.

This "middle ground" is rarely the same for all patients since they, their situations, and their underlying diseases are very heterogeneous (e.g., different metabolism, body sizes, rates of exercise, exposure to sunlight, compliance, genders, ages, concomitant medications, races, and tolerance levels). Different patients may respond to a given dose in different ways. Some will improve more and faster. Some will suffer worse or more frequent side effects. In general, the more heterogeneous the response, the more difficult it is to find acceptable balances of safety and efficacy.

Such heterogeneity can make assessing the risk–benefit ratio complicated. Simply calculating the mean or median risk–benefit ratio for each dose may not be enough, since the risk–benefit ratio may differ for different patients. Knowing the risk–benefit ratio distribution for each dose (e.g., the standard deviation, the 10th and 90th percentiles) is important. Ideally, you should be able to generate a histogram of risk–benefit ratios for each tested dose (Figure 10.1) and identify such parameters as the 10th and 90th percentiles. Moreover, quantifying the risks and benefits can be tricky. Is a moderate response equal to half of a full response?

Is one severe adverse event equal to 5, 10, or 15 mild adverse events? Clinical trials are good at generating population level dosing data, but you must then use this data to determine doses for individual patients.

When great heterogeneity exists, you may have to use any number of methods to make heterogeneous responses more homogeneous:

- *Customizing doses*: Customizing doses is the most common method and involves varying the dose by a parameter that drives heterogeneity (e.g., if you find that drug response varies by patient weight, you may have to give heavier patients higher doses than lighter patients).
- *Titrating to an endpoint*: An alternative method is choosing a relevant clinical endpoint (i.e., outcome) and adjusting the dose for each patient until the endpoint reaches a certain value (e.g., changing the medication dose until a certain blood pressure is achieved).
- *Dosing by subpopulation*: Another method is to identify subpopulations that may respond differently to the drug and giving each subpopulation a different appropriate dose (e.g., men may receive higher doses than women or African Americans may require different doses than Latinos, patients with liver failure may only tolerate lower doses). In some cases, the drug may not be indicated as safe for certain subpopulations.

Convenience and *practicability* are extremely important but often underappreciated facets of choosing the right dose regimen. The optimal dose from a pure risk–benefit standpoint is not necessarily convenient or practical. For example, many oral medications would be more effective and less toxic if given intravenously, since intravenous administration delivers the drug directly to the bloodstream. However, taking oral medications is much more convenient and requires significantly less time and effort. Similarly, frequently titrating the dose to a patient's daily fluctuations in body weight, temperature, blood pressure, fluid intake, and urine output could improve the risk–benefit ratio of a medication but would be confusing and not practical for a patient to do. (Many patients have difficulty just remembering to take a pill, let along having to perform self-measurements and alter their doses accordingly and frequently.) In general, to be practical and convenient, a dose should be:

- *Given as infrequently as possible*: The more often a patient has to receive an intervention, the more likely he is to miss a dose, the more likely administration errors and problems can occur, and more onerous and time consuming the intervention becomes. Remembering to take a pill once a day is much easier than remembering to take one four times a day. Going to psychotherapy sessions three times a week is much more time consuming and taxing on a patient's schedule than going once every two weeks. Being stuck with a needle once a day causes greater discomfort and potential harm than being stuck once a week.

- *Easily administered, preferably self-administered*: Minimizing the time, effort, and resources involved in administering an intervention is important. Oral and transdermal (i.e., skin patch) medications are the easiest to administer, followed by rectal and vaginal medications. Injections are much more difficult to administer and frequently require assistance. Anytime administration requires health care personnel, the cost, inconvenience, and effort required significantly increase.
- *Nondisruptive*: If possible, interventions should not interfere with daily activities such as sleeping, eating, and working. Anything that requires patients to wake up in the middle of the night, skip meals, or miss important activities will either impede their quality of life or deter them from getting proper treatment.
- *Reasonably cost-effective*: Do your best to minimize costs without sacrificing science and patient benefit. Avoid doses that are prohibitively expensive. An intervention will be useless if patients cannot afford it.

10.2.3 Design Issues

Remember that protecting the patient is paramount. All dose-testing trials should proceed carefully and cease before patients are subject to significant harm. Administering an intervention to patients before enough is known about its safety is an inherently risky endeavor. Do not escalate to a higher dose until you have collected extensive data and are convinced that the lower dose is safe.

Dosing investigation comes in several phases, each fraught with different challenges. *Phase I studies* define acute toxicities, aim to generate enough data about the drug, and escalate the dose carefully to the maximally tolerated dose. When the maximally tolerated dose cannot be reached, the highest dose should be comfortably above the anticipated target dose. Phase I studies include *single ascending dose (SAD)* and *multiple ascending dose (MAD) studies*, which we discuss later in this chapter. *Phase II studies* further investigate the dose to establish biological activity and the dose most likely to be useful. Typically you select 2–4 doses from the tested and tolerated doses in the SAD and MAD to be used for Phase II. Phase II studies aim to establish the dose(s) for the *Phase III study*. Both Phase I and II studies usually include pharmacokinetics. In most cases, you select the dose by the time you reach Phase III studies, which therefore mainly confirm the right dose. Phase III studies might include population pharmacokinetic studies to better characterize the effect of covariates such as age or sex on different pharmacokinetic parameters. *Phase IV studies* often investigate additional dosing regimens or formulations.

Usually in early phase studies, patients should not be taking concomitant medications (i.e., medications other than the intervention being studied) to minimize confounding due to drug interactions. However, during later stage studies, it is often important to either conduct specific studies with commonly used concomitant medications or include such patients in the clinical studies.

Although the goal of clinical trials is to identify a *target dose*, you must have a rough idea of what that dose might be before you even start Phase I trials. Otherwise, you may not even test that dose. So before starting clinical trials, use animal data (i.e., convert the target doses in animals using body surface area scaling factors, which we discuss later in this chapter) and knowledge of pathophysiology to select a possible target dose and make sure it falls inside your range of tested doses. Also, remember to account for potential variability (e.g., variation in absorption and bioavailability can significantly change the potential target dose).

10.3 PHARMACOKINETICS

10.3.1 Concepts

Pharmacokinetics is the study of the way drugs are absorbed, distributed, metabolized, and eliminated by the body (i.e., the relationship between dosing regimens and a drug concentration in body fluids over time). *Pharmacodynamics* is the study of the action of a drug on the body over a period of time (i.e., the relationship between drug concentration over time and drug effects on the body). Putting it another way, pharmacokinetics looks at what the body does to a drug, and pharmacodynamics looks at what a drug does to the body.

There are five possible phases in a drug's lifespan in the human body:

- *Administration*: You give the patient the drug through one of a variety of possible routes, such as oral, intravenous, intramuscular, vaginal, rectal, and subcutaneous. (We will discuss routes of administration later in this chapter.)
- *Absorption*: The drug moves from where it is administered into the bloodstream (i.e., systemic circulation).
- *Distribution*: The drug spreads throughout the body.
- *Metabolism*: The body alters the chemical structure of the drug.
- *Elimination*: The drug is excreted from the body.

Drugs can be *systemic* (i.e., enter the bloodstream and subsequently spread throughout the body) or *local* (i.e., confined to a certain part of the body). Systemic medications include those directly delivered into the bloodstream (e.g., intravenous) and those that enter other organs or tissue first and then are absorbed into the bloodstream. For example, systemic oral medications must get absorbed by the stomach or intestines before entering the bloodstream. Examples of local medications include many topical creams, joint injections, rectal suppositories for hemorrhoids, antacids, and eye drops. Even local medications can have some unwanted absorption into the bloodstream, sometimes causing toxicity. Local medications can have significant absorption into the bloodstream when administered incorrectly (e.g., accidentally injecting the medication into a blood vessel).

Absorption involves the medication crossing a series of semi-permeable cell membranes by any of the following possible mechanisms to reach the bloodstream (delivering drugs intravenously skips the absorption step):

- *Passive diffusion*: This is the movement of the drug from a region of high concentration (e.g., GI fluids) to a region of low concentration (e.g., blood). Passive diffusion occurs faster when the *gradient* (the difference in concentration between the two regions) is larger and the absorptive surface area is increased (e.g., intestines have very large surface areas from the many villi). Passive diffusion is also increased when the drug is more lipid-soluble (since the cell membranes are composed largely of lipids), consists of smaller (vs. larger) molecules, and exists in nonionized forms (which are lipid-soluble) rather than ionized forms (which are water-soluble).
- *Facilitated passive diffusion*: Even though there is a gradient across the cell membrane, the drug (especially ones that are not lipid-soluble) may require a special molecule to carry the drug across the cell membrane. Facilitated passive diffusion is analogous to getting on boat and riding it downstream without any energy expenditure.
- *Active transport*: Active transport is analogous to riding a boat upstream (i.e., against a concentration gradient). The process requires energy and involves carrying the drug across the membrane against a concentration gradient.
- *Pinocytosis*: In a process requiring energy expenditure, cell membranes can invaginate and engulf the drug into the cell.

The *absorption rate constant* quantifies absorption:

$$\text{Absorption rate constant} = \frac{\text{Rate of drug absorption}}{\text{Amount of drug remaining to be absorbed}}$$

Bioavailability is the degree to which or the rate at which the active portion of a drug reaches the systemic circulation:

Bioavailability = Amount of drug absorbed/Drug dose

Two drugs have *chemical equivalence* when they contain the same amount of the same active compounds (inactive ingredients may be different). When given to the same patient with the same dosing regimen, two drugs have:

- *bioequivalence* when they result in the same blood and tissue concentrations;
- *therapeutic equivalence* when they have the same positive and negative effects.

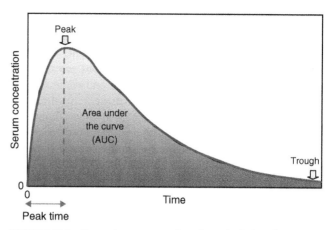

FIGURE 10.2   Serum drug concentration after a single drug dose.

Many factors can decrease bioavailability:

- *Decreased time at the absorption site*: In order to be absorbed, the drug has to remain at the appropriate location long enough to be absorbed adequately. For example, oral drug can pass too quickly through the stomach and intestines. Surgery, illnesses, stress, diet, physical activity, and the drug formulation and composition can affect the speed at which the drug goes through the stomach and intestines (i.e., gastrointestinal motility).
- *Poor penetration of cell membranes*: As mentioned previously, drugs that are not very lipid-soluble or exist largely in ionized forms do not penetrate cell membranes well.
- *Chemical reactions before reaching the systemic circulation*: The body, microorganisms, other drugs, and food may bind to, alter, or break down drugs before they reach their targets. For example, stomach acid, bacteria in intestines, and enzymes can affect oral drugs. Sometimes metabolism of a drug will occur (e.g., in the liver) before the drug reaches the systemic circulation (i.e., *first-pass metabolism*).

Graphing the plasma drug concentration over time characterizes the bioavailability of the medication (Figure 10.2). Such a graph can help ascertain several common measures of bioavailability: the *maximum (peak) plasma drug concentration*, the time at which this peak occurs (*peak time*), and the *area under the plasma concentration–time curve (AUC)*. Of these, the AUC is usually the most reliable measure. Peak plasma drug concentration informs you about the extent of absorption (the greater the absorption, the higher the peak); peak time tells you about absorption rate (slowing absorption delays the peak time); the AUC provides information about both extent and rate. The AUC reveals the total amount of drug that reaches systemic circulation. Two drugs that produce the same plasma concentration vs. time curves are bioequivalent.

After reaching the bloodstream, the drug spreads (or distributes) throughout the body occupying a certain total space or volume in the body called the *volume of distribution* (V_d). Drugs tend to go to areas where blood flow is high, cell membranes are permeable, and the drug binds to the tissue. A drug that stays in only a small portion of the body has a small V_d. So drugs that remain largely in the bloodstream (e.g., drugs that are water-soluble or bind heavily to plasma proteins) and do not readily spread into body tissue occupy small V_d. When traveling through the bloodstream, a percentage of the total drug amount is bound to blood proteins (e.g., albumin, lipoproteins, or hemoglobin).

This percentage varies depending on the drug and the serum pH. Only unbound drug can move out of the blood into the tissue to exert its effects. So it is often useful to calculate the *percentage or fraction of unbound drug*:

$$\text{Unbound fraction} = \frac{(\text{Plasma concentration of unbound drug})}{(\text{Plasma drug concentration})}$$

So, a drug that binds tightly to plasma proteins will have a V_d of around $0.05\,\text{L/kg}$, the volume of plasma in the human body. A drug that remains largely unbound but does not enter cells will have a V_d of around $0.2\,\text{L/kg}$, the total extracellular water volume. By contrast, a drug that spreads widely throughout the body has a large V_d. This includes drugs that are lipid-soluble or bind to tissue proteins so that they easily move from the bloodstream to various body tissues. A drug that enters cells freely has a V_d of around $0.55\,\text{L/kg}$, the total body water volume. Drugs that bind tissue have extremely high ($>10\,\text{L/kg}$) V_ds.

An analoguous situation with biologics occurs with neutralizing antibodies. Most biologics cause some degree of antibody formation. For example, infliximab causes anti-infliximab antibodies in a significant number of patients. These antibodies bind to the drug and neutralize some of the drug so that the effective concentration is lower than the total concentration. Unlike with traditional small molecules, neutralizing antibodies often do not eventually release the drug or equilibrate. In such cases, the drug can be considered to be eliminated once it binds to the neutralizing antibody although it may still be in circulation.

To understand how to calculate the V_d, picture the V_d as a bottle. Administering a drug to the body is like pouring it into the bottle. The concentration of drug in the bottle is then the drug dose divided by the bottle volume or:

$$\text{Drug concentration} = \text{Drug dose}/V_d$$

So to calculate the V_d, rearranging the equation yields:

$$V_d = \text{Drug dose}/\text{Drug concentration}$$

Typically you will know the drug dose and measuring the serum drug concentration is straightforward. For an individual patient, V_d is usually expressed in liters. For a group of patients, V_d is usually expressed in volume units per body mass unit (e.g., L/kg) since V_d increases with weight and body size.

There are two common routes by which drugs exit (i.e., are "eliminated from") the body: being excreted through urine or being metabolized (i.e., altered or broken down) first before being excreted. Water-soluble drugs usually leave directly through the urine while lipid-soluble drugs must first go through the liver to be metabolized into water-soluble metabolites that may be excreted through the urine. Although drugs may be excreted through the biliary system, intestines, saliva, sweat, breast milk, and lungs, most drug excretion occurs through the kidneys (i.e., renal or urinary excretion). Renal excretion decreases with age. Bound drugs remain in the blood as only unbound drug can be renally excreted. Unionized forms of drugs and their metabolites may filter into the urine but the kidneys then reabsorb them back into the blood circulation. Urine pH helps determine whether the drugs and metabolites are ionized and therefore affects renal excretion and re-absorption. The second most common excretion route is bile. The biliary tract tends to excrete drugs that are larger (drugs with molecular weight $>300\,\text{g/mol}$), lipid-soluble, and conjugated (i.e., connected to chemical groups such as glucuronic acid).

The liver handles most drug metabolism, breaking down or transforming drugs into metabolites that may or may not be pharmacologically active. In fact, sometimes a drug (called a *prodrug*) is not active until it is metabolized into active substances. Metabolism can involve a variety of possible chemical reactions such as oxidation (adding oxygen), reduction (removing oxygen), hydration (adding H_2O), dehydration (removing H_2O), hydrolysis (breaking down in H2O), conjugation (combining), isomerization (differing in the arrangement of the same atoms), *Cytochrome P_{450}* is a key liver enzyme system that helps oxidize many drugs. A number of substances can either stimulate (e.g., phenobarbital, rifampin, and carbamezapine) or inhibit (e.g., erythromycin, cimetidine, and omeprazole) cytochrome P_{450} enzymes and, in turn, affect the therapeutic effect of drugs. Liver (i.e., hepatic) metabolism rates decrease with age. Immediately after birth liver enzymes do not fully function yet, so newborns may struggle with metabolizing some drugs. Certain diseases (especially liver problems that decrease liver function and heart problems that impede blood circulation to liver) and other drugs also can reduce hepatic metabolism.

The rates at which urinary excretion and metabolism occurs is directly proportional to the amount of active drug in the body (i.e., first-order kinetics) until the capacity of each is reached. If D_B is the *amount of active drug in the body* and dD_B/dt is the change in the amount of active drug in the body per unit time (i.e., the *elimination rate of the drug from the body*) then:

$$\begin{aligned} dD_B/dt &= -k_e D_B - k_m D_B \\ &= -(k_e + k_m)D_B \\ &= -k_{el} \times D_B \end{aligned}$$

where k_e is the urinary excretion rate constant, k_m is the metabolism rate constant, and k_{el} is the final elimination rate constant ($=k_e + k_m$).

This elimination rate constant is equal to:

$$\text{Elimination rate constant} = \frac{\text{(Rate of drug elimination)}}{\text{(Amount of drug in body)}}$$
$$= \text{Clearance/Volume of distribution}$$

Once the metabolism capacity is reached (i.e., all the metabolic enzymes are saturated), the metabolism rate is no longer proportional to the amount of active drug present, that is metabolism no longer proceeds via first-order kinetics. The metabolism rate becomes fixed and no longer depends on the amount of drug present (zero-order kinetics).

The *clearance rate (Cl)*, which usually increases with patient weight, is the volume of blood or plasma completely cleared of a drug per unit time:

$$\text{Clearance rate} = \frac{\text{(Amount of drug cleared from the blood per unit time)}}{\text{(Plasma drug concentration)}}$$

You can use the clearance rate to calculate the AUC:

$$\text{AUC} = \text{Dose/Clearance}$$

Renal Clearance Rate (RCR) of a drug is:

$$\text{RCR} = \text{Amount of drug excreted in urine}$$
$$\text{per unit time/Plasma concentration}$$

The *metabolic clearance rate* of drug metabolized per unit time is:

$$\text{Metabolic clearnace rate} = \text{Rate of drug metabolism/}$$
$$\text{Plasma drug concentration}$$

The total rate of elimination is then:

$$\text{Rate of elimination} = \text{Renal clearance rate} +$$
$$\text{Metabolic clearance rate}$$

In order to calculate the percentage or fraction of drug not metabolized but excreted directly through the urine, use the following formula:

$$\text{Fraction excreted unchanged} = \frac{\text{(Rate of renal excretion of drug)}}{\text{(Rate of drug elimination)}}$$

When administering a drug, you aim to achieve a certain concentration of drug (i.e., *target concentration*) in the blood (or urine or other relevant body fluid). When there is no urgency, you can start giving the medication either by continuous infusion (e.g., intravenously) or at regularly scheduled intervals until the target concentration is achieved (Figures 10.3 and 10.4). When the medication is administered by continuous infusion, the serum concentration first increases rapidly but then more and more slowly until it reaches a *steady state*.

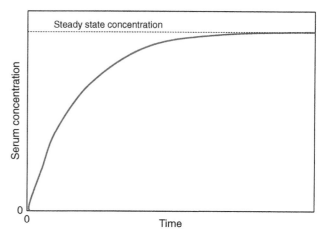

FIGURE 10.3 Serum concentration over time for a drug given by intravenous infusion.

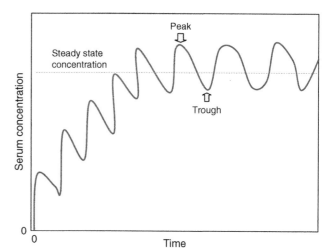

FIGURE 10.4 Serum concentration over time for a drug given at intervals.

The following formula calculates this *steady state concentration (C_{ss})*:

$$C_{ss} = \text{Infusion rate/Clearance rate}$$

To calculate the infusion rate needed to achieve a certain C_{ss}, rearranging the above formula results in the following:

$$\text{Infusion rate} = (\text{Target } C_{ss}) \times (\text{Clearance rate})$$

However, when there is urgency (e.g., treatment for stroke, severe infection, or seizure), you often need to give the patient a *loading dose* (i.e., a higher initial dose) to quickly achieve the target concentration. To calculate the size of the loading dose, use the following equation:

$$\text{Loading dose} = (\text{Target concentration}$$
$$- \text{Current measured concentration}) \times V_d$$

where V_d is the volume of distribution (to be explained later).

If there is currently no drug in the patient's body, the equation simplifies to:

$$\text{Loading dose} = (\text{Target concentration}) \times V_d$$

Giving an oral medication at a regularly scheduled interval will achieve a *steady state concentration* (C_{ss}) represented by the following equation:

$$C_{ss} = \text{Dosing rate/Clearnace} = \\ (\text{Bioavailability} \times \text{Dose})/ \\ (\text{Clearance} \times \text{Dosing interval})$$

Rearranging this equation gives you an equation to calculate the dosing regimen needed to achieve a target concentration:

$$\text{Oral dose} = (\text{Target } C_{ss} \times \text{Clearance} \times \\ \text{Dosing interval})/\text{Bioavailability}$$

Once you stop a treatment, you may want to know how long the drug remains in the body, especially if the drug is causing side effects:

$$\text{Plasma concentration} = (\text{Dose}/V_d) \times e^{-kt}$$

where k is the elimination rate constant and t is the time after the dose.

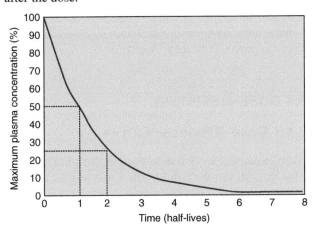

FIGURE 10.5 Decrease in plasma drug concentration over time after a single intravenous bolus.

This equation allows you to calculate the time it takes for the drug concentration to decrease by 50% (i.e., the biological half-life of the drug). Replacing "Plasma concentration/ (Dose/V_d)" with 0.5 and rearranging the equation yields the following:

$$\text{Biologic half-life} = \log_e 0.5/-k = 0.693/ \\ \text{Elimination rate constant}$$

Figure 10.5 shows what happens to drug concentration after an intravenous dose is delivered. After one half-life, the plasma concentration is 50% the initial concentration; after two half-lives, the plasma concentration is 25%; after three half-lives the plasma concentration is 12.5%, etc. (Figure 10.6).

10.3.2 Factors Affecting Pharmacokinetics

Many factors can affect pharmacokinetic parameters. Patient age can be an important factor. Two special age groups merit special consideration:

- *Neonates*: Compared to children and adults, neonates have a greater proportion of water per kg of body weight and, therefore, relatively higher volumes of distribution for water-soluble drugs (e.g., aminoglycoside antibiotics). They also have lower drug binding to albumin and alpha-L-acid glycoprotein (an "acute phase reactant" that is released in response to inflammation and trauma). Renal clearance is very low at birth and then rises dramatically over the first 2 weeks before stabilizing. Hepatic metabolism is also low for neonates, since their enzymes are not yet fully functional.
- *Elderly*: Compared to children and younger adults, the elderly have a greater proportion of fat per kilogram of body weight and, therefore, relatively higher volumes of distribution of fat-soluble drugs (e.g., diazepam). They also have lower drug binding to albumin but may have higher drug binding to alpha-L-acid glycoprotein, especially if they have chronic diseases. Renal clearance and hepatic metabolism decrease with age.

The half-life for a Drug P is 4 hours. The desired peak concentration is 10 mg/L and the desired trough concentration is 2 mg/L. The dosing interval should then be no-longer than 8 hours, because:

4 hours (or one half-life) after the peak, serum concentration = 10 mg/L/2 = 5 mg/L
8 hours (or two half-lives) after the peak, serum concentration = 5 mg/L/2 = 2.5 mg/L
12 hours (or three half-lives) after the peak, serum concentration = 2.5 mg/L/2 = 1.25 mg/L

In general, the dosing interval should be:

$$\text{Desired Trough} = \text{Desired Peak} \times (1/2)^{\text{Dosing Interval/Half-Life}}$$

FIGURE 10.6 Choosing the dosing interval.

Heavier patients usually require higher doses, which is why many drug doses are expressed in terms of medication per unit of patient body weight (e.g., mg/kg). The relevant type of body weight depends on the medication: "ideal body weight" or lean body mass may be more appropriate for highly water-soluble drugs that have limited fat distribution and total body weight may be more appropriate for highly lipid-soluble drugs. Usually gender differences in pharmacokinetics are too small to affect dosing, but pregnancy can significantly change a number of important physiological parameters and add a number of potential side effects. Keep in mind that the fetus will be exposed to most things that the mother receives. Also, women undergo some physiological changes during and after menopause which may affect pharmacokinetics.

Certain genetic differences can influence drug absorption, distribution, and elimination. Genetic variability (polymorphism) can lead to different levels of activity in important enzymes. Examples of such enzymes include cytochrome P450 (which helps metabolize many anti-arrhythmic, antidepressant and anti-psychotic drugs) and P-glycoprotein (which is an important transporter protein for digoxin).

Record all the medications (including prescription, over-the-counter, and herbal medications) and food that a patient is taking since some can affect the pharmacokinetics of the intervention that you are studying. Medications can stimulate or decrease the activity of liver enzymes and in turn hepatic metabolism, facilitate or impede intestinal absorption (e.g., antacids and milk products can interfere with tetracycline absorption and penicillin alters intestinal bacteria), promote or inhibit drug distribution, affect renal clearance, and change bile flow (e.g., probenecid can impair renal clearance of many antibiotics). Medications may be nephrotoxic (i.e., damage the kidneys) or hepatotoxic (i.e., damage the liver). Medications can bind other medications, receptors, and proteins.

The presence and severity of co-morbid diseases (diseases aside from the one being treated by the intervention) can affect pharmacokinetic parameters. For example, gastrointestinal disease can impair intestinal absorption of oral medications. Renal and hepatic disease can impair metabolism and elimination. Congestive heart failure (CHF) can decrease circulation and renal clearance (due to the decreased blood flow to the kidneys). Finally, diet can affect drug metabolism, such as grapefruit affecting P450 metabolism and green vegetables affecting coumadin efficacy by replacing vitamin K.

10.3.3 Therapeutic Drug Monitoring

Therapeutic drug monitoring, TDM (i.e., serially measuring medication levels in blood), is important in not only clinical trials but also sometimes in clinical practice. In medications with narrow therapeutic indices, TDM is essential to avoid insufficient levels (which can result in treatment failure or the development of drug resistance) and excessive levels (which can cause toxicity). Such monitoring is routine when using gentamicin, phenytoin, valproic acid, lithium citrate, pimozide, clozapine, and digoxin. Most commonly drug concentrations come from blood or serum samples. When blood is difficult to obtain (e.g., children), saliva samples can provide unbound drug concentrations.

Record the time between the dose and sampling time, the dosage history (i.e., how many doses the patient has received so that you know whether the steady state has been achieved), and the patient's response. The timing of sampling is important. You should allot enough time for a dose to be absorbed and distributed before measuring concentrations. Drug concentrations do not stay constant, but fluctuate between high (peak) and low (trough) levels. Whether to measure peak levels, trough levels, or both depends on the drug and situation. When drug concentrations must stay above a certain threshold to maintain protective effects (e.g., prevent seizures) tracking the trough levels may be important. When drugs begin to have significant toxicity above a certain threshold, following peak levels is important. Following peak levels is also important with "concentration-dependent" antibiotics, where the kill rate is solely dependent on the height of the peak concentrations. Sometimes the total time that drug concentrations remain above or below a certain threshold is important. For example, when antibiotics are "time dependent," they should be above an MIC as long as possible. Calculating the AUC can give you a patient's overall exposure to a drug over time. Recall that since AUC is equal to the dose divided by the clearance, reducing a patient's clearance by 50% doubles the patient's exposure to the same drug dose.

10.4 DOSE–RESPONSE

10.4.1 Dose–Response Curves

A *dose–response curve* is an *x–y* graph that plots the dose (or the logarithm of the dose) on the *x*-axis and the response (which can be any measure/endpoint) on the *y*-axis. Figure 10.7 illustrates a typical dose–response curve. Commonly, the *x*-axis plots the dose (in units of intervention per unit mass of test subject) or dose function (the log of the dose) and the *y*-axis plots the percentage of the population that exhibits the response (e.g., desired effect or toxicity). The more powerful the intervention, the steeper the curve becomes. The clinical generates data points to plot the dose–response curve. In general, the clinical trial should provide as many data points as possible to draw an accurate curve.

By plotting a dose–response curve in which response is the desired effect of the intervention, you can determine a number of important efficacy parameters. Figure 10.7 illustrates some of these parameters. The *threshold dose* is the lowest dose at which there is any response. This is the point at which the vertical height of the dose–response curve

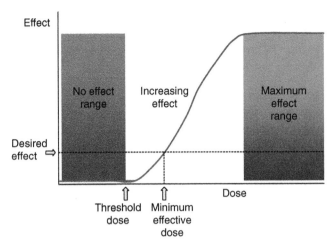

FIGURE 10.7 Dose–response curve.

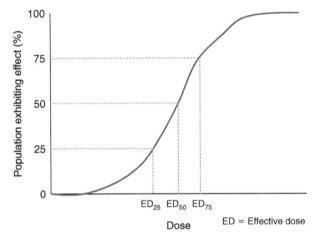

FIGURE 10.8 Median effective dose (ED50).

first starts to rise above zero. So if you were using a dose–response curve to demonstrate the effectiveness of a blood pressure medication, the threshold dose would be the dose at which any decrease in blood pressure in any test subject occurs. Usually slightly higher than the threshold dose is the *minimum effective dose* (*MED*), the lowest dose that will generate a specific effect. If the specific desired effect is lowering the blood pressure by 20mmHg, then the MED will be the dose at which at least one test subject's blood pressure decreases by at least 20mmHg. Finding a minimally effective dose is especially important when toxicity is of concern (e.g., small molecule drugs which tend to have toxicities at almost all doses or completely novel drugs that must be developed quickly to fill an important unmet need). For small molecules, the minimally effective dose tends to be the dose where the efficacy and safety curves diverge the most.

Plotting the percentage of the population exhibiting a response on the *y*-axis (Figure 10.8) can show the *median effective dose* (*ED50*), the dose that produces the specified effect in 50% of the population (e.g., half of the test population exhibits at least a 20mmHg decrease in blood pressure).

The *minimum curative dose* (*MCD*) is the lowest dose that can cure at least one subject. So if cure is defined as transforming a hypertensive patient into a nonhypertensive patient, then the MCD is the dose at which at least one hypertensive patient becomes normotensive. The *median curative dose* (*CD50*) is the dose that cures 50% of the subjects (e.g., 50% of the hypertensive patients become normotensive).

Similarly, plotting a dose–response curve in which response is toxicity can help determine a number of important safety parameters. The *tolerance dose* is the highest dose that will not cause any harm, that is the point right before the dose–toxicity curve height rises above zero. The *minimum toxic dose* is the lowest dose that will cause toxicity in any subjects. The *toxic dose for 50% of the population* or *median toxic dose* (*TD50*) is the dose that causes a toxic effect in half of the population. The *maximum dose* is the largest dose that can be safely administered. The *minimum lethal dose* (*MLD*) or the *minimum fatal dose* is the lowest dose that will kill at least one subject. The *lethal dose for 50% of the population* or *median lethal dose* (*LD50*) is the dose which kills half of the population. The *maximal tolerated dose* (*MTD*) is the highest dose that does not produce unacceptable toxicity, which is no toxicity in many cases but may be some toxicity when the intervention is for severe, life-threatening disease.

Some terms apply specifically to animal studies. The *lowest observed adverse effect level* (*LOAEL*) is the lowest dose tested that causes adverse effects in an animal species. The *no observed adverse effect level* (*NOAEL*) is the highest dose that does not significantly increase the incidence of adverse effects compared to the control group. The *no observed effect level* (*NOEL*) is the highest dose that causes no effects (positive or negative) in an animal species. The *pharmacologically active dose* (*PAD*) is the lowest dose that has the intended pharmacological activity in an animal species.

You may encounter other dosing terminologies depending on the situation or intervention being studied. When a total dose is given in portions over a period of time, each portion is called the *fractionated dose*. This commonly occurs in radiation therapy treatment. The clinician must decide not only the total dose of radiation to deliver but also over how many sessions to give this total dose (e.g., 1000Gy of radiation can be delivered in two sessions of 500Gy each or four sessions of 250Gy each). When toxicity is cumulative (e.g., radiation), determining the *maximum permissible dose* (*MPD*), that is the largest total cumulative dose that a subject may safely receive over a specified period of time, is important. Sometimes you may be interested in the dose (*target organ dose*) that a specific part of the body receives, for example, the *skin dose* (*SD*) when administering radiation. When the intervention is infective organisms, it is useful to know the *median infective dose* (*ID50*), that is the amount that will infect half of susceptible subjects. When evaluating vaccines, the *median immunizing dose*, that is, the vaccine dose that will confer immunity to 50% of the subjects, is important.

In general, the number after any dosing terminology is the percentile of the study population. So CD_{25} is the dose that cures 25% of the population, ED_{10} is the dose that produces a given effect in 10% of the population, and LD_{100} is the dose that kills the entire population.

From the efficacy and safety parameters, you can calculate the *therapeutic index* (otherwise known as *therapeutic ratio* or *margin of safety*), that is the ratio of the dose that causes toxic effects divided by the dose that generates the desired therapeutic effects. Commonly this is equal to:

$$\text{Therapeutic index} = LD_{50}/ED_{50}$$

The lower the therapeutic index, the narrower the therapeutic range is. Administering interventions with narrow therapeutic ranges, that is little difference between toxic and therapeutic doses, requires close monitoring (e.g., use TDM protocols), since slight changes in doses can mean the difference between helping and harming a patient. Examples of drugs with narrow therapeutic ranges include digoxin, lithium, theophylline, vancomycin, amphotericin B, gentamicin, and vancomycin.

Most responses are dose-dependent (i.e., changing the dose will change the degree and/or frequency of response), which allows you to plot a dose–response curve. Since the response (efficacy or toxicity) is usually monotonic (i.e., the response increases, or decreases depending on how you define response, over the entire dose range), the slope of this curve usually remains either >0 or <0. By contrast, the slopes of nonmonotonic dose–response curve (NMDRC) reverse (i.e., goes from >0 to <0 or <0 to > 0) as the dose increases. Some NMDRC are shaped like U's or inverted U's, which we will discuss later in this section.

The relationship between dose and effect is typically assumed to be continuous. Clinical trials generate dose–response points and a curve is drawn or extrapolated between these points, allowing you to predict responses for doses not tested (e.g., if a 4-mg and 5-mg dose were tested, the line between these points would predict the response for a 4.5-mg dose). Since the relationship is continuous, you normally can treat doses as a continuous variable, using them to perform mathematical manipulations and modeling.

However, some responses are not dose-dependent and therefore do not conform to a dose–response curve. It can be difficult to detect such situations, since the assumption during dose selection is that the response is dose-dependent. Classic examples of nondose-dependent responses are the toxicities agranulocytosis and Stevens Johnson Syndrome which can occur at any dose and are neither more likely nor more severe at higher doses.

Dose–responses curves can assume almost any shape, since there are many potential steps between administering an intervention and seeing a clinical outcome. For example, an oral medication must first be absorbed and reach the bloodstream. Once in the bloodstream, the active ingredients must

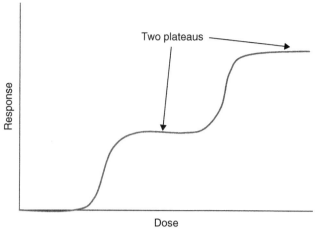

FIGURE 10.9 Bi-phasic response.

reach the target organ and bind the appropriate receptors. Binding the appropriate receptors then must trigger a cascade of chemical reactions that result in a clinical outcome. The greater the number and complexity of steps involved, the more complicated and unpredictable the dose–response curve may be.

However, despite many potential complex pathways, most biological phenomena and medications exhibit S-shaped (sigmoidal) dose–response efficacy and toxicity curves (Figure 10.11). At low doses, the pharmacological effect is slight; then at a certain dose range, the effect increases at a rapid rate; at a higher dose range, the effect plateaus; and at even higher doses, there is no further increase in the pharmacological effect. The Hill slope or the slope factor quantifies the steepness of the curve. A standard curve has a Hill slope of 1.0. A steeper curve has a slope factor >1.0. A shallower curve has a slope factor <1.0. A downhill curve has a slope factor <0.0.

Most interventions have a monophasic response, that is the dose–response curve has a single plateau. This is because above some point the receptors that mediate the response become saturated. Further increases in dose only means that more medication or units of the intervention wait around for the appropriate receptors or go unused (e.g., are excreted in the urine).

Some interventions have bi-phasic (there are two plateaus in the dose–response curve as in Figure 10.9) or multi-phasic responses (i.e., two or more plateaus). This occurs if the mechanism and/or effects of the intervention change as the dose increases. For example, some antibiotics just inhibit the replication of bacteria (bacteriostatic) at low concentrations (i.e., above the *minimum inhibitory concentration (MIC)*) but actually kill existing bacteria (bactericidal) at higher concentrations (i.e., above the *minimum bacteriocidal concentration (MBC)*). Therefore, testing an adequately wide range of doses is important. Looking at a limited range may reveal only the first plateau and not subsequent plateaus.

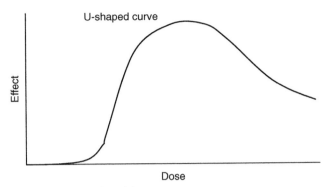

FIGURE 10.10 U-shaped dose–response curve.

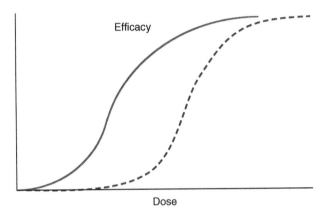

FIGURE 10.11 Standard model.

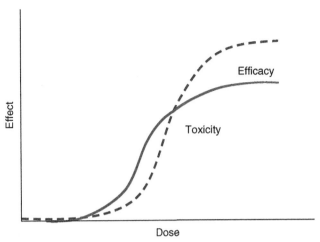

FIGURE 10.12 Crossing efficacy and toxicity curves.

Less commonly, the dose–response curve is U-shaped, that is as you increase the dose, the effect increases until a peak is reached and then the effect decreases (Figure 10.10). The low dose stimulation and high dose inhibition phenomenon that generates U-shaped curves has been termed *hormesis*. Hormesis manifests when overstimulation of a desired response causes a breakdown of normal body function or balance (i.e., homeostasis). This is reminiscent of the saying "too much of even a good thing is not good." Too much exercise can damage the body. Lower doses of radiation can destroy tumor cells but much higher doses can harm normal tissue. Very low and very high cholesterol levels are unhealthy. U-shaped curves also result when interventions have agonist (i.e., promotes the effect) activity at certain levels and antagonist (i.e., blocks the effect) activity at other levels (e.g., phytoestrogens are aromatase inhibitors at low concentrations but estrogenic at higher concentrations).

10.4.2 The Standard Model

When initially planning your dose selection strategy, you usually assume that the efficacy and toxicity curves will follow the simplified standard model depicted in Figure 10.11. The area where the efficacy and toxicity curves exhibit the greatest separation (maximal hysteresis) usually defines the therapeutically appropriate dose, unless high efficacy is required and

some toxicity is tolerable, as is the case with some oncology drugs. When the efficacy curve is always higher than the toxicity curve, the wider the separation between the two curves, the better the therapeutic index is. Insufficient separation or reversed curves (i.e., the toxicity curve is higher than the efficacy curve) usually means that the intervention is not useful therapeutically. (This is not always true. Sometimes you are willing to accept high toxicity in exchange for the benefits as in some chemotherapeutic agents.) When the curves cross as in Figure 10.12, the intervention may be beneficial at lower doses. Of course, depending on the degree of unmet medical need, the type of efficacy, alternative available therapies, and the type of toxicity, the drug may or may not be of use.

This standard model of efficacy and toxicity is obviously a simplification. Although useful as a starting point, this model has major limitations and relies on some important assumptions. Specifically, the model assumes that:

- *Efficacy and toxicity are dose-dependent.*
- *There is no significant variability in response.* Different patients in a population can have very different response and toxicity curves. When there is high variability, look for a wider separation between the efficacy and toxicity curves before deeming the intervention therapeutically acceptable. For example, if the threshold for cardiotoxicity is fixed at a 10 mg/kg dose, a 9 mg/kg dose would be safe. If there is significant variability in this threshold (e.g., the threshold varies from 5 mg/kg to 15 mg/kg), giving a 9 mg/kg dose would not be as safe.
- *The risk–benefit tradeoff is fixed.* In actuality, the risk–benefit tradeoff depends on the type of intervention, disease, and toxicities. You may be less willing to risk a toxic effect if the disease is not life-threatening, there are many alternative interventions, or the toxic effect is severe. Conversely, you may be more willing to risk a toxic effect if the disease is life-threatening, there is a dearth of alternative treatments, or the toxic effect is mild. For example, in evaluating a blood pressure medication, your

tolerance for a severe toxic effect like fulminant liver failure is very low. So the average toxicity curve is not very helpful. Instead, you want to identify the dose at which you are 99.999% sure that fulminant liver failure will not occur. On the other hand, for a medication treating acute myocardial infarction, the acceptable risk of intracranial hemorrhage toxicity may be higher (such as 1%).

- *The dose–response curve remains constant over time.* This is not always the case. Patients may develop tolerance (i.e., the effects of the same dose decrease over time) to the intervention. The intervention may have an additive or cumulative effect, that is, as more doses are given, the effects of each dose increases (e.g., the risk of pulmonary fibrosis increases with more doses of amiodarone). The initial doses of an intervention may have a "priming" effect, making subsequent doses more effective (e.g., after crossing below a certain concentration, bacteria may be easier to eradicate).

Successful dose selection and exploration should achieve certain criteria (i.e., performance criteria). It should produce dose–response curves that are detailed (i.e., many data points) and wide (i.e., explores a large range of parameters such as age, renal function, etc.) and define a space with good separation between safety and efficacy (even while accounting for individual variation) while maximizing convenience.

At first glance, the easiest way to define the safety and efficacy curves would be simultaneously testing a large number of different doses. Imagine performing dose selection and exploration for a new statin medication. Why not test 20 different doses of the medication from a low dose of 1 mcg to a high dose of 5 g? You could give each different dose to several thousand patients for 5 years to generate plenty of data points to fully define safety and efficacy dose–response curves.

Unfortunately, this approach would encounter several significant problems (i.e., constraints):

- *Exposure to toxic doses*: Immediately using a full range of doses could expose many patients to toxic doses. Therefore, the first step in dose selection is usually careful *dose escalation*: testing low doses first and then slowly raising the dose once you are convinced that it is safe.
- *Logistic and economic challenges*: Such a large and lengthy study would be very costly and difficult to coordinate. Therefore, earlier and medium stage studies exploring doses are often conducted with surrogate endpoints and/or enriched patient populations that will allow for an estimate of the dose–response curve with smaller sample sizes and shorter timeframe.
- *Heterogeneity*: As we mentioned previously, patients can have very heterogeneous responses to a given dose, and you often have to customize, titrate, or tailor (for different subpopulations) doses, especially for interventions with narrow therapeutic margins. Therefore, rather than immediately giving flat doses to many patients, using a careful *iterative* approach may be wiser. You can try a

low dose on patients and determine what factors affect their response. If in this first iteration you were to find that heavier or thrombocytopenic patients respond poorly to the drug, the second iteration could tailor the doses by weight and platelet count. The second iteration may find additional factors that affect response, such as liver function or age. You can then incorporate these factors into customizing dosing and continue the iterations until all relevant factors are elucidated. Sometimes it is impossible to find acceptable therapeutic windows until doses are adequately customized, titrated, or tailored.

Because of these constraints, dose selection and exploration usually proceeds in three stages:

- *Initial establishment of the safety window*: This corresponds to Phase I of clinical development and involves discovering the range of safe doses.
- *Dose exploration (sometimes iterative)*: This corresponds to Phase II of clinical drug development and
- *Final dose- and hypothesis-testing*: This corresponds to Phase III of clinical development and involves demonstrating the effects of these are consistent with the classic Phase I, II, and III divisions in drug development, and indeed dosing is a major driver for those divisions.

10.5 COMPONENTS OF DOSING

10.5.1 Types of Dosing

There are three general types of dosing.

Flat Doses

As we discussed earlier in this chapter, a flat dose (i.e., the same dose for all patients) is acceptable for interventions with wide therapeutic windows or for situations with limited heterogeneity. When possible, flat doses are preferable because they are relatively simple and convenient to administer. An example of a flat dose medication is Tylenol. Everyone takes the same dose, despite their weight, age, height, ethnicity, or gender. If you cannot seem to identify an acceptable flat dose, sometimes changing the way you measure intervention quantity can help. For example, there may be a single dose concentration, peak concentration, target concentration, or AUC that can be used for all patients. Therefore, plotting such measures against response could be useful. When you still cannot find an acceptable flat dose (or flat dose concentration, etc.), you must customize doses by either adjusting the dose based on some baseline characteristic or titrating the dose to a certain response.

Let us return to our pants shopping analogy. A flat dose is like a one-size fits all pair of pants. When conditions are more flexible (e.g., casual situations where pants do not have fit

Pitfall: Confounding

To establish a true concentration-response relationship, simply correlating serum drug concentration with effect is not enough. You have to establish a relationship between dose and serum concentration. Otherwise, you cannot rule out the presence of confounding factors.

Example: You are developing Oral Drug X for Crohn's disease and administer placebo, 10 mg, and 20 mg doses of the drug in a clinical trial. Patients who achieved the highest serum drug concentration had markedly better outcomes. However, there was no correlation between dose and outcomes. How could this be?

Explanation 1: The drug is effective. Oral Drug X Absorption is highly variable. The better the absorption, the more effective the drug is.

Explanation 2: Patients with severe Crohn's disease may poorly absorb Oral Drug X and therefore have lower serum drug concentrations. Patients with severe Crohn's disease also will tend to have poorer outcomes.

FIGURE 10.13 Pitfall: confounding.

perfectly) or the population is very homogeneous, finding a single size and style of pants for everyone is easy. When conditions are less flexible (e.g., in business meetings or formal dances the pants may have to fit well) or the population is very heterogeneous, you have to customize the pants to different individuals. There are two general ways to customize pants. The first way is identifying the characteristics that determine the fit of pants (e.g., people's waist sizes, leg lengths, color preferences, ages, genders, or jobs) and then adjusting the pants based on these characteristics. For example, if you find that people's jobs affect the fit of their pants, then you can have one set of pants for lawyers, one set for models, and one set for electricians. The second way is identifying some important relevant responses (e.g., compliments from friends, ability to bend over, and job promotions) and then titrating the size and type of pants to optimize these responses. For example, if compliments from friends are an important response, for each person you can do the following: test one pair of pants, see if she gets enough compliments, and try a different pair if she does not get enough compliments. Eventually you will be able to find a pair that elicits the optimal number of compliments.

Dosing Based on a Baseline Characteristic

The most common method of adjusting a dose is to use a physiological parameter (*physiology-based dose*) such as weight (e.g., total weight, lean weight, or estimated weight), body surface area, sex, age, and other physiological parameters. The choice of the physiological parameter depends on the drug and patient characteristics and the efficacy and toxicity parameters (e.g., using total weight rather than lean weight may be better for a drug that distributes largely into fat). With each of these parameters, you can either give tailored doses to each individual patient (e.g., the dose is 5 mg/kg) or have specific doses for each stratum or tier of patients (e.g., 10 mg for patients under 70 kg, 15 mg for patients >70 kg but <100 kg and 20 mg for patients 100 kg and above). The second most common way of adjusting dose is by metabolism, distribution, or excretion parameters that may affect a drug's therapeutic effects. Adjusting doses for renal or hepatic function (e.g., decreasing doses when either or both are impaired) is relatively common. For highly protein-bound drugs, adjusting doses for serum albumin levels may be important. A third way of adjusting doses is by disease severity or subtype. More severe forms or different manifestations of a disease may require higher doses. Finally, drug doses may need adjustment in the presence of other drugs because of potential drug–drug interactions. Remember the administered dose not necessariy represent serum concentration (Figure 10.13).

Titrated/Adaptive Dosing

Titrated or adaptive dosing involves following a certain parameter and altering the dose to achieve a target value of the parameter. This would be similar to fitting pants on someone whose needs are constantly changing. You have to check the situation repeatedly and then alter the pants selection accordingly. At 4 pm she is at work, so looser fitting slacks may be warranted. At 7 pm she is at a party, so a tighter pair of jeans may be in order. At 12 midnight, she is at home, so a very loose and comfortable pair of sweatpants could be appropriate. Once she has a clear work and recreation regimen, you can establish a set pants schedule. Titrated/adaptive dosing can avoid the pitfall or confounding that can result when a correlation is drawn between PK or PD paramaters and an endpoint in nontitrated dosing studies (Figure 10.13).

There are three general ways of titrating doses:

- *Pharmacokinetics-based dose*: When simple physiological parameters such as weight cannot predict a drug's pharmacokinetic activity, you can monitor plasma or serum drug concentrations (e.g., peak, trough, or average) and alter your doses to achieve certain ranges. In fact, this iterative process of repeat measurements and making necessary dose alterations may continue until the drug reaches a steady state concentration. Even after a steady state is achieved, periodic measurements can check if fluctuations in disease or physiological activity warrant further dose changes.

- *Pharmacodynamic-based dose*: Pharmacokinetic parameters may not adequately predict clinical effect or toxicity. There can be a time lag or other factors between achieving a certain concentration and seeing the effect. Measuring pharmacokinetic parameters such as plasma concentration may not be possible or practical (e.g., warfarin). In such situations, you can measure and titrate doses to a pharmacodynamic parameter [e.g., titrating doses of coumadin to the international normalized ratio (INR), heparin to the partial thromboplastin time, or thrombolytics to fibrinogen depletion). Since pharmacodynamic endpoints are surrogate endpoints, you must validate them. Sometimes the validation is straightforward (e.g., 80% platelet aggregation inhibition is a well-validated surrogate endpoint for acute coronary events and can serve as a pharmacodynamic parameter for IIb/IIIa inhibitor dosing). Sometimes validation is much more difficult. For example, what should be the target inhibition range for adhesion molecule inhibitors? 90% saturation? 95% saturation? Higher or lower? It may be very difficult to establish a clear relationship between the pharmacodynamic parameter and clinical effect. Even if you establish this relationship, significant variability can occur. Two patients may have 90% saturation, but each may have a rather different clinical effect. You can use pharmacodynamic parameters for both efficacy and safety dosing (e.g., titrating thrombolytic doses to fibrinogen levels, since low levels of fibrinogen portend an increased risk of bleeding).
- *Clinical effect-based dose*: Clinical effects or response can guide dosing (e.g., titrating analgesic doses to pain levels) for both efficacy and safety (e.g., titrating medication doses to liver function test elevations or nausea) if they are immediately apparent, easy to monitor, and reversible (since you can only titrate doses to something that can change). However, the vast majority of clinical endpoints do not fulfill these requirements (e.g., atherosclerosis progression is asymptomatic and difficult to monitor, stroke is irreversible, and osteoporosis takes a long time to manifest). The endpoint also can be the probability of an event instead of the event itself (e.g., coronary event risk instead of absence/presence of a coronary event).

10.5.2 Dosing Interval and Duration

The timing of doses usually depends on the drug's half-life, therapeutic index, absorption speed, and dose-dependent toxicities and can profoundly affect the drug's efficacy and safety profile. The *dosing frequency* is inversely proportional to the *dosing interval*:

$$\text{Frequency (times per day)} = 24 \text{ hours/Dosing interval}$$

$$\text{Frequency (times per week)} = 24 \text{ hours} \times 7 \text{ days/Dosing interval}$$

The dosing interval should be less than or equal to several times the half-life of the drug. Smaller, more frequent doses are preferable to larger, less frequent doses for interventions with shorter half-lives (e.g., small molecule drugs usually have shorter half-lives than biologics), narrower therapeutic windows, and dose-dependent toxicities. When the half-life is very short, the therapeutic window is very narrow, and toxicities are significant, continuous IV dosing might be necessary (e.g., epoprostanol [Flolan]).

The treatment duration depends on the timing and length of the illness and symptoms. Acute and self-limited conditions (e.g., infections and injury) require only *short-term dosing* (e.g., most oral antibiotic courses last between 2 and 14 days). Diseases that flare and remit (i.e., worsen and improve like gout and asthma) may call for *intermittent dosing* (i.e., interventions are admitted during the disease flares and discontinued when the flares resolve). Some conditions or normal body functions fluctuate at regular, predictable intervals (e.g., menstrual cycle) and lend themselves well to *cyclic dosing* or treatments corresponding to these regular fluctuations or cycles (e.g., oral contraceptive pills). Diseases that persist and cannot be easily cured (i.e., chronic diseases such as hypertension) may necessitate *chronic dosing* (i.e., treatment for very long periods of time).

Treatment frequency and duration are not necessarily constant. Treatment frequency can depend on specific pharmacodynamic parameters or outcomes (e.g., increase or decrease the frequency of coumadin doses depending on whether the INR is below or above the target range, respectively; and increase frequency of pain treatments when pain increases). The duration of some conditions can be quite variable (e.g., post-operative pain or constipation), and in such cases, treatment continues until symptoms and the condition resolve. Sometimes the patient or patient's caregiver can decide when and how long to administer the treatment (i.e., the treatments are given *pro re nata* or *p.r.n.* or on an "as needed" basis). *PRN medications* (e.g., Tylenol, laxatives, Ambien, Ativan, and Gravol) usually are relatively safe and straightforward to administer.

There are situations where you need to halt treatment for a specified period of time, that is, implement a *drug holiday* (or *drug vacation* or *structured treatment interruption*). Drug holidays may be *planned* or *unplanned*. Sometimes drug holidays allow another body mechanism to take place that assists the effects of the intervention (e.g., in HIV therapy, temporarily withdrawing medications may allow the body's immune system to attack the virus). Sometimes patients will develop tolerance to a continuously or repeatedly administered treatment (e.g., nitrates). This tolerance may disappear after the treatment is withheld for a while. Drug holidays can also reduce the risk of, or offer patients a respite from, intervention side effects (e.g., anti-depressants and Ritalin).

Initiating treatment can be simple or complex. The first dose (or first several doses) can be the same or different from subsequent doses. As we mentioned earlier in this chapter, giving a higher initial dose or *loading dose* of a medication is indicated when you need to achieve a target concentration quickly. The disease may be progressing too rapidly (e.g., heparin and clopidogrel during a myocardial infarction; procainamide for an abnormal cardiac rhythm) or symptoms may be too severe (e.g., morphine) to wait for regular doses. Sometimes patients are at high risk for an event (e.g., seizure) so a preventive intervention should be given as quickly as possible (e.g., phenytoin). Loading of a medication can occur over short or longer period of time. When side effects are associated with loading (e.g., dofetilide may cause QT prolongation and *Torsades de Pointes*), rapid loading over several days in a hospital setting where the patient can be monitored may be preferable to loading over several weeks in an outpatient setting. Giving a lower *test dose* is warranted when the intervention is associated with significant side effects or may not be effective. Treatment can continue if the test dose indicates that the patient will benefit or not suffer toxicity. A lower initial dose can also help a patient become accustomed to an intervention (*conditioning dose*). After giving a lower dose for any reason, you may either jump to the regular dose or gradually increase the dose (i.e., dose escalation).

Discontinuing interventions may or may not be trivial. *Withdrawal effects* are possible when the patient becomes physically or psychologically dependent on an intervention. Typically withdrawal signs and symptoms are the opposite of the intervention's effects (e.g., severe pain when withdrawing from pain killers) and can appear as soon as the effects of the intervention dissipate. Opiates, selective serotonin reuptake inhibitors (SSRIs), and benzodiazepines commonly cause withdrawal when stopped abruptly. *Rebound effects* (e.g., the rapid and severe appearance of a symptom or problem the intervention was treating) also may occur after discontinuing an intervention (e.g., rebound headaches after stopping migraine medications, rebound hypertension after stopping clonidine, and rebound depression after discontinuing anti-depressants). Rebound effects come from the body's regulatory mechanisms. Chronic use of an intervention often will suppress certain mechanisms in the body (e.g., prevent the release of a neurotransmitter) that overreact (e.g., a sudden surge of built-up neurotransmitter is released onto receptors that are not used to seeing the neurotransmitter) once the intervention is no longer present.

There are two ways of preventing withdrawal and rebound effects. One is to discontinue the intervention gradually (e.g., slowly decreasing the dose frequency and/or size) to allow the body to become acclimated. The second is to initiate a similar but less potent intervention after discontinuing the initial medication (e.g., starting oral oxycodone when stopping intravenous morphine).

10.5.3 Routes of Administration

The route of administration is the path by which an intervention enters the body and reaches its destination. Changing the route of administration can drastically change an intervention's effects and dramatically influence the pharmacokinetic properties of drug (e.g., absorption, distribution, and elimination). Several considerations dictate an intervention's route of administration:

- *Convenience*: Some routes are more convenient (i.e., require less time, effort, discomfort, equipment, and personnel). More convenient routes usually result in better patient compliance.
- *Urgency*: Emergent situations (e.g., stroke, heart attack, trauma, and seizures) require the intervention to be administered and reach its target as quickly as possible.
- *Practicality*: Certain formulations and, in turn, certain routes of administration are currently not possible (e.g., you cannot administer most antibiotics through a skin patch).
- *Therapeutic index*: The narrower the therapeutic index, the more control you must have over the intervention (e.g., intravenous administration allows you to alter the plasma concentration quicker and more precisely).
- *Access*: Not all routes are accessible (e.g., intravenous routes are impractical for patients with very poor venous access, vaginal formulations do not work for men, and not everyone can take oral medications).
- *Bioavailability*: Some routes do not offer high enough bioavailability (e.g., it would take dozens of pills to get plasma concentrations above the target level).
- *Disease location*: Interventions usually work best when applied as close as possible to the disease location (e.g., creams for skin disease, enemas for rectal disease, and joint injections for arthritis).

The *oral route* is the most convenient, inexpensive, and safest route. Oral medications must have a wide therapeutic window because bioavailability is relatively low and extremely variable compared to other routes. An oral medication may have to overcome a number of obstacles including acidic environments, various gastrointestinal secretions and enzymes, and food just to reach the site of absorption. Therefore, the drug must be stable and hardy enough to be administered orally (e.g., oral formulations of peptide drugs such as insulin are not practical). Moreover, patients must be compliant and able to swallow and eat.

Transit time, pH, bacteria, absorptive surface area, thickness of the epithelium, bile, mucus, food, and blood perfusion all affect absorption. The oral mucosa has good blood perfusion and thin epithelium, so placing a drug between cheek and gums (*buccal administration*) or under the tongue (*sublingual*) is possible for some medications (e.g., nitroglycerin, buprenorphine, and testosterone). However, absorption via these routes is usually inadequate and erratic since most drugs cannot stay in the mouth long enough.

Most oral medication absorption takes place in the intestines, in particular the small intestines, which have a vast surface area and comparatively thin and permeable epithelial lining. Many oral medications become absorbable only after being broken down and dissolved (*dissolution*). Undissolved medications pass through the gastrointestinal tract without being absorbed. Dissolution may start in the mouth. The stomach helps break down medications, but medications usually do not stay in the stomach long enough to penetrate its thick mucous layer. Factors that slow the rate of medications leaving the stomach (e.g., food, especially fatty food, or drugs that impair parasympathetic activity) can delay the medication from reaching the intestines and thus slow absorption. Food can either enhance (e.g., griseofulvin) or impair drug absorption. The remainder of dissolution takes place in the intestines. The formulation of the drug (e.g., salt, crystal, or hydrate) affects the dissolution rate and, in turn, the absorption. Gastrointestinal disorders that cause inflammation (and reduce the permeability of the intestinal lining) or increase gastrointestinal motility (so that everything passes through quicker) can reduce absorption.

The next most common route is *parenteral* (by injection). You can inject a medication beneath the skin (*subcutaneous*), into a muscle (*intramuscular*), into a vein (*intravenous*), into an artery (*intraarterial*), or into the cerebral spinal fluid (*intrathecal*). Intravenous and intraarterial drugs reach the blood circulation immediately. Other parenteral medications can take minutes, hours, or even days to reach the circulation. Subcutaneous or intramuscular injections must either cross cell membranes or travel through the lymphatic system (e.g., intramuscularly injected protein drugs with a molecular mass >20,000 g/mol) to reach the blood circulation. Enzymes in the tissue and the lymphatic system can metabolize some of these drugs before they reach the systemic circulation. Increasing local blood perfusion (e.g., exercise) will increase absorption. Beware that some medications can irritate and even damage soft tissue when injected subcutaneously. The intramuscular route allows you to inject larger volumes of medication than the subcutaneous route but necessitates a longer needle to reach below the subcutaneous tissue into the muscle. The upper arm, thigh, and buttocks are common sites for intramuscular injections. Intramuscular injections can cause pain, bleeding in anti-coagulated patients, and elevations of creatine kinase and other components of muscle. The intrathecal route is an option for drugs that should rapidly reach the brain, spinal cord, or related structures.

Most *topical drugs* (i.e., applied directly to the skin) are for treating skin disorders and consist of an active ingredient mixed in an inactive ingredient (*vehicle*). *Ointments* have the highest oil to water content, followed by *creams*, and then *lotions*. More oil helps lubricate and moisturize skin and improve absorption (i.e., an ointment is more potent than a cream which is more potent than a lotion with the same drug concentration). However, messiness and greasiness increase with oil content (e.g., it is easier to apply lotions to hairy skin). *Solutions* contain drugs dissolved in water, alcohol, propylene glycol, polyethylene glycol, or some other liquid and tend to dry and may irritate skin. *Gels*, which are effectively solutions gelatinized by nonoily and nonfatty substances, do not provide good absorption and may irritate the skin. *Baths* and *soaks* are effective in treating skin disorders affecting large areas of the body but are not appropriate for drugs with narrow therapeutic windows, since controlling absorption is difficult. *Powders* (dry medications) can protect areas subject to a fair amount of friction (e.g., armpits and beneath the breasts) or at risk for damage.

The skin also can serve as a route for systemic medications (*transdermal*) using a skin patch infused with the medication (e.g., nitroglycerin, nicotine, selegiline, scopolamine, and estrogen). The patch slowly and continuously delivers medication into the skin, and in turn, into the bloodstream and can maintain relatively constant serum drug concentrations. However, the skin patch can be irritating and cannot deliver large doses. To be delivered transdermally, a drug must be able to penetrate skin adequately and be fairly potent (since absorption is slow and limited).

The *rectum* has a relatively thin lining and good blood perfusion, which allows for fairly rapid drug absorption, and can serve as a route for many medications, especially if the patient cannot take oral medications (e.g., anti-nausea medications or patients about to have surgery) or has a condition specifically affecting the rectum (e.g., hemorrhoids or Crohn's disease). Rectally administered medications can be local or systemic and come in three general formulations: enemas, suppositories, and topical creams/gels. An enema is a liquid drug solution that can be delivered up the rectum using a rectal bulb, a syringe, or tubing (e.g., corticosteroid and mesalazine enemas for inflammatory bowel disease). A suppository is a solid mixture of a drug and a waxy substance that dissolves once it is placed in the rectum (e.g., anti-emetics or laxatives). Creams and gels treat local problems confined to the rectum (e.g., hemorrhoids and rectal itching).

Most *vaginally* administered medications treat problems that in some way affect the vagina (e.g., yeast infections, bacterial infections, and menopause-associated vaginal wall thinning). Such medications may exist as solutions, tablets, creams, gels, or suppositories. Absorption through the vaginal wall is slow.

The respiratory system is another potential route for medications as long as the medications can be *atomized* (i.e., converted into droplets suspended in air). When administered through the nostrils, atomized medications can enter the bloodstream rapidly through the nasal mucous membranes (e.g., nicotine). The *nasal route* can deliver a limited amount of drug and may result in nasal irritation. By comparison, *inhalation* can deliver greater drug quantities. Inhalation requires drugs to be atomized into smaller particles and given through the mouth. The smaller the particles, the deeper into the lungs the particles can reach. In the lungs, the particles enter the bloodstream. Inhalation is the route of choice for many general anesthetics and anti-asthmatic medications. Many aerosolized formulations of drugs are in development.

The *ocular route* (i.e., applied directly to the eyes) is the route used for most eye disorder treatments. Formulations of ocular medications include liquids, gels, ointments, and solid inserts that slowly release drugs. Gels and ointments are better than liquids at holding the medication to the eye surface longer. Although most ocular drugs are for local treatment, some can enter the bloodstream in significant quantities, causing side effects.

The development of different *drug delivery devices and technologies* has helped overcome some important dosing challenges. They include devices or drug formulations that gradually release medication over a long period of time (*slow-release*) or at specified times (*controlled-release*) as well as *implantable* (i.e., placed inside the body) devices or drug formulations. Such technologies do one or several of the following:

- *Deliver the drug close to its target.* Reducing the distance that the drug has to travel to reach its target helps increase the drug's potency and reduce its toxicities (by limiting the drug's interaction with other organs). Examples include *drug eluting stents* that gradually release drugs into the arterial walls and *implantable infusion pumps* that release drugs into a blood vessel or body cavity.
- *Provide a relatively constant level of medication.* Similar to intravenous infusions, slow-release and controlled-release formulations can provide a relatively constant concentration of medication, helping reduce dosing frequency and fluctuations in plasma drug concentrations. This is especially useful for drugs with short half-lives and durations of effect. *Oral controlled-released drugs* consist of a substance (e.g., water-insoluble material, a matrix, or ion exchange resin) that slowly releases the drug while the pill travels through the gastrointestinal tract. The colon subsequently absorbs most of the medication. Many transdermal skin patches work similarly.
- *Overcome patient noncompliance.* Patients with implanted pumps or skin patches do not have to remember to take their medications.
- *Temporally match release with biological or physiological patterns.* Many clinical phenomena cycle or fluctuate. Controlled delivery devices can deliver different doses at specific times when the doses would be most useful and effective. Examples include insulin pumps that can deliver higher doses of insulin after a meal and patient controlled analgesia (PCA) pumps that patients can trigger when they feel pain.

10.6 PHASE I DOSE STUDIES

10.6.1 Starting Dose

Before administering an intervention to patients for the first time in a clinical trial, you have no idea what the intervention will do to the patient. So start with a very conservative dose. Using data from animal studies choose a dose that will definitely not produce any positive or negative effects (i.e., typically, 1/25th to 1/100th of the no-effect dose seen in animals). The *maximum recommended starting dose* (*MRSD*) is the highest recommended initial dose for a clinical trial and should not cause any adverse reactions. There are five steps to calculating the MRSD as follows.

Determine the NOAEL for Each Animal Species

Use all available animal data to determine a NOAEL for each animal species tested. In this context, the NOAEL is the highest dose level that does not significantly increase adverse effects (including biologically significant adverse effects that are not statistically significant) compared to the control group. Do not confuse the NOAEL with the NOEL, the highest dose at which no positive or negative effects (not just adverse effects) are seen. Also, the NOAEL should be lower than the LOAEL, the dose at which adverse effects are seen, and the MTD. Usually these adverse effects are clinically evident (i.e., symptoms or a change in body function), but sometimes nonclinical findings, such as appropriate surrogate markers (e.g., rise in serum liver enzyme levels), histopathological signs (e.g., microscopic lesions), and exaggerated pharmacodynamic effects, can represent adverse effects. In some situations, data on bioavailability, metabolism, and distribution can help choose the NOAEL (e.g., if maximum absorption occurs at a certain dose, use that dose to calculate the human equivalent dose (HED). Even though higher doses may not produce any adverse effects, higher doses will not be beneficial because they will not result in higher plasma concentrations).

Convert the Animal NOAELs to the HED

If giving an animal a dose X produces effects A, the *HED* is the dose Y that will produce effects A in humans. The common method of converting the animal NOAELs to HEDS is *normalizing* the NOAEL to *body surface area*. Normalizing the NOAEL to body surface area means converting the NOAEL, which is in dose units per body weight

TABLE 10.1 Examples of a Single Ascending Dose (SAD) Study and a Multiple Ascending Dose (MAD) Study

Patient group	SAD	MAD		
		At 0 h	At 4 h	At 8 h
1	1 mg once	1 mg	1 mg	1 mg
2	3 mg once	3 mg	3 mg	3 mg
3	5 mg once	5 mg	5 mg	5 mg
4	7 mg once	7 mg	7 mg	7 mg
5	10 mg once	10 mg	10 mg	10 mg

(e.g., mg/kg), to dose units per body surface area (e.g., mg/m^2). This method assumes that a given dose per body surface area has similar effects across different animal species. To make this conversion, multiply the NOAEL by the constant k_m appropriate for the animal species (Table 10.1). So if the NOAEL for a ferret is 5 mg/kg, then:

$$HED = 5 \text{ mg} \times (k_m \text{ for a ferret})$$
$$= 5 \text{ mg/kg} \times 7 = 35 \text{ mg/m}^2$$

Normalizing to body surface area is not always the appropriate method to calculate HED. Normalize the NOAEL to concentration (e.g., mg/area of application) or *amount of drug (mg) at the application site* instead when the dose is limited by local toxicities rather than systemic toxicities (e.g., skin problems for topical drugs, nasal irritation for intranasal medications, and soft tissue and muscular toxicities for intramuscular drugs). When a drug does not enter the systemic circulation but remains in a small part (compartment) of the body like the bladder, CSF, or eye, normalize the NOAEL to the *compartment's volume* and *drug concentration in that compartment*.

Scaling by *body weight* (i.e., assuming that the HED (mg/kg) = NOAEL (mg/kg)) will result in a significantly higher HED (e.g., 12-fold higher if the NOAEL is from mice) than normalizing by surface area. However, scaling by body weight is appropriate for large protein (Mr > 100,000 Da) drugs that are administered intravascularly. You also may scale by body weight if the NOAEL (in mg/kg) is relatively constant among many different animal species.

Use the HED Calculated from the Most Appropriate Animal Species

The next step is to choose the most appropriate animal species. This should be the animal species most similar to humans with regards to the intervention being tested, that is, the most similar absorption, distribution, metabolism, excretion, toxicity profile, and relevant structures, enzymes, and receptors. The most appropriate animal species for one intervention may be completely different from the most appropriate species for another intervention. In many cases, prior studies have shown that certain animal species are most appropriate for certain drug classes (e.g., when taking phosphorothioate anti-sense drugs, monkeys experience similar toxicities to humans). Once you have selected the most appropriate animal species, use the HED derived from the NOAELs of that species. If you cannot identify the most appropriate species, then use the most sensitive species (i.e., the species with the lowest HED).

Use the Safety Factor to Calculate the MRSD from the HED

The toxicity of an intervention can differ greatly between animals and humans. Humans can exhibit different absorption, distribution, elimination, and toxicity manifestations. You may not know when animals are suffering certain symptoms, such as pain, psychological disturbances, headaches, or sensory deficits. Therefore, the first dose in human should be more conservative than the HED derived from animals. Dividing the HED by a safety factor can help account for these possible differences and ensure that the first dose in humans will not cause adverse effects:

$$MRSD = HED/Safety \text{ factor}$$

Typically, the safety factor should be at least 10. Any situation that may raise risk or concerns about the animal data should increase the safety factor such as:

- severe, poorly detectable, or irreversible toxicities;
- unexplained mortality;
- significant variability (e.g., variable bioavailability or dose–response);
- steep dose–response curve;
- nonlinear pharmacokinetics;
- inadequate dose–response data;
- inappropriate animal models;
- novel therapeutic targets.

Several conditions may justify using a safety factor less than 10:

- mild, easily detectable, easily monitored, and reversible toxicities;
- intervention is from a class of interventions that is well understood and well characterized;
- shallow dose–response curve;
- high quality and quantity dose–response data;
- animal toxicity studies had a longer duration of follow-up than the planned duration for human studies.

Compare the MRSD to the Calculated PAD

Sometimes the PAD is a better indicator of potential toxicity. When the PAD comes from *in vivo* studies, you can use the body surface area conversion factor to convert the PAD to an HED. If this HED is lower than the MRSD, decreasing the clinical starting dose may be appropriate, especially for certain drug or biological classes (e.g., vasodilators, anti-coagulants, monoclonal antibodies, or growth factors) that exhibit toxicity from exaggerated pharmacological effects.

10.6.2 Dose Escalation

The goals of dose escalation (i.e., gradually increasing the dose in a clinical trial) are to establish a relationship between dose and response, identify doses at which toxicities appear, and establishing a safety window (i.e., the dose range that is relatively free of toxicity) and therapeutic window. You should establish a therapeutic window before proceeding with each phase of development and before putting a drug on the market.

As we mentioned earlier in this chapter, Phase I studies consist of SAD and MAD. A SAD study follows the following procedure:

1. Start by giving a single dose to a small group of subjects (usually 3–6 patients). This starting dose should be multiple orders of magnitude lower than the expected efficacious or toxic doses (see Section 10.9 for details on choosing a starting dose). You can also give placebo to 1 to 2 patients.
2. Monitor the group for side effects and measure various pharmacokinetic and pharmacodynamic parameters. If the data indicates that this starting dose is safe, give a slightly higher dose to a second small group of subjects (also usually 3–6 patients). You can also give placebo to 1 to 2 more patients.
3. Every time you deem a dose level to be safe, raise the dose (*dose escalation*) and give it to a new group of patients. Continue this iterative dose escalation process until you either reach maximum safe doses as predicted by pharmacokinetic calculations or start to see intolerable side effects (i.e., the dose is the *MTD*).

Once the SAD is completed, you may initiate a MAD study. A MAD study is similar to a SAD, except that each group receives a dose multiple times at some subchronic interval over a period of time. The frequency and duration of dosing as well as the length of follow-up after dosing depend on the anticipated dosing schedule in clinical practice, the nature of the disease, anticipated onset of action, and potential for rebound effects, long-term toxicity, and long-term benefit. In Phase I MAD, giving the drug for 4–5 half-lives is typical, but if a drug has a very long half-life, then 10–14 days is common. Table 10.1 shows an example of a SAD and a MAD. The minimum length of follow-up for SAD and MAD is at least 4–5 half-lives of the drug. The follow-up should be longer for drugs that have long-lasting effects (e.g., drugs that are sequestered, accumulate, or have persistent biological effects).

Before testing any doses, establish dose escalation rules: what dosing levels you plan to give and how you will decide whether and when to move to a higher dose level. The disease, potential toxicities, and dose–toxicity curves in animals help determine your dose escalation plan. Faster escalation may be appropriate for severe life-threatening diseases with relatively few treatment options. Dose escalation should be much more gradual when there are potentially severe toxicities. In general, remember that even during clinical trials you want to avoid giving patients unnecessary, ineffective treatments. So the goal of a Phase I study is to identify a Phase II dose while employing the minimum number of patients and the fewest number of escalations.

Typically, dose escalation involves making large dose jumps early on when doses have no effects and making the jumps smaller and smaller as the doses start causing biological effects. For example, if you see no effect at 1 mg, you may jump to 5 mg. If there is still no effect, you could jump to 10 mg. Seeing some effect at 10 mg suggests that the next dose jump should be more cautious (perhaps to 12 mg).

Listed below are a number of different dose escalation schemes (see also Table 10.2). In each case n represents the starting dose:

- *Doubling method*: In this commonly used scheme, the next higher dose level is always twice the previous dose. In other words, if n is the starting dose, then the next dose level is $2n$, followed by $4n$, then $8n$, and so forth. This is rather rapid dose escalation and minimizes the number of patients who receive ineffective dose levels. However, this scheme's aggressiveness can overshoot the MTD and lead to severe toxicities.
- *Modified Fibonacci search*: Although the modified Fibonacci method may give a very high number of patients low ineffective doses, it is the most commonly used method of dose escalation because of its excellent safety record. This method is especially useful for interventions with steep dose–toxicity curves. The dosing multiples come from the mathematical Fibonacci

TABLE 10.2   Dose Escalation Methods

Dose step	Equally spaced	Doubling	Modified Fibonacci	Log scale
1	1n	1n	1n	1n
2	2n	2n	2n (100%)	10n
3	3n	4n	3.3n (67%)	100n
4	4n	8n	5n (50%)	1000n
5	5n	16n	7n (40%)	10,000n
6	6n	32n	9n (29%)	100,000n
7	7n	64n	12n (33%)	1,000,000n
8	8n	128n	16n (33%)	10,000,000n

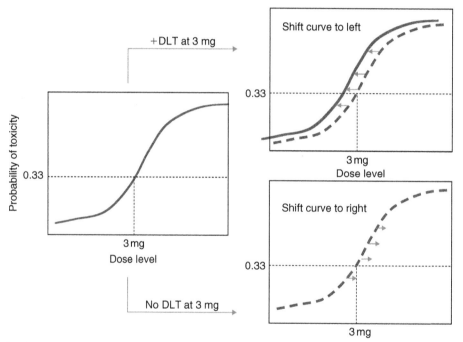

FIGURE 10.14   Continual re-assessment method (CRM).

sequence (1, 2, 3, 5, 8, 13, 21, …). So if the first dose is n, the second dose is 2n, the third dose is 3.3n, the fourth dose is 5n, the fifth dose is 7n, the sixth dose is 12n, the seventh dose is 16n, and so forth. As you can see dose levels increase more slowly than in the doubling method.

- *Log scale*: In this scheme, the dose increases logarithmically: if n is the starting dose, then the next dose level is 10n, followed by 100n, then 1000n, and so forth.
- *Continual re-assessment method (CRM) or modified continual re-assessment method (MCRM)*: Figure 10.14 illustrates the steps in CRM. First, use animal toxicology data to plot an estimated dose–toxicity curve. Choose the predicted MTD. For example, assuming that 33% is the maximum tolerable toxicity probability, give a single patient the dose that should yield this

probability (in this example, 3 mg). If the patient suffers a dose-limiting toxicity, then shift the predicted dose–toxicity curve to the left and then give another patient a slightly lower dose (e.g., 2.8 mg) and repeat the steps until you identify the MTD. If the patient does not suffer a DLT, then shift the curve to the right and then give another patient a slightly higher dose (e.g., 3.2 mg). This method is more complicated than other escalation methods and exposes patients to relatively high doses very quickly, raising safety concerns. These safety concerns have spurred others to develop modified versions of CRM, which we will not cover here. While CRM/MCRM methods do not save the overall time and number of patients a Phase I trial requires, they do get you close to the MTD quicker and decrease the number of patients receiving ineffective doses.

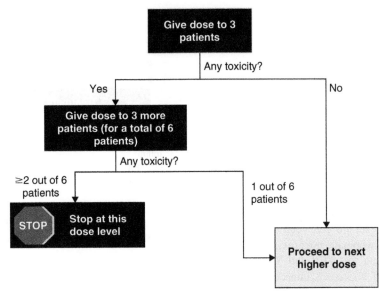

FIGURE 10.15 The traditional escalation rule (TER).

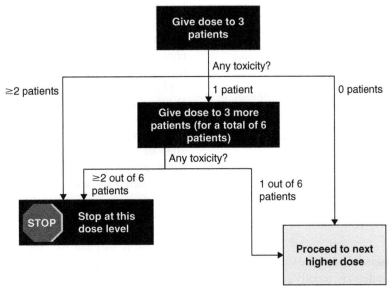

FIGURE 10.16 The strict traditional escalation rule (STER).

- *Accelerated titration design*: In accelerated titration design I, each dose level is 40% higher than the preceding dose level. In accelerated titration design II, each dose level is 100% higher than the preceding dose level. In either design, each dose level is given to a single (different) patient. When you detect a DLT, give that dose level to a total of three patients. Then escalate the dose by smaller increments.
- *Pharmacologically guided dose escalation*: The method sprung from the observation that the AUC at the LD10 (or MTD) for mice equals the AUC at the MTD for humans. So for each dose level, determine the AUC

which in turn determines the next dose escalation (assuming the agent has linear kinetics). Using this method requires real-time pharmacokinetic calculations and can lead to more aggressive dose escalations.

Many investigators (especially in oncology where doses used are high and a certain amount of toxicity is acceptable) use the "3 + 3 rule" to decide whether to stop at a dose level or proceed to a higher dose level. Two versions of the "3 + 3 rule" are the traditional escalation rule (TER) and the strict TER (STER) shown in Figures 10.15 and 10.16. In many cases, testing each dose level on one or two

Dose	Toxicity	
1 mg	None	
2 mg	None	
3 mg	None	
4 mg	None	
5 mg	None	
6 mg	None	
7 mg	None	Maximum tolerated dose (MTD)
8 mg	Yes	

FIGURE 10.17   Maximum tolerated dose.

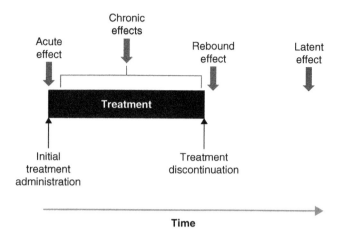

FIGURE 10.18   Temporal relationship between dose and response.

patients will suffice as long as no Grade 3 or repeated Grade 2 adverse events have occurred. When there is a sufficient risk of adverse events, you should give each dose level to a minimum of three patients who have not previously received the intervention. As you can see, TER and STER assumes that a >33% incidence of toxicity is unacceptable. Some situations may justify raising (e.g., the intervention is for a severe disease so that higher risk of toxicity is tolerable) or lowering (e.g., the toxicity is so severe or the disease is mild and not life-threatening) this threshold.

The dose level at which you stop by definition exceeds the MTD. Therefore, the MTD is one level lower than this dose (Figure 10.17). You should test the MTD on at least 6 patients, so if needed, once you identify the MTD, you should go back and test it on 3 more patients.

When no toxicity emerges even at high doses, it is reasonable to stop 2 logs beyond the expected effective dose/target dose. Also, make sure you stop dose escalation before reaching a dose that is 1/5th to 1/25th of the no-toxicity dose in animals.

10.7 RESPONSE PARAMETERS

10.7.1 Issues

The most critical parameter in dose selection is safety. Recognize that clinical studies are usually powered only to detect frequent, dose related toxicities. Detecting rare idiosyncratic (i.e., that are not dose related) toxicities without a large Phase IV type trial usually is impossible.

The timing of responses relative to treatment (i.e., *temporal relationship to intervention administration*) significantly affects clinical trial design. The trial duration must be long enough to capture all relevant positive and negative effects. Figure 10.18 shows the different times responses may occur. Responses that are contemporaneous with treatment may be either acute or chronic. *Acute responses* occur during (e.g., infusion reactions and nausea) or shortly after intervention administration. Delays in drug absorption and distribution can delay the appearance of acute responses. Acute single dose studies often can detect acute responses. *Chronic* contemporaneous responses appear only after treatment has occurred for a while. Responses may be too

low to detect early during treatment (e.g., a patient may not recognize nerve damage until it is severe enough to affect daily activities) or not manifest until the patient has had extended exposure to the intervention (e.g., suppressing red blood cell production may not cause anemia until several weeks have elapsed). The frequency and timing of chronic responses can be highly variable. Sometimes chronic effects do not materialize until patients are exposed to something else (e.g., an infectious agent or another medication) or subject to psychological or physical stress. Discussed earlier in this chapter, *rebound effects* may transpire after the intervention is discontinued. *Latent effects* appear after some time (i.e., a *latent period*) has elapsed after treatment completion. It may take decades before latent effects emerge (e.g., malignancies after exposure to psoralen long wave ultraviolet light (PUVA) psoriasis therapy).

Most drugs have a continuous and constant risk of toxicity over time (e.g., adverse event risk for treatment over 6 months is half the risk for treatment over 12 months). During treatment, the risk of a side effect may be 1% per month regardless of whether the patient has been receiving the intervention for 1 month, 5 months, or 20 months.

However, the risk of some effects can change during the course of treatment. Interventions can have a *first dose effect*, that is, the effect occurs the first time a patient is exposed to an intervention but declines or disappears with subsequent exposures. The patient's body may not be ready or used to an intervention. This is similar to jumping into a pool of cold water for the first time. After the initial shock wears off, the water no longer feels as cold. An example of a first dose effect is the dizziness that results from the sudden drop in cerebral blood flow when first taking blood pressure medications. Some effects (*re-treatment effects*) arise only when an intervention is re-started after being stopped for a while. An example is anaphylactic reactions. The initial treatment induces an immune response. During a hiatus from the treatment the immune system prepares a

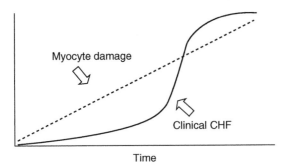

FIGURE 10.19 Relationship of myocyte damage and clinical CHF with continued adriamycin dosing.

response (e.g., manufactures antibodies). When the treatment is started again, the immune system is ready to mount a severe response.

Cumulative dose effects are different from *exposure–response effects*. An exposure–response effect depends solely on the length of time a patient is exposed to an intervention. In other words, what matters is how long and not how much (e.g., a patient taking 10 mg daily doses over 2 weeks will have the same risk of side effects as a patient taking 20 mg daily doses over 2 weeks). Usually the chances of an exposure–response effect increases the longer a patient is exposed to an intervention. Decreasing the dose will not change exposure–response effects. The only recourse is a drug holiday. By contrast, cumulative dose effects depend on the total amount of intervention a patient receives. In other words, what matters is how much and not how long (e.g., a patient taking 20 mg daily doses over 2 weeks will have a greater risk of side effects than a patient taking 10 mg daily doses over 2 weeks). Since the total cumulative dose matters, dividing the dose into smaller but more frequent doses will not make a difference (e.g., 10 mg daily doses over 2 weeks is the same as 5 mg twice a day doses over 2 weeks). Examples of cumulative dose effects include cardiotoxicity from adriamycin, pulmonary fibrosis from amiodarone, and cancer risk from radiation. Cumulative dose effects manifest when the intervention effects finally overcome the body's defense, repair, compensatory, or autoregulatory mechanisms. For example, when adriamycin first causes heart muscle damage at low doses, the remaining healthy heart muscle can work harder to compensate (Figure 10.19). More and more doses of adriamycin damage more and more cardiac muscle. Eventually, too much muscle is affected, the heart can no longer compensate, and CHF results.

10.7.2 Safety, Efficacy, and Convenience Parameters

Plotting efficacy and safety dose–response curves requires defining the efficacy parameters you want to maximize and the safety parameters you want to minimize, respectively.

Any number of endpoints can serve as efficacy or safety measures. See Chapters 4 and 7 for details. Commonly used endpoints include:

- *Clinical endpoints.*
- *Pharmacokinetic endpoints*: Pharmacokinetic measurements should include concentrations of the drug and its metabolites and bound and unbound drug.
- *Pharmacodynamic endpoints*: Pharmacodynamic effects can persist beyond the time drug is cleared from the blood. Also pharmacodynamic measurements can be less variable (e.g., the serum concentration may fluctuate significantly) and easier to measure (e.g., measuring a molecule's ability to inhibit cell trafficking may be easier than measuring the serum concentration of the molecule) than pharmacokinetic measurements.
- *Laboratory and surrogate endpoints.*
- *Harbinger signs*: For example, minor gum bleeding during anti-coagulant use may presage serious intracranial bleeding.

The target dose and acceptable toxicity levels may be different for different endpoints. For example, acute toxicity is more important for a drug given for a very short time. Cumulative toxicity is more important for a drug given over a long period of time.

In defining the efficacy dose–response curve, it is important to define what elements of efficacy you want to maximize. For example, you may want to find the dose that maximizes the intervention's ability to:

- *Cure a disease*: For example, resolve pneumonia.
- *Eliminate symptoms*: For example, headache.
- *Decrease time to resolution of symptom*: For example, length of oral herpes symptoms.
- *Prevent symptoms or disease*: For example, cardiovascular event or death.
- *Delay onset of symptoms or disease*: For example, atrial fibrillation or death.
- *Change symptoms or disease*: For example, decrease pain or blood pressure.
- *Take effect quickly (i.e., speed of onset of action)*: For example, time to improvement of headache.
- *Maintain effects (even after discontinuation)*: For example, resolve pneumonia.
- *Induce remission*: For example, treat cancer without return of malignancy.
- *Continue without tachyphlaxis.*

One important aspect of dose selection is that many dose related responses, such as pharmacokinetic and pharmacodynamic, are not stochastic. There is enough reproducibility and low enough variability so that deterministic methods can be used with some pharmacokinetic and pharmacodynamic parameters. This is clearly different from the vast majority of endpoints used in clinical trials, and permits someone to perform different types of analysis.

Remember that many factors may affect response, and tracking these factors is important in building dose–response relationships. For example, anything that can alter drug absorption, distribution, metabolism, or elimination may influence the dose–response curve. Also, various forms and metabolites of a drug may have different biological effects (e.g., change response, cause toxicity, or affect metabolism). Different conditions or factors may act as *effectors* (i.e., potentiate or increase the effects of the drug). The status and level of drug substrates or targets can affect response (e.g., vitamin K levels will affect the impact of coumadin).

As we mentioned before, convenience is also important. Key convenience parameters include:

- *Dosing frequency*: Taking medications three times or more per day can be difficult for patients to do. Very rare doses (e.g., once a week) can be easy to forget without appropriate reminders.
- *Customized vs. flat dosing*: Flat dosing is more convenient for patients and physicians.
- *Dosing with or without food*: Drugs that can be given either on full or empty stomach, without altering dose, offer the most convenient dosing regimen.
- *Route of administration*: Oral doses are significantly more convenient than subcutaneous doses. Most oral medications can be taken by the patient with professional assistance. Many subcutaneous medications require either professional (e.g., nurse) assistance or significant training to administer. Intramuscular (IM) injections are more difficult and frequently more painful than subcutaneous injections. Subcutaneous administration is usually preferable over IV or IM, especially since it can more easily administered at home.
- *Monitoring requirements*: Interventions that need monitoring (e.g., heparin and coumadin) are less convenient to use.
- *Setting*: Interventions that can be given at home, particularly via self-administration, are more convenient than ones that can only be administered at a clinic or hospital.

Population pharmacokinetics can be used in cases where frequent sampling is not possible and later in the program. Population pharmacokinetic relies on random or semi-random measurements, and mathematical modeling to estimate the pharmacokinetic curve.

10.8 POPULATION PHARMACOKINETICS AND PHARMACODYNAMICS

10.8.1 Variability

Remember that population averages and medians can be misleading. They do not represent the significant variability that exists among individuals. In general, the shapes of individual dose–response curves are different from the population (group) average dose–response curve. For example, Figure 10.20 shows that the individual dose–response curve is usually steeper than the population dose–response curve. So even if the therapeutic margin appears large, it may be much smaller for an individual patient. Small changes in doses can result in larger changes in response than expected (e.g., for the entire population, increasing the dose of blood pressure medication by 1 mg may lower blood pressure by 1 mmHg, but for a given individual, a 1 mg dose increase may lower blood pressure by 5 mmHg). So proceed carefully when titrating doses in individual patients.

A *mixed-effects model* attempts to explain this variability by breaking it down into two general categories: *random effects* and *fixed effects* (Figure 10.21). Some of the variability among individuals is random, that is, there is no clear cause. In other words, you cannot identify clear factors or variables (*covariates*) that explain this variability. The variability may be due to random statistical fluctuation (i.e., due to *random effects*) and does not occur consistently in one direction (e.g., the response is higher in some and lower in others). Some of the variability is due to identifiable factors. Certain covariates have so-called *fixed effects*. The magnitude of each covariate's effect differs. Some covariates may cause large variability (e.g., in Figure 10.21, older patients have a much lower

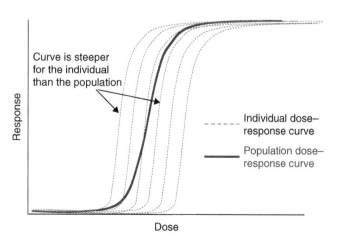

FIGURE 10.20   Individual vs. population dose–response curves.

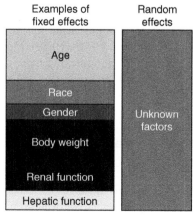

FIGURE 10.21   Mixed effects in explaining variability.

response than younger patients). Some covariates may have a relatively small effect (e.g., in Figure 10.21, there is not much difference between men and women).

Population pharmacokinetics (PK) and pharmacodynamics (PD) is the study of inter- and intra-patient variability in PK/PD parameters and how different demographic, pathophysiological, environmental, and therapeutic factors (e.g., body weight, metabolism, and concomitant medications) affect this variability. In other words, population PK/PD analyzes the distribution and behavior of different PK/PD parameters throughout the entire target population. This involves profiling PK/PD in a drug target population, identifying the covariates that influence PK/PD, delineating the magnitude of inter- and intra-patient variability, and analyzing PK/PD in special populations such as children, the elderly, and patients with various types of organ dysfunction. From this information, you can build predictive models that will help you to design dosage regimens for different individuals and extrapolate PK/PD parameters from even relatively sparse or suboptimal study subject data. It also allows you to predict PK/PD for subpopulations that you did not study.

For example, say you wanted to determine if peak and steady state drug concentrations differ significantly from patient to patient. Population PK involves identifying the degree of this variation and what factors may affect this variation (e.g., body weight and age). This will allow you to predict the peak and steady state concentrations for a 35-year old, 100-pound female.

Population PK/PD is playing an increasing role in drug development in defining the optimal dosing strategy for different populations, subpopulations, and individuals. It is particularly useful when a drug's target population is very heterogeneous and the therapeutic window is narrow. At different phases in drug development, population PK/PD can help design subsequent studies, generate additional safety and efficacy information, and provide information on special subpopulations.

10.8.2 Constructing the PK/PD Model

The two most common population PK/PD methods are the *two-stage approach* and the *nonlinear mixed-effects modeling approach*. While we will not discuss these methods in detail here; there are a couple of key differences between these two methods. The former requires more extensive PK/PD measurements, so the latter is more appropriate when data is less abundant (i.e., data-sparse situations). Also, the nonlinear mixed-effects modeling approach is better than the two-stage approach at estimating random effects. Population PK/PD involves several steps:

1. *Obtaining the data.*
2. *Analyzing the data (exploratory data analysis)*: This step involves using graphical and statistical techniques to reveal and describe possible patterns in the population

data. Flexibility and thoroughness are important as unexpected patterns may emerge.
3. *Developing the population PK/PD model*: Checking the reliability of results is important.
4. *Validating the model.*

There are three general ways of collecting PK/PD data:

- *Single trough sampling design*: This commonly used design is fraught with limitations but simple to perform. After obtaining a single drug concentration trough sample from each patient, you plot a frequency distribution histogram of these trough levels for your sample population. This method requires a large enough sample size, minimal assay and sampling errors, identical dosing and sampling regimens, patient compliance, and the drug to be dosed to steady state. Simple statistical procedures (e.g., multiple linear regression) can determine the drug clearance, how different patient characteristics correlate with trough levels and clearance, and how these PK-relevant covariates differ among subpopulations. However, this design reveals little about some other important parameters such as inter-individual and residual variability, volume of distribution, and half-life.
- *Multiple trough sampling design*: This design involves taking two or more trough samples from each patient and, therefore, provides information about inter-individual and residual variabilities. While this design bears many of the weaknesses of the single trough design, obtaining more samples per patient means that fewer subjects are required and greater precision in determining the relationship between patient characteristics and trough levels.
- *Full population PK sampling design (experimental population pharmacokinetic design or full pharmacokinetic screen)*: This design involves taking multiple blood samples at multiple times (usually 1–6 timepoints) from each subject. While more complicated than the above-mentioned trough designs, this design clearly yields a lot more data for each patient. This will allow you to calculate many more parameters.

10.9 DOSE–RESPONSE STUDY DESIGN

10.9.1 Choosing Doses

Choosing a target dose can be very subjective and challenging (Figure 10.22). Different physicians and different regulatory agencies can look at the same set of data and derive different target doses. Moreover, the situation and the goals help determine the choice. Table 10.3 shows the conditions that suggest a relatively high starting dose (i.e., one on or near the plateau of the dose–response efficacy curve) vs. a relatively low starting dose. A dose that is too high may have toxicity that thwarts people from receiving the intervention. A dose that is too low would not be as effective as it could be.

- Target dose is dose that yields best clinical efficacy:safety ratio.
- Usually, use clinical endpoints to choose target dose, but in rare instances, can use surrogate endpoints (e.g., blood pressure or blood glucose levels).
- If efficacy and safety curves separate sufficiently, select minimally effective dose (generally dose at beginning of plateau in standard dose-response curve) as target dose.
- When efficacy does not need to be so high, can select a lower dose.
- If efficacy and safety curves do not separate cleanly, exercise clinical judgment and choose dose that gives appropriate balance between safety and efficacy.
- Not possible to test every potential dosing regimen.
- Systematic bias toward underestimating safety signal in small studies.
- Iterative process during drug development:
  - Initial doses in Phase I are selected on basis of animal data and escalated carefully to assess initial safety.
  - Phase II doses selected on basis of Phase I safety information and in iterative clinical program, on basis of data generated in earlier Phase II studies.
  - Phase III doses selected on basis of Phase II data.

FIGURE 10.22   Choosing the target dose.

TABLE 10.3   High vs. Low Starting Dose

Quality	High starting dose	Low starting dose
Separation between effective and toxic dose ranges	Large	Small
Pharmacokinetic and pharmacodynamic variability	Low	High
Life-threatening disease	Yes	No
Rapidly evolving disease that requires rapid intervention	Yes	No
Salvage or alternative treatment	No	Yes

10.9.2 Dose–Response Trial Design Options

For the most part, dose-testing study design options are the same as for other trials (see Chapter 6) for more details on trial design). However, because dose-testing studies are usually smaller and generate data that will be re-tested later, you should use designs that conserve the number of patients and doses tested. Figure 10.23 and Table 10.4 list the four most common designs.

The *parallel dose–response* design entails randomly assigning patients to one of several groups and giving all patients in each group a specific fixed dose. You may either start the patient on the final or maintenance dose immediately or gradually titrate up to the final dose (in a scheduled forced titration). Demonstrating a positive-sloped dose–response curve suggests that the drug has an effect, even without a comparison placebo group. But you really need a placebo group (or some other type of appropriate comparison group) to delineate the actual magnitude of the drug effect. Moreover, when you do not test a wide enough dose range, the dose–response curve might not have a positive slope and only including an adequate control group will reveal that the intervention has an effect.

The *factorial trial* design may be useful when evaluating a treatment that involves giving more than one intervention simultaneously, especially when the interventions have the same effect (e.g., several different blood pressure or antidepressant medications given simultaneously) or one intervention is supposed to reduce the side effects of another intervention. The design is very similar to a parallel dose–response design except that each group receives different combinations of doses (e.g., Group 1 receives 5 mg of drug A and 10 mg of drug B, Group 2 receives 5 mg of drug A and 5 mg of drug B, Group 3 receives 10 mg of drug A and 10 mg of drug B). This design can demonstrate the contribution of each intervention to the response and the dose–response relationship for each intervention separately and together.

The *crossover dose–response* design gives each patient group one dose for a specified duration followed by a different dose for the same duration. Therefore, each patient receives more than one dose level, allowing you to estimate individual and population dose–response curves. This design also requires fewer patients than a parallel group design. However, this design is not ideal for interventions that cause very slow or irreversible responses and for disease that change over time.

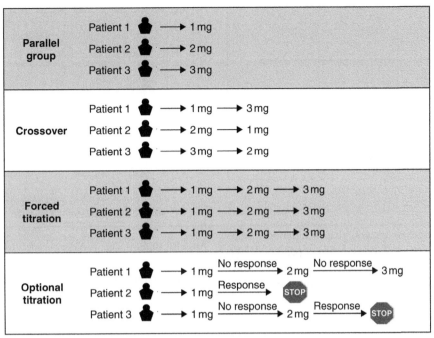

FIGURE 10.23 Common dose–response study designs.

TABLE 10.4 Comparison of Dose–Response Study Designs

Study design	Description	Advantages	Disadvantages
Parallel	Randomly assign each patient to one of several groups Give all patients in each group a specific fixed dose	Better for diseases that change over time Better for time-dependent responses	No information on individual dose–response curve May require large number of patients
Crossover	Give each patient group one dose for a specified duration followed by a different dose for the same duration Each patient receives more than one dose level	Can estimate individual dose–response curve Requires fewer patients than parallel	Not ideal for very slow or irreversible responses Not good for disease that change over time
Forced titration	Give each patient a stepwise progression of dose escalations Often controlled with a parallel placebo group	Can estimate individual dose–response curve Requires fewer patients than parallel Looks at wide range of doses	Response may be due to time on drug therapy or cumulative dose instead of increasing dose Not ideal for slow or delayed responses Not good for disease that change over time Patient drop-outs can be a problem
Optional titration (placebo-controlled titration to endpoint)	Give each patient increasing doses until you see a specific response (favorable or unfavorable)	Can estimate individual dose–response curve Requires fewer patients than parallel Looks at wide range of doses	Not good for slow/delayed or irreversible responses May yield a misleading inverted "U-shaped" curve (because poor responders titrated to highest dose)

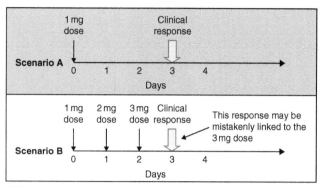

FIGURE 10.24 Titration study for a delayed or very slow response.

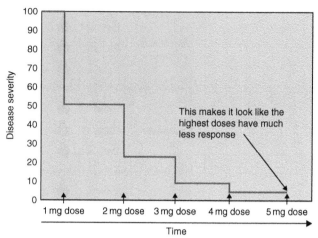

FIGURE 10.25 Ceiling or basement effect in dose titration.

In the *forced titration* design, you give each patient a step-wise progression of dose escalations. Often, a parallel design placebo groups serve as control groups. In the *optional titration (placebo-controlled titration to endpoint)* design, you also give each patient increasing doses but only until you see a specific favorable or unfavorable response (e.g., a PK, PD, or clinical endpoint). For reasons that will be explained later, you should always include a concurrent placebo group.

There are four main reasons why the forced dose and optional dose titration designs are most frequently used. First, practicing physicians often titrate doses (e.g., a physician will move the dose of an anti-hypertensive medication up or down depending on the patient's blood pressure). Second, the two titration designs use much fewer patients than the parallel or crossover designs, which is especially important when recruiting patients is difficult (e.g., the disease is rare or the intervention causes toxicity). Third, giving the same patient multiple doses will allow you to plot individual dose–response curves (in addition to population dose–response curves) and is important when inter-patient variability is high (i.e., different patients tend to have different responses). Finally, titration studies can identify dose levels for subsequent parallel or crossover studies.

However, the titration designs have several important drawbacks. Time-dependent effects can confound results. Distinguishing among dose–response (i.e., due to dose level), exposure–response (i.e., due to length of time on a treatment), and cumulative dose (i.e., due to total cumulative dose) effects can be very difficult. Diseases that change over time can cause problems as well. (For example, is the better response due to the disease naturally improving or the increased dose?) Moreover, the titration designs do not work well with delayed or very slow responses. For example, Figure 10.24 illustrates a titration study for a drug that requires 3 days to take effect. Unless you wait for at least 3 days before moving to higher dose (Scenario A), you will not be able to link the response to that dose level (Scenario B). Finally, as shown in Figure 10.25, lower doses may result in such improvement in the disease that there is no longer any more room for improvement with higher doses. As a result, you may underestimate the apparent effect of higher doses.

The optional titration design has a particularly important bias. Since patients who are not likely to respond will get higher doses, the design may spuriously raise the target or suggested dose. As a result, higher doses will always have deceivingly high response rates. False positive responders (i.e., patients who appear to have a response but really do not) will stop dose escalation too early. False negative nonresponders (i.e., patients who do not appear to respond but really do respond) will continue dose escalation for too long. Therefore, comparing the study group is important and will help identify patients who are less likely to respond to the intervention.

10.10 SPECIAL POPULATIONS

10.10.1 Pregnant Patients

A number of physiological changes take place during pregnancy, many of which may change the pharmacokinetics and pharmacodynamics of an intervention. For example, body weight, extra-cellular fluid, total body water, many cardiovascular parameters (e.g., cardiac output, stroke volume, heart rate, and blood flow to different organs), and renal clearance all increase. Body fat composition and liver enzyme activity change. Albumin levels, drug–protein binding, gastric emptying rates, and gastrointestinal transit rates all decrease. Such changes make it often inaccurate to extrapolate data from nonpregnant patients to pregnant patients. Moreover, physiological changes and disease activity may progress or fluctuate during pregnancy, necessitating you to modify doses for pregnancy and during the course of pregnancy (e.g., dose requirements may go up or down as the pregnancy progresses).

Therefore, sometimes there is no choice but to conduct pharmacokinetic studies on pregnant patients, as long as appropriate pre-clinical studies (which included pregnant animals) and clinical studies (which included nonpregnant women) have been completed and the risk to the fetus is minimal. Minimal risk means that the study intervention would pose no greater risk to the fetus than routine procedures usually performed on similar pregnant patients. PK studies of pregnant woman can occur either during clinical development (e.g., nested within a larger safety and efficacy trial) or after a drug has reached the market.

Dosing studies in pregnant patients aim to answer three questions:

- Is it safe and effective to give pregnant patients the intervention?
- Should pregnant patients receive the same doses as non-pregnant patients?
- How should dosing change during and after pregnancy?

Claiming that no dosage adjustment is needed for pregnancy requires demonstrating that relevant PK/PD measurements for pregnant patients are not statistically different from similar nonpregnant patients. For example, if the 90% confidence interval of ratios of different PK measurements (e.g., $AUC_{pregnant}/AUC_{control}$ or (maximum concentration-$_{pregnant}$/maximum concentration$_{control}$) fall within 80–125%, you may deem that pregnancy has no impact on PK.

Ideally, PK/PD measurements should take place before pregnancy to establish baseline levels and during all three trimesters, but since most subjects are already pregnant when enrolled in a clinical trial, making measurements during the second and third trimesters and baseline measurements after the patient has given birth is acceptable. Methods of dating pregnancy should be consistent and well documented. When deciding when to take baseline post-partum (after birth) measurements, remember that many pregnancy-associated physiological changes persist weeks to months after giving birth and, if possible, avoid the period when the patient is lactating. If you must include patients who are breast-feeding, understand how the drug may be excreted into breast make and the potential effects on the child (which may require a lactation study). Take necessary safety precautions. PK/PD studies of drugs that are employed exclusively during the peripartum period (i.e., at the time of labor and birth) should occur during and only during the peripartum period.

A longitudinal study design is the most common study design, especially for chronic medications used throughout and after pregnancy. Each pregnant patient serve as her own control: you compare PK/PD measurements on the same patient when she is in different trimesters and the post-partum period. Since physiological changes take place gradually through each trimester, you should choose specific time windows (e.g., 20–24 weeks) during each trimester to make measurements. If the drug is discontinued post-partum (e.g., treatments for pregnancy-induced hypertension or gestational diabetes), you can perform a single dose post-partum PK/PD study, which can be extrapolated to the multiple dose steady state PK if the PK are linear. Longitudinal designs are not always feasible. If patients do not take a medication throughout different trimesters, a multi-arm study design

comparing different pregnant patients who are at different stages of pregnancy and after pregnancy may be more appropriate.

Population PK/PD can be very helpful. First of all, performing an initial investigational population PK/PD study can help decide if there are enough differences between pregnant and nonpregnant women to warrant a PK/PD study of pregnant women. Population PK/PD can help determine the characteristics to consider when enrolling pregnant patients in PK studies and reduce the number of PK/PD measurements. You can also see how different maternal characteristics (e.g., age, gravity, parity, race, weeks or trimester of gestation) and concomitant medications affect PK/PD.

Using pregnant women to study interventions that have no intended direct therapeutic benefit (e.g., studies used to better clarify drug absorption, metabolism, and distribution) is reasonable as long as there is minimal risk to the fetus and the study can provide information that is generalizable to pregnant women. Only employ interventions that are known to be safe during pregnancy. Minimize exposure to the non-therapeutic intervention. Give only single doses of the intervention, no more than once during pregnancy and once during the post-partum period. As a result, the study design is usually nonlongitudinal (e.g., one cohort receives the dose in the second trimester while another cohort receives it during the third trimester). If possible, do not give interventions during the first trimester. Minimize the dose size and the number of drugs that the pregnant patient receives.

10.10.2 Other Special Populations

A special population is any population of patients that may have significantly different PK, PD, effects, or toxicities. The population may have pre-existing diseases (e.g., patients with bleeding disorders likely will have different responses to anti-coagulants) and special habits (e.g., take medications or regularly eat food that can interact with your study intervention). You should perform dose testing on any subpopulation that may have different dosing requirements (based on pathophysiology or animal studies) and comprise a relatively sizeable proportion of the people who will receive the intervention once it is on the market. Additionally, severe potential toxicities or narrow therapeutic windows lower the threshold for conducting dose-testing studies on different subpopulations. Such dose testing should either demonstrate that the subpopulation does not merit dose adjustments (relevant PK/PD measurements for the subpopulation patients are not statistically different from similar general population patients) or generate dose adjustment recommendations. Such studies may suggest that the intervention is contraindicated in that subpopulation.

As we mentioned, dose adjustments may be necessary in patients with either liver (hepatic) or kidney (renal) dysfunction. Since renal and hepatic dysfunction can significantly affect drug concentration levels, a narrow therapeutic index calls for dose testing to be done on hepatically impaired patients and renally impaired patients. You also should dose test on hepatically impaired patients any drug that is significantly (i.e., greater than 20%) metabolized by the liver or will be used in populations that have a high prevalence of hepatic dysfunction. You should dose test on renally impaired patients any drug that is excreted primarily through the kidneys or will be used in a population with a high prevalence of renal dysfunction.

Designing dose-testing studies on patients with hepatic or renal dysfunction entails some special considerations. A dose-testing study on hepatically impaired patients should include at least 6 patients from Child-Pugh's Class A, B, and C and a control group of age- and gender-matched patients from the target population. If P450 polymorphisms significantly affect the drug's metabolism, then match patients for P450 polymorphisms as well. A single dose study often is sufficient unless you anticipate either non-linear or time-dependent pharmacokinetics. A dose-testing study on renally impaired patients should include patients with mild (creatinine clearance of 50–80 mL/min), moderate (30–50 mL/min), and severe (<30 mL/min) renal dysfunction and patients on dialysis. While the variability of the pharmacokinetic and therapeutic windows will determine the sample size, the sample population should be large enough to detect statistically significant differences that would justify a reduced dosing schedule. As with hepatic studies, a single dose study is sufficient if the PK is linear and not time dependent. In addition to measuring levels of the parent drug, make sure you measure concentrations of metabolites, free drug, and bound drug. Population PK/PD may augment or, in some cases, replace formal studies on hepatic dysfunction and renal dysfunction patients.

The elderly patient population may present a variety of dosing challenges. Blood circulation, renal clearance, and hepatic clearance decrease with age. The incidence of co-morbid conditions increases. As a result, other disease processes and medications can interfere with your study intervention effects. Elderly patients may have lower tolerance for toxicity (i.e., nerve impairment may be more debilitating for an elderly patient than a teenager). Moreover, convenience and compliance issues may be different for the elderly. It may be tougher for elderly patients to receive certain interventions that require extensive procedures, difficult body positioning, swallowing, or opening pill bottles. In general, the pharmacokinetic profile in the elderly can be obtained by population pharmacokinetic or screening in the course of the program. In lieu of this, a formal pharmacokinetic study in the elderly can be performed. Most of the issues with the drug in elderly have been the result of altered pharmacokinetic, not pharmacodynamic, except in cases where the pharmacodynamic effect was due to conditions associated with age, such as decreased renal clearance or polypharmacy. If, however, a pharmacodynamic effect is expected – that is no difference in pharmacokinetic but a difference in clinical effect or pharmacodynamic effect, then those should be measured.

Chapter 11

Epidemiology, Decision Analysis, and Simulation

11.1 PROBABILITY

11.1.1 Simple Probability

Nobody is always a winner, and anybody who says he is, is either a liar or doesn't play poker.

Amarillo Slim

Few things in life and nature are 100%. Even if you are fairly certain that something will happen, there is always a chance that it will not occur. *Probability* is the measure of the likelihood of an event. If you were to stand outside during a rainstorm without an umbrella, there is a high probability that you will get wet and a small probability that you will remain dry. The wind patterns could blow the raindrops away from you, or you could be so oily that the raindrops bounce off of you. The chances of these events occurring are very low. Similarly, in any experiment, there is a chance or probability of different possible outcomes occurring. No intervention is guaranteed to work.

A probability is a number from 0 to 1 or 0% to 100%. An event that has 0 (or 0%) probability of occurring will never ever occur. An event that has a probability of 1 (or 100%) of occurring will always occur. A probability of 0.5 (or 50%) means that the event has the same probability of occurring as a coin flip turning up heads. A probability that is greater than 0.5 means that the event is more likely to occur than not occur.

How do you calculate probability? If you place a hundred balls (numbered 1 to 100), in a bin, what is the probability of randomly choosing the number 15 ball? The answer is one in a hundred or 1%. What is the probability of randomly selecting a ball numbered between 1 and 10? The probability would be 10/100 or 10%. What is the probability of blindly picking an odd-numbered ball? Since there are 50 odd-numbered balls and a total of 100 balls,

then the probability would be 50/100 or 50%. In general, the simple probability of an event is:

$$p(\text{Event}) = \frac{\text{Number of possible ways the event can occur}}{\text{Total number of possible outcomes}}$$

11.1.2 Conditional, Joint, and Cumulative Probabilities

A *conditional probability* (Figure 11.1) is the likelihood of an event occurring provided that another event has occurred. Probabilities often depend on prior events. For example, your probability of getting wet in a rainstorm is much less if you have an umbrella than if you do not have one. (Well, technically, you have to open and hold up the umbrella to change your probability of getting wet.) It also depends on the severity of the rainstorm, the presence of trees and other cover, and perhaps your oiliness.

The notation used for conditional probability is $p(\text{B}|\text{A})$, which reads "the probability of B, given A." In other words, when A has already happened, what is the chance of B happening? So, $p(\text{Diabetes}|\text{Male})$ would be the probability of having diabetes given that the patient is male:

$$P(\text{Diabetes}|\text{Male}) = 15/55 = 27.3\%$$

	Male	Female	Total
Diabetes	15	5	20
No diabetes	40	40	80
Total	55	45	100

FIGURE 11.1   Joint vs. conditional probabilities.

p(Diabetes|Female) would be the probability of having diabetes given that the patient is female:

$$p(\text{Diabetes}|\text{Female}) = 5/45 = 11.1\%$$

So in general, for two events (A and B):

$$p(B|A) = p(AB)/p(B)$$

where $p(AB)$ is the joint probability of A and B occurring at the same time. For three events (A, B, and C):

$$p(C|AB) = p(AC)/(p(A) \times p(B|A))$$

where $p(ABC)$ is the joint probability of A, B, and C occurring at the same time.

A *joint probability* is the likelihood of two (or more) events happening at the same time. The joint probability of Events A and B occurring is written $p(A,B)$. Note that this is different from the conditional probability. The joint probability of having diabetes and being a woman [p(Diabetes, Woman)] would be:

$$[p(\text{Diabetes, Woman})] = 5/100 = 5\%$$

By contrast, the conditional probability of a patient having diabetes if this person is female, that is p(Diabetes| Female) = 5/45 is 11.1%. Conditional and joint probabilities have different denominators. A joint probability is the chance of a combination of events (e.g., Event A and Event B) with the whole population as the denominator. A conditional probability is the chance of an event (e.g., Event B) within a subset of the population (e.g., only among people who already have experienced Event A).

The following equation calculates the joint probability of two events (A and B) occurring:

$$p(\text{Event A and Event B}) \equiv p(AB) = p(A) \times p(B|A)$$

The joint probability of three events (A, B, and C) occurring is:

$$p(A,B,C) = p(A) \times p(B|A) \times p(C|AB)$$

Two events are *independent* from each other when the occurrence of one event does not make the other event more or less likely to occur. Examples of independent events are coin flips or dice rolls. Getting "heads" on one coin flip does not change the chances of getting "heads" on the next coin flip. So, when A, B, and C are independent events then:

$$p(B|A) = p(B) \text{ and } p(C|AB) = p(C)$$

This means that the presence or absence of A does not affect the probability of B, and the presence or absence of A and B do not affect the probability of C. As you can see, when A, B, and C, $p(A, B, C)$ simplifies to the equation below:

$$p(A,B,C) = p(A) \times p(B) \times p(C)$$

Remember *"and"* is the operational word for joint probabilities. All of the following statements are examples of joint probabilities and have the word *"and"* in them:

- *Of all the people in clinical research, how many have a medical degree and a law degree?* To count, the person must have both medical and law degrees.
- *What is the chance of finding the right companion and the right job in the next month?* You may be asking for a lot to find both in 1 month.

By contrast, the operational word for *cumulative probabilities* is *"or."* A cumulative probability is the chance of any one of several events occurring. So examples of cumulative probabilities would be:

- *Of all the people in clinical research, how many have either a medical degree or a law degree?* Anyone who is a physician or a lawyer will qualify.
- *What is the chance of finding either the right companion or the right job in the next month?* This is clearly more realistic. Tackle one problem at a time.

By definition, a cumulative probability is greater than a joint probability. The cumulative probability of two events:

$$p(\text{Event A or Event B}) = p(A) + p(B) - p(A,B)$$

We have to subtract the joint probability of A and B occurring at the same time to eliminate double-counting. As Figure 11.2 shows $p(A,B)$ is already included in the probability of A and the probability of B. Similarly, the cumulative probability of three events is:

$$p(A \text{ or } B \text{ or } C) = p(A) + p(B) + p(C) - p(A,B) \\ - p(A,C) - p(B,C)$$

Events are *mutually exclusive* when they cannot occur at the same time. For example, someone cannot be over 65 years old and under 21 years old at the same time (although many try to be). By definition, when Events A and B are mutually exclusive,

$$p(AB) = 0$$

So when Events A and B are mutually exclusive, the cumulative probability of A or B simplifies to:

$$p(A \text{ or } B) = p(A) + p(B)$$

When Events A, B, and C are mutually exclusive:

$$p(A \text{ or } B \text{ or } C) = p(A) + p(B) + p(C) - p(AB) \\ - p(AC) - p(BC)$$

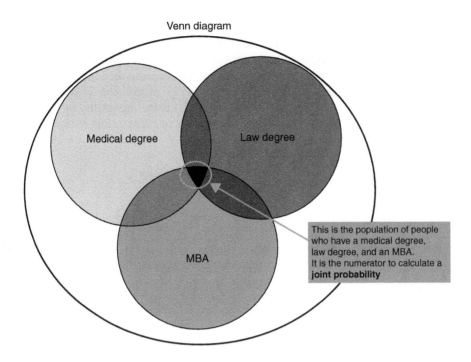

Venn diagram

Medical degree

Law degree

MBA

This is the population of people who have a medical degree, law degree, and an MBA. It is the numerator to calculate a **joint probability**

FIGURE 11.2 Venn diagram demonstrating joint probabilities.

So the cumulative probability of a coin turning up heads or tails during the next flip is:

$$p(\text{Heads or Tails}) = p(\text{Heads}) + p(\text{Tails})$$
$$= 0.5 + 0.5 = 1.0$$

In other words, there is a 100% chance that the next coin flip will be either heads or tails.

We can use a random draw from a deck of 52 poker cards to illustrate each of the probability concepts that we have discussed:

- *Cumulative probability: What is the probability of randomly drawn card being either a Spade or a Club?* $p(\text{Spade or Club}) = p(\text{Spade}) + p(\text{Club}) - p(\text{Spade}, \text{Club}) = 13/52 + 13/52 + 0 = 26/52 = 0.5$.
- *Conditional probability: What is the probability of a randomly drawn card being an Ace if the randomly drawn card is a Spade?* $p(\text{Ace}|\text{Spade}) = p(\text{Ace}, \text{Spade})/p(\text{Spade}) = (1/52)/(13/52) = 1/13$.
- *Joint Probability: What is the chance of drawing a card that is an Ace and a Spade?* $p(\text{Ace}, \text{Spade}) = p(\text{Ace}) \times p(\text{Spade}|\text{Ace}) = (4/52) \times (1/4) = 1/52$.

11.1.3 Probability in Sequential Events

The probability concepts that we just introduced can apply to *successive* or *sequential events*. The deck of cards example is good way of explaining the concept of *replacement*. Suppose you make two successful draws from the deck of cards.

What is the joint probability of both draws being Spades? Well, the answer depends on whether you put the first card back into the deck. If you do (i.e., replace the card):

$$p(\text{First card a Spade, Second card a Spade})$$
$$= p(\text{First card a Spade})$$
$$\times p(\text{Second card a Spade}|\text{First card a Spade})$$
$$= (13/52) \times (13/52) = 1/4 \times 1/4$$
$$= 1/16$$

If you do not put the first card back into the deck for the second draw:

$$p(\text{First card a Spade, Second card a Spade})$$
$$= p(\text{First card a Spade})$$
$$\times p(\text{Second card a Spade}|\text{First card a Spade})$$
$$= (13/52) \times (12/52) = 1/4 \times 12/51$$
$$= 1/17 \text{ (which is less than } 1/16)$$

As you can see, replacement makes a difference. So when calculating the probabilities of successive events always take into account whether or not replacement is occurring.

Let us assume that replacement occurs, and calculate the chance of getting a Spade on two successive draws. Remember, the answer would be:

$$p(\text{Spade on 1st draw } and \text{ Spade on 2nd draw})$$
$$= p(\text{Spade on the 1st draw})$$
$$\times p(\text{Spade on the 2nd draw})$$
$$= (1/4) \times (1/4) = 1/16$$

How about the chance of getting a Spade on either of the first or the second draw? This would be a cumulative probability:

p(Spade on 1st draw *or* Spade on 2nd draw)
= p(spade on the 1st draw)
  + p(Spade on the 2nd draw)
  − p(Spade on 1st draw and Spade on 2nd draw)
= (1/4) + (1/4) − (1/16)
= 7/16

Another way of attacking this same problem is to ask what is the probability of not drawing a Spade on both the 1st and 2nd draws? In other words, what is probability of drawing a Heart, Club, or Diamond on the 1st draw AND a Heart, Club, or Diamond on the 2nd draw:

p(Heart, Club, or Diamond on both draws)
= p(Heart, Club, or Diamond on 1st draw)
  × p(Heart, Club, or Diamond on 2nd draw)
= (3/4) × (3/4)
= 9/16

Then you can say that the probability of getting a Spade on either the 1st or 2nd draw is:

p(Spade on 1st draw *or* Spade on 2nd draw)
= 1 − p(Heart, Club, or Diamond on both draws)
= 1 − (9/16)
= 7/16

If the probability of a certain outcome is α whenever an event occurs, the probability of seeing that outcome at least once when the event occurs k times is:

$$= 1 - (1 - \alpha)^k$$

So if the probability of an adverse event is 10% every time you perform a certain surgery, the probability of seeing that adverse event at least once in 10 surgeries is:

$$= 1 - (1 - 0.10)^{10}$$
$$= 1 - (0.9)^{10}$$
$$= 1 - 0.349$$
$$= 0.651$$

As you can see, the probability of at least one adverse event is very high.

11.1.4 Binomial Distribution

An event is *dichotomous* when there are only two possibilities, that is, no third, fourth, or more options. Examples of dichotomous events are coin flips (either heads or tails), pregnancy (you are either pregnant or not pregnant), and

survival (a patient either survived or did not). When dichotomous events are mutually exclusive (e.g., if it is heads, it cannot be tails; a nonpregnant woman cannot be pregnant), random, and independent, you can use the binomial distribution to calculate the chances of different combinations of outcomes occurring. If $p(r)$ is the probability of an outcome occurring r times when an event occurs N times and the probability of the outcome for each event is π then:

$$p(r) = [N!/(r!(N - r)!)] \, \pi^r (1 - \pi)^{N-r}$$

$$(\text{NOTE: } N! = 1 \times 2 \times 3 \times ... \times N)$$

So for example, if there is a 10% chance of an adverse event every time you perform a surgery, the chance of the adverse occurring exactly five times in 10 surgeries would be:

$$p(5) = [10!/5!(10 - 5)!] \times (0.10)^5 \times (1 - 0.10)^{(10-5)}$$

The chances of the adverse event occurring at least five times would be:

$$p(\geq 5) = p(5) + p(6) + p(7) + p(8) + p(9) + p(10)$$

11.2 EPIDEMIOLOGICAL CONCEPTS

11.2.1 Risk

Epidemiology is the study of the determinants and distribution of diseases and conditions in a population. Epidemiology entails looking at data from a population and determining the likelihood of different outcomes and attempting to draw relationships between different factors and outcomes. Epidemiological techniques cannot establish definitively whether something *causes* a disease. Instead, these techniques can demonstrate *associations* between different variables (i.e., mathematical changes in one variable tend to occur when mathematical changes in another variable occur). In other words, an association is a mathematical relationship between two or more variables but does not necessarily mean that changes in one variable causes changes in another variable. For example, if every time you see certain celebrities like Madonna on television you develop nausea, you can say that nausea is associated with seeing Madonna. Does Madonna actually cause nausea? To prove that Madonna causes nausea, you would have to run some more rigorous experiments (e.g., performing laboratory experiments that look at the molecular mechanisms induced by Madonna). An association is the same thing as a correlation, which we discussed in Chapter 3.

Things associated with a disease may or may not be parts of the disease's *causal pathway*. The causal pathway is the sequence of events that eventually leads to the onset of a disease. Anything on the causal pathway is a cause or *etiology* of the disease. A disease may have multiple alternative causal pathways. Something is a *necessary cause* if it must be present for the disease to occur (e.g., HIV is a necessary cause of AIDS). A *sufficient cause* is a set of factors that are enough to cause a disease. For example, eating a rotten apple is sufficient cause for diarrhea. No other factors need to be present to cause the diarrhea. By contrast, the presence of streptococci is not sufficient cause for a skin infection. Streptococci are omnipresent but most people do not develop any skin infections. Some other cause(s) must be present additionally to result in a skin infection (e.g., a wound or immune disorder). A necessary cause is not always a sufficient cause.

Risk is the probability of an individual developing a disease or condition during a specific period of time. A *risk factor* is any attribute, exposure, or condition that changes the probability of developing the disease or condition. When the risk factor is a characteristic of the individual, we call it an *attribute*. When an individual encounters a risk factor in the environment (i.e., external to the individual), he or she is *exposed* to the risk factor (e.g., interacting with a co-worker with an infectious disease, alcohol intake, exposure to sunlight, or inhaling a toxic chemical). The time between exposure to a risk factor and the onset of a disease in an individual is the *induction period*. Induction periods can be very short (e.g., fire takes only a few seconds to cause burns) or very long (e.g., the induction period between radiation exposure and development of cancer can be decades). When the induction period is very long, linking the risk factor with the disease can be difficult. Many conditions remain hidden for a while before becoming clinically evident (e.g., manifesting signs and symptoms). This lag period is termed the *latent period*. Infectious diseases with long latent periods (e.g., HIV infection) can spread rapidly in a population since many individuals will not be aware that they have the disease and continue to spread it to other people.

Diseases usually have a variety of associated risk factors. For example, high cholesterol, smoking, and diabetes are all risk factors for heart disease. When studying a certain risk factor, there will be *competing risks*, that is other risk factors that may cause or accelerate the outcome that you are studying. For example, if you are studying the relationship between smoking and heart disease, high cholesterol and diabetes will be competing risk factors. Some risk factors are *modifiable,* the risk factor can be mitigated or eliminated (e.g., you can quit smoking). Other risk factors are not modifiable (e.g., a patient's family history cannot be changed). Beware of mistaking a *risk marker* for a risk factor. A risk marker does not cause a clinical outcome but instead indicates the presence of a risk factor. (For example, working in a bar may be a risk marker for lung disease. The act of working in bar does not cause lung disease. However, bars may be filled with smoke from cigarettes, which is a known risk factor for lung disease.)

A big role of epidemiology is determining how different risk factors affect the probability of developing disease. A risk factor that is consistently associated with an increased probability of a disease may play a pivotal role in causing that disease. There are many ways of quantifying the relationship between a risk factor and the risk of disease. For example, you can calculate a risk factor's *attributable risk (AR)*, the increase in risk associated with a given risk factor:

$$AR = \text{Probability of disease when exposed to risk factor} - \text{Probability of disease when not exposed to risk factor}$$

The *population AR* or *etiologic fraction* is another measure:

$$\text{Population AR} = (\text{Patients with the disease and the risk factor})/(\text{All patients with the disease})$$

In other words, the etiologic fraction is the proportion of the population that would not have developed the disease if the risk factor was not present. A commonly used measure is the *relative risk (RR)*:

$$RR = \text{Risk among patients exposed to risk factor}/ \text{Risk among patients } not \text{ exposed to risk factor}$$

$RR > 1$ means that the risk factor is associated with an increased risk of disease. $RR=1$ means that there is no association between the risk factor and risk of disease. $RR<1$ means that the risk factor is associated with a decreased risk of disease.

When you remove a patient's risk factor for a certain outcome, you presumably reduce the patient's risk of developing the outcome. The effectiveness of this treatment (i.e., removing the risk factor) depends on the degree to which the risk is reduced. There are several measures of this type of treatment effectiveness. The absolute risk reduction (ARR) is:

$$ARR = \text{Frequency of outcomes with risk factor exposure} - \text{Frequency of outcomes } without \text{ risk factor exposure}$$

The relative risk reduction (RRR) is:

$$RRR = (\text{Frequency of outcomes with risk factor exposure} - \text{Frequency of outcomes } without \text{ risk factor exposure})/(\text{Frequency of outcomes with risk factor exposure})$$

Another important measure is the *number needed to treat (NNT)*. Removing a risk factor from a patient (which we will call treating a patient) will reduce the patient's risk of developing a disease or having an outcome. The NNT is the number of different patients that you would have to "treat" to prevent one case of the disease or one outcome. If the treatment is 100% effective, then the NNT would be 1. In general:

$$\text{NNT} = 1/\text{Absolute risk reduction}$$

How do we determine if an association between a risk factor and an outcome is indeed a causal relationship? Finding the following strongly suggests that an association may be indeed a cause and effect relationships:

- *Biological plausibility*: A biological mechanism connects the risk factor together with the outcome (e.g., cigarette smoke has been found to damage lung tissue).
- *Strong association*: Risk factors that are strongly associated with an outcome are more likely to be the causes (e.g., smokers are a lot more likely than nonsmokers to develop emphysema).
- *Dose–response effect*: Increasing the dose or magnitude of the risk factor increases the risk of the outcome (e.g., the more you smoke, the more likely you are to develop emphysema).
- *Consistent association*: The association should be present under different conditions and in different situations (e.g., smoking is associated with emphysema regardless of the patient's country, diet, or gender).
- *Temporal effect*: Occurrence of the risk factor must precede the outcome (e.g., emphysema develops after smoking).
- *Intervention effective*: Mitigating or eliminating the risk factor reduces the risk of the outcome (e.g., smoking cessation leads to a decreased risk of emphysema).

11.2.2 Disease Outcomes

Different proportions, rates, and ratios measure disease outcomes. Table 11.1 shows how these terms are often confused. We admittedly misuse the term "rate" in this chapter mainly because in some cases the term has been misused so long that it has become convention. Many outcome measures in epidemiology come in the following general form, which is a proportion, not a rate:

= [Number of patients experiencing an event (e.g., death, illness, or side effects)]/[Study population (i.e., "at risk" population, anyone who could experience the event)]

But people often refer to the crude death rate, which is calculated as follow:

= Annual deaths/Size of study population (during midpoint of year)

As you can see, this is actually a proportion, not a rate.

One of the most commonly used rates in epidemiology is the *incidence*. Incidence is the frequency at which *new* cases of a disease develop in a population:

Incidence = Number of new cases/Duration of time

The *cumulative incidence* (or *incidence proportion*) is the proportion of a population that develops the disease over a specific period of time:

Cumulative incidence = Number of new cases over period *T*/Study population over period *T*

TABLE 11.1 Distinguishing proportions, rates, and ratios

Proportions, Rates, and Ratios

Often these three terms are confused and misused. In fact, we "misuse" these terms in this chapter (mainly because their misuse has been so frequent to become a convention. For example, attack and case-fatality "rates," are not really rates but proportions.

Proportions and ratios can be confused as well. A proportion is a fraction. Every member in the numerator must also be in the denominator (e.g., proportion of physicians who are women).

By contrast, a ratio is just the size of one group divided by another. The groups are usually separate and mutually exclusive (e.g., ratio of physicians to patients).

Term	Range	Numerator	Denominator	Dimensions
Proportion	0.0 to 1.0	Number of patients with event or characteristic	Total number of patients	None
Rate	0.0 to ∞	Number of events	Duration of time	Number of individuals/Unit time
Ratio	$-\infty$ to $+\infty$	One group of patients	Another different group of patients	None

If everyone in the study population develops the disease during the time period, the cumulative incidence is 1.0 or 100%. If no one does, the cumulative incidence is 0%. One weakness of cumulative incidence as a measure is that the study population may change in size overtime because of *competing risks*, that is other factors that can remove patients from the study population. For example, patients may die or dropout of the study. In such a situation, the *incidence rate* is a better measure:

$$\text{Incidence rate} = \text{Number of new cases over period } T/\text{Total person} - \text{Time of observation}$$

The number of *person-years* each patient contributes to the denominator is the number of years that patient remains in the study population (e.g., a patient who remains in the study for 1 year contributes a single person-year; a patient who drops out after 6 months contributes 0.5 person-years).

The *case fatality "rate"* is the cumulative incidence of deaths in a population:

$$\text{Case fatality "rate"} = \text{Number of deaths over period } T/\text{Study population over period } T$$

The *attack "rate"* is the proportion of patients exposed to a certain risk factor for a disease that end up developing the disease:

$$\text{Attack rate} = \text{Patients who develop disease}/\text{Patients exposed to risk factor for disease}$$

It is common to use attack rates with infectious diseases. The denominator is everyone exposed to someone with the infection (i.e., a *primary* or *index* case), and the numerator is everyone who develops the infection after an incubation period has elapsed. However, attack rates can also apply to noninfectious diseases, as long you are looking at a specific risk factor and a disease believed to result from that risk factor (e.g., heart disease and diabetes, mesothelioma and asbestos exposure, and side effects and a medical procedure).

Two very commonly used measures of disease outcomes are morbidity and mortality. *Morbidity* is the proportion of patients in a certain population that develop a certain specific condition (e.g., myocardial infarction among patients with coronary artery disease). *Mortality* is the proportion of patients in a certain population that die over a given period of time (usually a year). You can express morbidity and mortality as percentages or number of patients per population unit (e.g., per 1000, 10,000, 100,000, etc. patients). Since the size of the population may change overtime, the denominator is commonly the population size in the middle of the time interval.

Prevalence is the percentage of patients in a population who have a certain condition or disease at a specific moment in time:

$$\text{Prevalence} = \text{Patients with disease or condition}/\text{Total population}$$

Prevalence is most relevant for chronic, low mortality diseases but less useful for diseases that have very short durations or high mortality. A cross-sectional study can establish disease prevalence.

11.3 TESTING

11.3.1 Test Performance

A *test* is a measure that provides evidence about a physiological process, a psychological state, a disease or condition, or the effects of an intervention. A test can be a laboratory assay, an imaging procedure, a history or physical exam technique, a machine administered procedure, etc. A *screening test* is analogous to filter through which you pass a population to catch any patients that may have a certain condition or disease. Most of the patients receiving a screening test will be symptom-free. By contrast, you use a *diagnostic test* to determine whether a patient suspected of having a disease indeed has the disease. A test is considered a *"gold" standard*, *reference standard*, or a *definitive test* if it can confirm whether a patient has a disease with a high level of certainty. In many cases, an autopsy or other invasive procedure like surgery is the gold standard. Most gold standards are too expensive or risky to perform routinely. Therefore, clinicians frequently rely on less definitive tests.

The *information gain* from a test is the quantified impact of the test results on decision making:

$$\text{Information gain} = \text{Probability of disease with test result} - \text{Probability of disease without test result}$$

The information gain from a positive test result is frequently different from that of a negative test result. For example, finding a mass on a breast exam significantly raises the probability that a patient has breast cancer. However, not finding a mass lowers the probability that a patient has breast cancer but not by the same magnitude. In other words, finding a mass raises concern to a much greater degree than the degree to which a normal breast exam alleviates concern.

Few tests are 100%. There is almost always uncertainty about a test result. A positive test result does not necessarily mean the patient has the disease. A negative test result does not eliminate the possibility that the patient has the disease. Tests provide evidence rather than definitive diagnoses. Tests vary in the strength of the evidence that they can provide. Changes on an electrocardiogram can suggest that a patient has coronary artery disease. An abnormality on a nuclear stress test can provide stronger evidence. But neither of these test results is as convincing as findings on a coronary angiogram.

Even very direct tests can be wrong. Suppose you are buying either a suit or a dress. Trying on the suit or dress in the fitting room tests the fit and look of the item. But how many times have you been satisfied with an item while in the store, only to change your mind when you get home? Testing an item in the store is not 100%.

Figure 11.3 show several common measures of a test's *performance*, that is a test's ability to rule in or rule out the presence of a disease. The more *sensitive* a test, the more likely a patient with the disease will test positive. Diagnostic tests should be relatively sensitive since missing the disease could be disastrous. Highly sensitive tests serve as good *rule-out tests* (i.e., a negative result makes the disease very unlikely). The more *specific* a test, the more likely a patient without the disease will test negative. Screening tests should be relatively specific. A highly specific test

	Disease	No disease
Positive test	a	b
Negative test	c	d

False negative (FN) = c = Negative test when the individual actually has the disease
False positive (FP) = b = Positive test when the individual does not have the disease
True negative (TN) = d = Negative test and individual is disease-free
True positive (TP) = a = Positive test and individual has disease

Measure	Description	Probability	Formula	Alternative formula
Positive predictive value (PPV)	Given a positive test, what is the chance that the patient has a disease	p(Disease|Positive test)	$a/(a + b)$	TP/(TP + FP)
Negative predictive value (NPV)	Given a negative test, what is the chance that the patient has a disease	p(No disease|Negative test)	$d/(c + d)$	TN/(TN + FN)
Sensitivity	Given a patient with disease, what is the chance that the patient will have a positive test	p(Positive test|Disease)	$a/(a + c)$	TP/(TP + FN)
Specificity	Given a patient with no disease, what is the chance that the patient will have a negative test	p(Negative test|No disease)	$d/(b + d)$	TN/(TN + FP)
Apparent Prevalence (Test prevalence)	Proportion of positive tests among all the test results.	Total positives/Number of all test results	$(a + b)/(a + b + c + d)$	(TP + FP)/ (TP + FP + TN FN)
Negative likelihood ratio (−LR)	How much should a negative test result shift our belief that the patient does not have the disease	p(Negative test|Disease)/p(Negative test|No disease)	$[c/(a + c)]/[d/(b + d)]$	(1 − Sensitivity)/ Specificity
Positive likelihood ratio (+LR)	How much should a positive test result shift our suspicion that person has the disease	p(Positive test|Disease)/p(Positive test|No disease)	$[a/(a + c)]/[b/(b + d)]$	Sensitivity/ (1 − Specificity).

FIGURE 11.3   Common measures of test's performance.

is a good *rule-in test* (e.g., a positive test strongly suggests that the disease should remain as a possibility). A test *threshold* is value at which a test goes from being negative to positive. Raising the threshold for a positive test will raise the sensitivity of a test (e.g., patient's cholesterol has to be over 220 instead of over 200 to be at risk for coronary artery disease). This is analogous to having more stringent admission standards to a college. The more stringent the standards, the more likely a student or graduate of the college is of good quality. In other words, there will be fewer "admissions mistakes." However, increasing the threshold will also decrease specificity. In the college admissions analogy, very stringent admissions standards may accidentally exclude some very qualified candidates. In other words, there will be more "admissions misses." As you can see, raising a test's sensitivity will lower its specificity and vice versa.

Plotting a *receiver operator characteristic (ROC)* curve can help set the optimal test threshold. The ROC curve plots the true positive rate (i.e., the sensitivity) against the false positive rate (i.e., $1-$specificity) for different test threshold value (Figure 11.4). A ROC curve illustrates the tradeoff between sensitivity and specificity. The area under the curve measures the *accuracy* of the test (we discussed accuracy and precision in Chapter 4). The greater the area under the curve, the more accurate the test is. So moving the curve closer to the upper left corner increases the accuracy of the test. Also, the slope of the curve at a certain threshold is the likelihood ratio (LR) of the test using that threshold.

The prevalence and severity of the condition being measured affect the predictive values of a test. If most patients have very severe forms of a disease, the false positive and the false negative rates will decrease, that is there will be fewer borderline or equivocal cases. Increasing the

prevalence of the condition will decrease the false positive rate (i.e., increase the PPV) and increase the false negative rate (i.e., decrease the NPV). To understand this phenomenon, suppose you are trying to guess if people are married by observing certain aspects of their behavior. If you observe a college campus population where the majority of people are not married, a guess that a given person is not married is more likely to be true. If you observe workers in a company where most people are married, a guess that a given person is married is more likely to be true.

11.3.2 Bayes' Theorem

A simple clinical study easily can determine the sensitivity of a test, that is p(Positive test|Disease): administer the test to a group of patients with the disease, and see what proportion of them have a positive test. However, in clinical practice, we use a test because we do not know whether a patient has a disease. The challenge is interpreting the test result. What does a positive test mean, that is what is the positive predictive value of the test? How confident are we that a positive test means that the patient has the disease? *Bayes' Theorem* allows us to calculate $p(A|B)$ from knowing $p(B|A)$:

$$p(A|B) = \frac{p(B|A) \times p(A)}{[p(B|A) \times p(A)] + [p(B|A') \times p(A')]}$$

A' is the *complement event* of A, that is Event A not occurring. So, $p(A')$ is the probability of Event A not occurring, and $p(B|A')$ is the probability of Event B given that Event A does not occur.

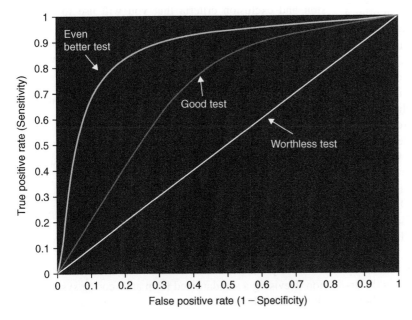

FIGURE 11.4   A receiver operator characteristic (ROC) curves plots the true positive rate against the false positive rate for different test threshold value.

So, for example,

$$p\!\begin{pmatrix}\text{Disease}\,|\\ \text{Positive \textbackslash test}\end{pmatrix} = \frac{\begin{array}{c}p(\text{Positive test}\,|\,\text{Disease})\\ \times\, p(\text{Disease})\end{array}}{\begin{array}{c}[p(\text{Positive test}\,|\,\text{Disease})\\ \times\, p(\text{Disease})] + [p(\text{Positive test}\,|\\ \text{No disease}) \times p(\text{No disease})]\end{array}}$$

This can be re-written as:

$$\begin{aligned}\text{Positive predictive}\atop\text{value} &= \frac{\text{Probability of disease}}{\text{given a positive test}}\\ &= \frac{(\text{Prevalence} \times \text{Sensitivity})}{\begin{array}{c}[(\text{Prevalence} \times \text{Sensitivity})\\ + ((1 - \text{Prevalence})\\ \times (1 - \text{Specificity}))]\end{array}}\end{aligned}$$

11.4 META-ANALYSIS

11.4.1 Effect Size

Suppose you want to answer the following question: How effective is Drug A? A literature search unearths a handful of studies that have addressed this question, but their answers vary significantly. One trial shows that Drug A cures 80% of people. Another trial shows that it is 60% effective. As you pore through the different studies, more and more different answers emerge. Which one do you believe? Different trials have different study population sizes and different conditions. How do we reconcile these differences? How do we answer the question?

A *meta-analysis* is a statistical technique that involves analyzing, combining, and summarizing relevant previous studies to answer a specific research question. In other words, a meta-analysis pools different studies with varying quantitative "answers" into one large study that can offer a single quantitative answer. A meta-analysis answers questions that have the following general form: What is the *effect size*? The effect size is magnitude of a clinical phenomenon. In general, effect sizes are either the mean differences between groups (e.g., what is the difference in survival between patients that did and did not receive the drug) or the correlations between variables (e.g., how strongly does taking vitamins correlate with a reduction in disease rates). Studies may report effect sizes in different ways, which may require you to convert one effect size into another.

The biggest drawback of a meta-analysis is comparing apples and oranges problem. Studies may be too different to combine into one large study, especially if the results of individual studies vary significantly. The quality of a meta-analysis depends heavily on how the procedure is performed. As you will see, many steps depend heavily on the people performing the meta-analysis. Setting different selection criteria and differing opinions on what should be included can substantially alter the results of the meta-analysis. Finally, since new studies are always emerging, a meta-analysis can quickly become outdated.

11.4.2 Steps

The first step in a meta-analysis is to collect all relevant studies. This potentially enormous and time consuming task entails doing exhaustive searches of the medical literature (using databases such as Medline) to identify all the studies that may have addressed your research question. Finding all important studies can be a lot more challenging than it initially appears. Knowing how to search a database takes skill and experience (e.g., knowing the right keywords to use in your searches of electronic databases). Some studies, especially ones that are older or in a foreign language, do not appear in traditional databases such as Medline. You will also need to locate so-called *fugitive literature*, publications that escape the purview of traditional databases, such as dissertation theses, drug company studies, and government documents. Searching the bibliographies of important articles and experts in the field can unearth important studies. Contacting some of these experts can also help locate unpublished trials as well. Since the body of studies continues to grow, clearly establish cutoff dates (e.g., your meta-analysis only includes studies conducted between January 1, 1970 and October 2, 2007). Try to make the cutoff date as recent as possible. Otherwise your meta-analysis will quickly become out-of-date.

Paring Down Studies

Once you have collected a big library of different studies, the next step is to whittle the library down to the group of studies suitable for the meta-analysis. Delineate the inclusion and exclusion criteria that you will use to winnow down the studies. The selection criteria should include measures of study quality (i.e., exclude poor quality studies). Examples of selection criteria include the following:

- Study design (e.g., RCT)
- Study population size (e.g., frequently very small studies are excluded)
- Length of follow-up
- Years that the study is conducted
- Patient characteristics (e.g., gender or age distribution)
- Intervention characteristics (e.g., specific doses or routes of administration)
- Study setting (e.g., outpatient vs. inpatient, geographic location)
- Language of the article

Clearly state the rationale behind each selection criterion. Devising a standardized form and scoring system usually is helpful, so that you may score each study's quality.

Skimming through titles and abstracts may eliminate a large percentage of studies. The closer you get to your final group, the harder it becomes to eliminate studies and the closer you have to scrutinize what's remaining. Carefully document every step in your meta-analysis including your search strategy, your inclusion and exclusion criteria for studies, and any potentially controversial decisions. Your documentation should be extensive enough for anyone to reproduce your meta-analysis if necessary.

Data Abstraction

Data abstraction, that is pulling the relevant information from each study and entering it into a database, comes next. Having multiple reviewers (at least two independent reviewers and a third to resolve any discrepancies between the first two reviewers) assess the results and abstract data from each study will reduce errors (e.g., misinterpretation of data and data entry mistakes). To ensure that data abstraction is performed properly, each reviewer can first practice data abstraction on several articles before embarking on the whole set of studies.

Publication bias is a significant problem with medical literature. According to this bias, studies that show statistically significant effects are more likely to appear in journals than studies that show no effect or insignificant results. For example, which one is more likely to be accepted by a journal: a study demonstrating that jellybeans significantly inhibit a person's ability to work or a study that shows chocolate chip cookies really have no effect on work productivity? Studies that have an interesting or dramatic revelation have greater public appeal. In this way, the medical literature is similar to the lay press such as daily newspapers, magazines, and television news. Dramatic and sexy headlines will displace boring, mundane information. Therefore, studies gleaned from the medical literature may tend to overstate

an intervention's effects or risks. The studies that showed a smaller effect may remain unpublished and unnoticed. While completely overcoming publication bias is impossible, several strategies can minimize it. First, always keep in mind the potential role of publication bias. Secondly, do your best to find all relevant studies inside and outside the medical literature. Finally, construct a funnel plot (Figure 11.5). A funnels plot graphs effect size along the *x*-axis and study population size along the *y*-axis. The magnitude of an intervention's effects should decrease the larger the study population size, that is the funnel plot should resemble a traffic cone and not an ice cream cone. Testing an intervention on 10 people may reveal wide variation of effects that lead to a large average effect. Testing an intervention on 1000 people is likely to reveal a smaller average effect: the extreme cases will be balanced by the majority of cases that have more modest effects. Seeing anything different suggests that publication bias is strong (Figure 11.6).

Analysis

The type of analysis you perform depends on the *homogeneity* vs. *heterogeneity* of the studies. Combining studies that are relatively homogeneous (i.e., the studies are comparable in study design, characteristics, and study population) seems to be more reasonable than combining studies that are apparently heterogeneous (e.g., significant differences among different studies).

In analyzing the results of a meta-analysis, you can use a fixed effects model or a random effects model. (The details of putting together each statistical model is beyond the scope of this chapter.) *A fixed effects model* assumes that there is little inter-study variability (i.e., the studies are similar enough to be lumped together) and that the body of studies can determine the effect size. The fixed effects model jumps right to the question: What is the effect size?

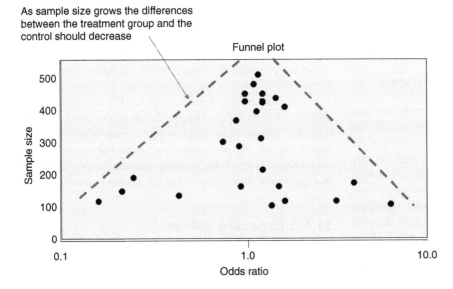

FIGURE 11.5 A funnel plot when publication bias is not strong.

- **Separating very different study types:** When study types are significantly different, clumping different study types (e.g., RCT vs. non-RCT) and reporting effect sizes for each group may be more accurate than just reporting one general effect size. Study designs may so different that they lead to very different effect sizes.
- **Selecting multiple publications from same study:** Many times a large study will generate multiple publications. Remember, in this case, each publication is not a separate study. They should all be treated as a single study.
- **Choosing the wrong effect?:** Many times a study will generate multiple measurements and endpoints. It may show different effects and report effects within different subgroups of the study population. Make sure that the effect comes from a study design or population that fulfills your selection criteria (e.g., if you exclude children, do not take a result that comes from a population with children)

FIGURE 11.6   Potential pitfalls in meta-analyses.

The *random effects model* is more cautious and first asks: Is there so much inter-study variability that this body of studies cannot properly answer the question? If the body of studies can answer the question, what then is the effect size? By analogy, a fixed effects model assumes that we are dealing with all oranges and simply tests how good the oranges are. A random effects model asks at the same time are we dealing with apples and oranges, can we combine apples and oranges, and how good are the fruits?

Of course, if the studies in your meta-analysis are homogeneous, the fixed effects and random effects models should yield very similar results. Since the random effects models involve more work, when studies are relatively homogeneous, a fixed effects model is more appropriate. However, when the studies are heterogeneous, fixed and random effects models can generate vastly different results.

Performing a *sensitivity analysis* can be helpful. As with other types of sensitivity analyses, this involves altering different factors and seeing how they affect results. In the case of meta-analyses, you can see how changing the types of studies included in your group of studies alters your results (e.g., only including studies with men, only including studies with women).

11.5 DECISION ANALYSIS

11.5.1 Decision Making and Uncertainty

Decisions are a big part of health care, medicine, science, research, and life. Some decisions are relatively easy: for example, should you eat the salmon or that pile of lint in the corner; should you fix the flat tire on the car or junk the car? However, many decisions are much more difficult: which job should you take or career path should you pursue; should you get married; whom should you marry; which medical treatment should you give? Decisions are often difficult to make because the outcomes and the implications of the decisions are unknown. In other words, there is uncertainty about the outcomes and consequently about the optimal decisions to make. If we all knew for certain how each career choice would turn out then decision making would be easy. Take that Job 1 and you'll be successful and happy; take Job 2 and you'll be miserable and have no friends. Gee, which job would you choose?

One of the big challenges of decision making is predicting the possible outcomes. How many times have you said long after a decision, "I had no idea that could have happened"? Each decision has a range of possible outcomes. If you choose a particular job, you could stay in the job until retirement and be satisfied, stay in the job until retirement and be miserable, quit after different lengths of time, be laid off after different lengths of time, be fired after different lengths of time, etc. Many decisions have a seemingly infinite number of alternative outcomes. Knowing the entire universe of outcomes is impossible. Therefore, when making decisions, we try to limit the range of achievable outcomes to a finite number. Otherwise, decision making would be unfeasible. The dizzying array of infinite outcomes would paralyze us. So when deciding to marry someone, perseverating over every consequence of your decision (e.g., what if that person nags me, what if that person loses his or her job, what if that person betrays me, etc.) could prevent you from making a decision. But simplifying the set of outcomes may make the decision easier: "After 30 years will I still be married and happy?"

Each outcome has a probability of occurring. Some outcomes are very unlikely. The probability of getting married and then separated the next day is usually very low (unless you are a celebrity like Britney Spears or Carmen Electra). Other probabilities are higher. For example, the chance of being dissatisfied after 2 years of marriage is higher than being separated after 1 day. Ideally you would like the probabilities of favorable outcomes (e.g., being satisfied and content after 2 years of marriage) to be high enough to justify getting married.

11.5.2 Expected Values

Probabilities alone do not govern decisions. The *rewards or payoffs* of outcomes also are very important. Most people

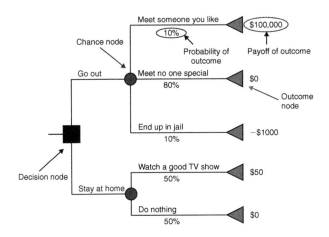

FIGURE 11.7 Examples of a decision tree depicting an important decision.

are willing to risk more if the potential payoff is high. Would you rather have a 50% chance of getting $2 or a 10% chance of getting $1000? A majority of people would choose the latter. The payoff of each outcome can be any kind of cost, reward, or both (we discussed these issues in Chapter 8), such as dollars, life years saved, quality-adjusted life years (QALYs), or utilities.

The *expected value* combines probabilities and payoffs. The expected value of each outcome is its reward multiplied by the probability of that outcome. So for a situation with n possibleD outcomes:

$$\text{Expected value} = (\text{Probability}_{\text{Outcome 1}} \times \text{Payoff}_{\text{Outcome 1}})$$
$$+ (\text{Probability}_{\text{Outcome 2}} \times \text{Payoff}_{\text{Outcome 2}})$$
$$+ (\text{Probability}_{\text{Outcome3}} \times \text{Payoff}_{\text{Outcome 3}})$$
$$+ \ldots + (\text{Probability}_{\text{Outcome } n} \times \text{Payoff}_{\text{Outcome } n})$$

Situation 1: In a situation where you have a 10% chance of earning $1000, a 50% chance of earning $10, and a 40% chance of earning $0:

$$\text{Expected value} = (0.10 \times \$1000)$$
$$+ (0.50 \times \$10) + (0.40 \times \$0)$$
$$= \$100 + \$5 + \$0$$
$$= \$105$$

Situation 2: In a situation where you have a 5% chance of earning $1000, an 85% chance of earning $10, and a 10% chance of earning $0:

$$\text{Expected value} = (0.05 \times \$1000)$$
$$+ (0.85 \times \$10) + (0.25 \times \$0)$$
$$= \$50 + \$8.50 + \$0$$
$$= \$58.50$$

As you can see the expected value for Situation 1 is greater than for Situation 2. This suggests that Situation 1 is preferable to Situation 2, even though Situation 2 has a

smaller chance of netting you $0. The chance of earning $1000 overpowers the risk of earning you nothing.

11.5.3 Decision Trees

Decision trees can represent decision problems. Figure 11.7 shows examples of a decision tree depiction of an important decision. The first picture represents a decision with two choices: go out vs. stay at home. The square is called a decision node. Each of the branches of this tree represents a choice. At the end of each branch is a *chance node* (represented by a circle). The chance node represents several different events, each has a certain probability of happening. So in this case, if you go out, one of three possible things may happen:

- You meet someone you like. There is a 10% chance of this outcome occurring. This will have a payoff of $100,000.
- You do not meet anyone. This is the most likely outcome (80% chance) and has a neutral result of $0.
- You end up in jail. This has a 10% chance of happening and would cost you $1000.

As you can see, each branch in the chance node has a probability of occurring and a corresponding payoff. "Rolling back" the chance node, that is calculating the expected value of this chance node, will generate the chance node's expected value:

$$\begin{aligned}\text{Expected value} \atop \text{of going out} &= (0.10 \times \$100,000) + (0.80 \times \$0)\\ &\quad + (0.10 \times -\$1000)\\ &= \$10,000 + \$0 + -\$100\\ &= \$9900\end{aligned}$$

You can roll back the other chance node associated with the decision of *staying home*:

$$\begin{aligned}\text{Expected value of} \atop \text{staying home} &= (0.50 \times \$50) + (0.50 \times \$0)\\ &= \$25 + \$0\\ &= \$25\end{aligned}$$

As you can see, the EV of *going out* far outweighs the EV of *staying home*. Therefore, you should go out even though you may end up in jail.

Figure 11.8 shows the roll back of an even more complicated decision tree. This decision tree depicts several sequential decisions. The probabilities after each chance node are conditional probabilities, that is the probabilities given the fact that you made the decisions to the left of the chance node. A decision tree can be complex as you make it, having multiple arborizations (branches), decision nodes, and chance nodes. In theory, you could represent any set of decision with a decision tree, as long as the number of decisions and choices are finite.

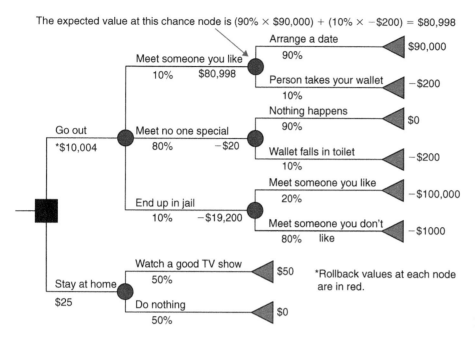

The expected value at this chance node is (90% × $90,000) + (10% × −$200) = $80,998

FIGURE 11.8   Rolling back a decision tree.

11.6 LINEAR PROGRAMMING

A *linear function* is any equation that comes in the following general form:

$$y = a_1 x_1 + a_2 x_2 + a_3 x_3 + \dots + a_n x_n$$

where a_n are constants and x_n are independent variables. The equals ("=") sign may be replaced with a greater than (">"), or combination sign ("≤","≥").

Many situations have multiple *linear constraints*, that is several linear equations have to be satisfied at the same time. For example, suppose you have only $1000 to recruit patients for a study. Successfully recruiting each man costs $50. Successfully recruiting each woman costs $40. It takes three study personnel to follow each man and four study personnel to follow each woman. You have a total of 100 study personnel. What is the maximum number of patients you will be able to recruit? Several parameters and linear constraints can represent this problem:

Maximize: Men + Women
Subject to the constraints: Men ≥ 0
Women ≥ 0
($50 × Men) + ($40 × Women) ≤ $1000
(3 Personnel × Men) + (4 Personnel × Women) ≤ 100 Personnel

The solution to this problem is the largest numbers of men and women that still satisfy both equations. This is an example of a linear programming problem. In other words, you want to maximize or minimize a linear function (also called the *objective function*, which, in this example, is

Men + Women) that is subject to several linear constraints. Men ≥ 0 and Women ≥ 0 are examples of *nonnegativity constraints*. Without these constraints, you could get an answer like −7 men, which would not make sense. The rest of the constraints are *main constraints*. Not all linear programming problems are solvable. Sometimes no solution will satisfy all the constraints, that is the problem is *infeasible*. Linear programming problems that have answers are *feasible*.

11.7 SIMULATION AND MODELING

11.7.1 Role of Simulation

Simulation is any method or technique that imitates a real life system or situation. Simulations can use real people, physical models, or computer models. A fire-drill is an example of a simulation. No real fire occurs, but everyone acts as if there were a real fire. Practice sessions in sports or dress rehearsals in acting are simulations as well. Simulations provide a "dry-run" of a situation or process and allow you to predict how smoothly things will progress, identify factors that may affect operations, and run virtual experiments to test the effects of changing different parameters. Computer simulations can depict very complicated and complex systems or situations.

Remember that simulations are approximations of real life. No simulation will ever be able to capture all of the nuances and uncertainties of a real situation. Dress rehearsals, practices, and drills all lack the same elements of the "real thing." The goal of simulations is to supplement and support rather than replace real experiments. A simulation will not provide definitive answers but may raise important questions.

Simulation is becoming increasingly popular in clinical research. Current and potential roles include:

- Predict the pharmacokinetic and pharmacodynamic properties of a medication.
- Plan the logistics of patient recruitment and clinical trial operations.
- Help to determine the design and parameters of a clinical study.
- Extrapolate clinical study results to other populations and situations.
- Extend animal data to human data when planning human experiments.

Without simulation, we would have to run many more real life experiments and rely more heavily on "trial-and-error." Without practice or dress rehearsal, players, actors, and actresses would suffer many poor performances before finally "getting it right." Trial-and-error is costly, time consuming, and in the case of clinical research potentially dangerous.

11.7.2 Deterministic vs. Stochastic Models

A model is *deterministic* if it provides the same answer every time you run the model. In other words, the model parameters are *fixed*, that is, constant or the same each time. Simple arithmetic formulae are examples of deterministic models. For example, the formula $y = 5x + 10$ is deterministic. Every time you enter $x = 1$, you will get $y = 15$. Every time you enter $x = 2$, you get $y = 20$. There is no chance or uncertainty involved.

Does real life operate this way? Usually not. There are few incidences where you know exactly what you are getting. There is always a chance that something will occur differently from expected. Each time you get a haircut from the same barber or hairdresser, there is some variation. Even a trusted barber or hair stylist could mess up your hair if he or she is having a bad day or conditions are not right. Therefore, deterministic models may be limited.

Stochastic (probabilistic) models incorporate uncertainty into the model. In a stochastic model, key parameters are not constants and instead uncertain and may change every time you run the model. For example, the following formula would be stochastic:

$$Y = ax + 10$$

where a = (Distribution with mean = 5 and standard deviation = 1).

Entering $x = 1$ does not always give you $y = 15$ because the parameter that you multiply x by is no longer fixed. Instead, it is a number drawn from a distribution:

Sometimes, the formula will be $y = 4x + 10$, which will mean $y = 14$. Other times, the formula will be $y = 5.5x + 10$,

yielding $y = 15.5$. After running this "model" multiple times, the mean of y should be close to 15 (most answers will be close to $y = 15$), but individual cases will vary.

A stochastic model, in effect, makes certain parameters like "dice rolls," that is, every time you run the model, you may get a different answer. With a few runs, the answers may be wildly variable. However, after running the model many times, you may start to see clear patterns. The answers may start to *converge* on an answer (e.g., y has a mean of 15 and a standard deviation of 1), which means that a large percentage of the answers are clustered around a certain value. This does not always happen. When answers do not converge, either the model is incorrect or the phenomenon that you are modeling is inconsistent.

This example of a stochastic model is a *Monte Carlo simulation*. This type of simulation derived its name from the city of Monte Carlo, home to world famous casinos that offer a panoply of games of chance. In a Monte Carlo simulation, key variables are sampled from a probabilistic distribution (as seen in the example of a stochastic model above). Since different variables come from a probabilistic distribution, the answers also come in the form of a distribution.

11.7.3 Model Validation

As with measures and instruments, *validation* is important with models. You should provide evidence that the model is simulating what it is supposed to simulate. Model validation involves checking face validity (which we discussed in Chapter 4) and testing the model on known data. For example, if you know that increasing cholesterol and blood pressure increase heart attack risk, a simulation of heart disease should show this same result.

11.8 PROBABILITY DISTRIBUTIONS

11.8.1 Types of Distributions

An important part of designing a simulation is to choose the *probability distribution* for each relevant parameter. A probability distribution is a frequency at which the parameter assumes different values. The most common distribution for biological phenomena is the normal distribution, which we discussed in Chapter 3.

Figure 11.9 illustrates some common probability distributions. The *probability density function* is the mathematical formula that can generate the given curve for a given probability distribution.

11.8.2 Bootstrapping

When you do not know the probability distribution of a sample, *bootstrapping* is an option. When you bootstrap, you sample from within a sample. Suppose you are trying to determine the favorite football teams in the United States. In a random sample of 1000 people, 40% say the Pittsburgh Steelers, 30% say the Dallas Cowboys, 20% say Philadelphia Eagles, and 10% say the St. Louis Rams. How sure are you about these numbers? Will the distribution change in Southern California vs. Texas vs. New Jersey?

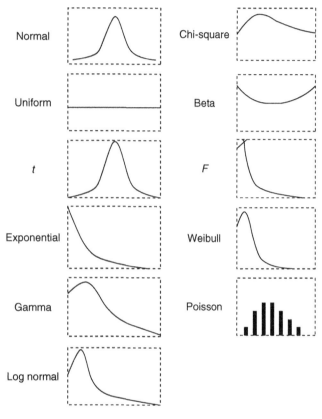

FIGURE 11.9　Examples of common probability distributions.

One way to answer these questions is bootstrapping. You can take multiple random samples of varying sizes from your original sample of 1000 people. For example, you can randomly sample 50, 100, and/or 110 people from within your sample of 1000 people. Each of these samples may have differing distributions of favorite teams (e.g., Sample 1 may be 50% Steelers, 10% Cowboys, 10% Rams, and 30% Eagles). You can then determine the variations among the different samples and, consequently, the accuracy of your 1000-person sample. If the distribution of favorite teams among the different subsamples fluctuates wildly, the results of your 1000-person sample may not be very accurate. If the distribution of favorite teams among the different subsamples is relatively constant, the results from your sample may be quite accurate. In other words, bootstrapping can unearth the variability within your main sample.

Remember that your subsamples should be samples of the original sample *with replacement*. In other words, if you take a sample of 50 people from the 1000-person sample, you should put those 50 people back into the mix when taking your next subsample. People in each subsample should be equally eligible to be part of subsequent subsamples.

11.9 TYPES OF MODELS

11.9.1 Compartment Models

A compartment model (Figure 11.10) divides a population into different mutually exclusive groups (i.e., compartments). The groups are logical divisions of the population (e.g., well, sick, and recovered; or susceptible to infection, infected, and resistant). Each person in the population is a member of one (and only one) of the groups. As time passes, the individuals can change classifications from one compartment to another. Mathematical equations govern their chances and rates of moving from one compartment

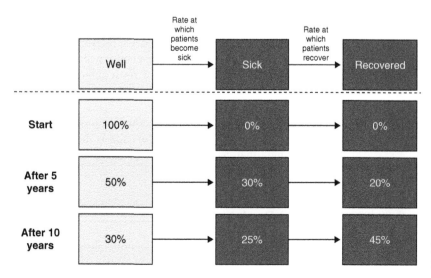

FIGURE 11.10　A compartment model divides a population into different mutually exclusive groups.

to another. So, for example, 100% of the people may start off in the "well" compartment. With time, a fraction of the people will move to the "sick" compartment and then a fraction of them will move on to the "recovered compartment. So after 5 years, you may have 50% in the "well" compartment, 30% in the "sick" compartment, and 20% in the "recovered" compartment. After 10 years, 30% may be in the "well" compartment, 25% in the "sick" compartment, and 45% in the "recovered" compartment.

There are multiple applications of compartment models in clinical research. For example, the gastrointestinal tract, the blood circulation, the body tissues, the liver, and the urinary system can all be different compartments for a model of drug distribution, pharmacokinetics, and pharmacodynamics. A compartment model can simulate the movement of drugs through these different body components. Another example would be using a compartment model to simulate progression of patients through different stages of a disease.

The classic compartment model is an infectious disease epidemic compartment model dubbed at SIR model. This model has three compartments: Susceptible (S), Infectious (I), and Resistant (R). All patients begin in the susceptible (S) compartment. A limited number become infected and then turn infectious, move into the I compartment. The infectious patients then infect some more patients in the S compartment. After being infectious for a while, patients will move to the R compartment, where they are immune or resistant to the disease.

11.9.2 Discrete Event Simulation

Discrete event simulation is a technique that can model the operation of a dynamic system over time. This technique can simulate nearly any type of process. The manufacturing industry has used discrete event simulation for years to simulate assembly lines and product delivery and distribution. The transportation industry has employed this technique to better understand air traffic control, train scheduling, and highway traffic patterns. Certain biological and physiological processes, medical interventions, and health care operations can be the subject of discrete event simulation (e.g., organ function, surgery, and emergency room operations).

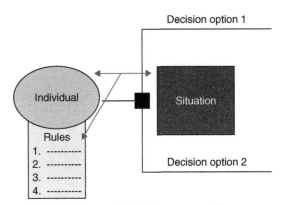

Each agent individually assesses its situation and makes decisions on the basis of a set of rules.

FIGURE 11.11   Schematic of an agent-based model.

11.9.3 Agent-Based Modeling

An *agent-based model* (Figure 11.11) contains programmed computer agents that each has decision making power and can take independent actions. Each *agent* may represent a person, group of people, animal, object, molecule, or drug: any entity that may face options and take actions based on those options. Each agent is imbued with its own set of characteristics and preferences. For example, if Agent 1 is faced with Situation 1, it may have a 70% probability of taking Action A and a 30% probability of taking Action B. By contrast, Agent 1 facing the same situation may have a 10% probability of taking Action A and a 90% probability of taking Action B.

Some researchers (including one of the authors of this book) have used very large and complex agent-based models to simulate people in a city or country. Each agent is a person that moves throughout the city during the day and night, making decisions, and taking actions. Each agent has different probabilities of certain choices and occurrence of certain events (e.g., the agent may get sick, be hospitalized, or die). Agent-based models can simulate a variety of different things in clinical research. For example, you can conduct a virtual clinical trial with agents representing individual study subjects.

Chapter 12

Study Execution

12.1 BACKGROUND

Study execution represents the practical aspect of clinical trial medicine, and involves activities such as protocols being written, drugs being shipped, IRB approvals being secured, patients being enrolled and treated, and data being gathered and collated. It is an exciting period. It is also a period fraught with risks. The study may not receive the appropriate approvals from the regulatory agencies and IRBs. The drug may not be available. The study may run over budget. Worst of all, patients may be injured. Second worst of all, the results of the study may be uninterpretable because of protocol violations, waivers, dropouts, poor study design, improper randomization, or other factors.

There are many things that are important in conducting clinical trials, but there are two cardinal goals during study execution. The most important goal is to protect patient safety. The second is to ensure integrity of the data.

The safety of the patient is protected by several mechanisms, including the IRB, informed consent, and most importantly, by the continuous monitoring of the study by the medical monitor.

The data integrity is ensured by standardized procedures, fully documented and audited processes, and strict adherence to GCP.

12.2 PROJECT AND PROGRAM MANAGEMENT

12.2.1 Overview of Project Management

Conducting a clinical trial is a complicated endeavor under any circumstances, but conducting a multi-center, multi-national, long-term trial is extremely complicated. There are many different people, many different functions, multiple organizations, and myriad activities that must be coordinated carefully.

In most organizations, *project management* is used to coordinate these activities. The discipline of project management started in the 1950s in the U.S. Department of Defense (DOD) to manage complex projects, and DOD has often been at the forefront in this field since then. Project management is the discipline of defining the project scope, planning the timeline/budget, controlling the budget and timelines, and ultimately, delivering the deliverables on time and on budget.

The steps in project management are as follows:

1. Establish goals and scope
2. Establish teams
3. Set timelines and budget
4. Decide on how to implement the study
5. Implement and monitor the study
6. Respond to unexpected or expected challenges, deviations, and problems
7. Perform assessment after the project on lessons learned.

Program Management and Project/Study Management

In drug development, there are multiple clinical trials for any given molecule, starting with Phase I and continuing through Phase IV. In addition, there are many important nonclinical activities such as manufacturing scale up. The entirety of activities that are required in order to bring a drug to registration and market is called a *Development Program*. The development program encompasses all clinical and nonclinical studies and activities that will be required to bring a drug to approval. These include the following.

Clinical studies
* Phase I
* Phase II
* Phase III
* PK studies in elderly, renal impaired, hepatic impaired
* Fed/Fast study
* Immunogenicity/Immunocompetence studies
* QTc studies

Pre-clinical work
* Toxicology
* Immunotoxicity/Immunogenicity
* Reproductive toxicology
* Long-term mutagenicity

CMC
* Pre-formulation and formulation
* Assays and assay development
* Stability
* Scale up

Pharmacoeconomics

Commercial
* Positioning and market research
* Thought leader advocacy

FIGURE 12.1   Components of a development program (not all-inclusive).

The goals and activities that are required to manage this development program are to:

* maximize the likelihood of success (registration) for the drug;
* if the drug is destined not to succeed, to discover that as early as possible and terminate the program with the least number of exposed patients and cost as possible:
  – remove as much of the uncertainty and risk around the program as early as possible;
* identify the correct set of indications for the drug;
* develop the drug as rapidly and as cost effectively as possible;
* protect patient safety;
* develop a drug that will meet an unmet medical need.

The activities making up the program management includes:

* constructing the target product profile of the drug;
* developing the proposed regulatory path;
* assessing the timeline and cost of development;
* assessing the scientific data and likelihood of clinical, regulatory, and commercial success;
* assessing the unmet medical need (market size) and competition;

* selecting the indication(s);
* constructing the correct series of clinical studies to support the proposed indications;
* establishing clear Go/No-Go criteria for the critical milestone and clinical study results;
* project managing the individual clinical trials to success.

Project management is obviously very important if you want to coordinate all of these pieces of clinical development. But it is also important at lower levels: project or clinical study level. Project level involves coordinating all the functions – data management, CMC, commercial, preclinical, toxicology, regulatory, clinical development, clinical operations, statistics, quality control, medical writing, pharmacoeconomics – that are necessary to conduct the clinical study successfully.

Here is an example of the components of a clinical study:

Medical
* Protocol development
* Medical monitoring
* Final report writing

Statistical and data management
* Statistical design
* Sample size calculation
* Statistical analysis plan (SAP)
* Case report form (CRF) design
* Database design
* Interactive voice response system (IVRS)
* Data entry
* Data cleaning
* Database lock
* Table listing
* Analysis

CMC
* Clinical supplies

Pharmacoeconomics

Clinical operations
* Site qualification, selection, initiation
* Monitoring visits
* Oversight of clinical research organization (CRO)
* Data cleaning/queries
* Contracts with sites
* Central laboratories

PK/PD

Regulatory
* Regulatory strategy
* Investigational new drug (IND) filing
* Regulatory package filings

FIGURE 12.2   Components of a clinical study.

A clinical study must be managed carefully if it is to:

- be completed in the projected timeline;
- be completed on the projected budget;
- protect patient safety;
- follow all the regulations and laws;
- generate reliable data;
- answer the scientific question being asked;
- lead to the next clinical trial in the development program.

Management consists of:

- assembling the team;
- coming to a common understanding at the beginning of the project what the desired outcome is;
- dividing up the roles and responsibilities among the team members;
- mapping out all the required activities and the dependencies;
- writing the procedures and processes for performing the required activities;
- developing contingency plans for things that could go wrong;
- developing a budget;
- tracking the study to ensure that the following are being done properly:
  - budget,
  - timeline,
  - adherence to the procedures, processes, regulations, and laws,
  - corrective action plans,
  - documentation;
- communicating the status of the project to stakeholders.

It is only by this process that you can minimize the number of disasters, such as finding out a week before the start of the trial that drug labeling, which can take 6–8 weeks, has not started, or realizing after patients have started enrolling that the appropriate blood sample tubes have not been dispatched to the sites.

Here is a pyramid that outlines the levels of project management:

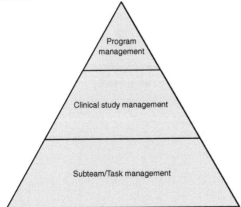

FIGURE 12.3   Levels of project management.

12.2.2 Target Product Profile

The very first step in clinical development is development of the target product profile (TPP). Between the TPP and the clinical development plan, the goal for the clinical program should be well characterized.

A TPP is the core document that outlines the anticipated profile of the drug once it is made available to patients. In essence, it is a condensed package insert that is anticipated. There are many different ways of writing a TPP. The specific format is less important than making sure that it clearly defines what the ultimate deliverable for the program is. Examples are given on the next page.

The TPP is critical because the clinical development plan and the regulatory plan are built around achieving the TPP. The development organization is accountable for delivering a product that meets the TPP.

The TPP is also critical because the assessment of unmet medical need/market forecast is also built on the basis of the TPP.

The TPP ties together and integrates scientific and commercial ends of the drug development endeavor. It is the document by which the decision whether to develop a drug or not is based. It is also the document with which different decisions regarding which drugs to develop are based.

We should note that the internal TPP that we are talking about in this section is *not* the TPP that is shared with the Food and Drug Administration (FDA). The term "TPP" has been adopted by the FDA recently to refer to what is essentially a draft package insert (PI) outline. (See draft guidance, "Target Product Profile – A Strategic Development Tool" on fda.gov.) This TPP is essentially an outline form of the draft PI, with annotations indicating what study and data set support the statements and/or claims in the TPP. It is a useful document, and should be used, but not the same as the internal document we discussed above.

The elements of an FDA TPP include the following:

- Description
- Clinical pharmacology
- Indications and usage
- Contraindications
- Warnings
- Precautions
- Adverse reactions
- Drug abuse and dependence
- Overdosage
- Dosage and administration
- How supplied
- Animal pharmacology and/or animal toxicology
- Clinical studies

	Indication	Efficacy	Safety	Dosing/Administration

Optimistic	• Moderate to severe RA
	• Approved as first-line therapy
	• Claims
	  ◦ Reduction in signs/symptoms
	  ◦ Inhibition of structural damage
	  ◦ Improvement in physical function
		• ACR20: 70%
		• ACR50: 50%
		• ACR70: 25%
		• Onset of response in 25% of patients (ACR 20) – occurs as early as 48 hours from first treatment, and in most almost always by 2 weeks
			• No increase in serious infections compared to control and lower than TNF inhibitors
			• No increase in malignancy compared to control
			• No significant Ab formation
			• Combination w/other DMARDs/biologics – no increase in safety signals
			• No immunosuppressive
				• SC injection once a month, nonweight-based

Target	• Moderate to severe RA
	• Approved as first-line therapy
	• Claims
	  ◦ Reduction in signs/symptoms
	  ◦ Inhibition of structural damage
	  ◦ Improvement in physical function
		• ACR20: 70%
		• ACR50: 50%
		• ACR70: 25%
		• Onset of response in 25% of patients (ACR 20) – occurs as early as 1 week from first treatment, and in most almost always by 2 weeks
			• Slight increase in serious infections but lower than TNF inhibitors
			• No increase in malignancy compared to MTX alone
			• No significant Ab formation
			• Combination w/other DMARDs/biologics – no increase in safety signals
				• SC injection every other week

Minimal	• Moderate to severe RA
	• Approved DMARD failures
	• Claims
	  ◦ Reduction in signs/symptoms
	  ◦ Inhibition of structural damage
	  ◦ Improvement in physical function
		• ACR20: 60%
		• ACR50: 40%
		• ACR70: 20%
		• Onset of response in 25% of patients (ACR 20) – occurs as early as 1 week from first treatment, and in most almost always by 2 weeks
			• Slight increase in serious infections but lower than TNF inhibitors
			• No increase in malignancy HAHA <10%
			• Mild, reversible hypertension in 5% of patients, not requiring treatment
			• Combination w/other DMARDs/biologics – no increase in safety signals
				• SC injection once a week

FIGURE 12.4   Sample TPP 1:

Description	Antibody against gd1 surface antigen
Mechanism of action	Induction of apoptosis in tumors cells
Indications	Non-small cell lung cancer, Stage IIIa/IIIb, front line (initial)
	Solid tumors (later)
Dosage	1 mg/kg every 4 weeks
Background therapy	Carbotaxol and Avastin
Pre-medication	None
Safety	Well tolerated, adverse event rates similar to control arm, no bone toxicity
Contraindications	Allergy to goodimab
Warning	Long-term toxicity has not been established
Precaution	5–10% rate of infusion reactions
Drug/food interaction	None
For impaired renal function	No need to adjust dose
For impaired hepatic function	No need to adjust dose
Effect of age	No need to adjust dose
Effect of race	No need to adjunct dose
Pregnancy and lactation	Do not use in pregnancy
Storage	Room temperature

FIGURE 12.5   Sample TPP 2: Product profile for Goodimab.

12.2.3 Clinical Development Plan

A clinical development plan is a document that maps out the proposed series of clinical trials that will allow the drug to reach the market with the characteristics outlined in the TPP. It will often also include the preclinical work to support the plan, as well as a CMC plan to support the clinical studies and to meet market needs.

It usually lays out the rationale for the drug, including scientific rationale for why the drug might work, the unmet medical need, the current therapeutic options, regulatory path, and clinical studies.

12.2.4 Flowcharting, Project Scoping, and Gantt Charts

One of the first steps in project management is to put together the team. This is described below. The second is to map out the timelines and the dependencies. Drug

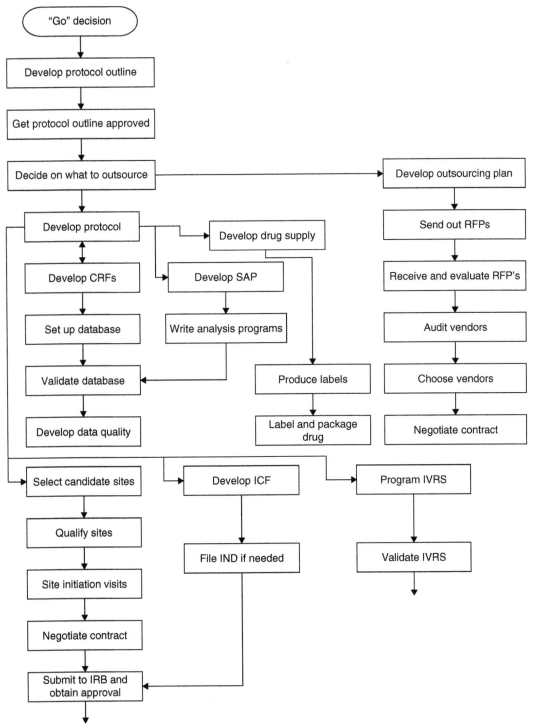

FIGURE 12.6 Flowchart of clinical study process.

FIGURE 12.6 (*Continued*)

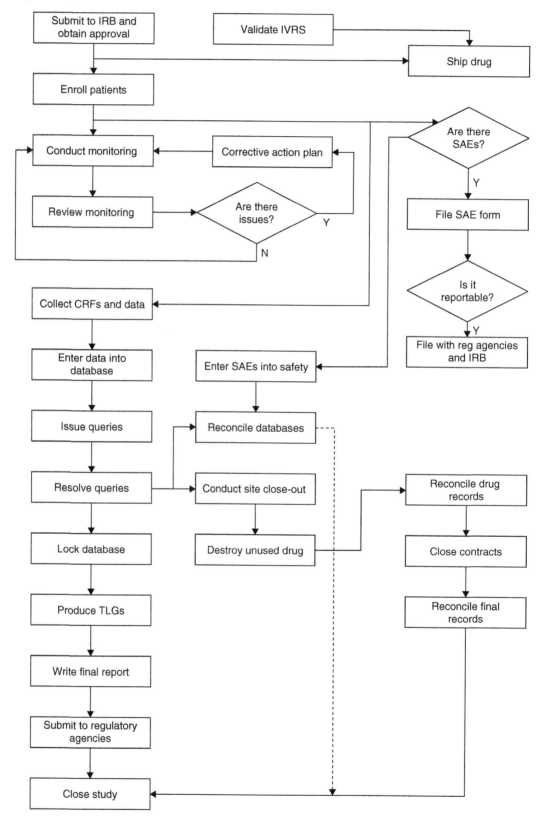

development is a complicated process, and it is critical to map out all the steps several years in advance.

The simplest first step is to draw up a flowchart, as below. Often, there will be a template flowchart that can be used, already developed for the company or organization.

Concurrent with the flowchart, most organizations will require that a project scope document be prepared that outlines the rationale for the study, the anticipated cost and timelines, and other pertinent information. An example is given below:

The second step is to construct a detailed Gantt chart that includes all the major tasks. Next, the critical path

there will be a new critical path, and the process should be repeated to then shorten that critical path.

12.2.5 Key Players, Organizations, and Teams

There are many functions and organizations involved in designing and executing a study. Some of the key players and organizations are listed below:

Sponsor: This is usually the organization funding the study. Typically, it would be corporations, government

---

Project Identifier
Project Number: 1234

Project Title: Randomized, Placebo-Controlled, Double-Blind, Parallel Group Phase II Study Comparing Examplamab vs. Placebo in Patients with Moderate Asthma

Submission Date: June 2, 2003
Approval Date: June 7, 2003
Prepared by: Someone
Approved by: Bigwig

Goals and Objectives
Description: This is a 200 patient study to determine whether we should proceed to Phase III.

Objectives:
1. Determine whether Examplamab is effective and safe in reducing exacerbations in patients with asthma
2. Enable the Go/No-Go decision into Phase III

Deliverables:
1. First patient enrolled by September 30, 2003
2. Last patient out by September 30, 2005
3. Enable Go/No-Go by October 15, 2005
4. Final Study Report by December 15, 2005

Rationale:
1. This study is necessary before moving onto Phase III
2. The clinical review committee has determined that the design is appropriate
3. This study is necessary to meet the corporate goals.

Timeline
Initiations: 48 hours from approval
Completion: 30 months from initiation
Stretch Timeline: completion 24 months from initiation
Worst Case Timeline: completion 48 months from initiation

Business Investment
Total Budget: $6,000,0000
  Internal Headcount: 5
  Outside Spending: $3,000,000
  Allocated Overhead: $1,000,000

Stretch Budget: $5,500,000
Worst Case Budget: $10,000,000

Amount already in the current approved project budget: $6,000,000

Approach
Monitoring: NexCRO
Statistics and Data Management: internal
Safety monitoring: internal

Alternate approaches:
1. Perform entire study internally
2. Not perform the study

Risks and Contingency Plans

Attachments
Protocol
Clinical Review Committee Minutes
Detailed Budget

FIGURE 12.7 Project Scope Document.

should be identified. The critical path is the sequence of tasks that are rate limiting. In other words, there will be a set of tasks that together determine the length of the project because other tasks must wait for those tasks to be finished. Attention should be directed toward reducing the length of time required for those tasks, with the goal of removing some of the tasks from the critical path. Once this is done,

(NCI, NIH, etc.), or a nongovernment organization such as American Diabetes Association. Sponsor is distinguished from a *sponsor–investigator* who designs and conducts his own study such as at his own clinic. Definition in the CFR states:

[Sponsor is a] person who initiates a clinical investigation but does not actually conduct the investigation, that is the test article

is administered or dispensed to or used involving a subject under the immediate direction of another individual.

21CFR50.3(e)

Sponsor means a person who takes responsibility for and initiates a clinical investigation. The sponsor may be an individual or pharmaceutical company, governmental agency, academic institution, private organization, or other organization. The sponsor does not actually conduct the investigation unless the sponsor is a sponsor–investigator.

21 CFR 312.3 (b)

As a general rule, the organization that files the IND or the equivalent is usually the sponsor, although the regulations provides that someone who finances a study and directs it may be considered to be a sponsor as well. There may be more than one sponsor for a study.

Clinical Research Organization (CRO): This is an organization hired by the sponsor to conduct a trial or part of a trial. Per FDA,

Contract research organization means a person that assumes as an independent contractor with the sponsor, one of more of the obligations of a sponsor, e.g., design of a protocol, selection or monitoring of investigations, evaluation of reports, and preparations of material to be submitted to the Food and Drug Administration.

21CFR 312.3

Regulatory agencies: These include the national regulatory agencies such as FDA, regional agencies such as the EMEA, and similar bodies.

Institutional Review Boards (IRBs) and Ethics Committees (ECs): These are independent organizations responsible to making sure that patient rights and safety in clinical trial are protected. Most IRBs and ECs are associated with individual hospitals, universities, and other medical centers. There are also national ECs in Europe, as well as central commercial IRBs in the United States.

Key personnel involved in clinical study execution include:

Medical monitor: The sponsor representative who is responsible for assessing adverse events and overseeing the study to make sure that the protocol and GCP is being followed, and that patient safety is being protected.

Clinical research associate (CRA) or monitors: Sponsor personnel who is responsible for interacting with the clinical sites and ensuring that the study is being conducted properly.

Investigator or principal investigator (PI): This is the physician who conducts the study at his site. Typically is an MD or DDS. He is responsible for conducting or overseeing the conduct of the study at the clinical site, and is also responsible for safeguarding patient safety. The patient is under his or her care.

Investigator means an individual who actually conducts a clinical investigation. In the event an investigation is conducted by a team of individuals, the investigator is the responsible leader of the team.

21 CFR 312.3 (b)

PI usually refers to the investigator (see below). In some cases, PI can also refer to a specific PI who is overseeing the entire study or leading the study, and who typically authors the resulting publication.

Sponsor–Investigator: This is someone who acts as both the sponsor and the investigator. This is typically the case with small academic studies. Corporations, agencies, or other institutions do not qualify as sponsor–investigators. It must be a physician, acting as an individual on his own behalf.

Sponsor–Investigator means an individual who both initiates and conducts an investigation, and under whose immediate direction the investigational drug is administered or dispensed. The term does not include any person other than an individual. The requirements applicable to a sponsor–investigator under this part include both those applicable to an investigator and sponsor.

21 CFR 312.3 (b)

Subprincipal investigator: A physician working on a study under the auspices of the principle investigator.

Site clinical coordinator: The person, usually a nurse, at the study site who coordinates the study.

Subjects: Patients or volunteers enrolled in the study.

It should be stressed that although all the key organizations and key personnel interact extensively, the roles and relationships should not be confused. The investigator (usually the physician) is responsible for treating and interacting with the patient. There should be no contact or relationship between the sponsor and the patient. In most cases, the sponsor should not even know the names of the patients. The investigator has the relationship with the IRB in most cases, except in cases of regional IRBs or National ECs. The sponsor, if it is holding the IND, has the primary relationship with the FDA. The CROs act as sponsor's agent so far as regulatory issues go. The investigator, by the virtue of 1572, established a relationship with the FDA with regard to certain things, namely compliance, but it does not duplicate or overlap with the relationship that the sponsor has with the FDA.

12.2.6 Sponsor Teams

In general, there are several levels of teams in the sponsor organization for programs. It is good practice that every team reports to another team, so that lines of responsibility are clear.

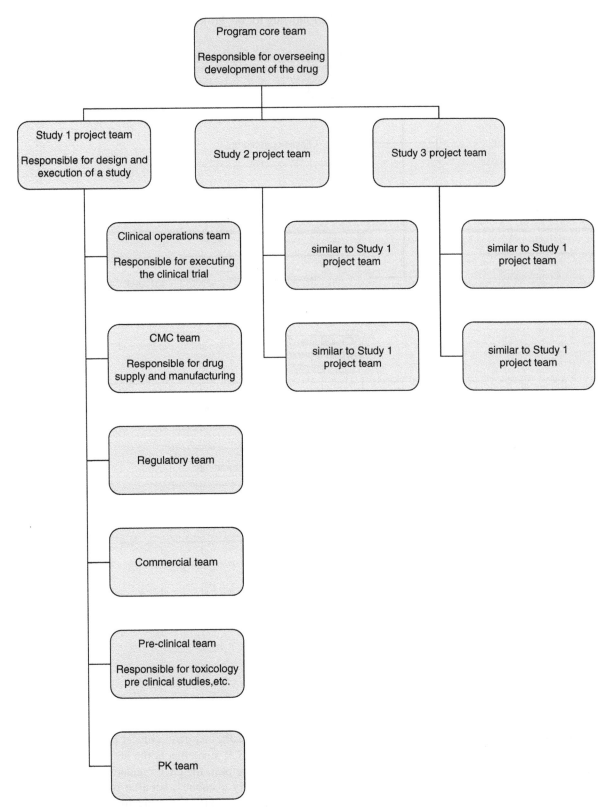

FIGURE 12.8 Typical Team Structure.

In a typical team, the team members will consist of the following for the Project Team:

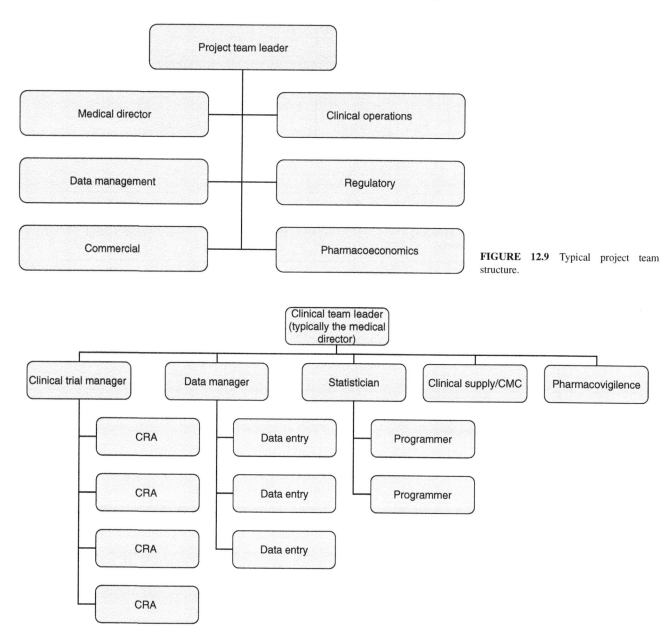

FIGURE 12.9 Typical project team structure.

FIGURE 12.10 Typical clinical team structure.

12.3 COMPLIANCE: GXP AND ICH GUIDELINES, OTHER LEGAL REGULATIONS

12.3.1 GXP Overview

There are several sets of regulations and laws that govern clinical trials.

The first are GXP regulations. GXP encompasses good manufacturing practice (GMP), good laboratory practice (GLP), and good clinical practice (GCP). We will focus on GCP, since that is the most applicable to clinical trials. In the past, the GCP regulations varied significantly from country to country, but after International Conference on Harmonization issued guidelines, the differences have largely been resolved. Although United States, European Union, and Japan are the members of ICH, most countries have now adopted the output from the conference. Nevertheless, the GCP regulations can and do vary a little bit from country to country.

In addition to GCP, there are other laws in each country that govern the conduct of clinical research. For the most part, they are minor variations, but there are some very important variations such as privacy laws specific to individual countries. These can be very serious and can impact the conduct of clinical trials in a major way.

In addition to regulations, there are nonregulations that are important. For example, the policy at most major medical journals that they will only publish studies that had been prospectively listed in a public clinical trial database.

GCP

GCP specifies how a clinical trial is performed. The purpose of GCP is to:

- protect patient safety and rights;
- ensure data integrity.

Specifically, GCP is meant to prevent careless errors, violations, fraud, and ethical issues.

GCPs are required and important because of the following:

- Clinical trials usually involve exposing patients to risk, by administering drugs of unknown efficacy and safety:
- The risk can be very severe and can include death.
- Decision (such as approval decisions) will be made on the basis of data from clinical trials that will affect health and safety of future patients who will receive the drug.

The definition of CGP from ICH Glossary is

> A standard for the design, conduct, performance, monitoring, auditing, recording, analysis, and reporting of clinical trials that provides assurance that the data and the reported results are credible and accurate and that the rights, integrity, and confidentiality of trial subjects are protected.

GCP is concerned with *how* the study is performed, not with *what* drug is being studied or *what* the results of the study are. It specifies how to conduct clinical trials safely, accurately, and responsibly. It is important to know that *even if nothing goes wrong, if GCP is violated, that is a serious problem*. For example, if a serious adverse event (SAE) is not reported, then that in and of itself is a violation of GCP and a major problem, even if no other patient is harmed because of this failure. It is a problem even if it eventually turns out that the adverse event was a mistaken diagnosis and there never was an event.

GCPs are similar to traffic laws that are meant to protect people and minimize risk, such as stopping at a red light or not going over a speed limit. Violating GCP is analogous to running a red light. You can still get a ticket even if you did not cause an accident. It is not sufficient to say that no one got injured as a result of not following GCP. GCP violation in and of itself is a cause for major concern.

The point is that you may not be reckless in how you conduct a study, even if you are lucky and nothing major goes wrong. It is against the law to conduct a study in a reckless (non-GCP compliant) fashion.

There are several key aspects of GCP. The first is the concept of *being in control*. This is composed of two aspects. First, you must have systems in place to detect problems when they occur. You must have, in other words, the quality systems and standard operating procedures (SOPs) (discussed below). For example, you must regularly check the drug supply at the sites to verify that they are being stored properly (secure, at correct temperature, etc.). Second, if problems are detected, you must take corrective action to ensure that the problem is abated and that the way you do business (processes) is modified as is reasonable to avoid the problem in the future.

If you do not have adequate mechanisms to know when things are going wrong, then you are by default in violation of GCP. This is true whether things actually go wrong or not. For example, if you are not regularly checking drug storage, this is a major problem, even if it turns out that the drug had been stored appropriately all along.

Once you put corrective actions into place, it is necessary to loop back at a later date and to close out the findings. One common mistake is to identify deficiency, but to never check to ensure that they have been addressed. Because of this, it is important to have a corrective and preventive action system (CAPA) in place that will track and monitor GCP findings and resolutions. This can be a sophisticated computer system or just a spreadsheet. A CAPA system tracks the violations, the investigations into the violations, and closeouts of the investigation and the issues.

How do you know if you are monitoring enough? How do you know if the corrective action plan is sufficient? The answer is that they are subjective. They need to be reasonable, and more importantly, it must be documented how the decision was taken. For example, if you decide that visiting sites every 6 months is enough, then you should document why you think that, beforehand. If it is not documented in advance, then it is very difficult to justify in retrospect.

The second key aspect of GCP is *ensuring patient safety and rights*. Because of this, informed consent is one of the most important aspects of GCP. The patients must be fully informed, and they must sign and date the informed consent forms. Someone else may not date the forms for them.

In addition, timely reporting of adverse events and proper follow-up is critical. It is very important that the unexpected SAEs be reported within the regulatory timeframe.

The third key aspect of GCP is that *responsibilities can be delegated but not transferred to CROs*. Often, sponsor will hire CROs to conduct studies for them. This is permissible. A "transfer of obligations" form is required in these instances, outlining which obligations the CRO undertakes. However, the title is a misnomer in that the document does not abrogate the responsibilities of the sponsor, so long as it holds the IND or the equivalent.

The fourth key aspect is that *documentation is critical.* If it is not documented, it wasn't done. The documentation should clearly state what and when the data was obtained, how it was obtained, and from whom and where it was obtained.

Where to Find GCP Regulations

Where do you find GCP? GCP can be found in several places. The main source is ICH guidelines that have been published. The ICH guidelines are adopted into law/regulation by individual countries or governments. In the United States, they are published in Federal Register. In the European Union, they are published by the EMEA and then adopted by individual countries by their lawmaking bodies.

In the United States they are found in:

- 21 CFR Part 11: Electronic records; electronic signatures
- 21 CFR Part 50: Protection of human subjects
- 21CFR Part 54: Financial disclosures by investigators
- 21 CFR Part 56: Institutional Review Boards
- 21 CFR Part 312: Investigational new drug application
- 21 CFR Part 314: Application for FDA approval to market a new drug

In ICH, GCP is found in E6 Document: Good Clinical Practice: Consolidated Guidelines:

1. Glossary
2. Principles of ICH GCP
3. IRB/IEC
4. Investigator
5. Sponsor
6. Clinical trial protocols and protocol amendments
7. Investigator Brochure
8. Essential documents for the conduct of a clinical trial

In addition, ICH E2A Document on clinical safety data management is also applicable.

There are some slight differences in the GCP regulations in different jurisdictions. Usually, the individual countries tailor the regulations to their specific circumstances. In the process, they will usually tighten the GCP regulations, not loosen them. For example, FDA has made it clear that in their view, the minimal number of patients in the safety database that ICH recommends is the minimal number, and that they will often require a larger database. In general, the most strict and conservative should be followed. In addition, you should remember that GCPs prescribe the minimal standards. There is nothing to prevent you from applying and following higher standards.

GCPs, compared to GMPs and GLPs leave much more to the discretion of the sponsors and investigators. For example, GMP regulations might specify "10 parts per million"

as the acceptable level of particulate matter in the air during the fill process, as opposed to saying "low enough level of particulate matter to prevent contamination of the drug vials." GCP regulations are much more likely to have requirements such as "adequate monitoring to ensure all SAEs are reported" rather than "at least one monitoring visit every 6 weeks."

GCPs are set of regulations – they are not laws *per se*, but have the force of laws. FDA and EMEA also put out guidelines. Guidelines are recommendations and fall below the level of regulations. In theory they do not have to be followed. In practice, they almost always are to be followed, though.

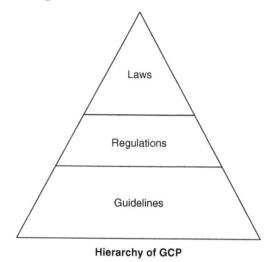

Hierarchy of GCP

FIGURE 12.11　Hierarchy of laws and regulations.

In addition, the FDA posts its internal policies and procedures on the web, including their procedures for reviewing applications, conducting audits, and so forth. These are just as valuable, if not more valuable, than the formal GCP regulations and guidelines. In particular, the *Compliance Program Guidance Manual for FDA Staff* which can be found in Appendix A and on the web at http://www.fda.gov/ora/compliance_ref/bimo/7348_811/default.htm is absolutely critical to read.

In addition, a very useful resource is CDER's Manual of Policies and Procedures (MaPPs). MaPPs are approved instructions for internal practices and procedures followed by CDER staff to help standardize the new drug review process and other activities. MaPPs define external activities as well. All MaPPs are available for the public to review to get a better understanding of office policies, definitions, staff responsibilities and procedures. MaPPs are found at http://www.fda.gov/cder/mapp.htm.

12.3.2 GCP Content

The GCP regulations are widely available on the web and as collections bound into books, so we won't reproduce them in this book. We will, however, give a brief overview. The regulations lay specific requirements on each person or entity involved in conducting clinical trials. The requirements are, as we mentioned above, designed to ensure patient safety and data integrity. As such, much of it is directed at:

- ensuring that people performing the studies are qualified and trained;
- ensuring that there are standardized procedures for various aspects of the study;
- ensuring that there is adequate monitoring and oversight of the study;
- ensuring that drug is stored properly and disposed of properly;
- ensuring that the protocol is followed and accurate data is collected;
- ensuring that any safety problems are detected and addressed as quickly as possible.

GCP is evolving, and will continue to change over time. Let's examine the responsibilities of each of the major entities.

Sponsor Responsibilities

- Selecting qualified personnel, training them, documenting their training, and refreshing their training
- Filing appropriate regulatory filings and keeping them updated
- Selecting qualified investigators and sites
- Allocating duties clearly
- Ensuring appropriate data management, data handling, record keeping
- Quality assurance/control
- Investigational drug accountability
- Informing investigators promptly of significant new data, particularly safety data
- Ensuring that informed consent is being obtained properly
- Ensuring that IRB approval is being done properly and that they are being kept informed properly
- Prompt safety reporting: FDA and investigators/IRBs
- Monitoring/Auditing
- Ensuring the investigators are following the protocol
- Selecting CROs and vendors who are qualified
- Documenting transfer of obligations
- Overseeing CROs and vendors properly

CRO/Vendor Responsibilities
The CROs/vendors have the responsibilities that are delegated to them by the sponsor. For those assigned responsibilities, they have as much responsibility as the sponsor.

Investigator Responsibilities

- Filling out appropriate regulatory forms
- Ensuring the staff are qualified and trained

- Submitting the protocol and informed consent form to the IRB
- Keeping IRB informed of pertinent information
- Keeping drug stored appropriately
- Following protocol
- Reporting any SAEs quickly and accurately
- Keeping records for the appropriate length of time

IRB Responsibilities

- Ensuring appropriate composition of the IRB
- Keeping written minutes
- Reviewing protocols and informed consent forms (ICFs) thoroughly and scientifically

12.3.3 Other Regulations

Health Insurance Portability and Accountability Act Guidelines

In addition to GCP, there are many other regulations. For example, there are strict privacy laws in many countries. In the United States they are HIPAA regulations. These were passed in 1996, and have very stringent requirements and penalties, including criminal penalties.

HIPAA applies to "covered entities" which are health care providers, health plan, and health care clearinghouses. A pharmaceutical company typically is not a covered entity. However, it can become a hybrid or a covered entity by doing certain things, such as, for example, collecting information from patients in an outreach or patient support programs.

The definition of protected health information (PHI) is:

- created or received by a health care provider, health plan, health care clearinghouse, or employer;
- relates to physical or mental health or condition, provision of health care, or payment for provision of health care;
- identifies or could be reasonably used to identify individual;
- electronic, paper, or oral;
- includes demographic data collected from an individual.

HIPAA applies to person for 2 years after death as well.

The penalties for negligent disclosures are $100–$25,000/person/year. For wrongful disclosure, the fine can be up to $250,000 and 1–10 years in prison.

For clinical research, HIPAA disclosures are required from the covered entity (e.g., the investigator) to the sponsor. Disclosures are allowable under one of the following.

- HIPAA authorization by patient;
- IRB/EC or Privacy Board waiver;
- de-identification of patients by either removing 18 prescribed data elements or statistical analysis and opinion.

In practice, de-identification is almost impossible. The 18 prescribed elements are:

- Name
- Geography (if lower than state level)
- Zip code
- Dates of birth, admission, discharge, death, etc.
- Age
- Telephone number
- Fax number
- Email address
- Social security number
- Medical record number
- Account numbers
- Health plan beneficiary number
- Certificate and license numbers
- Vehicle identification and serial numbers
- License plate numbers
- URIs
- IP address number
- Finger and voice prints and other biometric identifiers
- Face photos and similar images
- Other unique identifiers

In order to transmit PHI, you will generally obtain an HIPAA consent. This is often part of the ICF or attached to them. It notifies the patients of HIPAA rights, and obtains their consent for transfer of the information. The consent must be clear on whom the transfer will be to, and that once it is transferred that it may no longer be protected. In addition, if there is an agreement between a covered entity and a business partner, it may be transferred to the partner.

The authorization/release of HIPAA must be for a specific study. It cannot be for an unspecified future use, except for creation of repository or a database (e.g., a recruitment database). In certain states such as California, the authorization must expire after a period of time. The required "core elements" of authorization to use or disclose PHI are as follows:

- Description of PHI to be used or disclosed
- Persons authorized to make the use of disclosure
- Person to whom the PHI is being sent
- Purpose of the use or disclosure
- Expiration date (or "none")
- It must also include statements
  - Right to revoke authorization plus exceptions
  - How authorization or lack thereof will affect treatment, enrollment, payment, etc.
  - That PHI may no longer be protected under HIPAA once it's been disclosed

The authorization must be signed and dated by the patient, must be in plain language, and the patient must receive a copy of the authorization.

Under certain circumstances, a limited data set can be transferred or disclosed without authorization, but the type of data that can be released under this is very limited.

In addition, information that is collected in order to fulfill a regulatory requirement, such as AE reporting, is exempt from HIPAA.

Covered entities must keep written or electronic records of items that need to be documented. The records must be kept for 6 years after the date of creation or last date in effect.

European Union Clinical Trial Directive

The EU Directive was first published by the EMEA in 2001. The purpose was to harmonize the initiation and conduct of clinical trials in the European Union. Among other things, it was also designed to:

- protect patients, especially incapacitated and minors patients;
- standardize applications for starting trials;
- standardize EC process;
- standardize pharmacovigilance data handling;
- allow information exchange between European Union countries;
- mandate GCP inspections.

The directive applies to all medicinal trials that are interventional. It applies to both commercial and noncommercial trails, although the standards are slightly looser for noncommercial trials.

The directive does not automatically become effective across European Union. Each country must implement it by passing laws enacting them. They can add more detail during the implementation.

Now, there are five detailed guidance documents associated with the directive:

1. European clinical trial database (EudraCT).
2. The request for authorization of a clinical trial on medicinal products for human use to the competent authorities, notification of substantial amendments and declaration of the end of the trial.
3. The application, format and documentation to be submitted in an application for an EC opinion.
4. The European database of SUSARS (Eudravigilance).
5. The collection, verification, and presentation of adverse reaction reports.

The terminology of the directive is as following:

- The Agency: EMEA
- Competent Authority: country's regulatory body
- Member State: country within the European Union
- Commission: body that drafts the European laws

The directive requires that for a clinical trial application, the following must be submitted to a competent authority:

- Application form with the Eudract number
- Protocol
- Investigator's brochure (IB)
- Investigational medicinal product number
- Country specific information

For submission to the EC, the directive standardizes the material and process. The following are required:

- Application form and Eudract number
- Protocol
- IB
- Recruitment arrangements
- Subject information and consent
- Insurance and indemnity details
- Financial arrangements

Now, you should know that in addition to the European Union countries, there are non-European Union countries that follow European Union regulations. These currently include Iceland, Norway, Liechtenstein, and Switzerland, Russia, Croatia, Georgia, Ukraine, and Yugoslavia.

There are specific things that should be pointed out:

- E2B requires electronic submission of SUSAR reports
- EC and CA must be notified of study completion and final reports

European Union Data Protection Directive

This directive applies to personal data, including any data about living individuals who can be identified either directly or indirectly from that data of that data combined with other information in possession of the data controller. This applies to data that is on a computer or in a similar strctured form.

It is important to note that this directive applies not just confidential data but any personal data. It also applies to physicians, not just to patients.

Data controller: Entities that determine the purpose and means of processing. Usually sponsor or in some cases the investigator.

Data processor: Any entity that processes personal data on behalf of the controller, including CRO, IVRS vendor, etc.

With regard to the question of which country's law applies, if the controller is in European Union, then the laws of that country apply. If not, then the local laws apply.

The data protection says that personal data must be:

- processed fairly and lawfully;
- collected for specific explicit legitimate purposes;
- adequate, relevant, and not excessive;
- accurate;

- not kept for longer than necessary;
- secured.

In order to be able to process personal data, it must be done under certain circumstances, one of which is under consent. The consent must include the following:

- Identity of controller and representative
- Purpose
- Recipients of data
- Whether the replies are voluntary or obligatory and the impact of failure to reply
- Existence of right to access to and to correct data
- Additional information necessary to guarantee fair processing

Of course, this means that the subject has the right to the data, and in addition, has the right to know what data is being processed and whom it is being disclosed to, and the right to correct data and to rectify data that doesn't comply with the directive.

The controller must protect the data from accidental destruction or loss, unauthorized changes, or unauthorized disclosure/access. Controller must ensure that the processors will have the security measures in place and will only process the data on instruction from the controller. This must be in writing, in a contract.

Also, the personal data can only be transferred outside European Union if the country has adequate safeguards on personal data, or if consent is obtained from the subject. United States does not qualify, so the subjects must consent to the transfer.

U.S. Financial Disclosure Regulations

21 CFR Part 54 was enacted to minimize bias that could be caused by financial conflict of interest on the part of investigators in clinical trials. It calls for disclosure of potential financial conflict of interest on the part of the investigators with the financial outcome of the product or financial interest in the sponsor.

Most clinical trials are covered but the following are not:

- Phase I and PK studies
- Large open-label safety studies at multiple sites
- Treatment protocols
- Parallel track protocols

Financial conflict of interest is defined as follows:

- Any financial arrangement where the amount of investigator's compensation is tied to the outcome of the study.
- Any payment over $25,000 (cumulative) beyond which is part of the site contract for the study and is appropriately paid for services.
- Any proprietary interest (royalty, etc.) in the product or drug.
- Any equity above $50,000 in sponsor's stock.

Most of these apply from beginning of study to 1 year after completion of the study. It is critical to have a system for tracking payments to the investigator over the entire period of the study because the $25,000 limit is cumulative. The tracking system must cover payments not just from the clinical group but from marketing group, sales group, etc. because it applies to all payments from the sponsor.

Remember to collect financial disclosure form not just at the beginning of the study but also at the end, a year past the completion of the study.

Publication and Disclosure

In September 2004, the International Committee of Medical Journal Editors (ICMJE) published a joint editorial requiring that clinical trials be registered before the enrollment of the first patient. The policy applies to trials that start recruiting after June 30, 2005. Trials in violation of this policy will not be published by the journals that have adopted this policy, which includes most of the major medical journals. The intent of the policy is to prevent sponsors from hiding data from negative trials.

Their definition of a clinical trial is:

> Any research project that prospectively assigns human subjects to intervention and comparison groups to study the cause-and-effect relationship between a medical intervention and a health outcome.

Phase I studies are excluded from the policy.

The registration must include the following data fields, called *Minimal Registration Data Set* (taken from http://www.icmje.org/clin_trialup.htm, accessed September 18, 2007):

TABLE 12.1 Minimal registration data set

Item	Comment
1. Unique trial number	The unique trial number will be established by the primary registering entity (the registry).
2. Trial registration date	The date of registration will be established by the primary registering entity.
3. Secondary IDs	May be assigned by sponsors or other interested parties (there may be none).
4. Funding source(s)	Name of the organization(s) that provided funding for the study.
5. Primary sponsor	The main entity responsible for performing the research.
6. Secondary sponsor(s)	The secondary entities, if any, responsible for performing the research.
7. Responsible contact person	Public contact person for the trial, for patients interested in participating.
8. Research contact person	Person to contact for scientific inquiries about the trial.
9. Title of the study	Brief title chosen by the research group (can be omitted if the researchers wish).
10. Official scientific title of the study	This title must include the name of the intervention, the condition being studied, and the outcome (e.g., The International Study of Digoxin and Death from Congestive Heart Failure).
11. Research ethics review	Has the study at the time of registration received appropriate ethics committee approval (yes/no)? (It is assumed that all registered trials will be approved by an ethics board before commencing).
12. Condition	The medical condition being studied (e.g., asthma, myocardial infarction, depression).
13. Intervention(s)	A description of the study and comparison/control intervention(s) (For a drug or other product registered for public sale anywhere in the world, this is the generic name; for an unregistered drug the generic name or company serial number is acceptable). The duration of the intervention(s) must be specified.
14. Key inclusion and exclusion criteria	Key patient characteristics that determine eligibility for participation in the study.
15. Study type	Database should provide drop-down lists for selection. This would include choices for randomized vs. nonrandomized, type of masking (e.g., double-blind, single-blind), type of controls (e.g., placebo, active), and group assignment (e.g., parallel, crossover, factorial).
16. Anticipated trial start date	Estimated enrollment date of the first participant.
17. Target sample size	The total number of subjects the investigators plan to enroll before closing the trial to new participants.
18. Recruitment status	Is this information available (yes/no)? (If yes, link to information).
19. Primary outcome	The primary outcome that the study was designed to evaluate description should include the time at which the outcome is measured (e.g., blood pressure at 12 months).
20. Key secondary outcomes	The secondary outcomes specified in the protocol. Description should include time of measurement (e.g., creatinine clearance at 6 months).

Most sponsors register the study at clinicaltrials.gov, but other registries are acceptable if they meet the following requirements (from the ICMJE statement):

- The registry must be accessible to the public at no charge.
- It must be open to all prospective registrants and managed by a not-for-profit organization.
- There must be a mechanism to ensure the validity of the registration data, and the registry should be electronically searchable.

12.3.4 International Data

In general, all studies including international studies must be performed under GCP. Most jurisdictions will accept data generated in other countries, though most have a preference for having at least some of the data come from patients within the country. As far as FDA regulations go, there are three ways of performing international studies:

1. Perform the study ex-United States only. An IND does not need to be filed with the FDA.
2. Perform the study in the United States and ex-United States, and place all the sites under a U.S. IND. In this case, FDA regulations must be followed for all the sites, in addition to the regulation of the country the sites are in.
3. Perform the study in the United States and ex-United States but only place the U.S. sites under the IND. Usually, this is accomplished by splitting the study into two studies or two sister protocols that are analyzed as one study at the end. In this case, only the U.S. sites are subject to FDA oversight.

FDA will accept data from foreign studies even if they are not performed under an IND if they meet the more stringent of

1. Declaration of Hensinki;
2. laws and regulations of the country of the sites.

12.3.5 Institutional Review Boards and Ethic Committees

IRBs are part of GCP but are covered in Chapter 2.

12.3.6 Quality System, SOPs and Training

As mentioned above, you must maintain control of the study at all times. In order to do this, you need a quality system. A quality system is composed of the following:

- Policy statement
- SOPs
- Guideline/Work instructions
- Training
- Monitoring of the processes (audits)

A policy statement is a general declaration that the studies will be conducted in compliance with GCP.

SOPs are documents that operationalize the policy statement by outlining how the tasks must be performed. It is the "recipe" for conducting various aspects of clinical trials. If done well, it will

- protect patient safety and rights;
- ensure integrity and quality of the data produced;
- ensure that GCP is being followed;
- allow you to document that GCP is being followed;
- establish consistency.

There is usually a hierarchy of SOPs. At the top level is the SOP on SOPs. This is the SOP that outlines how an SOP will be written, who authorizes/approves SOPs, when it becomes official/active, who can override or grant exceptions to the SOPs, how often SOPs will be reviewed, how soon and often people must be trained on SOPs, and so on. At the next level down, there are multi-functional SOPs that apply to many groups. At the bottom are SOPs that apply only to a limited number of people.

All SOPs must be dated, stated to whom it applies, and there must be a system for tracking versions of them. This is critical because when you are audited, you will be required to show not only the current version of the SOP but also the version that was in effect at the time a task was done, and you must show that the task was done according to that version of the SOP.

It is critical to make the SOPs comprehensive but at the same time as simple as possible. It is worse to have an SOP and not follow it than to not have one at all. For example, do not write, "Remove paper clips and file the document facing toward the forward of the file" but rather "file the document." Otherwise, if the auditor finds a paper clip on the document, that is a GCP violation.

It is also critical to make the SOPs not overly strict. The SOP should only mandate doing things a certain way only if it has to be done that way. For example, it should not state "the AE report must be photocopied in duplicate and a copy sent to the medical monitor" if in 10% of the time the report should be sent to the chief medical officer (e.g., while the medical monitor is on the road). It should say "the AE report must be photocopied and a copy sent to the medical monitor *or similar person*." Otherwise, you would be in violation 10% of the time.

Training

Of course, SOPs won't do much good unless the employees are trained. A formal training program must be in place. There should be periodic general GCP/GXP training (typically every 1–2 years). In addition, there should be a matrix that lists the SOPs required for each job family. For instance, CRAs and clinical operations personnel would be trained in one set of SOPs, statisticians in another, and so on.

The training must be documented, with signature and time. It should also ideally test for understanding, typically with a quiz at the end of each training session.

Typically, the SOP on SOPs should specify how long a new employee has until they must compete the training for his job family. IT should also state how long employees have from the time that an SOP is created or modified to train on it, and how often they need to re-train on it. Of course, there should be allowances specified as well on exceptions and extensions, such as when an employee is on maternity leave.

The SOPs should be kept in the employee's training file. The training file should also include other training that the employee has received, such as external training courses the employee has attended.

Other Records

Signed and dated CVs and job descriptions must also be kept. They should be updated at least yearly, and certainly when the job descriptions change. A current organizational chart must also be kept current, ready for inspections.

12.4 AUDITS AND CORRECTIVE ACTIONS

12.4.1 Overview

Per ICH, an audit is

A systematic and independent examination of trial related activities and documents to determine whether the evaluated trial related activities were conducted, and the data were recorded, analyzed and accurately reported according to the protocol, Sponsor's SOPs, and applicable regulatory requirements.

ICH 1.6

We discuss audits before discussing other aspects of study conduct because all activities performing in the course of the study should be performed with an eye to being prepared for an audit. If the study fails audit, all the work may be for naught.[1]

Before delegating responsibilities to a CRO or a vendor, an audit should be performed to ensure that they are capable to doing the task. Similarly, sites should be audited before they are selected. During the course of a trial, there should be periodic audits to ensure that the study is being conducted properly. The vendors should be audited, and the site should be audited (sometimes called co-monitoring) to ensure that the monitoring visits are being performed property. The frequency of audits will vary, and depend on the number of patients the site is enrolling, the number of queries, etc. The frequency and the criteria for audits should be outlined in advance, and be justified in advance, in a written form.

After the study is complete, audits should be conducted to verify that the conduct was appropriate. The highest enrolling sites should be audited, and the sites with the highest number of adverse events, as should the problematic sites (such as sites with numerous protocol violations). In general, the sites you want to audit are the sites that the regulatory agencies might audit.

Some of the other things that might trigger an audit include the following:

- Inconsistent or outlier data
- Data that is too perfect: no missed visits, no dropouts, no noncompliant patients, etc.
- Physicians practicing outside their expertise
- Too many studies at one site
- Very rapid enrollment
- Data inconsistent with other sites
- Complaints from subjects or employees

12.4.2 Preparing for FDA Audits

There are several types of audits that regulatory agencies perform. One is periodic routine audits. These are usually unannounced and can occur at any time. They will typically target a specific function, such as safety or data management system. Another is a for-cause audit. These are triggered by a specific event, such as a complaint, an unreported SAE, or some other occurrence. The third is a pre-approval inspection or audit. Typically, if a drug is about to be approved or may be approved, the agencies will conduct an audit to verify that the study was conducted properly.

The agencies may audit the sponsor, the CRO, the site, or any combination. They can audit within their jurisdiction or outside (e.g., in another country).

AS mentioned earlier, it is vital to become familiar with FDA's manual to its auditors for conducting audits (the BIMO guidance). They can be found at http://www.fda.gov/ora/compliance_ref/bimo/7348_810/48-810.pdf and is included in Appendix A.

It is critical to have an audit readiness plan at all times. If you have filed NDA or BLA, then it is critical to have inspection readiness plan as well. Of course, the appropriate people should be trained – it is of little use having a plan that no one can execute.

An audit readiness plan and pre-approval inspection plan should include the following:

- All the receptionists, including temps, should be trained what to do if an inspector arrives: ask for ID, call the lead audit host (typically, the head of regulatory group).
- There should be a lead audit host identified, and a backup.
- There should be a notification list that the receptionist or the lead host should use in case of an audit.

---

[1]Much of the material in this chapter is based on presentations by Firoz Nilam, given in various venues.

- There should be a defined procedure for how the audit will be handled: where the auditor will work, how to give him access to photocopying, etc.
- Part 11 compliance should be reviewed.
- All previous observations from previous audits should have been closed out properly.

The personnel involved should be trained in the process. They should have run-throughs. They should be trained in how to answer the auditor's questions. The two key aspects of training should be:

1. always be truthful;
2. never volunteer more information than asked for.

Most importantly, there should be periodic mock audits. There are former FDA and EMEA inspectors who provide mock audit training services.

For routine, unannounced audits, the process should be along the following lines:

- Inspector arrives and announces himself.
- Receptionist asks for identification, and calls audit host.
- Audit host notifies people on the notification list or asks someone to notify them.
- Audit host welcomes the auditor.
- Auditor explains the purpose of the audit.
- Audit host shows auditor to the appropriate place, and notifies appropriate personnel. For example, if the inspection is on safety systems, the head of safety will be called to be the audit co-host. The host or co-host should remain with the auditor at all times, typically.
- The auditor performs interviews, asks for documents, asks questions.
- Auditor has a closeout meeting with the audit host to go over the findings, if any.

For the pre-approval audits, you (if the sponsor is being audited) or the site will often get several days' advance notice. This is especially true of foreign sites. As soon as the site gets notified they should notify the sponsor. As soon as it is known that an audit will occur, a team should be dispatched (or if at the sponsor, the team should be assembled) and prepare for the audit. This includes double-checking all the documents, ensuring that they are assembled and accessible readily, re-training the personnel, etc. In cases where there are deficiencies, it should be noted as appropriate and either a corrective action plan put into place or an appropriate documentation be filed. For example, if an IRB approval letter is missing, a duplicate should be secured, and filed along with a note to file indicating that it is a duplicate and that the deficiency was found and corrected. During this process, *do not perform source verification against the case report forms (CRFs) or the data sets if the database has already been locked*. If a discrepancy is found during the source data verification (SDV) process, the database might need to be unlocked, relocked,

tables recreated, and amendment to the study reports and NDA/BLA may be necessary. The sponsor is permitted to be present during clinical site audits (as an observer), and often, that is advisable, though not required.

12.4.3 Sponsor Audits

The audits of sponsors focus on conduct of the study to ensure that the regulations were followed, that patient safety was protected, that data integrity has been protected, that the sponsor exercised control over the study (detecting and correcting GCP violations), that there is no fraud. According to the FDA's internal compliance/audit manual, they focus on the following sponsor duties:

1. Obtain agency approval, where necessary, before studies begin.
2. Manufacture and label investigational products appropriately.
3. Initiate, withhold, or discontinue clinical trials as required.
4. Refrain from commercialization of investigational products.
5. Control the distribution and return of investigational products.
6. Select qualified investigators to conduct studies.
7. Disseminate appropriate information to investigators.
8. Select qualified persons to monitor the conduct of studies.
9. Adequately monitor clinical investigations.
10. Evaluate and report adverse experiences.
11. Maintain adequate records of studies.
12. Submit progress reports and the final results of studies.

The audits can cover a wide variety of areas, but they will include the following:

- Review of who does what: job descriptions, organizational charts, CVs, qualifications, and training records:
  - to check that personnel are qualified;
  - to check that they are current, that they have been current for all employees present and past.
- Review of what has been transferred to CROs and whether it was performed review properly:
  - how the CRO was selected;
  - whether transfer of obligations was clear;
  - review of CRO oversight, including selection records, oversight plan, transfer of obligations, meeting minutes, etc.
- Review of investigator selection and oversight:
  - review of investigator qualification and selection process and criteria;
  - review of monitoring reports and follow-ups, review of audits records (though not of audit reports themselves which are privileged);

- review of investigator selection, including qualification of the investigators, making sure they are not debarred, etc.;
- review of clinical trial supplies, including shipping, return records/destruction records.
- Review of monitor (CRA and medical monitor) selection, qualification, and oversight.
- Review of subject data and CRF:
  - review process for SDV;
  - review process for data cleaning.
- Review of processes, quality system, and SOPs:
  - review of QA system, audit system, CAPA system;
  - that SOPs cover the essential processes, that they are up to date, that versions have been tracked properly, and that study was conducted according to the SOPs in effect at the time;
  - that personnel have been trained in SOP, that they know it, and follow it (they will interview the personnel to verify).
- Review of AE and SAE collection, clarification, and reporting system.
- Review of drug supply, accountability, and disposition.
- Review of other regulatory records.
- Review of investigator files including correspondence and teleconference minutes.
- Review of protocols including consistency with the CRF.
- Review of IB including how often they are updated.
- Review of protocol waivers and deviations.
- Review of SAEs, including upgrade/downgrades, and monitoring for trends, and documentation thereof, and Safety Data Exchange Agreements.
- Notes to File.
- Review of document tracking, archiving, and storage, including Part 11 compliance, privacy protection.
- Review of actions taken on any fraud or product complaints and documentations thereof.

12.4.4 CRO Audits

The most common, and the most important finding with respect to audits of CROs and CRO oversight is the oversight itself. As a rule, most sponsors do not exercise enough oversight of the CRO. Management of CRO is discussed in the later section.

Some of the most common findings are as follows:

- Inadequate task ownership matrix
- No routine audit of CRO
- Failure to follow up on audit findings
- Inadequate system to oversee the CRO
- CRO not qualified
- CRO SOPs not reviewed and approved
- CRO failure to be GCP compliant
- Conflicting SOPs in different parts of the CRO

12.4.5 Investigator Audits

During investigator site audits, here are some common findings:

- Sloppy or improper procedures:
  - the PI does not supervise the study adequately;
  - CRAs don't get a chance to meet the PI;
  - staff is not trained and qualified;
  - site lacks SOPs or more importantly, not following their SOPs;
  - someone other than the patient dates the ICFs for them;
  - improper versions of protocol, ICF, or other forms are used (either out of date, or before IRB/EC approval);
  - study is started before IRB approval;
  - query resolution forms are improperly completed or completed too late;
  - protocol not followed, or amendments not followed, or amendments followed before IRB/EC approval:
    - patient visits or procedures outside specified time window,
    - data not collected,
    - violations of inclusion/exclusion criteria,
    - prohibited medications;
  - improper changes made data already entered on the CRF data (in some cases, this can constitute fraud);
  - failure to review all documents to ensure that all data is being collected (e.g., emergency room charts, clinic charts from other specialists, etc.);
  - not compliant with Part 11;
  - CRA unable to access electronic health records;
  - receipt of drug and temperature monitor not documented properly;
  - pharmacist not trained properly;
  - drug not stored properly;
  - drug not properly prepared and the preparation documented properly;
  - drug not destroyed properly at end of study;
  - drug supply logs incomplete;
  - wrong drug given or right drug given but from wrong kit;
  - IVRS or EDC password shared among personnel.
- Lack of documentation or improper/incomplete/out of date documentation:
  - incomplete screening logs or lack of screening logs;
  - no documentation that patients were asked about AEs;
  - study records or source documents missing, or not signed and dated;
  - IRB/EC documents (minutes, membership list) inadequate or outdated;
  - 1572 or financial disclosure forms not filled out before initiation of the study;
  - 1572 not updated when personnel changes;

- IRB letter, IB, protocols, amendments, are not signed and dated properly;
- CRF forms not filled out properly and timely;
- lack of documentation that items not acted upon were reviewed and considered not significant, such as abnormal laboratory values;
- documents signed by wrong people or people not listed on the Delegation of Responsibilities form.
- Lack of follow-up:
  - SAE not reported;
  - ICF not updated with IND safety updates, and without documentation of reason for not updating it;
  - IRBs not notified timely manner of amendments or IND safety updates without documentation why;
  - sponsor not notified about changes in local regulations;
  - laboratory abnormality not reviewed and followed up in a timely manner;
  - CRF not modified to match protocol amendments;
  - withdrawals not followed;
  - pregnancies not followed to term.
- Inadvertent mistakes:
  - unblinding:
    - due to frank true unblinding,
    - due to laboratory results,
    - due to blinded assessor talking to primary PI.

A word about source documentation: source document is any original document where the information is first recorded. It can be the patient chart, but if the information is first written down in a worksheet, paper napkin, lab coat sleeve, or back of someone's hand, that is the source document. Those items (obviously, it will be hard with someone's hand) must be persevered and be available for audits.

Among these findings, the most important are the ones that affect patient safety and rights. To that end, ICF is very important. They should be signed and dated by the patient. They must be explained clearly to the patient in advance and this discussion must be documented. They must be filed properly. The correct version must be used. They must be updated if there are pertinent changes in the safety profile or other important information.

SAEs must be reported in a timely manner.

The third most important aspect is inclusion/exclusion criteria.

Next is the dosing, that patients received the intended dose and the proper doses.

12.4.6 Other Considerations

You should note that the quality and experience of the auditors will vary. FDA audits in the United States, in particular, may be conducted by generalists who are not necessarily experts in drugs. It will sometimes be necessary to

educate them gently. Foreign audits by the FDA are usually performed by more senior, experienced personnel.

For foreign audits (FDA auditing ex-U.S. or ex-U.S. regulator auditing U.S. sites, etc.), it will often be helpful to arrange for housing and logistics, including contacting the site as well as locating an independent translator. Please be mindful that the travel and lodging expenses may be constrained for many regulatory agencies when arranging for them. You cannot pay for those expenses, so you should make sure they are not overly burdensome. It is a good idea to ask them what kind of accommodations they would prefer.

The outcome from the audit may be one of the following:

- No significant findings (unusual, but the best outcome).
- 483s – these are forms on which significant findings or deficiencies are noted.
- Warning and untitled letters.
- Re-inspection.
- Termination of an exemption (IND, IDE, INAD).
- Refusal to approve or license.
- Withdrawal of approval (PMA, NDA, NADA).
- Determination of not substantially equivalent or recission of a 510(k) for devices.
- Implementation of the Application Integrity Policy.
- Initiation of stock recovery – see Regulatory Procedures Manual Part 5, 5–00–10.
- Seizure of test articles.
- Injunction.
- Prosecution under the FFDCA and other Federal statutes, that is, 18 U.S.C. 2, 371, 1001, and 1341.
- Referral of pertinent matters with headquarters' concurrence to other federal, state, and local agencies for such action as that agency deems appropriate.
- Debarment or closure of the site, facility, or the company-wide activities (the most severe).

For any significant findings there must be a response, outlining how the deficiencies will be corrected. If the findings are to the site, the sponsor should help the site craft responses to the findings.

The clinical site will often devote a great deal of time to an audit if it occurs. Though not always standard, it is advisable to include a provision for reimbursing the site for the time and effort they spend on audit preparedness and audit itself.

12.4.7 Corrective Action

There will be, after almost every audit, findings. They are generally classified into the following:

- Critical – extremely serious findings that must be corrected right away, or in some cases, require immediate cessation of the study.

- Major – serious finding that may have significant impact.
- Minor – less than serious findings.

Obviously, any issues that impact patient safety must be investigated and corrected right away.

Having findings *per se* is not a cause for major concern; so long as there are not so many that it throws into question whether there is an effective compliance system in place. What is a cause for major concern is if there are findings that were previously noted and have not been corrected. Let us repeat: it is not a sin to make a mistake, but it is a major sin to make the same mistake more than once. Auditors are not very forgiving – nor should they be – of repeated, uncorrected violations.

To that end, the most important part of an audit is the follow-up. The follow-up should consist of the following:

1. *Response*: This takes each finding one by one and responds to it. The finding may be accepted, with a corrective action (with a target date) identified or the finding may be disputed (with the rationale).
2. *Root cause analysis*: For each major or critical finding (and in some cases, minor findings as well), there should be a root cause analysis. The root cause analysis identifies gaps in the process that allowed the mistake to occur. It is important that the root cause identified is a process not a person. IT is not a process for finding who's at fault – it is for finding out what process is at fault.
3. *Corrective action implementation*: This should address correcting the mistake itself (e.g., training records out of date) and more importantly, should address the root cause (e.g., no system in place for tracking training records on a regular basis).
4. *Reassessment of effectiveness of corrective action*: If the corrective action was not effective, then a new corrective action plan should be put into place.
5. *Closeout of the audit findings*: All finding should be closed out.

Of course, all these should be documented.

12.4.8 Fraud

Fortunately, fraud in investigations is rare, but it does happen. For example, investigators might make up a study patient. They might not collect the data and make up the data. There must be an SOP to deal with fraud. Fraud must be investigated immediately and thoroughly. If there is fraud, then the regulatory agencies should be notified right away, the site must be closed down, and the IRBs should be notified.

Generally, there will be a committee made up of senior executives to investigate all allegations of fraud. Any fraud found should be reported to the IRB and to the regulatory agencies.

12.5 PROTOCOL DEVELOPMENT AND MEDICAL MONITORING

12.5.1 Role and Requirements of a Medical Monitor

Each study must have a *medical monitor* (MM). In most cases, the medical monitor is a physician, although in some cases he may be a dentist, pharmacist, or other qualified personnel. Because the most important duty of the medical monitor is to safeguard patient safety, it is often difficult for other personnel to serve as the medical monitor, although it can be done with appropriate experience and backup by a physician. In some cases, the medical monitor is called *medical director*, *study physician*, or simply *monitor* – or combination of these names.

Per FDA guidance,

> Physicians, veterinarians, clinical research associates, paramedical personnel, nurses, and engineers may be acceptable monitors depending on the type of product involved in the study. A monitor need not be a person qualified to diagnose and treat the disease or other condition for which the test article is under investigation, but somewhere in the direct line of review of the study data there should be a person so qualified.

A medical monitor is the person in charge of the study and who has the primary responsibility for ensuring that the safety of the patients in the study, as a whole, is protected. He is responsible for all the patients in the study. This is in contrast to the investigator, who has responsibility for the safety of the patients in his particular practice. While the MM has no direct contact with individual patients – he doesn't have the opportunity to do physical examinations or take history from them – he is in a unique vantage point in that he can see the adverse events from all the patients in the study, and therefore can interpret new AEs in context of previous AEs and can find patterns. For example, a nosebleed in and of itself may not cause concern to the investigator, but if the MM knows that the two previous patients with nosebleeds subsequently developed disseminated intravascular coagulation, he would know to take action right away. Therefore, the most important role of the MM is to monitor adverse events closely, and to ensure that patient safety is being protected.

In some cases, the pharmacovigilance group will process adverse events, and there is some debate over whether the MM or the pharmacovigilance physician should be responsible for the safety of the study patients. On the one hand, the MM knows the study better than anyone else. On the other hand, the PV physician has the vantage point of seeing all adverse events across multiple studies of the drug and related drugs. There are also some who argue that the PV physician is more independent because it is not "his study." Either way is acceptable, but in general, it is preferable to have the MM hold the primary responsibility over safety because knowledge of the study and the drug almost always is more important in assessing events. Also, PV is usually no more independent since they are still employees of the same sponsor.

The second major role of the MM is science. He is generally responsible for designing the study and for interpreting the results at the end of the study. As part of these duties, he is responsible for understanding the drug, the target indication, other drugs for the target indication, past regulatory and development history for the field, and so on.

The third major role of the MM is oversight of nonsafety issue during the study. He is responsible for protocol waivers/ deviations, for interacting with investigators, for leading or participating in the interactions with regulatory agencies, and so on. In some companies, the MM is also responsible for managing other personnel on the study project, including CRAs, statisticians, data managers, and so forth.

12.5.2 Protocol Development

The protocol serves several functions:

- Outlines scientific rationale and objectives.
- Pre-specify primary endpoint and statistical analysis.
- Serves as handbook and background for investigators.
- Specifies the procedures, visits, and other things that need to be done in the course of the study.
- Specifies the data to be collected.

The key principles for a protocol are clarity, brevity, specificity, and accommodation.

Above all, a protocol needs to be clear. It should specify if systolic blood pressure is required, if diastolic blood pressure is required, whether leg cuffs are acceptable, etc. Otherwise, it will generate lot of questions from investigators regarding which way to perform the procedure, and even worse, may result in their performing the procedure inappropriately.

A protocol should be explicit about data that must be collected in a certain fashion and those that do not. For example, if the urine collection absolutely needs to be collected 3–6 hours after a drug is administered, it should be specified as being required, but if 7–8 hours is acceptable, then, 3–6 hour window should be a recommendation, with the broader window being the requirement. A protocol specifies what is acceptable and unacceptable data, and if a specimen is collected even 1 minute after 6 hours, then it is a protocol violation. If in fact a specimen that is collected at 6 hours, 0 min, 1 second would be useless, then the protocol should impose a limit of 6 hours, but if not, then it should leave it as a recommendation rather than a requirement. A protocol needs to be specific about what is important and what is not important to do in a particular way.

It should also anticipate any unusual situations or exceptions and have instructions for it. For example, it should give instructions on what to do if a patient misses a visit, or if the ECG is uninterpretable, etc.

A protocol should be brief – the last thing you need is a protocol that is so long that the investigator is discouraged from reading it.

A protocol should be parsimonious. If a measurement is not required, it should not ask for it. Respiratory rate, for example, is a common piece of data that is collected but is almost never necessary. This does not mean that data that is needed should not be collected. It means that data generally should not be collected unless it is known what the data is for. While in some cases, the data may be useful later for data mining, in practice the data is never used, and the amount of resources on collecting the data and cleaning it is tremendous. Excess data collection threatens the integrity of the study.

Below is an outline of a typical protocol.

Protocol

Title
Site
Investigators
IRB
Summary
Background
Rationale
Objectives
Patients
Study design
Treatment definition
Concurrent treatment
Clinical and laboratory measurements
Planned data analysis
Dose rationale
Administrative aspect
Labeling
Preparation of drug
Record retention
Informed consent
Confidentiality
Adverse reactions
Signatures

12.5.3 Informed Consent

Because clinical trials are typically conducted with drugs of unestablished safety and efficacy, and because the goal of the trial is not to benefit the patients in the study but rather future patients, an ICF is an important requirement of any clinical trial. Both the content of the ICF and the way that it is obtained are important.

The required elements for ICF are outlined in ICH E6 and 20 CFR 50, and are largely similar. ICH calls for following elements:

(a) That the trial involves research.
(b) The purpose of the trial.

(c) The trial treatment(s) and the probability for random assignment to each treatment.

(d) The trial procedures to be followed, including all invasive procedures.

(e) Those aspects of the trial that are experimental.

(f) The expected duration of the subject's participation in the trial.

(g) The reasonably foreseeable risks or inconveniences to the subject and, when applicable, to an embryo, fetus, or nursing infant.

(h) The reasonably expected benefits. When there is no intended clinical benefit to the subject, the subject should be made aware of this.

(i) The anticipated prorated payment, if any, to the subject for participating in the trial.

(j) The alternative procedure(s) or course(s) of treatment that may be available to the subject, and their important potential benefits and risks.

(k) That the monitor(s), the auditor(s), the IRB/IEC, and the regulatory authority(ies) will be granted direct access to the subject's original medical records for verification of clinical trial procedures and/or data, without violating the confidentiality of the subject, to the extent permitted by the applicable laws and regulations and that, by signing a written informed consent form, the subject or the subject's legally acceptable representative is authorizing such access.

(l) That records identifying the subject will be kept confidential and, to the extent permitted by the applicable laws and/or regulations, will not be made publicly available. If the results of the trial are published, the subject's identity will remain confidential.

(m) The compensation and/or treatment available to the subject in the event of trial-related injury.

(n) The person(s) to contact for further information regarding the trial and the rights of trial subjects, and whom to contact in the event of trial-related injury.

(o) That the subject's participation in the trial is voluntary and that the subject may refuse to participate or withdraw from the trial, at any time, without penalty or loss of benefits to which the subject is otherwise entitled.

(p) The foreseeable circumstances and/or reasons under which the subject's participation in the trial may be terminated.

(q) The anticipated expenses, if any, to the subject for participating in the trial.

(r) That the subject or the subject's legally acceptable representative will be informed in a timely manner if information becomes available that may be relevant to the subject's willingness to continue participation in the trial.

(s) The approximate number of subjects involved in the trial.

The FDA regulations call for following basic elements of informed consent:

1. A statement that the study involves research, an explanation of the purposes of the research, and the expected duration of the subject's participation, a description of the procedures to be followed, and identification of any procedures which are experimental.

2. A description of any reasonably foreseeable risks or discomforts to the subject.

3. A description of any benefits to the subject or to others which may reasonably be expected from the research.

4. A disclosure of appropriate alternative procedures or courses of treatment, if any, that might be advantageous to the subject.

5. A statement describing the extent, if any, to which confidentiality of records identifying the subject will be maintained and that notes the possibility that the FDA may inspect the records.

6. For research involving more than minimal risk, an explanation as to whether any compensation and an explanation as to whether any medical treatments are available if injury occurs and, if so, what they consist of, or where further information may be obtained.

7. An explanation of whom to contact for answers to pertinent questions about the research and research subjects' rights, and whom to contact in the event of a research-related injury to the subject.

8. A statement that participation is voluntary, that refusal to participate will involve no penalty or loss of benefits to which the subject is otherwise entitled, and that the subject may discontinue participation at any time without penalty or loss of benefits to which the subject is otherwise entitled.

Additional elements of informed consent: When appropriate, one or more of the following elements of information shall also be provided to each subject, per FDA regulations:

1. A statement that the particular treatment or procedure may involve risks to the subject (or to the embryo or fetus, if the subject is or may become pregnant) which are currently unforeseeable.

2. Anticipated circumstances under which the subject's participation may be terminated by the investigator without regard to the subject's consent.

3. Any additional costs to the subject that may result from participation in the research.

4. The consequences of a subject's decision to withdraw from the research and procedures for orderly termination of participation by the subject.

5. A statement that significant new findings developed during the course of the research which may relate to the

subject's willingness to continue participation will be provided to the subject.

6. The approximate number of subjects involved in the study.

Essentially, the goal is to make sure that the patient understands exactly what he or she is signing up for. The ICF should be written as much as possible in nontechnical language so that an average person is able to read it. It will sometimes include additional information than what is outlined above, but should never include less.

An ICF is a form that formalizes the relationship between the patient and the investigator. The investigator will modify it as needed and send it to the IRB for approval. Some sponsors will review the ICF after modification; others will only review it if the "key provisions" have been changed. The sponsor will usually let the investigator aware of what constitutes the "must have" sections of the form.

The ICF is also a legal document, in that it reduces claims for liability for the sponsor under certain circumstances. This is why it is typically reviewed by the legal department as well as the clinical department.

For minors, there is a similar document called an *assent form*. This is written for older minors, and they will typically review and sign it. Of course, an ICF needs to be signed by their guardian as well.

For certain studies, namely studies for emergency indications where it is not possible to have an ICF signed, there are some special procedures that can be followed that obviates the need for an ICF, but these are very rare. An example would be if you were studying defibrillation for sudden death patients, where ICF would not be feasible and there is a very short window before the therapy must be administered. In such cases, you would publicize the study among the public and would need to demonstrate that you have received "community consent." In addition, you would need to put into place certain additional safeguards such as involving an independent physician to provide oversight.

As important as the content of the ICF is how the patient consent is obtained. It is not sufficient to have the patient just sign the form. The patient must truly be informed of the risks. This can take some time, and it can be particularly difficult in countries where there is a very different power relationship between the physician and the patient such as the patients almost always does what the physician asks. For patients who do not speak English, a certified translation (the ICF has to be translated and then back translated and compared against the original document) is required. For patients who are illiterate, it used to be that a verbal consent could suffice, but the regulations around this has been becoming more and more onerous and it is not straight forward to do this any more.

The patient or the guardian/representative must sign and date the form (the date cannot be entered by someone else).

Below are the requirements regarding the consent process, from CFR:

Sec. 50.27 Documentation of informed consent.

(a) Except as provided in Sec. 56.109(c), informed consent shall be documented by the use of a written consent form approved by the IRB and signed and dated by the subject or the subject's legally authorized representative at the time of consent. A copy shall be given to the person signing the form.

(b) Except as provided in Sec. 56.109(c), the consent form may be either of the following:

1. A written consent document that embodies the elements of informed consent required by Sec. 50.25. This form may be read to the subject or the subject's legally authorized representative, but, in any event, the investigator shall give either the subject or the representative adequate opportunity to read it before it is signed.

2. A short form written consent document stating that the elements of informed consent required by Sec. 50.25 have been presented orally to the subject or the subject's legally authorized representative. When this method is used, there shall be a witness to the oral presentation. Also, the IRB shall approve a written summary of what is to be said to the subject or the representative. Only the short form itself is to be signed by the subject or the representative. However, the witness shall sign both the short form and a copy of the summary, and the person actually obtaining the consent shall sign a copy of the summary. A copy of the summary shall be given to the subject or the representative in addition to a copy of the short form.

Remember that in light of any significant new information, especially safety information, the IRB must be notified, the ICF updated, and in some cases, the patient may need to be re-consented with the new form.

12.5.4 Investigator's Brochure

The Investigator's Brochure is an important document that is essentially the "reference book" for the investigator. It contains the information, both clinical and pre-clinical, that may be important or relevant for the investigator to know. The sections in an IB are specified by ICH and include the following (taken from ICH E6).

Title Page

This should provide the sponsor's name, the identity of each investigational product (i.e., research number, chemical or approved generic name, and trade name(s) where legally permissible and desired by the sponsor), and the release date. It is also suggested that an edition number, and a reference to the number and date of the edition it supersedes, be provided.

Confidentiality Statement

The sponsor may wish to include a statement instructing the investigator/recipients to treat the IB as a confidential document for the sole information and use of the investigator's team and the IRB/IEC.

Table of Contents

The table of contents should list the sections in the IB.

Summary

A brief summary (preferably not exceeding two pages) should be given, highlighting the significant physical, chemical, pharmaceutical, pharmacological, toxicological, pharmacokinetic, metabolic, and clinical information available that is relevant to the stage of clinical development of the investigational product.

Introduction

A brief introductory statement should be provided that contains the chemical name (and generic and trade name(s) when approved) of the investigational product(s), all active ingredients, the investigational product'(s') pharmacological class and its expected position within this class (e.g., advantages), the rationale for performing research with the investigational product(s), and the anticipated prophylactic, therapeutic, or diagnostic indication(s). Finally, the introductory statement should provide the general approach to be followed in evaluating the investigational product.

Physical, Chemical, and Pharmaceutical Properties and Formulation

A description should be provided of the investigational product substance(s) (including the chemical and/or structural formula(e)), and a brief summary should be given of the relevant physical, chemical, and pharmaceutical properties.

To permit appropriate safety measures to be taken in the course of the trial, a description of the formulation(s) to be used, including excipients, should be provided and justified if clinically relevant. Instructions for the storage and handling of the dosage form(s) should also be given.

Any structural similarities to other known compounds should be mentioned.

Nonclinical Studies

Introduction

The results of all relevant nonclinical pharmacology, toxicology, pharmacokinetic, and investigational product metabolism studies should be provided in summary form. This summary should address the methodology used, the results, and a discussion of the relevance of the findings to the investigated therapeutic and the possible unfavorable and unintended effects in humans.

The information provided may include the following, as appropriate, if known/available:

- Species tested.
- Number and sex of animals in each group.
- Unit dose (e.g., mg/kg).
- Dose interval.
- Route of administration.
- Duration of dosing.
- Information on systemic distribution.
- Duration of post-exposure follow-up.
- Results, including the following aspects:
  - nature and frequency of pharmacological or toxic effects;
  - severity or intensity of pharmacological or toxic effects;
  - time to onset of effects;
  - reversibility of effects;
  - duration of effects;
  - dose response;
  - tabular format/listings should be used whenever possible to enhance the clarity of the presentation.

The following sections should discuss the most important findings from the studies, including the dose response of observed effects, the relevance to humans, and any aspects to be studied in humans. If applicable, the effective and nontoxic dose findings in the same animal species should be compared (i.e., the therapeutic index should be discussed). The relevance of this information to the proposed human dosing should be addressed. Whenever possible, comparisons should be made in terms of blood/tissue levels rather than on an mg/kg basis.

a. Nonclinical Pharmacology

A summary of the pharmacological aspects of the investigational product and, where appropriate, its significant metabolites studied in animals, should be included. Such a summary should incorporate studies that assess potential therapeutic activity (e.g., efficacy models, receptor binding, and specificity) as well as those that assess safety (e.g., special studies to assess pharmacological actions other than the intended therapeutic effect(s)).

b. Pharmacokinetics and Product Metabolism in Animals

A summary of the pharmacokinetics and biological transformation and disposition of the investigational product in all species studied should be given. The discussion of the findings should address the absorption and the local and systemic bioavailability of the investigational product and its metabolites, and their relationship to the pharmacological and toxicological findings in animal species.

c. Toxicology

A summary of the toxicological effects found in relevant studies conducted in different animal species should be described under the following headings where appropriate:

- Single dose
- Repeated dose
- Carcinogenicity
- Special studies (e.g., irritancy and sensitization)
- Reproductive toxicity
- Genotoxicity (mutagenicity)

Effects in Humans

Introduction

A thorough discussion of the known effects of the investigational product(s) in humans should be provided, including information on pharmacokinetics, metabolism, pharmacodynamics, dose response, safety, efficacy, and other pharmacological activities. Where possible, a summary of each completed clinical trial should be provided. Information should also be provided regarding results of any use of the investigational product(s) other than from clinical trials, such as from experience during marketing.

a. Pharmacokinetics and Product Metabolism in Humans

A summary of information on the pharmacokinetics of the investigational product(s) should be presented, including the following, if available:

- Pharmacokinetics (including metabolism, as appropriate, and absorption, plasma protein binding, distribution, and elimination).
- Bioavailability of the investigational product (absolute, where possible, and/or relative) using a reference dosage form.
- Population subgroups (e.g., gender, age, and impaired organ function).
- Interactions (e.g., product–product interactions and effects of food).
- Other pharmacokinetic data (e.g., results of population studies performed within clinical trial(s).

b. Safety and Efficacy

A summary of information should be provided about the investigational product's/products' (including metabolites, where appropriate) safety, pharmacodynamics, efficacy, and dose response that were obtained from preceding trials in humans (healthy volunteers and/or patients). The implications of this information should be discussed. In cases where a number of clinical trials have been completed, the

use of summaries of safety and efficacy across multiple trials by indications in subgroups may provide a clear presentation of the data. Tabular summaries of adverse drug reactions (ADRs) for all the clinical trials (including those for all the studied indications) would be useful. Important differences in ADR patterns/incidences across indications or subgroups should be discussed.

The IB should provide a description of the possible risks and ADRs to be anticipated on the basis of prior experiences with the product under investigation and with related products. A description should also be provided of the precautions or special monitoring to be done as part of the investigational use of the product(s).

c. Marketing Experience

The IB should identify countries where the investigational product has been marketed or approved. Any significant information arising from the marketed use should be summarized (e.g., formulations, dosages, routes of administration, and adverse product reactions). The IB should also identify all the countries where the investigational product did not receive approval/registration for marketing or was withdrawn from marketing/registration.

Summary of Data and Guidance for the Investigator

This section should provide an overall discussion of the non-clinical and clinical data, and should summarize the information from various sources on different aspects of the investigational product(s), wherever possible. In this way, the investigator can be provided with the most informative interpretation of the available data and with an assessment of the implications of the information for future clinical trials.

Where appropriate, the published reports on related products should be discussed. This could help the investigator to anticipate ADRs or other problems in clinical trials.

The overall aim of this section is to provide the investigator with a clear understanding of the possible risks and adverse reactions, and of the specific tests, observations, and precautions that may be needed for a clinical trial. This understanding should be based on the available physical, chemical, pharmaceutical, pharmacological, toxicological, and clinical information on the investigational product(s). Guidance should also be provided to the clinical investigator on the recognition and treatment of possible overdose and ADRs that is based on previous human experience and on the pharmacology of the investigational product.

12.5.5 Medical Monitoring, Documentation, and Line Listing Review

In the course of a study, the MM should continually review data to ensure that the study in on track. He should review line listings, which are listing of recent data by patient and visit. The listing should be reviewed for abnormal data, missing data, and potential safety signals. If the MM notices that there are inconsistencies or missing data in the listings, he should notify the study personnel so that corrective action could be taken. For example, the instructions for the CRF may be confusing or wrong.

The MM should also review monitoring visit reports on an ongoing basis, to ensure that no site is in serious GCP violation, that patient safety is being protected, and that findings are being closed out in a timely fashion.

MM will often be in contact with various sites and investigators. He should document all significant contacts with the sites in writing and maintain a file. This should include emails and telephone calls.

The MM will also make decisions on difficult or ambiguous data management issues if a medical input is required. For example, he may be asked to decide whether a patient who missed 2 visits out of 10 should be counted as a major protocol violator and be excluded from the per-protocol analysis. Or he may be asked to decide whether myocardial infarction (MI) secondary to trauma should be mapped to MI or not in the course of adverse event coding.

12.5.6 Protocol Deviations and Waivers

Ideally, a protocol should be so well written, and should anticipate all contingencies so well that there is no need for a protocol amendment or any waivers in the course of the study. In such as case, the integrity and interpretability of the study is maximal. However, this is rarely the case.

There are multiple reasons for protocol changes and deviations in the course of the study. The types of deviations/changes include the following:

- Protocol deviations and violations:
  - major violations:
    - authorized by the sponsor as a waiver,
    - not authorized by the sponsor as a waiver;
  - minor violations:
    - authorized by the sponsor as a waiver,
    - not authorized by the sponsor as a waiver.
- Protocol amendments.
- Protocol administrative changes.

Sometimes the assumptions regarding the protocol initially are not valid; other times they change due to external circumstances. Sometimes it's not possible to define in advance every contingency. There are limitations on how much can be specified in writing. For example, patients with age over 90 may be excluded in the protocol, but a healthy 90 year old might be perfectly fine to include in the study.

Sometimes the enrollment is too slow because the inclusion and exclusion criteria are overly strict.

A protocol deviation and protocol violations are essentially the same thing – both occur when there is a variance between the protocol and the activity. In other words, whenever an investigator does not follow the instructions outlined in the protocol, there is a protocol violation.

The exact wording of the protocol determines whether there is a violation or not. For example, if the protocol specifies that a urine sample must be collected within 24 hours, and it is collected 24 hours and 10 minutes after the drug is given, then it is a protocol violation. If the protocol specifies that the urine sample must be collected at 24 ± 6 hours, then it is not a violation. Often, a protocol is poorly drafted in such a way that it is almost certain to generate needless violations. For example, if the protocol specifies that each patient must return for a follow-up visit once a month ±2 days for 12 months, it is almost certain to result in a protocol violation. It would be better to write that a monthly visit is expected ±2 weeks (unless it is indeed critical to have the visit exactly on a monthly basis).

Protocol violations can be classified as major or minor.

A major violation

- results in harm to patient, either actual or potential;
- impacts integrity of the data;
- is due to willful or knowing misconduct;
- the investigator or staff commits other serious of continuing noncompliance with federal, state, or local regulations.

A minor violation

- has little or no effect on the risk to the research subjects;
- does not materially affect integrity of the data;
- is not due to willful or knowing misconduct.

In many cases, the distinction between major and minor violations is subjective. With respect to the threat to the integrity of the data, violations that affect the type of patients enrolled (inclusion/exclusion criteria), the storage/dosing/blinding of the drug, or primary endpoint of the study tends to be major violations.

Major violations need to be recorded when discovered, tracked, and corrective action steps must be instituted in response to them. In some cases, the IRB should be notified. If violations that affect the safety of the patients recur, then the study might need to be placed on hold until the issues leading to the violations can be corrected.

Impact of Protocol Violations

Major violations can have a major impact on the interpretability of the study. For example, if a significant number of patients did not meet the inclusion/exclusion criteria, then the study may be uninterpretable, because the analysis with those patients included may differ from the analysis with those patient excluded. Sensitivity analysis with and without major protocol violators should be performed at the end of all studies to verify the robustness of the results.

It is extremely important to note that even minor protocol violations are serious, because every violation degrades the quality of the study. Multiple minor violations suggest poor design/draftsmanship of the protocol and/or poor operationalization of the study, both of which portend poorly for the reliability of the results. Furthermore, each protocol violation is a violation of GCP, and each violation must be addressed.

Causes of Protocol Violations

There are multiple causes of protocol violations. Some of the most common are listed below.

Unclear instructions can be a major source of violations. For example, an inclusion criterion that excludes patients with recent MI's can lead to much confusion if the cutoff for "recent" is not defined. Instruction to exclude patients with documented ulcers can be confusing because "documented" can mean documented in the chart to some physicians, and documented by EGD to others.

Difficult–to–carry–out instructions can also be a major source of violations. For example, instruction to administer the drug within 1 hour of patient presentation to the hospital if the inclusion criteria include a serum pregnancy test may lead to frequent protocol violations since the turnaround time for such tests may be more than an hour at many hospitals.

Simple errors can lead to protocol violations. In the course of a long, complicated study, some errors are unavoidable.

Of note, in cases where it is necessary to violate the protocol in order to protect patient safety, the safety of the patient is paramount.

Protocol Waivers

As mentioned above, it is not possible to anticipate everything that might occur in a clinical trial; and as a result, protocol waivers may be necessary in some circumstances. In general, protocol waivers should be reserved for situations that are expected to happen once, or rarely, since if it is expected to occur frequently, a protocol amendment should be instituted instead. In some cases, where an amendment is planned, but the process of putting the amendment in place is expected to take a significant amount of time, it is appropriate to issue protocol waivers until the amendment has been instituted.

Protocol waivers are permission for the investigator to violate the protocol. In general, they can be issued only by the medical monitor on the trial, and the request for the waiver, the rationale for the waiver, and the action on the waiver request must be clearly documented.

Some possible reasons for issuing the waiver are as follows.

Inclusion/Exclusion Criteria Wrongly or Poorly Drafted

In most cases, it would be better to institute a protocol amendment, but as a short-term measure or in extraordinary circumstances, a waiver of the inclusion/exclusion criteria may be acceptable. For example, the exclusion criteria might specify no episode of prior MI, but if the MI was a small non-Q wave MI from hypotension at age 20 secondary to toxic shock syndrome, then the intent of the exclusion criteria may not be met.

Waiver for Trivial Things

The protocol might specify a CT scan within 30 days of drug administration, and the earliest timeslot available for the CT scan may be 31 days after drug administration.

Waiver for Mistake

Some laboratories' upper range of normal might be different than specified in the protocol. The intent of the protocol might have been to exclude patients with abnormally high WBC counts, and the way it is written, patients with high normal levels would be excluded. This should be corrected with an administrative change but in the short term, waivers may be appropriate.

Caveats

We should emphasize that protocol waivers create risk. This goes double for waivers given not because of scientific reason, but because of enrollment pressures or need to maintain relationship with investigators. If the study doesn't enroll the intended patients, or if the drug is not given consistently, or if the endpoint measurements are unreliable, then it becomes very difficult to interpret the result. This can result in FDA and other regulatory agencies rejecting the study data. Specifically, waivers:

- can change the original intent of the study, different population than intended, different dose than intended;
- can increase the variability of the study to make it more difficult to interpret;
- can put results at risk – if sensitivity analysis reveals different results for patients with waivers and those without.

Amendments

Protocol amendments are a necessary evil in the course of many trials. Generally, the amendments can be divided into the following categories: amendments due to poor draftsmanship/incorrect assumptions; amendments due to information from the study; amendments due to logistic considerations; and amendments due to external factors.

Some amendments are due to poor draftsmanship or poor planning/assumptions. These are amendments that could have been prevented, and often occur when the sponsor enters an unfamiliar area. For example, the study might call for a complicated test that can only be performed at a few sites. Or the assumptions regarding event rate turns out to be incorrect.

Some amendments are due to information obtained in the course of the study that could not have been obtained otherwise. Amendments due to safety events fall into this category. The majority of amendments are due to logistic considerations, such as enrollment rates. Finally, external factors can necessitate an amendment. An example is a competing drug becoming available partway through the trial.

Amendments require a tremendous amount of work, and often require re-consenting of the patients in the trial. Any time there is a significant change that can impact the procedure that the patient has to go through, potential risks or benefits, the consent needs to be rewritten. Therefore, the amendments should be carefully considered before being presented to approval.

All the caveats that apply to waivers can apply to protocol amendments, although amendments are instituted in a more consistent manner so that the risks generally tend to be less.

Administrative Changes

Administrative changes are those that arise during the course of the study but do not require a formal amendment, especially if they do not affect patient population, dosing, or endpoint. An example would be changing the MM or his telephone number. Another would be clarifying minor wording in the protocol that may be unclear.

12.5.7 Safety Monitoring

Clinical trials are inherently risky and (to patients) dangerous endeavors. It is only because of tremendous potential benefit to society that they are tolerated. Because of this risk, monitoring the study to ensure patient safety is of paramount importance.

In particular, the Phase I studies are the most risky studies, from the safety viewpoint. The drug is unknown, and potentially catastrophic adverse events can occur, as happened in the infamous FIAU study. The only period of clinical development that comes close to the Phase I studies in terms of risk is Phase IV, shortly after launch of a new drug, when sufficient number of patients become exposed to the drug to uncover rare but SAEs.

The MM must pay attention to both individual adverse events as well as the aggregate adverse event profile. He must be attuned to subtle signs, such as somewhat higher rates of liver enzyme elevations, which might presage more serious hepatic failures. He must also proactively review line listings assiduously to keep current on the pattern of adverse events that may not be serious enough to warrant expedited reporting but may still be of clinical significance.

SAEs and Signals

There are very specific reporting requirements for serious unexpected adverse events. The specific rules are described in Section 12.8.3, and the mechanics of collecting the data and submitting it is usually handled by ancillary personnel in the pharmacovigilance units. However, the MM is responsible, usually, for reviewing the report, assessing the seriousness and relatedness, and for signing off on the submission. MM should also, in especially serious or significant cases, call or visit the site to review primary documents, including radiographic and pathology data. The MM is also responsible for flagging especially important cases to his superior, to the Chief Medical Officer, or the Drug Safety Committee, according to the prevailing internal procedures.

For very serious or important cases, most companies have procedures for escalating the cases for assessment and discussion via peer review. Typically, there is a Drug Safety Committee made up of senior personnel who are responsible to assessing the adverse event, and taking appropriate action. The action can include placing the study on hold, canceling the study, or withdrawing the drug from the market. Ultimately, the Chief Medical Officer is responsible in most organizations for making such a decision.

The MM must also be prepared to assist the investigator in case of SAEs, as the situation warrants. For example, he may be required to give advice in case of overdoses. If there are specific agents or procedures that can reverse the drug effects, such as activated factor VII or plasmapheresis, the MM should be prepared to offer knowledge and advice to the investigator.

12.5.8 Final Analysis and Report Writing

The MM is also responsible for overseeing the analysis, and more importantly, interpretation of the study results. The MM will typically review the SAP with the statisticians at the beginning of the study, collaborate with the programmers in setting up the mock tables and listing, and setting up the zero draft reports with the medical writers.

Though the statisticians and the programmers are responsible for the technical aspects of data analysis, the MM should provide input on the analysis strategy and also on checking of the assumptions behind the analysis. And of course, the interpretation of the data is mostly a clinical task.

Clinical Study Report

A clinical study report (CSR) is a report of the study. It follows standard scientific report format, with introduction, methods, results, and discussion. In order to facilitate the writing of the report, a "zero draft" report is typically written during the study. A zero draft report is a shell report with as much of the report pre-written so that once the results are available, the report can be finished as quickly as possible.

The text of CSR should be brief, since very few people will read it, and most of the critical data is in the tables and graphs. It should be written as would any other scientific report, following practices for good report writing such as being careful about making conclusions that are only clearly supported by data are widely known.

Filing NDA/BLA

If a Phase III study is positive, then the results will usually be filed as an NDA/BLA/MAA. The MM will typically write or oversee the writing of the CSRs and large sections of the regulatory submission. He will also present the data to FDA Advisory Committees.

In writing the reports, the key is to be succinct, clear, and scientifically rigorous. The reports should be considered to be scientific documents, and should exercise similar level of scientific prudence that you would put into a journal article. The conclusions should be conservative and supportable by data. The regulators do not have much time to read the reports, and they do their own analysis anyway, so there is little point in making the reports long. They should hew closely to the facts, with moderate number of tables, and the discussions should be succinct. Other than the regulators, few if any, other persons will read the reports.

All significant studies should be published, even if the results are negative. There is an ethical obligation to publish, since patients volunteered for the study with the understanding that the results will benefit other patients. The publications should be rigorous, and once again, be supportable by the scientific data.

12.6 CLINICAL OPERATIONS

12.6.1 Role of a CRA

The CRA and other members of the clinical operations, such as clinical trial manager, clinical project manager, and other similar persons play a critical role in the conduct of a study. They are responsible for ensuring that the clinical sites have been selected properly, that contracts are in place, that regulatory documents have been collected, that the site has drug, that the protocols are being followed, that data is being collected properly, and a multitude of other tasks. The CRAs are the most hands-on people in the entire conduct of the study, from the sponsor's side.

The counterpart to the CRA is the clinical site coordinator (CSC), who performs complementary functions from the investigator's side. A detailed description of the CSC's role is beyond the scope of this book, but their role is discussed at the end of this section.

The most important of the numerous tasks that a CRA performs are (1) ensuring that the site is following the protocol properly and (2) ensuring that the data being sent into the sponsor by the site is accurate. Both of these tasks usually require on-site visits and indeed, the CRAs spend a significant portion of their time on the road. In addition to these formal tasks, the CRA is usually the most important liaison between the site and the sponsor and is responsible for building and maintaining the relationship. A good CRA can have an enormous impact on the success of a study.

In addition, in some organizations, a CRA or CTM may also serve as the project manager or project leader. In this capacity, they may assume many of the tasks outlined in Section 12.1.

12.6.2 Budgets, Funding and Impact of Economics

The CTM usually manages the budget for the study.

Depending on the type of study and the source of funding, budgets might vary from few thousand dollars to hundreds of millions of dollars. Many early, small trials and post-approval small trials are often funded by the individual investigators or by small grants from government and industry. Much of the larger Phase II and III trials are funded by industry, with the rest being funded by government, or nongovernmental organizations (NGOs) such as World Health Organization and Bill and Melinda Gates Foundation. The government agencies include U.S. National Institute of Health (NIH) and its branches such as National Eye Institute (NEI) and National Cancer Institute (NCI), Cancer Research United Kingdom (CRUK), U.S. Department of Defense (DOD), Centers for Medicare & Medicaid Services (CMS), and so on.

At the beginning of a study, a budget needs to be constructed. Typically, the budget is based on previous experience of the CRA or CSC. However, past experience may not be a good indicator of what a study should cost for two reasons. First, the cost of clinical research is climbing rapidly, at approximately 20% or more per year. Second, the costs of clinical trials vary widely in industry, and to a lesser extend in academia. This is because there is little standardization in how tasks are done and how much the vendors charge. The standard deviation for clinical trial costs usually exceeds the mean cost. In other words, depending on which vendor you select, you will probably see up to 3–5 fold difference in costs.

The bulk of the cost of clinical trial is personnel costs. The payments to internal personnel, payments to investigators, payments to cover cost of contractors, etc. consume much of the budget. Drug development is a capital-intensive industry, but little of it goes toward physical capital investments.

Typically, as a rule of thumb, costs can be broken down as follows: one-third to the site, one-third to the CRO, and one-third for internal costs. Of course, depending on how much work is outsourced, this ratio will change.

A detailed budget should include all internal and external costs, including cost of drug, cost of internal personnel, cost of insurance, cost for CROs, costs for DSMB members, cost for procedures at sites, payments to sites, and so forth. As a general rule, most studies do not come in under budget, and it is not uncommon for studies to exceed budget by 100% or more. This is particularly true when there are inexperienced personnel in charge. The most common reasons for large cost overruns include the following:

- Trial last longer than expected, typically due to slower than planned enrollment. Since personnel costs drive most of the costs, lengthening the trial will have a large impact on the trial.
- Change orders and amendments, which can significantly increase costs, especially if a CRO is involved. Just as in building a house, changing the specifications of a trial will result in change orders from the CRO that can be substantial.

Because there will always be unforeseen events, most of which result in increased costs rather than decreased costs, budgets should allow for 10–20% overruns unless the CTM is very experienced and competent.

There are services that will provide an estimated project budget, such as Fasttrack. Fasttrack uses data they directly obtain from sponsors and tend to be very accurate.

Once the budget has been created, the CTM should work with the finance organization to ensure that the actual spending can be mapped accurately to the budget numbers and that up-to-date numbers will be available in the course of the study. Otherwise, it will be very difficult to manage the study to the budget.

12.6.3 CRO and ESP Selection and Management

Rationale for Outsourcing

While there are some companies that perform all clinical trials with internal employees, it is very common for sponsors to contract with contract research organizations (CROs) and other vendors to conduct part or nearly all of the study. A CRO can be either a clinical operations specialist, responsible for the clinical operations services or full service CRO, which serves as a general contractor that manages not just the clinical operations work but also provides or coordinates other services. The other vendors, sometime called external service providers (ESPs) are generally providers that provide a specific service, such as IVRS or clinical supplies.

The outsourcing is due to several reasons. One common reason is that because the workload associated with clinical trials are lumpy – there are times of high activity, such as during Phase III clinical trials, punctuated by times of low activities. Most companies do not want to hire dozens of people only to lay them off months or couple of years later.

Another reason is capabilities or capacity. Some small companies do not have the skills or infrastructure (such as databases, electronic submission capabilities, presence in foreign countries) to be able to conduct clinical trials. Sometimes, the company does not have the expertise to conduct the trial, or to devise a regulatory strategy, etc. and will often hire a CRO or consultants for the expertise.

Another reason can be cost. Although in general, it is more expensive to hire a CRO to conduct studies than to perform them internally (rule of thumb is that it doubles costs to outsource), it may be less expensive in certain cases, particularly if the CRO can amortize the costs over multiple projects, such as maintaining presence in multiple countries.

Selection of CRO

Typically, CRO selection starts with a request for proposals (RFP). This is a document that outlines the intended study and solicits bids for the project. It will outline the number of patients, the study design, the size of the CRF, number of countries, and so forth. In general, the RFPs are very general, particularly compared to other industries. Ideally, it should include the final protocol, final CRF, as well as the terms of the contract (such as whether the payment will be fee-for-service of by earned value).

Once the proposals come in, the evaluation begins. This includes assessment of not just the costs but more importantly the capabilities and capacity. The industry is nonstandardized and the quality varies significantly between CROs. As might be expected, the costs vary significantly as well, since some CROs are much more cost efficient than others. By law, the CROs are prohibited from communicating about their bids with their competitors, but the quotes will often be close.

You will find that though the quotes are often similar, the final price for the study will be very different at the end of the study, depending on the quality of the CRO and their procedures for how much change orders are worth. In general, most studies come in at about 20–100% over the original budget. Two primary drivers for the increase in costs are change orders – such as when the sponsor changes the protocol or the scope of the project – and enrollment misprojection. As with building a house, a small change order can result in a very large change in price. The length of the trial drives much of the cost of a clinical trial, and most enrollments err on the side of optimism rather than pessimism.

The industry as a whole is moving from fee-for-service model to an earned value model. Previously, the CROs often charged by the hour for the work they did. Because of escalating costs, and because of the fact that CROs are becoming better in terms of quality of work, management skills, and talent, the ability to assess and assume risk of clinical trials are becoming better in the CROs. The combination of the two has resulted often in arrangements where the CROs are paid not for time but for delivering milestones, such as number of CRF pages, the number of patients enrolled, etc. The industry is moving from cost-plus contracts to fixed-price contracts. It is highly recommended that fixed price (earned value) be used wherever possible.

As part of the assessment, the qualifications and experience of the CRO personnel should be reviewed. The experience of the personnel and the CRO in conducting the particular type of trial – the indication, the geography size, phase, etc. – should all be considered carefully. For special studies such as Phase I studies, there are specialty CRO's that specialize in those studies.

Also, it is important to recognize that most CROs have multiple clients. They will of course give highest priority to largest clients. The more business you concentrate in one CRO, the better service you will likely receive. This is reflected in the trend toward preferred provider programs at many companies. More importantly, if you're a small company, you will often be assigned less than the best team from a large CRO.

Once the choices are narrowed down, then the top 2–3 CRO's should be formally audited, to check their SOP's, documentation, physical plant, and so on.

In parallel with the CRO selection, the terms of the contract should be negotiated. In particular, clear specifications outlining which tasks will be performed by the CRO and which by the sponsor should be enumerated. The terms by which pricing of change orders will be determined should also be specified. The team that will be assigned by the CRO to the project should be specified.

This is important, because once the CRO has been selected, since all negotiation leverage is lost. As a rule of thumb, in order to manage the CRO appropriately, you will need one sponsor personnel for every 5–10 CRO personnel. You should be reviewing a sample of monitoring reports, AE reports, regulatory packet, and other similar material. You should co-monitor at least 5% of the sites. You will also need to continue periodic audits of various parts of the study.

You should keep in mind several caveats about working with the CRO. Hiring a CRO to perform a large, multi-million dollar, multinational clinical trial involving unknowns is analogous to building a house. There are many things that can go wrong, that are unpredictable, and the interests of the sponsor and CRO will be somewhat misaligned.

It is important to make a CRO selection carefully. Conducting a clinical trial is difficult, and many CROs do not have the capabilities or capacity they claim to have (or believe themselves to have). The CRO must be qualified.

In addition, clinical development is a service business, and it is currently at a "cottage industry" status. This means that the processes are not well standardized, and the quality of the work depends to a great deal on the quality of the team performing the task. It is therefore important to determine which particular personnel will be working on the project. The "pitch team" that comes to solicit the business is usually not the "work team" that will actually conduct the study, and it is rare that the quality of the latter exceeds or even meets the quality of the former. For this reason, many sponsors insist on "key personnel" clauses into the contract, specifying by name the personnel who will be assigned to the project by the CRO.

Managing and Monitoring a CRO

After CRO selection, there are two critical things to do, right at the beginning of the study. The first is to prepare and approve the vendor oversight plan. This is an internal document that specifies how the sponsor will satisfy itself that the CRO is performing adequately and how the sponsor will ensure that the CRO is upholding GCP. We must stress that the plan must be robust enough to proactively detect GCP violations. The sponsor cannot wait until the CRO tells them about problems. There must be a systematic way of monitoring the CRO – for example with periodic visits, regular reports, regular audits, regular verification of data – that performance is as expected. All these things should be specified in the vendor oversight plan. The plan must be in place at the beginning of the study, since it would be a violation of GCP to start the study before the control mechanisms were in place.

The second important task is to transfer the obligations of the sponsor to the CRO. This is conducted with a document called *Transfer of Obligations*. The FDA regulations specify that

> A sponsor may transfer responsibility for any or all of the obligations set forth in ... part [312] to a contract research organization. Any such transfer shall be in writing and, if not all obligations are transferred, shall describe each of the obligations being assumed by the contract research organization. If all obligations are transferred, a general statement that all obligations have been transferred is acceptable. Any obligation not covered by the written description shall be deemed not to have been transferred.

> A CRO that assumes any obligation of a sponsor shall comply with the specific regulations in this chapter applicable to this obligation and shall be subject to the same regulatory action as a sponsor for failure to comply with any obligation assumed under these regulations. Thus all references to "sponsor" in this part apply to the CRO to the extent that it assumes one or more obligations of the sponsor.

While a CRO may assume any of the sponsor's responsibility, it should be emphasized that the transfer does not relieve the sponsor from responsibility for study. In other words, the sponsor is still responsible for compliance even if the obligation has been transferred. Filing the Transfer of Obligations with the FDA does not change the fact that the sponsor, as the holder of the IND, is responsible for ensuring that the study is done in a compliant fashion.

The obligations should be outlined in a task ownership matrix, which will largely reflect the similar list in the contract.

Below is a sample.

Transfer of Obligations

Pursuant to 21 CFR 312.52, Sponsortech Inc. will transfer to Superior CRO Inc. certain sponsor obligations, as identified below. Superior CRO, Inc. agrees to perform such transferred obligations.

TABLE 12.2 Sample Transfer of Obligations

Task	Superior CRO	Sponsortech
Protocol writing		X
Preparation of CRF	X	
Filing of regulatory documents	X	
Site qualification visit	X	

As with building a house, the CROs need to be managed and communication is very important. Regularly scheduled meetings are critical, and ideally, collocating a sponsor representative at the CRO or a CRO representative at the sponsor is recommended.

The CRO will usually have their internal SOPs. The study can be conducted following either the CRO SOPs or the company SOPs, but this must be clearly defined in the beginning. If multiple CROs are being used, the sponsor SOPs will generally need to be used. Even if the CRO's SOPs are being used, there should be a process for exemptions (either systematic exemptions or one-off exemptions) because there will likely be times when the SOPs are not appropriate or conflict with the sponsor SOPs. The exemptions need to be put into place either before or contemporaneously with the tasks being performed, not in retrospect.

In general, for every 5–7 people assigned to the study by the CRO, the sponsor will need 1 person from the sponsor to oversee the CRO. Alternatively, there are CROs that specialize in managing other CROs, which can be a viable option if you don't have the personnel in house. The oversight includes many tasks, but can be broken down into:

- preparing the specifications and the budget;
- monitoring that CROs work is meeting the specifications and the budget;
- if the work is not satisfactory, preparing and instituting corrective action.

The specifications for the study, such as number of sites, number of monitoring visits, the activities to be performed on the visits, and so forth must be specified in detail. Otherwise, there is bound to be misunderstandings and conflicts later.

The monitoring should be performed through teleconferences, written reports, and in-person visits to the CRO and to the sites. There should be metrics set up in advance so that the performance can be tracked real time. Of course, the sponsor's team and the CRO team must work closely together and develop a good working relationship if the study is to proceed smoothly.

The corrective actions will normally be negotiated with the CRO. Every study will run into unanticipated issues and there will always be a need for corrective action in the course of a study.

The CRO will often subcontract aspects of the study out to another vendor. The sponsor should always retain the right to inspect and approve subcontractors.

12.6.4 Investigator/Site Selection

Selection of investigators and sites is a critical topic, and therefore is covered separately in the next chapter, in detail. Briefly, it consists of assessing three criteria: qualification, recruitment potential, and relationship needs.

The sites and the investigator must be qualified. They must have the appropriate experience in the indication (e.g., it would be inappropriate for a dermatologist to participate in an oncology study except for special circumstances), must have trained personnel including CSC, laboratory personnel if applicable, pharmacist if applicable, must have appropriate facilities (e.g., $-70°$ freezer if applicable unless it is to be supplied by the sponsor), must have other pertinent qualifications (e.g., if they need to overnight ship samples, they must have access to overnight courier service). Obviously, all investigators should be pre-screened to ensure that they are not on the FDA's debarment list. Ideally, the site and the investigator would have conducted previous clinical studies in the indication being studied, though obviously this cannot be an absolute requirement.

The site must also have access to the patients, either from their own practice or from referrals. Sites tend to overestimate their ability to recruit, so as a rule of thumb, whatever number they provide should be divided by 2. For every major exclusion criteria, the rule of thumb is to further multiply the site's estimated recruitment rate by 60%. For most studies of common indications such as rheumatoid arthritis or multiple sclerosis, average recruitment rate of between 0.25 patients per site per month to 0.5 is typical.

Finally, there are usually sites that are of importance because of relationships or strategic importance. These are usually academic sites with major opinion leaders whose participation in the study is important.

12.6.5 Recruitment and Minimizing Dropout and Drug Compliance

This topic is covered in the next chapter.

12.6.6 Site Monitoring and Compliance

Monitoring Plan

A monitoring plan outlines how the study will be monitored to ensure compliance with GCP. Per FDA guidance,

> A sponsor should establish written procedures for monitoring clinical investigations to assure the quality of the study and to assure that each person involved in the monitoring process carries out his or her duties. A single written monitoring procedure need not be developed for each clinical investigation. Rather, a standardized, written procedure, sufficiently detailed to cover the general aspects of clinical investigations, may be used as a basic monitoring plan and supplemented by more specific or additional monitoring procedures tailored to the individual clinical investigation.

Site Qualification

Before a site is selected for participation in the study, a qualification visit should be conducted to inspect the physical plant, to interview the site personnel to ensure that they are qualified, to inspect drug storage area, etc. Per FDA guidelines, a site qualification visit should ensure that the investigator:

- Understands the investigational status of the test article and the requirements for this accountability
- Understands the nature of the protocol or investigational plan
- Understands the requirements for an adequate and well-controlled study
- Understands and accepts his or her obligations to obtain informed consent in accordance with 21 CFR Part 50 (The monitor should review a specimen of each consent document to be used by the investigator to assure that reasonably foreseeable risks are adequately explained.)
- Understands and accepts his or her obligation to obtain IRB review and approval of a clinical investigation before the investigation may be initiated and to ensure continuing review of the study by the IRB in accordance with 21 CFR Part 56, and to keep the sponsor informed of such IRB approval and subsequent IRB actions concerning the study
- Has access to an adequate number of suitable subjects to conduct the investigation
- Has adequate facilities for conducting the clinical investigation
  - Has sufficient time from other obligations to carry out the responsibilities to which the investigator is committed by applicable regulations

Site Initiation

For site initiation, the site must submit the required regulatory documents, receive IRB approval of the protocol and ICF, have an executed contract with the sponsor, and have all other items in order (including validation of sample shipping if applicable, training on EDC as applicable). Typically, there will be an initiation visit where the CRA visits the site and demonstrates the procedures required by the protocol and answers any questions the site might have. In some instances, the investigator meeting includes enough training so that a separate initiation visit may not be necessary.

Site Monitoring

It is standard practice to visit and monitor each site after first patient has been enrolled, and then subsequently every 6–12 weeks. The exact frequency is driven by the complexity of the protocol and the number of patients enrolled at the site. On each visit, the CRA checks to ensure that the documents are in order, that the protocol is being followed, that the drug supply is in order, and that queries are being closed out. In addition, SDV is performed. The CRA will cross-check the information that was supplied by the site on the CRF to the source data (which is usually the patient's medical record) to check that the data is accurate. Some companies rely on CRA's to fill out the CRF's rather than the CRC from the site, which is usually not advisable (since it eliminates independent check by a second party). Many companies perform 100% source verification, which entails checking every piece of data in the CRF. This is almost always superfluous; and SDV of key data, such as inclusion/exclusion criteria, primary endpoints, and serious AEs, with spot checks of other data, is sufficient for most studies.

Per FDA guidelines, the purpose of a monitoring visit is to ensure that:

- the facilities used by the investigator continue to be acceptable for purposes of the study;
- the study protocol or investigational plan is being followed;
- changes to the protocol have been approved by the IRB and/or reported to the sponsor and the IRB;
- accurate, complete, and current records are being maintained;
- accurate, complete, and timely reports are being made to the sponsor and IRB;
- the investigator is carrying out the agreed-upon activities and has not delegated them to other previously unspecified staff.

Also per FDA guidelines, a monitoring visit should ensure that:

- the information recorded in the investigator's report is complete, accurate, and legible;
- there are no omissions in the reports of specific data elements such as the administration to any subject of concomitant test articles or the development of an intercurrent illness;
- missing visits or examinations are noted in the reports;
- subjects failing to complete the study and the reason for each failure are noted in the reports;
- informed consent has been documented in accordance with 21 CFR Parts 50 and 56.

After each visit, a monitoring report should be written that includes, as per FDA guidelines the following:

- The date of the visit.
- The name of the individual who conducted the visit.
- The name and address of the investigator visited.

- A statement of the findings, conclusions, and any actions taken to correct any deficiencies noted during the visit.

Below is a sample report. The MM should review each monitoring report.

Interim monitoring report
Protocol number
Protocol name
Site principle investigator
Site sub-PIs
Address and phone number
Monitor(s)
Site attendees
Patient status
- Screened
- In screening
- Randomized
- Active
- Completed
- Discontinued

Part I: Regulatory documents

Form 1572 (signed)	Present/Absent/Not applicable
PI and sub-PI CV, license, and financial disclosure	Present/Absent/Not applicable
Screening log	Present/Absent/Not applicable
Patient log	Present/Absent/Not applicable
ICF (signed and dated)	Present/Absent/Not applicable
Study correspondence	Present/Absent/Not applicable
Lab director CV	Present/Absent/Not applicable
Lab normal reference ranges	Present/Absent/Not applicable
IRB approval of ICF, ads, and revisions	Present/Absent/Not applicable
IRB roster, minutes, reports	Present/Absent/Not applicable

Part II: Serious adverse events

Any SAE since the last visit?	Yes/No/Not applicable
All SAEs reported in timely manner?	Yes/No/Not applicable
All SAE follow-ups performed correctly and in a timely manner?	Yes/No/Not applicable
If so, IRB notified of new INDs Safety Reports and acknowledgment from IRB filed?	Yes/No/Not applicable

Part III: Case report forms

CRFs complete, promptly signed, and dated?	Yes/No/Not applicable
Source documents available and verified?	Yes/No/Not applicable
All queries and discrepancies resolved?	Yes/No/Not applicable
CRFs collected?	Yes/No/Not applicable

Part IV: Drug accountability

Drug receipts and records filed?	Yes/No/Not applicable
Dispensing records match supply?	Yes/No/Not applicable
Storage conditions appropriate?	Yes/No/Not applicable
Expiration dates acceptable?	Yes/No/Not applicable
If drug was to be destroyed, done correctly and documented?	Yes/No/Not applicable

PartV: Laboratory

Samples stored properly and shipped properly?	Yes/No/Not applicable
Inventory and shipping records up-to-date?	Yes/No/Not applicable
Lab reports reviewed in a timely manner?	Yes/No/Not applicable
	Yes/No/Not applicable

Part VI: General

Action items from last visit completed?	Yes/No/Not applicable
Any changes in personnel or facility?	Yes/No/Not applicable
Any protocol violations?	Yes/No/Not applicable
Meet with PI?	Yes/No/Not applicable
Protocol being followed?	Yes/No/Not applicable

FIGURE 12.12 Sample monitoring report form.

Site Name

The visit started at 8 am on July 20, 2006. Jamie Top, the site coordinator was present. Dr. James and Dr. Smith were not present.

There is a new sub-PI. Eight patients were screened since last visit. Seven were screen failures, and 1 was enrolled. One patient has completed the study since last visit. There are 2 active patients at the site currently.

Regulatory Documents

There has been a new sub-PI since the last visit, Robert Smith, M.D. The regulatory binder has his CV (signed and dated July 2, 2006), his medical license (expiration date December 31, 2009), and financial disclosure form (signed and dated July 2, 2006). There are no other changes in personnel or facility. All ICFs have been signed dated properly.

SAEs

The IND safety report dated March 3, 2006 has not been submitted to the IRB. The site will submit it immediately.

CRFs

CRF for patient AF-334233 was not completed.

CRF for patient DD-334988 was reviewed. There is no IVRS screening confirmation for the patient in the file. The site will request the form from IVRS.

CRF for patient SJ-334002 was reviewed. The outstanding queries have been resolved.

Drug Accountability

There has been no change in storage conditions. The drug records match the supply. Expiration dates were checked.

Laboratory

The laboratory results are not being checked promptly. The site was reminded to do this. The PK samples have been stored properly and are being shipped properly, although two shipments were shipped several days late.

Action Items
Resolved:

New drug has been received.
Outstanding queries resolved.
Sub-PI financial disclosure form filed properly.

Not Resolved:

CRF for patient AF-334233 not completed.

New Items:

The IND safety report dated March 3, 2006 to be submitted to IRB.
IVRS confirmation for patient DD-334988 to be requested and filed.
Laboratory results to be checked promptly.

Site Closeout

At the end of the study, or if site is to be terminated early, a site closeout visit should be performed. At this visit, all the documents are checked to make sure they are in order, final SDV is performed, all the queries are closed out, all follow-up on SAEs are closed out, and the drug is reconciled and typically retrieved from the site for destruction.

12.6.7 Study Conduct Report

In many companies, the CRA, along with the MM, will write a study conduct report, summarizing how the study was monitored, enumerating significant GCP deviations, protocol violations, corrective actions, and the like. This report is an internal document for process improvement, and not part of reports submitted to the regulatory agencies. In most cases, they are protected documents, like audit reports, and not subject to inspection by the FDA.

12.6.8 Clinical Study Coordinator

The clinical study coordinator (CSC) is the project manager at the clinical site. Typically a nurse, a CSC may be fully dedicated to clinical studies or may devote only part of her time to it, the rest of his or her time being devoted to nursing or other tasks.

A CSC has numerous responsibilities. A CSC often prepares forms necessary for the site, files and maintains the study files and records, coordinates the submission of the protocol and ICF to the IRB, often receives and stores the drug, and so on. She is often also responsible for scheduling the patient visits, instructing the patients, coordinating with the pharmacist to prepare drug, calling the IVRS to receive the randomization codes, filling in the CRFs, hosting the CRA on-site visits, and other innumerable tasks.

A CSC is also usually responsible for preparing the site budget, and often participates in the contract negotiation with the sponsor. For single site investigator sponsored studies, the CSC is often responsible for managing the entire site budget, and often for coordinating correspondence with the regulatory agencies.

The CSC is also usually responsible for compliance at the site, and often writes and manages the SOPs at the site.

12.7 STATISTICS AND DATA MANAGEMENT

12.7.1 Statistical Analysis Plan

Prior to unblinding of the data, a statistical analysis plan should be finalized. An SAP is a document that specified the type of analysis that will be performed on the study data set, defines the data set parameters, describes imputation methods for incomplete data, defined sensitivity analyses, and generally describes, prospectively, the set of analysis that will be performed. It adds detail to the brief description of the statistical analysis that is described in the protocol.

For pivotal studies, the plan should be reviewed with the FDA and their agreement as to the appropriateness of the plan be obtained in advance of the study.

The importance of finalizing the SAP prior to unblinding is that once the data has been unblinded, it is impossible not to introduce a bias in designing the analysis plan. Almost inevitably, the analysis will be biased to show a positive result. The reason for this is that there are many judgment calls that have to be made with regard to the population to be included in the final analysis, imputation of missing values, etc. that can have an impact on the final results. And of course, once the data has been unblinded, it is always possible to design an analysis that will make the results look positive. In effect, a *post hoc* SAP turns a prospective study into a retrospective study, and makes it impossible to use the study to ascribe causality.

Some investigators and companies prefer to finalize the analysis plan at the time of protocol writing, to minimize the possibility that the analysis plan could be influenced by the data generated during the study. Even for a blinded study, dropout rates, DSMB recommendations, anecdotal information, and unblinded patient data for unexpected SAEs may be available during the course of the study.

12.7.2 CRF and Database Design, Safety Database

Data from a clinical trial is collected in a CRF. These have traditionally been paper based, but most studies are now based on electronic data capture, described in the next section.

A CRF is a critical piece of the study. It defines the type of data collected, amount of data collected, and therefore directly impacts the cost of the study and the difficulty of monitoring the study. A study with a 20 page CRF is much easier to run and monitor than one with a 2000 page CRF.

The CRF should collect all the data that the protocol says will be collected. In most cases, it should collect little else. The key to CRF design is to be brutal about limiting the amount of data collected. Each additional page of CRF can add hundreds of thousands of dollars to millions of dollars of additional cost. If the data is not absolutely necessary, it should not be collected. To do otherwise is to waste time and resources of the patient, physician, CRC, CRA, data manager, and other personnel.

In general, it is desirable to limit open-ended questions, where the CRC can enter text. Check-boxes and fill-in questions are preferable. For example, rather than asking,

"Please describe any hospitalization," you should ask, "Was the patient hospitalized since the last visit? Yes/No."

To avoid confusion, try not to use negative or double negative questions, such as "Did the patient have no episodes of hemoptysis since the last visit?" Avoid ambiguous abbreviations. Avoid collecting same information in different ways or places.

Ideally, the CRFs should be developed from a standard template that is used across the company or across the various studies for that drug. This will minimize the required training, and will make development of the database easier.

There will typically be a CRF instruction manual that is distributed to the sites. Sometimes in lieu of this, instruction will be printed on the back pages of the CRF. Either is acceptable, but with the former, the advantage is that the instruction can be modified or updated without reprinting the entire CRF.

Database Design
For paper-based CRFs, the database will need to be designed. The data structure should be laid out to be as consistent as possible with the other studies. An annotated CRF, with the variable names mapped to each of corresponding data on the CRF should be developed and archived.

Data Entry
Double data entry is usually performed with clinical studies. Each piece of data is entered separately twice, so that they can be cross-checked against each other.

There are several methods of collecting the CRFs. The classic method is to use triplicate forms, with the physical forms being mailed to the sponsor. Another method is by forms that are faxed to the sponsor, either for subsequent data entry or for automated optical character recognition. The newest method is web-based electronic data capture.

12.7.3 Electronic Data Capture

Electronic data capture uses computers, and usually the Internet, so that the CRC enters data directly into the database. The advantages to EDC are many. First, it lowers error rate, since edit checks can be built into the interface. So if the CRC, for example, enters age as 210, then he can be queried immediately regarding the accuracy of the data.

Second, it lowers costs. It eliminates the cost of data entry. It reduces the number of queries.

Third, it reduces timelines in most cases. It certainly reduces the time between last patient out and database lock.

Fourth, it allows real-time monitoring of the data. This means that if a site is delinquent on entering data, or if there are data quality problems, then corrective action can be taken immediately.

Fifth, it allows true adaptive trials. Whereas in the past, there was a lag of months between a patient visit and data analysis, now the analysis can be available within hours.

This means that it is now possible to have true adaptive clinical trials, where the data can be used to change the study design on the fly. This is revolutionizing clinical trials.

The implementation of EDC requires development of a robust, user-friendly interface that will be usable by CRCs. It also requires ability to control user privileges so that only appropriate persons can enter or alter data, and it requires audit trails, so that if there are alterations, it can be easily tracked by person, date/time, and reason for the change. The system need to be fully validated and compliant with CFR Part 11.

12.7.4 Data Quality and Management Plan and Data Cleanup

In the course of collecting and entering data into the database, there will be errors. The process of correcting the errors is called data cleaning. Data cleaning consists of three steps. First, the data quality and management plan is developed. This plan specifies the algorithm for detecting errors, for correcting errors, and the final standard that the data has to meet before it is consider to be clean. The algorithms might specify the highest acceptable value for data, such as "age below 18 or over 100 should be flagged," or "if all the respiratory rate values from a site are 20, then query." Some of these are called edit checks – simple queries that are automatically generated as the data is entered, to reduce the rate of frank typographical errors. The plan also specified acceptable final error rate. It might, for example, specify that 99% of the outstanding queries be resolved before the database can be locked.

The query process starts with a query form, which specifies the questioned data point, such as "please verify that the patient visited the emergency room three times in two days." The query is sent to the site, and the site fills out the query form.

In general, most sponsors tend to over-query. The percent of queries that results in a change to the database should be greater than 50%, as a general rule.

Obviously, EDC allows easier data cleaning and faster, real-time data cleaning.

12.7.5 Data Monitoring Committee and Interim Analysis

In some cases, there might be a data cut partway through the study, to enable an analysis for the DMC/DSMB. A data cut is an analysis based on the database at a certain period of time, usually with data that has not been fully cleaned.

In some cases, there might be a "soft" database lock to enable an interim analysis. The data up to a certain date or up to a certain visit is cleaned to a standard that is high but not as high as the final analysis, and the data analysis is performed on this partially cleaned database.

12.7.6 Database Lock, Unblinding, and Data Listings

A database lock occurs once the data has been cleaned to the specifications in the data quality plan. The database is frozen, and no further changes are permitted. Data unblinding is typically performed next. There is no turning back after the unblinding. The unblinding is performed by matching the randomization codes to the data in the database. This allows analysis to be performed, and the tables to be generated.

As the first step in analysis, all data should be presented in tables, listings, and graphs (TLGs). This includes data by each visit, data by each patient, aggregate data, etc. Typically, the tables would include both standard deviations and confidence intervals. Means and standard deviations, or in nonparametric cases, medians and quartiles, should be presented.

The programming for the TLGs should be prepared and validated in advance. Validation typically requires two independent sets of programmers to program the TLGs and test/dummy data set to be run with the programs. The output should match each other, and should match the expected output.

Listings are lines of data, sometimes aggregate data, sometimes individual data and they should include the following.

Patient Dispositions and Drug Exposure

This summarizes the number of patients enrolled, the number of patients who were randomized, the number of patients who competed follow-up, the number of patients who discontinued along with reasons for discontinuation, etc. This is usually the first set of analysis because it frames the subsequent data and exposes any gross biases or inadequacies of the data. This section also might include number of patients enrolled by site, by geography, and so forth.

In addition, it is a good idea to prepare a table of major protocol violations, GCP violations, and similar limitations of the data. This is not currently the orthodox way of preparing the tables, but is highly recommended.

There is usually a table summarizing drug exposure and compliance.

Demographics and Baseline Characteristics

This summarizes the characteristics of the patients who were enrolled in the study, usually broken out by treatment groups. This is done in order to assess whether there were significant imbalances in the groups. These tables, in addition to sex, age, race, etc., will often also include baseline disease characteristics such as length of disease, severity of disease, prior medical history, concomitant diseases, etc.

Efficacy Endpoints

Typically, the primary efficacy endpoint is presented first. Then hierarchical primary endpoints, if any, are presented. Hierarchical endpoints are sometimes called contingent primary endpoints. In either case, these are primary endpoints that are nested, such that only if the first endpoint is successful will the second primary endpoint be tested. In this way, the alpha value is preserved.

In general, it is prudent to show the primary results graphically as well as with a table, to show the overall distribution of the data. A Kaplan–Meier curve is traditionally used for efficacy analysis of survival data.

Even for endpoints such as mean changes, it is advisable to use a figure, such as below (from FDA presentation on Raptiva, http://www.fda.gov/ohrms/dockets/ac/03/slides/3983S1_03_FDA-Efalizumab.ppt).

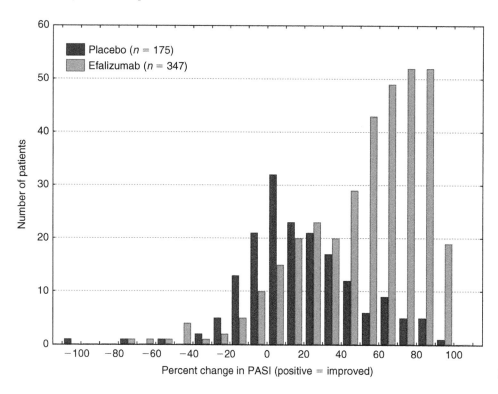

FIGURE 12.13 Efalizumab efficacy.

Or alternatively,

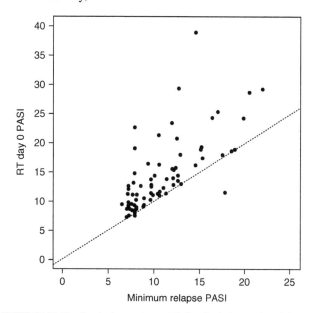

FIGURE 12.14 Psoriasis severity at RT day 0 relative to the minimum relapse PASI value.

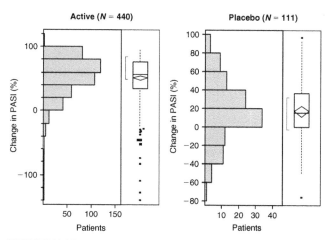

FIGURE 12.15 Percent change in PASI by treatment group.

(both from FDA, http://www.fda.gov/ohrms/dockets/ac/03/briefing/3983b1.htm)

This is followed by secondary endpoints, such as efficacy at different timepoints, secondary measures of efficacy, etc. For composite endpoints, individual scores are presented. For example, ACR20 might be presented at 6 months, followed by efficacy at 3 and 12 months, ACR50, ACR70, X-ray efficacy data, individual components of ACR, and so on. These analyses are meant to characterize the effect of the drug on various measures of efficacy, as well as to assess robustness of the results.

Sensitivity analysis is then presented, with different assumptions, different imputations of the data, and so on. For example, per-protocol analysis may be presented, or imputations using LOCF or other imputations may be presented. An important, but frequently misleading, analysis is to determine exposure–response relationship. This can be done by taking patients who had high levels of drug, or alternatively, free of neutralizing antibodies and examining their response. An analysis that is even more prone to misinterpretation is to look at pharmacodynamic vs. response relationship, where a pharmacodynamic marker is used to analyze response. This may be acceptable in some cases in Phase II studies, but must be interpreted carefully, as will be discussed in Chapter 16.

Subgroups are then often presented. These can be demographic subgroups, such as by race or age, and they can be by sites/geography, or they may be by pre-/post-amendment or by patients enrolled in the first half of the study vs. second half.

Exploratory analysis is then often presented, which must always be considered cautiously. Although nonstandard, it is a good practice to list all the analyses that were conducted, and note which tables were not presented. This, to a degree, addresses the potential for data-dredging by performing multiple analyses.

Response over time, and persistence of response or rebound after discontinuations should also be presented if possible.

Safety Data

Safety section usually starts with a table listing the incidence of any adverse events, followed by deaths, SAEs, common adverse events, and targeted events. Targeted events are events of particular interest, based on the mechanism of action of the drug, previously seen adverse events with the drug, or drugs of the same class, etc.

For example, if the drug prolongs QT, then there ought to be a table summarizing cardiac arrhythmias, sudden deaths, syncopes, etc.

Typically, there would be several levels of groupings – for example, pulmonary events, pneumonias, and viral pneumonias would be several levels of adverse events that should be presented, and an incidence of viral pneumonia

would be in all. Also, both pulmonary adverse events and infectious adverse events would capture viral pneumonia. Drug-related adverse events should also be separated from all adverse events. Dropouts should be analyzed carefully, to determine whether the dropouts were due to adverse events.

Adverse events by patients and by occurrence should also be separated. For example, there might have been 20 pneumonias but 3 patients might have had 2 episodes each, so 17 patients would have had pneumonias. In addition, incidence of adverse events over time should be presented. This is important to determine if there is a first dose effect, and more importantly whether there is cumulative toxicity. Many types of toxicities present only after a length of time, and the signal may not be apparent unless the results are segregated by time. This sort of analysis can also uncover ascertainment biases.

As with efficacy, the adverse events should be analyzed carefully with sensitivity analysis, with different assumptions, and imputations. In addition, there should be sensitivity analysis with different categorizations of diseases. Since any or most of adverse events are categorized retrospectively, it is important to make sure that categorization process doesn't hide signals by using too broad or too narrow categories. There should be a section or an appendix with detailed narratives of all the major or serious AEs.

Laboratory Data

Shift tables are generally used to analyze laboratory data. These are analyses that categorize the values as low, normal, or high (or sometimes very low, low, normal, high, and very high). The values that go from one category to another are captured.

A better way of analyzing the laboratory data is graphically. One helpful way of presenting the laboratory values is to graph pre- and post-drug values on the x- and y-axis. This makes it very easy to detect changes.

Immunogenicity, for biologics, is an important assessment to perform and a table summarizing anti-product antibodies, by total amount and neutralizing antibody amount should be presented. Overdoses are sometimes then analyzed as well as re-challenges – patients who had an adverse event when they received the drug and improved off the drug, and then were re-administered the drug.

12.8 OTHER SUPPORT FUNCTIONS

12.8.1 Regulatory

Interacting with the Regulatory Agencies

The regulatory interactions with the FDA and other agencies will typically be handled by the regulatory affairs personnel, but given that most of the reviewers at the agencies will be physicians, the physicians on the team will often play a significant role.

The keys to interacting with the agency personnel are to recognize the following:

- The reviewers do not know the drug as well as you does. They cannot be certain you are providing all the relevant information. Some sponsors can and do hide information from the FDA! The most critical thing in interacting with the FDA is to be absolutely upfront, because if they suspect you are not being completely transparent and upfront, then they have no choice but to assume that you are hiding things from them or trying to trick them. Therefore, in the filings, you should never bury issues such as safety issues. It should be stated upfront. If they find something buried in the middle of the IND, then they will go through the filing with a fine tooth comb. You should also be very careful about things that might appear to be an effort to trick them, such as placing information in the appendix or referencing nonpeer reviewed articles such as journal supplements or abstracts.
- Most reviewers and other people who work at the agencies are overworked, short-staffed, and short on resources. It is not uncommon for one reviewer to have dozens of drugs on his docket. It is not always easy for the reviewers to get ready access to photocopiers or to have time to photocopy large documents. They may not be in a position to just order journal articles at whim. Make it as easy as possible to them, by being considerate of their time, sending journal articles with submissions, etc.
- The reviewers are public servants and as such, they are the last line of defense when it comes to patient safety. They have an important duty and they take it seriously. The FDA is particularly sensitive to the number of patients who will be exposed to the drug. They are the ones likely to be hauled before Congress if something goes wrong. The reviewers are asking themselves the following questions:
  - What is the worst thing that could go wrong?
  - How many patients could be harmed?
  - How great is the unmet medical need?
  - How will I explain this at the Congressional hearing if this blows up?
- The reviewers are bureaucrats. They must follow procedures and they must tick off the appropriate boxes. Even if they want to help you, they cannot if you don't give them something to hang their hat on. For example, no matter how much they might want to approve a drug, they cannot approve it if it violates laws or regulations. You must provide them the data that will allow them to check the appropriate boxes.

- The European reviewers are also cognizant of the economic impact of the drug. If the drug is gong to increase the cost of health care without providing additional benefits, they will take that into consideration. They often see part of their duty to the public to assess the economic impact.
- The reviewers often have access to data from other companies you don't. They cannot share this data with you, but they may ask you to do additional pre-clinical or clinical studies that do not make sense to you.
- It is a good idea to give the reviewer advance notice of press releases or publications so that they do not get blindsided by them.

Preparing for FDA Meetings

With the FDA, and now more and more with the European regulatory agencies, you can request meetings to discuss development programs. These meetings are extremely useful, and in most cases vital. It is to both FDA's and your advantage to come to agreement on study designs, safety database sizes, manufacturing controls, and other critical matters before rather than after the work has been done.

There are three classes of meetings:

Type A meeting is for issues that are critical to resolve in order to proceed on a stalled development program. FDA should grant a meeting within 30 days of the request.

Type B meeting includes certain milestone meetings such as pre-IND, end of Phase II, and pre-BLA/NDA meetings. FDA should grant a meeting within 60 calendar days. Typically, the agency will grant one Type B meeting per landmark.

Type C meetings are all other meetings.

Below is a list of meetings and their types, taken from the FDA web site.

Meetings may be in person, telephonic, or by video conference. In general, an in-person meeting is almost always preferable. Most communication and correspondence with the FDA, including filing of an IND, is confidential. They are not subject to Freedom of Information requests. The documents that the FDA generates in the course of a review of an NDA or BLA are subject to FOI requests, though.

The sponsor should submit a request that includes the following:

- Purpose of the meeting
- Range of requested meeting dates
- Proposed agenda and length of meeting
- Proposed list of attendees from the sponsor
- List of proposed attendees from the FDA (optional), by function or by name
- Specific questions
- Time when supporting material will be sent to the FDA

TABLE 12.3 Types of FDA/sponsor meetings

Type	Name	Definition	FDA Code
A	CRITICAL PATH	A meeting which is necessary for an otherwise stalled drug development program to proceed (previously referred to as a "special considerations" meeting).	CP
A	SPECIAL PROTOCOL, MEDICAL	Applies only to the medical portion of the review. Under section 119 (a) of the Modernization Act, FDA is to meet with a sponsor or applicant for the purpose of reaching agreement on the design and size of clinical trials intended to form the primary basis of an effectiveness claim if the sponsor or applicant makes a reasonable written request for such a meeting. The special protocol should be submitted to the appropriate division with a cover memo clearly identifying it as a "Special Protocol for Review." FDA will review the special protocol in 45 days and send a written response to the sponsor. If, after review of FDA response, the sponsor decides that a meeting is necessary, the sponsor may submit a written request for a Type A meeting.	SPM
A	SPECIAL PROTOCOL, PHARM/TOX	Applies only to the pharmacology and toxicology portion of the review. Under section 119 (a) of the Modernization Act, FDA is to meet with a sponsor or applicant for the purpose of reaching agreement on the design and size of clinical trials intended to form the primary basis of an effectiveness claim if the sponsor or applicant makes a reasonable written request for such a meeting. The special protocol should be submitted to the appropriate division with a cover memo clearly identifying it as a "Special Protocol for Review." FDA will review the special protocol in 45 days and send a written response to the sponsor. If, after review of FDA response, the sponsor decides that a meeting is necessary, the sponsor may submit a written request for a Type A meeting.	SPX
A	SPECIAL PROTOCOL, CHEMISTRY	Applies only to the chemistry portion of the review. Under section 119 (a) of the Modernization Act, FDA is to meet with a sponsor or applicant for the purpose of reaching agreement on the design and size of clinical trials intended to form the primary basis of an effectiveness claim if the sponsor or applicant makes a reasonable written request for such a meeting. The special protocol should be submitted to the appropriate division with a cover memo clearly identifying it as a "Special Protocol for Review." FDA will review the special protocol in 45 days and send a written response to the sponsor. If, after review of FDA response, the sponsor decides that a meeting is necessary, the sponsor may submit a written request for a Type A meeting.	SPC
B	PRE-IND	Prior to the submission of the initial IND, the sponsor may request a meeting with FDA to review and reach agreement on the design of animal studies needed to support human clinical testing. The format of the IND and the scope and design of planned Phase I clinical studies may also be discussed (21CFR312.82).	P-IND
B	END OF PHASE I	The sponsor may request a meeting with FDA after completion of early Phase I studies (21CFR312 subpart E or 21CFR314 subpart H) to review the Phase I data and reach agreement on plans for Phase II program (21CFR312.82).	EOP1
B	END OF PHASE II/ PRE-PHASE III	The purpose is to review the Phase II data to determine whether it is safe to proceed to Phase III, to evaluate the plans for the Phase III program and protocols, and to identify any additional information necessary to support a marketing application for the uses under investigation (21CFR312.47). Additional guidance regarding End of Phase II meetings may be found in MAPP _____.	EOP2
B	PRE-NDA/SUPPLEMENT	The purpose is to acquaint FDA reviewers with the general information to be submitted in the marketing application, discuss appropriate methods for statistical analysis, discuss proposed format for data in the planned marketing application, to identify those studies that the sponsor is relying on as adequate and well controlled, and to discuss any major unresolved problems (21CFR312.47). Additional guidance regarding pre-NDA meetings may be found in MAPP _____).	P-NDA
C	OTC MONOGRAPH FEEDBACK	Any non-type A or non-type B meeting where feedbacks on OTC monographs are discussed.	560FB

(Continued)

TABLE 12.3   *(Continued)*

Type	Name	Definition	FDA Code
C	90 DAY	90 days after the submission of an NDA for a new chemical entity or major indication for a marketed drug, the applicant may request a conference with FDA reviewers. The purpose of the conference, which often is a teleconference, is to discuss the general progress and status of the application and to advise applicants of deficiencies that have been identified which have not been previously communicated (21CFR314.102(c)).	90DAY
C	ADVERTISING/ PROMOTION	Any non-type A or non-type B meeting where advertising or promotion issues are discussed.	ADPRO
C	BIOPHARM/ BIOEQUIVALENCE	Any non-type A or non-type B meeting where biopharmaceutical or bioequivalence issues are discussed.	BIOEQ
C	CHEMISTRY	Any non-type A or non-type B meeting where chemistry issues are discussed. Specifically excluded are END-OF-PHASE 2/PRE-PHASE 3, PRE-IND, AND PRE-NDA MEETINGS.	CMC
C	COMPLIANCE	Any non-type A or non-type B meeting where compliance issues are discussed.	COMPL
C	ELECTRONIC SUBMISSION	Any non-type A or non-type B meeting where electronic media submitted in support of an application is discussed, regardless of whether it is referring to methods or results.	ELECT
C	END OF REVIEW CONFERENCE	After FDA has concluded the review of an application and issued an approvable or not approvable letter, the applicant may request a meeting with FDA reviewers to discuss what further steps need to be taken by the applicant before the application can be approved (21CFR314.102 (d)).	EOR
C	FILING CONFERENCE	If FDA refuses to file an application, the applicant may request in writing, within 30 days of the date of the agency's notification, an informal conference with the agency about whether the agency should file the application. If following the informal conference, the applicant requests that FDA file the application (with or without amendments to correct deficiencies), the agency will file the application over protest (21 CFR 314.101).	FC
C	GUIDANCE	Any non-type A or non-type B meeting where guidance is discussed. An example of a guidance meeting is an endpoints meeting.	GUID
C	LABELING	Any non-type A or non-type B meeting where labeling issues are discussed.	LABEL
C	OTHER	Any non-type A or non-type B meeting that does not fit into a pre-defined type C category.	OTHER
C	PHASE IV	Any non-type A or non-type B meeting where Phase IV issues are discussed.	PH_4
C	PHARM/TOX	Any non-type A or non-type B meeting where pharmacology and toxicology issues are discussed.	PHTOX
C	SAFETY ISSUES	Any meeting other than a critical path meeting where safety issues are discussed.	SAFTY

The most critical portion of the request is the questions. The FDA will not in general agree to 100% firm commitments. So, the questions should be couched as:

"Does the Agency agree that the proposed number of patients (2000) exposed to the drug may be sufficient to support a filing?"

rather than

"Will the Agency approve the drug if there are at least 2000 patients in the safety database?"

Keep the questions specific to each function, and group them by function. For example, rather than combining a clinical and statistical question, separate them. Also, the questions should be asked such that they can be answered as a Yes/No, though this is not a requirement.

Completely speculative questions will not be answered. Questions regarding study design, statistical plans, interim analysis, comparator arms, and similar topics can be fruitfully asked.

The FDA must respond to the request for the meeting within 14 days. Please make sure you send the request to the appropriate person.

In general, the briefing package should arrive at the FDA 30 days before the meeting. For Type A meetings, it should arrive 14 days before the meeting. It should contain the following:

- Product name
- Application number
- Chemical name and structure
- Proposed indication
- Dosage form and route
- Purpose of the meeting
- Questions for the Agency
- List of sponsor attendees
- Proposed agenda
- Background preclinical data as appropriate
- Background clinical data as appropriate
- Background CMC data as appropriate
- Background references as appropriate

You want to make it concise and organized. You do not want to include too little information since that will raise questions from the reviewer; but you want to avoid including too much information since that might raise gratuitous questions from the reviewer. You don't want extraneous or spurious concerns to arise. You should be absolutely transparent and upfront. Do not hide any data or exclude information that is pertinent.

Make it as easy for the reviewer as possible. Include copies of articles as appropriate. You should keep in mind that you cannot discuss anything at the meeting that is not included in the package, since the FDA team will not have had time to consider it and to reach internal consensus on it.

Generally, you should request 60 minutes for the meeting, though you can request up to 90 minutes.

You should keep any presentation brief. It should not last more than 10 minutes total. FDA will in most cases have reviewed the material beforehand. You should arrive with enough time to get through security.

The FDA personnel will generally have their internal meeting beforehand to discuss the answers to the questions. Usually, the internal team will consist of the program manager, reviewer, team leaders for each function, division (deputy) director, and internal and external consultants.

In some divisions, the draft responses to the questions will be sent to the sponsor beforehand; in some others they will be handed out at the meeting; and in others they will not be shared with the sponsor.

At the meeting, the sponsor should have a point person, usually the regulatory affairs person, who will control the meeting from the sponsor's side, and decide who will answer the questions. It is not a good idea to allow everyone to speak freely, especially if the members of the team will contradict one another. You will usually want to have a practice meeting (or several) where answers to objections or questions from the agency are rehearsed. A golden rule is: never volunteer extra information that is not directly pertinent to the question being asked. At the end of the

meeting, the point person should try to summarize what was said or agreed to.

After the meeting, you should have an immediate debriefing session. People will often walk away from the meeting with different understandings of what was said. Also, as a courtesy, it is a good idea to send draft minutes to the agency personnel. They will often appreciate it, and in many cases, use it as a template for the official minutes.

Pre-IND Meeting

In the Pre-IND meeting, the planned pre-clinical studies, in particular the toxicology studies, are discussed. It is a good idea to have this meeting in advance of starting the studies, because you don't want to find out at the end of a 28-day study that you need to do a 6-month study. The FDA will need to understand the Phase I study design to weigh in on the proposal.

Some pre-IND meetings will also focus on or include discussion about the CMC issues. This is less common, despite the fact that the regulations seem to indicate pre-IND meetings are really for CMC rather than toxicology studies.

End of Phase II Meeting (EOP2)

There is typically an end of Phase II meeting (sometimes called pre-Phase III meeting). This is a critical meeting, where the sponsor and the FDA come to an agreement on the design of Phase III study or studies as well as other clinical and nonclinical work that must be done before a BLA or an NDA can be filed. For example, discussion to decide if special population studies must be done (elderly patients, immunocompetency study more CMC work, etc.) will be had.

The briefing package for the EOP2 meeting should include:

- proposed indication and in some cases, claims;
- Phase III protocol;
- summary of preclinical and clinical data to date;
- data analysis proposal.

For a special protocol assessment, additional information that might be requested includes:

- draft CRF;
- draft IDMC charter;
- draft SAP.

Pre-BLA/NDA Meeting

After a successful Phase III study or studies, you should hold a pre-BLA or pre-NDA meeting with the FDA. The meeting should agree on the format and content of the submission. You should come to an agreement on the content of the data set, types of data tables that will be generated, types of analysis, and so on. For example, the sponsor might propose to include certain safety data in the 120-day safety update, and might want to make sure that it wouldn't qualify as a major amendment that would trigger the resetting of the review clock.

It is also a forum for discussing the possibility of a priority review, although the agency will often not commit to it.

The meeting package should include:

- topline efficacy and safety data;
- description of the data set to be submitted;
- types of tables that will be submitted;
- indication and claims being sought.

Preparing and Submitting Regulatory Filings

Administering a new drug (or in some cases, devices) to patients for the first time is a risky proposition under the best of circumstances. It is, in fact, illegal in virtually all countries. In order to conduct first in man studies the sponsor must obtain a special exemption from the laws prohibiting such an action. The application to obtain such an exemption goes by different names in different jurisdictions. In the United States, it is called an IND or an Investigational Device Exemption (IDE). In the European Union, it is called Investigational Medicinal Product Dossier (IMPD).

There are three main parts to an IND. The first part is the clinical protocol being proposed and the target indication. It should also include a general outline of the clinical development plan, although this does not need to be extensive. This will tell the agency what you plan on doing with the drug.

The second part is the CMC section or the equivalent. It is nontrivial to manufacture a drug or a device that is consistent from batch to batch, does not degrade over time, and so on. This is particularly true for new drugs. The CMC section should describe the manufacturing and the quality control/assurance process used to ensure that you know what it is that you're administering to the patients.

The third part is the toxicology section. Before drugs are administered to patients, you must perform adequate and appropriate toxicology work to ensure that you have done reasonable things to identify major risks associated with the product.

It is highly recommended that you conduct a pre-IND meeting with the FDA before initiating the toxicology work.

The IMPD is similar to the IND, though with slightly different formatting requirements and slightly different sets of data.

The IND is sent in with *Form 1571*, which states that the sponsor will wait 30 days before beginning the study, will not begin or continue the study if placed on clinical hold, will ensure that the IRB will review and approve the study, and will conduct the study in accordance with all applicable regulatory requirements.

Regulatory Documents

Before the sites can begin enrolling, the sponsor must collect and submit "regdocs" to the FDA. The regdocs include several forms but in particular, a signed Form 1572 from the investigator which commits to the following:

- To conduct the study in accordance with the protocol
- To personally supervise or conduct the investigation
- To inform the subjects of the investigational status of the test article
- To report adverse events to the sponsor
- To read and understand the Investigational Brochure
- To inform all support personnel of the investigation requirements
- To maintain adequate records and make them available for inspection
- To assure that the IRB is in compliance
- To assume responsibility for initial and continuing review by the IRB
- To promptly report study changes and unanticipated risks to the IRB
- To make no changes in the research without IRB approval
- To comply with the requirements regarding the obligations of clinical investigators

Ongoing Regulatory Activities

In the course of the study, the regulatory group will typically ensure that the SAE forms are being filed, that annual IND updates are being filed, that the IB is being updated annually, and that all other filing requirements are being met.

NDA/BLA/MAA

Upon successful conclusion of a Phase III study, an application for approval will be submitted.

There are three ways of obtaining approval in the European Union: centralized procedure, de-centralized procedure and mutual recognition procedure.

12.8.2 Drug Supply, Labeling, and IVRS

One of the rate limiting steps in many clinical trials is drug supply and IVRS. Clinical drug supply must be appropriately labeled before it can be used. This can take 6 weeks or longer. The regulations require that the drug be labeled in the appropriate language, and that the label identify the product, the manufacturer, the study, and the investigator site (for Europe).

The easiest way to meet the language requirement is to use multi-lingual labels that include languages for all the countries concerned, rather than separate labels for each language. IT will reduce the amount of QC work.

The IVRS system is a generic term that is now used to refer to the method of randomization. It can be paper based, telephone based, fax based, or web based. The most sophisticated systems can handle dynamic randomization, and can be linked to drug shipment so that drug can be shipped automatically to replenish drug supply that is being used by the site. The IVRS system must be thoroughly validated (tested). It is unfortunately not uncommon for the system to be buggy. After all, it is software, and often it is custom-built software. It is, however, mission critical software, that can scotch the entire study if improperly programmed or configured.

The most common IVRS is voice based. Typically, the site will call a number, and will be walked through a set of prompts. The IVRS will ask for the caller's identification number, passcode, site identification number, confirmation of each inclusion and exclusion criteria (such as, "Is the patient over 18 years of age? Press 1 for yes, 2 for no."), questions on the stratification criteria (such as "press 1 if the patient has anterior MI, 2 if the patient has posterior MI"), and so on. At the end, the patient will be assigned a patient number and a drug kit number.

12.8.3 Pharmacovigilance

SAE *Reporting*

Since clinical trials are risky endeavors, there are strict rules on safety monitoring. They fall into two buckets: SAE reporting and trend detection.

Let's start with the definition of an adverse event. The standard definitions, which come from the FDA (http://www.fda.gov/CDER/GUIDANCE/3580fnl.htm) and ICH are as follows.

ICH *Definitions*

An *adverse event* (AE) or *adverse experience* (AE) is "any untoward medical occurrence in a patient or clinical investigation subject administered a pharmaceutical product and which does not necessarily have to have a causal relationship with this treatment." In other words, an AE is anything bad that happens to the patient.

An *ADR* has slightly different definition depending on whether it occurs in a pre-approval or post-approval setting. In the former, an ADR is "all noxious and unintended responses to a medicinal product related to any dose." In the latter, an ADR is "a response to a drug which is noxious and unintended and which occurs at doses normally used in man for prophylaxis, diagnosis, or therapy of disease or for modification of physiological function."

An *unexpected ADR* is an ADR, "*the nature or severity of which is not consistent with the applicable product*

*information (e.g., Investigator's Brochure for an unapproved investigational medicinal product)." You should note that severity of the reaction or different presentation of the AE can make it unexpected, if the IB or the product insert doesn't mention it in that manifestation. For example, a headache that lasts for an unusually long period of time (e.g., 2 months) may be considered to be unexpected, even if headache is mentioned in the IB. So may lupus cerebritis be considered unexpected even if lupus is expected. So may increased frequency of an AE.

An *SAE* is defined by ICH as follows:

Any untoward medical occurrence that at any dose that meets any of the following criteria:

- results in death;
- is life-threatening (*Note:* The term "life-threatening" in the definition of "serious" refers to an event in which the patient was at risk of death at the time of the event; it does not refer to an event which hypothetically might have caused death if it were more severe.);
- requires inpatient hospitalization or prolongation of existing hospitalization;
- results in persistent or significant disability/incapacity; or
- is a congenital anomaly/birth defect.

Medical and scientific judgement should be exercised in deciding whether expedited reporting is appropriate in other situations, such as important medical events that may not be immediately life-threatening or result in death or hospitalisation but may jeopardise the patient or may require intervention to prevent one of the other outcomes listed in the definition above. *These should also usually be considered serious.* Examples of such events are intensive treatment in an emergency room or at home for allergic bronchospasm; blood dyscrasias or convulsions that do not result in hospitalisation; or development of drug dependency or drug abuse.

A serious AE is different from a severe AE. ICH distinguishes between the two as follows.

To ensure no confusion or misunderstanding of the difference between the terms "serious" and "severe," which are not synonymous, the following note of clarification is provided: The term "severe" is often used to describe the intensity (severity) of a specific event (as in mild, moderate, or severe myocardial infarction); the event itself, however, may be of relatively minor medical significance (such as severe headache). This is not the same as "serious," which is based on patient/event outcome or action criteria usually associated with events that pose a threat to a patient's life or functioning. Seriousness (not severity) serves as a guide for defining regulatory reporting obligations.

FDA *Definitions*

FDA definitions have largely been harmonized with ICH definitions:

The term *adverse reaction* is used to refer to an undesirable effect, reasonably associated with the use of a drug that may occur as part of the pharmacological action of the drug or may be unpredictable in its occurrence. This term does not include all adverse events observed during use of a drug, only those for which there is some basis to believe there is a causal relationship between the drug and the occurrence of the adverse event. The term *adverse event* is used here to refer to any untoward medical event associated with the use of a drug in humans, whether or not it is considered drug-related.

In other words, anything that happens to the patient which is bad is an adverse event. If it may be related to the drug, then it is an adverse reaction. SAE is a specific regulatory term defined as follows by the FDA:

The phrases *serious adverse drug experience* and *serious adverse event* are used in this guidance to refer to any event occurring at any dose, whether or not considered drug-related, that results in any of the following outcomes:

- Death
- A life-threatening adverse experience
- Inpatient hospitalization or prolongation of existing hospitalization
- A persistent or significant disability/incapacity
- A congenital anomaly or birth defect.

Important medical events that may not result in death, life-threatening, or requiring hospitalization may be considered serious adverse drug events when, based upon appropriate medical judgment, they may jeopardize the patient or subject who may require medical or surgical intervention to prevent one of the outcomes listed in this definition. Examples of such medical events include allergic bronchospasm requiring intensive treatment in an emergency room or at home, blood dyscrasias or convulsions that do not result in inpatient hospitalization, or the development of drug dependency or drug abuse.

Cancer and overdose used to be considered SAE, but are no longer.

Reporting SAEs

When there are SAEs, the knowledge of that should be disseminated as quickly as possible. That knowledge may have an important impact on the safety of the patients in the study. Therefore, there are some very strict guidelines on how and how rapidly such events need to be reported.

All serious, unexpected, ADRs need to be reported in an expedited fashion. You do not have to report expected AEs. If it is listed in the IB, it is considered to be expected. There is some debate over whether an addendum to the IB can be used to make an unexpected AE into an AE so that the events need not be reported with each incident.

An AE that is considered to be unrelated to the drug need not be reported. Of course, it is a judgment call whether the AE is related to the drug. There will usually be an assessment by the treating physician and another by the MM. In general, if either considers the AE to be related to the drug, or possibly related to the drug, then it should be reported. There are many different ways of describing the degree of

likelihood: not related, possibly related, probably related, plausibly related, suspected to be related, definitely related, and so on. In general, only the ones that are definitely unrelated should be excluded from the reporting, although the regulations seem to allow a bit more latitude. In a safety reporting, it is always prudent to err on the side of caution.

In addition to traditional SAE triggered expedited reporting, there are instances, such as change in the rate of AEs, or new pre-clinical data, or other instances where expedited reporting may be required. Even lack of efficacy, in a life-threatening disease, may fall into this category in some cases.

Fatal or life-threatening, unexpected ADRs should be reported occurring in *clinical investigations* qualify for as soon as possible but no later than 7 calendar days after first knowledge by the sponsor. This should be followed by a complete (to the extent it is possible) report within 8 additional calendar days. Please note that the regulation doesn't say to report in 7 days – it requires sponsors to report as soon as possible, with maximal cap of 7 days. The regulatory agencies can be notified by telephone, facsimile transmission, or in writing.

Serious, unexpected reactions (ADRs) that are not fatal or life-threatening must be filed as soon as possible but no later than 15 calendar days after first knowledge by the sponsor.

It is extremely important to meet the reporting requirements. Failure to do so may not only result in regulatory sanctions but may jeopardize the health of patients in the study.

Minimum Criteria for Reporting

When does the clock start running for the reporting requirements? It starts running when the following minimum criteria are met:

- An identifiable patient.
- A suspect medicinal product.
- An identifiable reporting source.
- An event or outcome that can be identified as serious and unexpected, and for which, in clinical investigation cases, there is a reasonable suspected causal relationship.

The clock starts running if any employee of the sponsor becomes aware of the event – even if the employee is not involved with the study or is not in the clinical group, the clock starts running. This would, for example, include a salesperson hearing about an event on a sales call or an administrative assistant hearing about an event over the radio. The CRO and the CRAs employed by them are considered to be agents of the sponsor and the clock starts running when they are aware of the event.

How to Report

An SAE should be reported as soon as possible by the site to the sponsor. During the training of the investigators, this should be made absolutely clear to them. Because of the time lag traditionally associated with paper-based CRFs most sponsors have a separate, faster, process for SAE reports. A site will typically fax a special SAE form to the sponsor, but may in some cases use an EDC system.

Once the sponsor is notified, there should be a predefined process for processing the adverse events. The event should be logged in, and the data entered into a database. The SAE reports are typically submitted in a MedWatch format. There should be a clearly identified person who is responsible for each step of the processing and for each of the cases. There should be quality checks built into the system. There is usually a person assigned to query the site or to ask the CRA to query the site for additional information as needed. There should be follow-up with the site until the event has resolved.

The MedWatch form is preferred by the FDA for reporting of unexpected SAEs. The CIOMS-I form is also widely used.

The initial report may not contain all pertinent information. The form should be submitted with what data is available. Follow-up information should be actively sought and submitted as it becomes available. The report must include an assessment of the importance and implication of the findings, including relevant previous experience with the same or similar medicinal products.

Key data elements for inclusion in expedited reports of serious ADRs (from ICH)

Patient Details
Initials
Other relevant identifier (e.g., clinical investigation number)
Gender
Age and/or date of birth
Weight
Height

Suspected Medicinal Product(s)
Brand name as reported
International nonproprietary name (INN)
Batch number
Indication(s) for which suspect medicinal product was prescribed or tested
Dosage form and strength
Daily dose and regimen (specify units, e.g., mg, mL, mg/kg)
Route of administration
Starting date and time of day
Stopping date and time, or duration of treatment

Other Treatment(s)
For concomitant medicinal products (including nonprescription/OTC medicinal products) and nonmedicinal product therapies, provide the same information as for the suspected product.

Details of Suspected ADR(s)
Full description of reaction(s) including body site and severity, as well as the criterion (or criteria) for regarding the report as serious should be given. In addition to a description of the reported signs and symptoms, whenever possible, attempts should be made to establish a specific diagnosis for the reaction.
Start date (and time) of onset of reaction.
Stop date (and time) or duration of reaction.
De-challenge and re-challenge information.
Setting (e.g., hospital, out-patient clinic, home, nursing home).

Outcome
Information on recovery and any sequelae; what specific tests and/or treatment may have been required and their results; for a fatal outcome, cause of death and a comment on its possible relationship to the suspected reaction should be provided. Any autopsy or other post-mortem findings (including a coroner's report) should also be provided when available.
Other information: anything relevant to facilitate assessment of the case, such as medical history including allergy, drug or alcohol abuse; family history; findings from special investigations.

Details on Reporter of Event (Suspected ADR)
Name
Address
Telephone number
Profession (specialty)

Administrative and Sponsor/Company Details
Source of report: was it spontaneous, from a clinical investigation (provide details), from the literature (provide copy), other?
Date event report was first received by sponsor/manufacturer.
Country in which event occurred
Type of report filed to authorities: initial or follow-up (first, second, etc.).
Name and address of sponsor/manufacturer/company.
Name, address, telephone number, and fax number of contact person in reporting company or institution.
Identifying regulatory code or number for marketing authorization dossier or clinical investigation process for the suspected product (e.g., IND or CTX number, NDA number).
Sponsor/manufacturer's identification number for the case (this number must be the same for the initial and follow-up reports on the same case).

Special Considerations

In blinded studies, most sponsors will unblind the patient (while as much as possibly limiting the number of personnel who are privy to the unblinding) before submitting the report. They will generally not report unexpected SAEs that occur in the placebo patients. In some companies, the blind will not be broken, and the unexpected SAEs will all be reported to the agency as blinded report.

If an SAE is suspected to be related to another drug that the patient is exposed to, such as a comparator drug or a concomitant drug, then the sponsor must report the SAE to the regulatory agency or to the manufacturer of the comparator drug.

For products with different formulations or multiple indications, an SAE that is expected for another indication or formulation but not for the indication or formulation being studied is considered to be unexpected and is reportable. For example, if PML is an expected AE for multiple sclerosis for a drug but not for rheumatoid arthritis, and a PML AE occurs in a rheumatoid arthritis study, then it is considered to be unexpected.

An AE that occurs after a study has been finished may often be considered to be related and therefore reportable.

EC/IRB/Investigator

The unexpected SAE should also be distributed to the investigators, who then should notify the IRBs and ECs.

Signal Detection

In addition to specific AEs, the sponsors are required to monitor the overall pattern of AEs and if they see something unusual, are required to report it. For example, one or two pneumonias in and of themselves may not be significant, but multiple patients with pneumonias, bronchitis, and other related infections, in aggregate may indicate that a drug is increasing the risk of infections. Sponsors must perform *signal detection* real time to detect and to report such patterns.

Safety Committees

There are, in addition to the MM and the pharmacovigilance physician, often two committees charged with patient safety in trials. The first, the DSMB, has already been mentioned. The second is a Safety Committee that is found in many companies. This is usually made up of the CMO, head of pharmacovigilance, head of clinical development, and other senior personnel, who review both on a periodic basis and *ad hoc* basis, available safety data. They are usually charged with flagging any unusual patterns, investigating them, and if necessary, taking action to mitigate the risk.

Chapter 13

Site Selection and Patient Recruitment

13.1 SITE SELECTION

13.1.1 General Principles

Single Site

Clinical trials can take place at one or multiple sites (i.e., locations). Although the trend has been toward performing multi-center (i.e., multiple sites) trials, many clinical studies still occur at only one location. Often, a single site study will precede a multi-center trial. A single site study typically is much less costly and less complicated to run than a multi-site trial. Dealing with a single set of personnel, institutional review board (IRB) requirements, equipment, and facilities usually means less variability than a multi-site study. But enrollment and completion of the study may take much longer. Moreover, depending on the diversity of the patient population included, study results from a single site may be much less generalizable than results from a multi-center study. The single site may have a characteristic (e.g., unusual patient population or practice patterns) that significantly biases the results.

Multiple Sites (Multi-center Studies)

The trend has been toward performing multi-center (i.e., multiple sites) trials, since including many different locations increases the number and diversity of patients as well as enrollment speed. Having multiple centers decreases the likelihood of having a spurious result due to a systematic bias at one center or practice patterns peculiar to one institution or region (e.g., the use of IV nitroglycerin in acute myocardial infarction or coumadin after myocardial infarction varies considerably from region to region). Sites are analogous to colonies in an empire or subsidiaries in a large company. The more there are, the more complicated it is to manage them. Also, sites (like colonies or subsidiaries) may vary in quality, experience, and autonomy. The ideal site functions relatively autonomously, resolves problems quickly, follows instructions and directions, generates reliable and credible data, and needs little monitoring or oversight. Some sites require

significant "hand-holding" and monitoring. The greater the monitoring a site requires, the more cost and hassle it incurs. Typically, the more experience a site has, and more experience it has in the particular indication that you are studying, more likely it will be that things will go smoothly.

Therefore, choosing the right site is essential to conduct a successful study. Good site selection is not trivial. You must select sites that are qualified to perform the study, that have access to patients, that are not too expensive, and that don't have too many competing trials. In some cases, you also have to select sites that have physicians who are influential in the field. Carefully evaluating the site's physical layout, resources, personnel, and environment is a complicated and time-consuming process. Since running clinical trials can bring money, resources, and prestige to sites, sites may have incentives to "sell" and potentially "oversell" their capabilities. Separating a site's marketing "fluff" from reality can be challenging. Many businesses specializing in clinical trial site selection have emerged. If you choose to use a third party to find sites, make sure that the third party is legitimate and credible.

Rather than a one-step process, choosing sites is a multi-stage iterative negotiation. You will try to determine if the site has what your trial needs and if the price or cost is right. The site will try to ascertain whether it is worth hosting your trial. Highly desirable sites typically demand higher remuneration for their services, especially if there is intense competition for their services. Eventually if negotiations progress, both sides will put together a budget, which should be further scrutinized, negotiated, and adjusted. The budget should be detailed and account for unexpected events. This will minimize budgetary surprises after a trial commences.

International Sites

Clinical trials frequently employ sites from different countries for numerous possible reasons listed below:

- Certain diseases and conditions are more prevalent in (or even endemic to) certain regions of the world.
- More populous areas may make patient recruitment easier.

- Running clinical trials may be less expensive in certain countries.
- There may be fewer competing trials (i.e., less competition for resources and patients).
- Certain countries may have special scientific capabilities or resources.
- Prominent and experienced principal investigators (PIs) may be located abroad.
- Drug approval may be faster in other countries.
- Performing trials in other countries may expedite the approval and marketing of the intervention in those countries.
- Multi-national trials may help ensure a racially, ethnically, and culturally diverse population.

Using international sites has made site selection increasingly complex. Assessing the suitability of sites in different distant countries can be challenging. Local regulatory, political and scientific environments and concepts of trial suitability, safety, and operations may be drastically different. In some cases, political or economic climates may be unstable or unpredictable. Local disasters (e.g., severe weather, earthquakes, or disease outbreaks) can play havoc with your trial. Cultural and language barriers as well as the sheer distance can make communications difficult. Lack of infrastructure, for example for refrigerated shipping, may make trials more challenging and expensive. Privacy issue in some countries can hinder the ability to conduct trials or store tissue samples.

Clinical practice patterns, the definitions of diseases, and patient populations may vary significantly across different regions and countries. The diagnosis and treatment of the same disease can be different in Philadelphia, Tokyo, Berlin, London, and Shanghai. Some places rely more heavily on so-called complementary and alternative medicine treatments (e.g., herbal remedies or acupuncture). Other places which have limited technology and access to cutting edge medications may rely on older, more established diagnostic techniques and treatments. When selecting a site, experience with and thorough knowledge of the local/regional differences will help avoid surprises, poor recruitment, and trial problems.

13.1.2 Site Characteristics

Since potential sites may oversell or exaggerate their capabilities, always request documentation and objective measures of their claims. For example, the site may claim that it has enough people and experience to conduct the trial. But how many and what specific people will be available? What are their qualifications? How much time will they have? Sites and site personnel must meet International Conference on Harmonisation (ICH)/WHO Good Clinical Practice (GCP) standards for all of the site characteristics listed below. Please remember that in addtion to verbal answers, the sites must provide written documentation for many of the standards below. For example, the site must provide copies of

CV's and training records. In addition, a site qualification visit is necessary unless the site has been used by you in a previous study recently.

Accessibility

Patients and study personnel should be able to readily access the site. So geographically isolated (e.g., islands or tops of mountains), dangerous (e.g., country is at war), or difficult to find (e.g., must navigate a maze of tunnels) sites are undesirable. Poorly accessible sites may deter patients from participating and increase study administrative costs.

Regulatory Environment

The site's local regulations should be conducive to running a legitimate, credible, and efficient trial. Regulations can vary from being too lax to too stringent. Certain regulations can vary from city to city, state to state, and country to country. Make sure you are aware of all the local regulations germane to your trial (e.g., radiation safety if you are using radioactive isotopes). Also, be cognizant of impending regulation changes that may affect your trial.

Political Environment

Remember that the site is ensconced in a series of increasingly larger environments. Each environment has its own set of politics. The site (e.g., hospital or clinic administrators and departments) sits in a town or city (e.g., city councils and departments) which in turn sits in a state or province (e.g., state regulatory boards) which sits in a country (e.g., federal government). Instability or unrest in any of these environments can affect your trial (e.g., hospital mergers, civil wars, government upheaval, scandals, currency fluctuation, labor unrest, or legal problems). A tumultuous environment can threaten the trial and even endanger trial personnel.

Principal Investigator

Every site must have a principal investigator (PI), the person responsible for the conduct of the trial at that site. The PI is like the site manager, president, or overlord. The PI should have the appropriate education, training, qualifications, and experience. This includes the necessary licenses, board certifications, and Human Subject Training Certification. Check if the PI has had publications and clinical trial experience, especially in relevant related phases and therapeutic areas. The PI also should have enough available time to dedicate to the trial. (The percent effort is the percent of the PI's total time that can be allocated to the study.) A full-time clinician may not have enough time. Assess the potential PI's enthusiasm for and familiarity with the relevant therapeutic area, intervention, and experimental protocol. Make sure the PI has the necessary dedication to complete your trial. Make sure that there are no potential conflicts of interest (e.g., the PI holds a patent for a competing intervention).

Staff

A site should have sufficient committed staff (e.g., clinical research coordinators, data managers, and administrative staff) to conduct the trial. Ask for the organizational chart curriculum vitaes CVs, and the available time of potential research personnel. Ideally, there should be at least some dedicated research staff as part-time staff may not have as much time and enthusiasm as promised. Staff should have the necessary experience, licensure, and certification. They should be thoroughly knowledgeable about the intervention, protocol, relevant disease or condition, and GCP requirements, preferably having experience within the relevant therapeutic area. Staff should cooperate and work well together. Any sign of disharmony is a potential red flag. High staff turnover is also a red flag and can significantly increase costs (e.g., finding, hiring, training, and transferring data to new personnel) and inconvenience.

Facilities and Equipment

Proper facilities and equipment should be available, up-to-date, functioning, and amenable to clinical research. Even though facilities and equipment are present at a site, they may not be available (e.g., limited hours of operation, competition for their use, or out of service), facilities should be fully accessible (e.g., handicapped access) and reasonably comfortable for patients and research staff (e.g., adequate lighting, spaciousness, waiting areas, and bathrooms). Emergency, laboratory, and transportation services should be readily available in case the patient suffers an adverse event. The site should have adequate facilities to store and dispense the intervention (e.g., freezer for compounds that need to be frozen) safely and securely. When the intervention is a medication, the site should have an appropriate *investigational pharmacy* that stores, mixes, dispenses, and doses the drug as needed. A site should have facilities and equipment for the clinical (e.g., administering the intervention, performing and interpreting diagnostic tests, and treating side effects) and administrative (e.g., data entry, management, storage, and transmission) aspects of the trial. The facilities and equipment must be able to maintain patient privacy and confidentiality (e.g., secure FAX machines and enclosed spaces). Facilities must be able to accommodate and monitor potential regulatory body visits.

Institutional Review Board/Independent Ethics Committee

The site's IRB/EC (or the off-site IRB that the site uses) should be legitimate and properly accredited and credentialed.

As IRB's vary significantly in bureaucracy and administrative hassle, be wary of IRB's that have excessive administrative requirements that impede research. Protocols that fly through some IRB's could get caught in limbo in other IRB's. Know the IRB's, requirements, approval process, average turnaround times, deadlines, frequency of meetings, and potential fees. Politics within and around the IRB can wreak havoc. It helps if the PI is familiar with and can help navigate through the IRB. Be aware of any other local review committees as well such as Scientific Review Committees.

Operations

A site should be responsive, compliant to regulations and protocols, efficient, and rapid in initiating the study. It is important to determine how quickly they respond to calls, return questionnaires, submit regulatory documents, and initiate studies. Personnel should be available for monitoring visits and investigator meetings. Ask sites to provide copies of their standard operating procedures (SOP), quality assessment (QA) records, training logs, and record keeping forms. The SOP should include measures to prevent and detect errors. Having extensive record keeping capabilities in place is key.

Potential Subjects

For the most part, the sites and their immediate vicinities will be the locations from where subjects are recruited. Some medical centers are major referral centers and will get patients from around the world. Others will only draw from the local population. Have a good understanding of the site's typical and available patient populations. How stable and compliant is their patient population? Know their standard and potential recruiting methods.

13.2 PATIENT RECRUITMENT

13.2.1 General Strategies

Patient recruitment involves identifying patients eligible for your study and convincing them to participate. This process can be an extremely complicated, expensive, and initially overlooked bottleneck, preventing the timely initiation of a clinical study. In fact, people usually underestimate the challenges of patient recruitment and overestimate the number of potential patients available for participation, a phenomenon so prevalent that it has been dubbed "Lasagna's Law." A good rule of thumb is to divide the sites' entrollment estimate by fastor of 2 or 3.

Successfully recruiting patients requires a clear plan, an adequate budget, periodic monitoring of the recruitment process, and contingency plans in case recruitment does not go as smoothly as anticipated. When planning, overestimate the time and expense involved, as recruitment rarely goes as planned.

TABLE 13.1 Recruitment Personnel Compensation

Incentive structure	Advantages	Disadvantages
Flat salary	No incentive to use inappropriate or unethical means to induce patients to participate	No incentive to complete patient recruitment as soon as possible
Pay per patient screened	Incentive to screen as many patients as possible	Incentive to screen patients regardless of their suitability for trial
Pay per patient recruited	Incentive to recruit patients as quickly as possible	Personnel may use inappropriate or unethical means to induce patients to participate
Pay per patient successfully enrolled in trial	Incentive to recruit appropriate patients as quickly as possible	Whether a patient eventually is enrolled may be beyond a person's control. Therefore, person may not change behavior

Management Challenges

In many ways, patient recruitment is a complicated management challenge, involving different elements of strategy, operations, marketing, finance, and leadership. You must supervise a substantial number of personnel that may be in different locations. Tremendous variability in the motivation, experience, and ability of everyone involved may exist. Study personnel may misunderstand directions, make mistakes, fail to remain motivated and active, and even drop out during patient recruitment. Potential problems include interpersonal conflicts, noncompliance with directions, miscommunication, and differing agendas. Maintaining open communication among personnel is essential. A clear organizational structure can help operations. Personnel need to know whom to contact with questions or concerns.

Monitoring Recruitment Progress

Monitoring recruitment progress is important. You need to periodically determine how well recruitment is going, which strategies and locations have been successful, and how many more patients are needed. Poor recruitment progress may require modifying your recruitment strategies. Better-than-expected recruitment may allow you to curtail recruitment early, saving time and money. Criteria, procedures, and methods of monitoring recruitment progress should be in place before recruitment commences. Tracking the recruitment yield (e.g., % subjects enrolled/subjects screened; % subjects screened/total population) is helpful in determining if your recruitment strategies are too broad, too narrow, or targeting the wrong patients.

Recruitment Personnel Incentives

Recruitment personnel include people involved in advertising, administering screening, and referring patients for a clinical trial. Personnel may be volunteers or paid employees. While volunteers are less expensive, they may be more unreliable without financial incentives. They are not obli-

gated financially to be present, responsible, and work hard. However, simply paying personnel does not necessarily guarantee quality work. Properly structuring incentives can be important. Incentives should enhance but not significantly bias and hamper appropriate recruitment. Table 13.1 lists the advantages and disadvantages of different pay schemes. Of course, the overall available budget may leave you with little choice of how you pay personnel. When this occurs, be aware of the potential biases introduced and effects on the recruitment process. Please keep in mind that the payments for recruitment must not be so large as to constitute an undue inducement. In addition, it is illegal to pay referring physicians for referring patients to the study, although it is permissable to reimburse them for services rendered.

Patient Incentives

Deciding how much to pay patients is tricky. Figure 13.1 demonstrates the potential problems. Clinical trials can cause inconvenience and some degree of financial hardship on patients. Patients may have to miss work or school, hire babysitters and child care, or travel significant distances. Without any compensation, many patients may not want to participate. Naturally, the more you pay, the more willing patients are to participate. However, paying too much may attract and unduly influence patients who need the money. Cash-strapped patients may be reluctant to withdraw from the study even if they should (e.g., experiencing side effects). Financial incentives may motivate patients to lie during screening and the trial so that they can participate and remain in the trial. Once again, the size of the payments must not be large enough to cause inducement. In general, patient incentives are usually seen in Phase 1 trials.

Phase II Studies

Often, the ideal Phase I and Phase II study populations are different from the desired Phase III population. In order to make the study results as generalizable as possible,

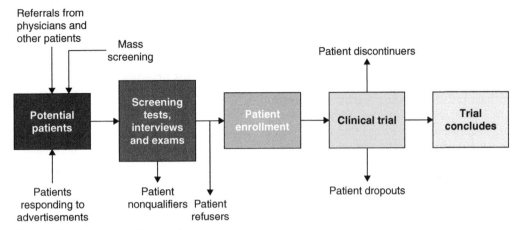

FIGURE 13.1   Outlines of the broad steps in the recruitment process.

the Phase III population should mirror the ultimate target population closely. However, for Phase II studies, you may choose a more homogeneous population of patients who are more likely to have events.

Because Phase II studies are generally smaller than Phase III studies, it is often impossible to adequately power the study without using an alternate endpoint and/or patient population. For example, in acute coronary syndrome (ACS), one might select troponin positive patients for Phase II since they are at the highest risk of having an additional coronary event. In an asthma trial, one might select patients with the highest number of exacerbations in the previous year. This type of patient population enrichment can lead to smaller Phase II studies.

An important caveat is that the patient population in Phase II must have a similar response to the intervention as the ultimate target population. For example, if troponin positive ACS patients had a disease that was fundamentally different in pathophysiology such that they respond to GP IIb/IIIa inhibitors while the patients who were troponin-negative did not, then Phase II can be very misleading.

A caveat regarding extrapolation of Phase II results to Phase III is that there will always be subgroups who respond better than others to therapy, purely by chance. Unless this subgroup has been pre-specified, it is most likely a spurious result. In addition, as the treatment paradigms change, the patient populations that enroll in later trials may be somewhat different from patients who enroll in earlier trials. Also, a positive Phase II trial in itself can change the willingness of patients to enroll in a trial, so that the characteristics of patients in Phase III study may be different solely due to the Phase II results.

13.2.2 Choosing a Strategy

Recruitment as Sampling

Patient recruitment is basically sampling. After identifying the sampling frame, you try to find an appropriate sample from that frame willing to participate in the trial. This sample is rarely truly random (even though in an ideal world, you would prefer a truly random sample). Even if you were able to pick patients randomly from a sampling frame, many may refuse to participate in or complete the study. Certain recruitment strategies are more likely to yield biased sample (e.g., choosing a limited number of clinics to recruit from will only select patients who go to those clinics).

So while making your recruitment sample truly random is usually impossible, you still want to make your sample as representative of the accessible study population as possible. Doing so involves comparing the characteristics of your "sample" (i.e., successfully recruited population) with the accessible population and then making extra efforts to recruit more members with the characteristics that your "sample" is missing (e.g., if the accessible population is 40% women and 5% Asian American and your recruited population has neither women nor Asian Americans, you may have to try to find more women and more Asian Americans). This is another reason why monitoring recruitment is important. Simply monitoring the number of patients is not enough. You have to monitor the types of patients you have recruited thus far, so that you may alter recruiting strategies to find the types of patients that you are missing.

Broad vs. Targeted Strategies

In the next section, we will discuss recruitment strategies in detail. Patient recruitment is analogous to fishing. A *broad recruitment strategy* is like throwing a large net into the ocean and seeing what the net catches. Such a strategy may catch many fish, but not catch the right fish if your desired fish is rare. Examples of broad recruitment strategies include mass media campaigns and mass screening. A *targeted recruitment strategy* is like putting on a scuba suit and searching a coral reef for your fish. You will not find as many fish, but most of the ones that you do find may be appropriate if you go to the right reef. An example of targeted recruitment strategies is using physician referrals or disease registries.

Understanding the Market

Choosing a recruitment strategy is in many ways similar to choosing a marketing strategy for a product or service. For example, to effectively sell basketball jerseys, you must know who is more likely to buy the jerseys (e.g., people who play or watch basketball, are young and healthy enough to stay physically active, and live in a city where there is a professional basketball team), where can I find such people (e.g., basketball courts, sporting goods stores, reading sports magazines, or watching sports programs), and how do I reach these people (e.g., post advertisements in sports magazines, run commercials during sporting events, and directly sell jerseys at basketball courts)? Many times a combination of strategies is effective since different potential customers may be found in different ways (e.g., a person may not play basketball but still watch it on television or vice-versa).

Similarly, when recruiting patients, you must know where to find the appropriate patients or risk wasting significant time and effort. Some strategies are obviously less effective for certain populations because physical, geographical, or social limitations may prevent the strategies from reaching the appropriate patients (e.g., posting billboard advertisements for visually impaired patients or setting up recruiting tables at an exclusive golf club to find patients of different ethnic, economic, or social backgrounds). The prevalence and incidence of the relevant disease or condition affects your choice of strategy. More rare diseases or conditions require more targeted recruitment strategies (e.g., mass screenings for a rare genetic disease would be less cost-effective than having specialty physicians refer the patients).

General public knowledge, concern, and acceptance of the disease or condition are important. Broad recruitment strategies may be better for diseases that are well known and well understood. More people may be aware of their conditions and be willing to seek treatment. Broad strategies can spawn secondary dissemination (i.e., someone who does not have the disease sees the recruiting advertisement and then notifies a friend or family member who does have the disease). Social stigma can either impede or help recruitment. Patients may be unwilling to reveal that they have an "embarrassing" condition. They may not be willing to accept that they have the condition. Some conditions can make patients pariahs or social outcasts (e.g., physically deforming diseases) and, in turn, make them very difficult to reach. In such cases, targeted recruitment may be more discrete and effective. On the other hand, patients may welcome the opportunity to interact with people who either have or understand their stigmatized condition. When conducted appropriately, broad strategies can help raise awareness and compassion for the patients.

Disease severity and the need for treatment can affect your strategy. Very debilitating conditions can prevent patients from going outside or participating in certain activities, limiting the effectiveness of broad strategies. Broad strategies are also less useful when diseases progress rapidly. Patients may be anxious to seek treatment and less likely to respond to advertisements that Patients may be anxious to seek treatment and less likely to respond to advertisements that do promise immediate effective treatment.

Reputation and Public Opinion

You will not be recruiting in a vacuum. How potential subjects and investigators view your study, intervention, and organization (e.g., company, academic medical center, or government agency) will affect your recruiting and, in turn, recruitment strategy. Preliminary results from your trial or other related trials can affect recruitment. Favorable results can encourage more patients to participate. Unfavorable results can deter patients from participating. Good experiences and impressions of your intervention, organization, or study sites can enhance recruitment. Your recruitment strategy may include answering questions or addressing concerns potential subjects may have about your trial. While you should never mislead patients, providing pertinent information can be very valuable.

Working with Limitations

Many different factors may limit your choice of strategies:

- *Budget constraints*: Some recruitment strategies are more costly than others. Understand all of the costs entailed (including hidden costs) and determine the cost-benefit (i.e., how much will you invest for each patient successfully recruited) of each strategy before making your choice. Anticipate and factor in potential problems when estimating costs.
- *Resource availability*: Not all strategies are possible. They may need equipment (e.g., television equipment to tape a commercial), people (e.g., web designers), or facilities (e.g., billboard space) that you do not have.
- *Access*: Some recruitment strategies require access to particular people (e.g., physician to refer patients), organizations (e.g., owners of disease registries), or places (e.g., the local government may not allow you to set up tables in public areas). Access may be impossible (e.g., for political reasons some physicians may not comply) or prohibitively costly (e.g., many organizations charge for access to their disease registries).
- *Geography, legal, and political environment*: Be aware of your recruiting environment. People in certain locations may oppose your recruitment (e.g., recruiting for patients with sexual problems in a very conservative town). Geographical (e.g., recruiting at the top of a mountain may not reach people at the bottom of the mountain) and political barriers may prevent your message from reaching potential subjects. Some strategies may be illegal in certain areas (e.g., using an electric sign in a place where the use of electricity is banned).
- *Timeline*: Some recruitment strategies may take too long.

- *Capacity*: Your personnel and trial must be able to handle the potential onrush of potential subjects after recruitment begins. If your capacity to handle inquiries and patients is limited, perhaps a more targeted approach is wise.

13.3 RECRUITMENT STRATEGIES

13.3.1 Broad Strategies

Mass/Community Screenings

Mass or community screens involve testing a large portion of the population for eligible patients. These can be very complex and expensive operations. Mass screenings may be appropriate in the following circumstances:

- *The condition and desired characteristics are relatively common*: Finding rare conditions and characteristics with mass screenings is like finding a needle in a haystack: too much effort, too much cost. Other more targeted approaches may be more cost-effective.
- *The screening test is relatively specific, inexpensive, and noninvasive*: A nonspecific test will miss many potential subjects. Painful or harmful tests may injure patients or deter them from participating.
- *Many people will benefit from the information gathered*: There is added incentive to do mass screenings that provide ancillary benefits to individual patients or the community at large (e.g., mass blood pressure or cholesterol testing will give patients information about their cardiovascular health). This is especially true when everyone undergoes screening benefits regardless of the findings or outcomes (e.g., knowing your cholesterol level is useful regardless of whether you qualify for the study).
- *Mass screening mechanisms are already in place*: Hospitals, health organizations, churches, insurance companies, and employers frequently sponsor and run health screenings to help identify patients at risk for certain conditions. Partnering with these pre-existing screenings will save money, time, and effort.
- *The population density is high enough*: The more people you screen, the more likely you are to find appropriate patients. As a result, sparsely populated areas are not amenable to mass screenings.
- *Local communities support the screening*: Mass screenings require cooperation of local leaders. Some screenings may conflict with other community initiatives or concerns. A community may be opposed to screening for a genetic or acquired condition that may impair a person's ability to find employment. Community members may be suspicious of your motivations or be concerned about who will have access to the screening information. They may worry that your screening will detract from their own screening and health initiatives.

There are several key considerations when planning a mass screening:

- *Appropriately publicize/advertise the screening*: We will discuss advertising in mass media strategies.
- *Be cognizant of concurrent health initiatives and screening*: Avoid competition for patients. Collaborating with other initiatives may reduce costs and avoid unnecessary repeat testing or procedures (e.g., patients will not have to be stuck by needles more than once). There is no sense in developing the infrastructure for a screening program when one is already in place. Moreover, pairing up with an existing and trusted initiative may dramatically aid patient recruitment. Patients are more likely to comply with mass screening if they know and trust the sponsoring organization.
- *Schedule the mass screening to enable maximum participation*: Be aware of potential weather, seasonal, work, and family life factors. Unless necessary, avoid scheduling a screening when the weather is bad. Unless screening occurs at the workplace, choose times (e.g., lunch hour, after work, and weekends) that will not conflict with traditional workplace and family life obligations. Keep in mind that in certain areas populations may fluctuate dramatically from season to season (e.g., ski resorts are relatively under populated during the summer; beach communities lose a lot of residents during the winter).
- *Choose locations that are central, visible, and convenient*: Location should be close to the population you will be screening and easily accessible. The more hassles a patient has to endure, the less likely she will be to participate. So be aware of all possible impediments such as lack of parking, waiting areas, or unclear directions. In some cases, you can bring the location to the patients. For example, vans with portable MRI's or DEXA scan machines can be moved from location to location.
- *Choose locations relevant to the condition and patient characteristics*: Patients with the specified condition should frequent the location. Night clubs may not be the best places to find elderly patients (depending, of course, on the night club). Beverly Hills may not be the best place to find patients of the lowest socioeconomic status (depending on how you define lowest socioeconomic status).
- *Provide minor incentives*: Patients will not travel or commit valuable time to screening without any perceived benefits. When designing screening, always consider what the patients have to gain from participating. Often the benefit is information (i.e., they learn whether they are at risk for certain conditions). Sometimes information is not enough. Financial incentives (e.g., reductions in insurance premiums), prizes, or food can greatly enhance participation. Coupling the mass screening with a social event is often an effective strategy.

- *Beware of potential biases from screening design and methods*: Your choice of screening location, time, and method can dramatically affect the types of patients you will encounter. For example, screening for patients at 2 pm on a weekday may be selected for patients that do not work. Screening in Iowa may not identify enough minorities. Screening at a health club located at the top of five flights of stairs may prevent those with limited mobility from participating.

Mass Media

Mass communication vehicles such as television, radio, print media (e.g., newspapers, magazines), and the Internet can be effective in attracting subjects. However, do not underestimate the effort required to create and execute a successful mass media recruitment campaign. More often than not, mass media recruitment is not cost effective. Remember that many large companies spend millions of dollars devising and implementing mass media marketing strategies. Potential general logistic considerations include:

- *Cost*: Each vehicle's effectiveness depends heavily on how much you are willing to spend. Typically greater spending will lead to more control over when and how vehicles are used (e.g., if you are willing to pay, you can dictate when a television commercial airs). More spending does not always make a campaign more effective. Media outlets and advertising firms may encourage you to purchase additional features that will have no impact on recruitment.
- *Second-order dissemination*: Any media communication may lead to unexpected additional publicity through other sources. News agencies may see your campaign as newsworthy and do a story on it. (e.g., posting recruitment signs on all city buses may lead to a news story about the signs). While this so-called second-order dissemination can help further disseminate your recruitment information, negative or improper second-order portrayal of your recruitment campaign actually can hinder recruitment. Usually you do not have much control over second-order dissemination, so reporters may inadvertently or deliberately misrepresent your recruitment campaign or clinical study (e.g., provide incorrect details or emphasize the dangers of your study intervention). Remember that media outlets frequently do not have enough knowledge about your study or subject area and are primarily interested in making a story newsworthy to attract more viewers or readers. Since controversial and dramatic news sells more than the mundane, they may add or alter information about your trial to spice things up.
- *Timing*: Timing is particularly important for television and radio. Unless you are willing to spend money to purchase highly coveted times (e.g., during prime-time spots such as weekday evenings or popular events such as the Super Bowl), public service announcements (PSA's) and

commercials may air at unpredictable and unusual times. Broadcasts that occur during very early morning hours or that compete with very popular shows on other channels may have relatively few viewers. The timing of the broadcasts may significantly bias the type of patient recruited (e.g., broadcasts in the middle of the day may select for people who do not work). Broadcasts during television shows oriented toward particular social demographic groups (e.g., some talk shows target certain genders, age groups, or ethnicities) will reach an overrepresentation of that particular group and an under representation of others. Timing can be an issue with other media vehicles as well. Internet and some print advertisements may only appear at certain specified times (e.g., rotating billboards).

- *Duration and frequency*: Announcements and advertisements may appear once or repeatedly in waves. Generally, the effectiveness as well as the cost of a recruitment campaign increases with the duration and frequency of these appearances. Repeated announcements and advertisements may be necessary when the pool of potential subjects changes frequently (e.g., cities with significant ingress, egress, and transient populations), the patient enrollment period is lengthy, or the trial criteria change.
- *Clear contact information*: Once viewers see an advertisement, they must know how to contact the recruitment coordinators. Repeating the contact information clearly (e.g., large, bright letters and numbers; well-paced voice with appropriate volume and enunciation) and in multiple formats is important. People are more likely to remember information that they both hear and see. Moreover, some patients may be hearing or visually impaired, far from the television, or watching with the volume muted.
- *Attention grabbers and memory triggers*: Careful use of marketing techniques such as musical jingles, catchphrases, and visual-stimulation can aid recruitment. Overuse may make your campaign appear too trivial, frivolous, or commercialized.
- *Cultural and language differences and barriers*: Ensure that your campaign is suitable for cultures and ethnicities that may be in your pool of potential subjects. Providing announcements in different languages will reach non-English speakers. Including pictures or images of people from different ethnicities and cultures will help more people identify and feel more comfortable with enrolling in the trial. Carefully consider the location of your campaign (e.g., not including Spanish and Chinese versions of advertisements may hamper recruitment in Southern California) and the disease and target population (e.g., Hebrew versions may help recruitment for a trial involving Tay Sach's Disease, more common among Ashkenazi Jews). Avoid advertisements that may offend certain cultures or social groups (e.g., pictures of breasts, even for a breast disease trial, may not be appropriate in a conservative town).
- *Anticipating and handling response*: Recruitment coordinators must be prepared to handle a surge of calls and

TABLE 13.2   Examples of Mass Media Vehicles

Vehicle	Examples	Advantages	Disadvantages	Considerations
Television	News story, talk show, public service announcement	Combination of visual and audio messages	Patients may miss or not pay attention to the segment	Time of day (e.g., prime time), day of week, channels (e.g., cable vs. network; local vs. national). Who should appear (e.g., celebrity, expert, real patients, or model)
Radio	News story, talk show, public service announcement	Usually less expensive than television. Can target people during commuting hours	Biased against hearing impaired. Lack of visual stimulus. Radio becoming less popular	Similar to television, except voice and vocal delivery (e.g., voice clarity, intonation, and speed) of message more important
Print media	Magazine or newspaper article, advertisement	Patients may read the information as often and as carefully as they want	Biased against visually impaired (unless in Braille)	Magazine's or newspaper's circulation and target audience. Who and what is depicted is important
Internet	Stand-alone web site, banner advertisement, Internet media sites, web portals	Potentially very wide audience, constant (24 h) advertising	Biased against patients without Internet access. Risk of fake imitators	Search engines and web portals can help guide patients to your web site

inquiries immediately after an announcement occurs. As infomercials have demonstrated, viewers are most likely to call impulsively right after they see information. Having recruitment coordinators available at all hours (or at least during key hours), a computer assisted telephone interviewing (CATI) system in place, or at least a voice mail message with detailed information will help catch potential subjects when they call.

- *Competition*: Unrelated advertising and similar clinical trial recruitment campaigns compete for the attention of potential subjects. While competition should not deter your efforts, be reasonably aware of its impact. If a much larger company or organization is advertising at the same time, consider delaying your recruitment or cooperating with the larger competitor.

- *Inadvertent messages*: Any media announcement or advertisement may have its untoward effects. Be aware of any messages you may unintentionally transmit (e.g., a picture of a Latino in a recruitment advertisement for a depression study may unfairly suggest that Latinos are more likely to be depressed).

- *Target audience*: Make sure that the typical audience of the media vehicle that you are using matches the study population that you are seeking (e.g., do not use MTV to recruit elderly patients, men's magazines to recruit women, or radio advertisements to recruit the hearing impaired).

Table 13.2 lists examples of mass media vehicles.

Door-to-Door Campaigns

Systematically visiting each person's house, apartment, or dormitory in a neighborhood is very labor intensive but can have relatively high yield. Such face-to-face recruiting can allow patients to ask questions and feel more comfortable with the study. Psychologically people also find it more difficult to reject a live person (e.g., on site car salespeople are usually more effective than a printed advertisement). While hiring the right personnel is essential in any recruitment strategy, it is especially important in door-to-door campaigns. The right people can mean the difference between effective recruitment and shutting down your trial (due to poor recruitment, complaints, and even lawsuits). The right person is a good communicator who handles rejection well (as most people will decline to participate). The wrong person may offend, frighten, or coerce potential subjects. Visits should occur during times when people are likely to be at home. When there is no answer, personnel may have to re-visit the home (or apartment) a specified number of times before giving up. Take appropriate measures to ensure your personnel's safety.

- Visit dangerous neighborhoods in groups and during the daytime.
- Personnel should be trained to recognize and react to dangerous situations.
- Personnel should understand what words and statements may be offensive or inflammatory.

Telephone or E-mail Campaigns

The telephone and e-mail can help you contact large numbers of people in a short amount of time. Many companies and organizations use both means to conduct surveys and polls. Businesses continue to use telemarketing (unsolicited and often unwelcome phone calls) and spam (unsolicited e-mails) to market and sell their products and services. Unfortunately the wide prevalence of these practices has hurt phone or e-mail patient recruitment. Many people have learned to avoid answering the telephone or reading e-mails from unrecognized senders. Many technologies and strategies designed to thwart telemarketers and spammers (e.g., caller ID or spam detecting programs), in turn, thwart patient recruiters.

Moreover, these recruitment strategies carry several inherent biases. They are biased against patients who do not have a telephone or Internet access and anyone with physical limitations that impair the use of a phone (e.g., hearing impairment) or computer (e.g., visual or typing impairment). They are also biased against patients with situations that keep them from answering the phone or e-mail (e.g., jobs with long working hours, extensive travel, or long periods of isolation). Conversely, patients with multiple phone numbers or e-mail accounts may be more likely to respond to these strategies. When using the telephone for recruitment, remember that some people do not have a telephone, answer their phones, or have listed phone numbers.

When using the telephone for recruitment, the phone book is a natural sampling frame. It provides a readily accessible study population from which you can sample. Also, the phone book's listings allow you to stratify by geographical region. However, the biggest problem with using the phone book as a sampling frame is unlisted phone numbers. This problem continues to increase as cell and Internet phone use increases. Most cell and Internet phone numbers are unlisted, and more and more people are using their cell phones as their primary phone numbers.

Random digit dialing (RDD) can overcome the problem of unlisted numbers. In RDD, patient recruiters call phone numbers generated at random, many of which will not normally be listed in the phone book. Of course, many randomly generated numbers may be business or invalid phone numbers. RDD is particularly effective in areas with many telephones (i.e., the number of invalid numbers will be low).

Often, patients will not answer their telephones, forcing you to either call again or leave a message on their answering machine or voice mail. In general, leaving a message is much less effective than speaking to the patient directly. Even patients who would be willing to participate may not expend the effort to return a phone call. Therefore, choose times when patients are likely to be home and answer the phone (e.g., evenings). Calling multiple times will increase the "hit" rate. Sending letters warning the patient of an upcoming phone call may convince them to answer or be available when the phone call occurs.

Devising telephone scripts will help standardize what the recruiter says to the patient, answering machine, or voice mail. Since recruiters may have varying levels of experience or ability, standardization is important and can

help recruiters deal with difficult situations and avoid saying anything controversial, insulting, unprofessional, or incorrect. Recruiters must be prepared to deal with rude, angry, depressed, or even abusive people. They must retain a professional tone and attitude without sounding like they are selling something or coercing someone.

In some cases, employing CATI may be appropriate. In CATI, a software program provides a script that changes depending on how the patient responds. The recruiter follows the script and enters the patient response in the computer, which then displays another script depending on the response. Alternatively, the computer actually makes the phone call and talks to the patient using recorded voices (e.g., "if you are interested in participating, please press 1 for further information"). This is similar to the phone routing systems that many businesses now use. Such a system cuts down the number of personnel needed but also reduces the human, personal element to the phone calls. Patients may be less willing to respond to or deal with a computer recording.

E-mail has several advantages and disadvantages over telephone recruitment. E-mailing usually is cheaper to implement, can be completely automated, and is not subject to the same variability seen amongst different telephone interviewers. You can also send e-mail at any time of the day and almost anywhere to patients who have Internet access. Potential subjects can carefully read and ruminate over the e-mail message, without feeling pressured to respond immediately. It is easier for patients to respond to e-mail messages. They do not have to worry about calling during business hours or being placed on hold. However, e-mail is not interactive (i.e., patients cannot have a conversation with the e-mail message). Getting potential subjects' e-mail addresses can be difficult. E-mail addresses can change frequently as people switch jobs or have their e-mail accounts clogged up and rendered useless by excessive spam. The wording of e-mails is extremely important, especially the subject header of the message. Many people will delete e-mail messages that have suspicious or uninteresting subject headers. Since responding to e-mail messages is easy, your staff must be prepared to deal with a massive influx of relevant and irrelevant questions or junk e-mail. Finally, e-mail messages from patients may contain sensitive health information that must be protected and kept confidential.

Posters, Billboards, and Fliers

Using posters, billboards, and fliers may be the least expensive mass recruitment strategy. It can be a very effective strategy for relatively low cost, depending on how well you address the following considerations:

- *Location*: Choose areas that are visible and frequented by patients with the relevant diseases, conditions, and characteristics (e.g., student centers for college students, busy freeways, or gyms for patients with sports injuries).

- *Competition*: Avoid areas that have too much advertising. Otherwise your advertisement may get lost in a sea of billboards and posters.
- *Timing*: Choose appropriate and high yield times to hand out fliers or post-advertisements.
- *Appearance*: Posters and billboards should be eye-catching but professional. Usually larger posters are more noticeable but more expensive.
- *Personnel*: Make sure that the people who post or hand out advertisements have proper directions and incentives. Otherwise they may not perform their duties appropriately.

13.3.2 Targeted Strategies

Advocacy Groups, Disease Registries and Databases

Advocacy groups are particularly helpful in small, niche indications such as Crohn's disease and anaplastic thyroid cancer. The advent of the internet has made the groups very well-connected and they can significantly assist in recruiting patients. Many individuals, groups, or organizations own databases of patients. Table 13.3 lists some examples. These databases can be very general (e.g., everyone admitted to a hospital or on a particular insurance plan) or very specific (e.g., patients with a certain disease). There are many reasons why such databases are maintained. When databases created to meet specific objectives (e.g., safety surveillance, epidemiological research, or outcomes research), they are called *registries*.

Such databases can help identify patients for your study. The utility of such registries have significnatly decreased with the advent of strict privacy laws, but in some cases can still be very helpful. They may be particularly useful if they indicate important patient health information (e.g., demographics, conditions, or medications). This will allow you to do targeted searches (e.g., women with diabetes, elderly taking metformin, or nurses who have visited the emergency room) for potential patients that match some of your study selection criteria.

When selecting a database to use, there are several important considerations:

- *Data mining*: Some databases are easily searchable. They may have built-in computer programs that allow you to quickly find patients with particular symptoms or conditions. Others are more cumbersome, requiring you to either design special computer programs or enlist the aid of many people to find particular patients.
- *Cost*: Many parties are in the business of selling data, charging a flat fee or per patient charge for access. Be fully aware of the fee structure and potential cost before using these sources.
- *Quality*: Assess the database quality before using it. The database should be complete, reasonably up-to-date, and accurate. Ask to see a sample dataset and documentation characterizing the data quality (e.g., publications generated by the dataset, rates of missing variables, and data collection procedure).
- *Patient Consent*: Confirm that the registry or database owners have properly obtained the patients' consent to have their information available for research recruitment.

TABLE 13.3 Examples of Databases

Database	Description	Limitations
Pharmacy databases	Lists patients that have filled prescriptions for medications as well as the types and quantities of medications	Disease information may be limited Contact information may be outdated Medications can have many different uses
Disease specific registries	Databases of patients that have specific diseases or conditions (e.g., CAPSure is a prostate cancer registry)	Relevance and completeness depends on the purpose of and who manages the registry
Insurance company databases	Information on all patients covered by particular insurance plans	Patients may switch insurances Only contains information relevant to insurance processing and reimbursement Does not include uninsured
Public health databases	Keep track of patients with reportable diseases (e.g., tuberculosis, sexually transmitted diseases)	Public health databases vary significantly in quality and completeness May only contain information relevant to public health officials
Electronic medical records (EMR)	All patients that visited or were admitted to a given health care facility (e.g., clinic, hospital, or emergency room)	Many EMRs are not designed for research use and may be very difficult to maintain

- *Permissions*: Clarify what can and cannot do with the data. Remember even if you are able to obtain patient information, you may not be authorized or allowed to contact the patients.
- *Privacy*: There should be procedures in place to safeguard patient privacy. If privacy rules are violated, the database and all projects stemming from it may be terminated and the personnel involved in privacy violations are subject to significant terms of imprisonment.

Physician and Other Health Care Provider Referral

Physicians and other health care providers can be effective sources of potential patients, especially when the study population is rare (e.g., oncologists can help find hairy cell leukemia patients). Health care providers have relationships with their patients, which confer several advantages. Knowing their patients' conditions, personalities, and treatment history helps health care providers identify patients most suitable for your study. Patients may be more likely to trust a study endorsed by their health care provider. Health care providers also can provide important information about the patients' health status that would otherwise be unavailable (e.g., patients do not always know their own health histories very well).

There are problems and challenges with using such referrals. Health care providers may demand financial reimbursement to refer patients. The amount of compensation depends on the scarcity of patients (e.g., a well-known specialist who is the sole source of patients with a rare disease may demand higher compensation) and the time and effort required. Of course, please keep in mind that the reimbursement must not be so large as to be an inducement. Health care providers may feel responsible for treating patients themselves. They may be overburdened, involved in a competing study, or resistant to assisting someone whom they do not know (e.g., some health care providers are averse to assisting any pharmaceutical companies). Sometimes administrators or executives of a health care facility may agree to help enroll patients without getting "buy-in" (i.e., agreement) from or even properly informing the individual health care providers who will actually be doing the referring. As a result, health care providers may be resentful and ignore instructions or even impede the process.

Additionally, health care providers could introduce important biases. They may selectively refer patients who are:

- *Difficult, emotionally needy, or noncompliant*: Clinical trials can provide treatment and attention to patients and, therefore, serve as a means for health care providers to unload their problem patients.
- *Treatment failures*: Health care providers may selectively refer patients that do not respond to their traditional treatments (i.e., "we've tried everything else, might as well try the clinical trial").

- *Disadvantaged (e.g., socioeconomically)*: Some patients cannot afford traditional medical treatment. The patients may be disadvantaged socioeconomically or have insurance that does not provide adequate coverage. Health care providers may see clinical trials as a means of getting patients free medical care.

Selecting the right health care providers is important. Health care providers should see an adequate volume of patients. Their patient population should be likely to include patients that match your selection criteria (e.g., if you want a racially diverse population, using only Beverly Hills physicians may not be the best strategy). If you want to catch patients before they are treated, understand where patients may receive treatment (e.g., a patient who is seeing a cardiothoracic surgeon probably has had a number of heart treatments already).

Portal of Entry

One common strategy is to recruit patients where they might seek help and treatment for the first time (e.g., the emergency room for patients experiencing a heart attack or stroke; the intensive care unit for septic shock patients; primary care clinics for a wide variety of problems). Potential locations include traditional (e.g., spine specialist clinics for backaches) and nontraditional health care settings (e.g., alternative medicine practitioners) as well as nonhealth care settings (e.g., gyms). Recruitment personnel stay at the recruitment site and on the lookout for any patients that match the inclusion criteria. For emergent interventions (e.g., thrombolytics for stroke; pressors for severe hypotension), recruitment personnel try to enroll patients immediately so that they may administer the study intervention on the spot. Since predicting when certain urgent conditions will occur (e.g., heart attack, massive bleed, or seizure), this may be the only viable strategy for emergent intervention.

This strategy can be labor intensive and logistically challenging. Recruitment personnel may have to be available for long periods of time, sometimes 24 h a day. They may have to recognize appropriate patients quickly and act. For emergent interventions, recruiting, obtaining patient consent, enrolling patients, and starting the trial all may occur quickly in very short period of time. Recruitment personnel must be appropriately aggressive to recruit patients but refrain from interfering with and obstructing the normal work flow of the clinic, emergency room, intensive care unit, etc.

Special Populations

It may be easier to recruit within certain subpopulations such as military personnel, health care workers, students, and members of other specific industries. Certain types of patients are more recruitable because they understand the importance of clinical studies, are easy to reach (e.g., are on e-mail distribution lists or have central gathering areas), enjoy contributing to science, or have a reasonable amount of free time. Do not confuse easily recruited with easily coerced. You should never coerce patients to participate in a study. They should participate completely on their own free will. Grades, evaluations, jobs, or financial gain should never be at stake. Some populations also may be more compliant with clinical study protocols. They may have more members who are familiar with the requirements of clinical studies (e.g., health care workers), disciplined (e.g., military personnel), or enthusiastic (e.g., students). However, avoid stereotyping. Every population has its range of personalities and experience. Moreover, every population has its potential disadvantages (e.g., health care workers are exposed to many patients and military personnel may be deployed to distant locations).

13.4 PATIENT SCREENING

13.4.1 Separating Qualifiers from Nonqualifiers

Once patients are recruited, you must screen each patient carefully. Carefully confirm that every patient truly fulfills selection criteria. This may involve re-checking records, verifying laboratory values and diagnostic test results, and re-interviewing and re-examining patients. Do not rely on "third-parties" for patient characteristics. For example, do not trust the physical exams of physicians not involved in the trial. Many physicians are busy, vary in skill and experience, and may not have been looking for the same physical findings as you are. Moreover, patient record transcription errors could have occurred (e.g., physical findings misreported). Diagnostic test interpretations and reports can be wrong as well. Whenever feasible, go back to the original data source (e.g., the actual radiograph film or echocardiogram) to have an expert from your study interpret the study. Sometimes having two separate experts review the same data may be necessary, especially when findings are subtle or equivocal.

Beware of changing characteristics. Patients may initially qualify for the study but as their conditions improve or worsen and their life situations change they may become *nonqualifiers* (i.e., those who do not meet the selection criteria). This may be a reason to exclude patients whose characteristics or measurements are volatile (i.e., rapidly changing or fluctuating). Therefore, checking measurements on multiple occasions and under different conditions may be important (e.g., measuring blood pressure during different times of day and on different days). It may be necessary to delineate the course of a patient's disease before patient screening and extrapolate whether the patient will

no longer qualify during the course of the study. (e.g., the patient's functional status decreased by 25% over the past year and may decrease by another 25% over the next year. If the trial requires the patient to be above a certain functional level for the next year, then the patient may have to withdraw from the study).

The quality of your screening techniques is of paramount importance. Poorly performed diagnostic tests can lead to erroneous patient inclusions and exclusions. Screening personnel should have adequate levels of training and experience. Afford screening personnel plenty of time to make the necessary assessments accurately. Screening equipment should be up-to-date and well maintained. Inattention to the details of the screening process can lead to significant hassle and problems later on in the study.

Patient screening is like the college admissions process or the professional sports draft. Some argue that top colleges simply select students who would succeed anywhere they go and that the key to building a winning sports team is selecting the right athletes. Clinical studies are the same way. The screening process can make or break a clinical study. An outstanding study design, gifted and hard-working study personnel, and creative analysis cannot make a study succeed without the right patients.

13.4.2 Identifying Noncompliant Subjects

The screening process is a two-way street. Not only are you trying to determine if patients qualify, but also you are helping patients decide if they want to participate in the trial. Patients often will respond to recruitment as the result of misconceptions of the trial. Many do not fully understand the requirements and potential benefits of the study.

Some common misconceptions include:

- *Everyone in the study will receive active treatment*: Patients frequently do not realize that they may receive no treatment, placebo, or a potentially less effective treatment. Ethically, this must be clearly explained to them.
- *The study has minimal risk*: All studies have risk. Sometimes the risk is substantial. Make potential study risks clearly evident to patients. Using medical jargon to describe risks may not adequately convey the nature of the risks (e.g., instead of myocardial infarction, say heart attack.)
- *The study will not interfere with the patient's daily schedule*: Clearly describe everything the patient will have to endure during the trial, including follow-up visits, lab tests, and paperwork. Patients should not underestimate how even required paperwork may disrupt their schedules and consume time.
- *The study physician will be the patient's regular physician*: Explain the roles of the study physicians and other health care providers. Some patients may see a clinical

study as an opportunity for free health care or access to "better quality" health care providers. The study physician may not be able to provide all of the care that the patient desires. The patient may still have to see other physicians for problems unrelated to the study.

- *The compensation and other benefits will be greater*: Delineate the potential benefits of the study including the monetary compensation. Some patients view clinical studies as a way to make money when in actuality monetary compensation should be designed simply to offset the hardships incurred by the trial.
- *Everything will be free*: Outline what services and materials will be provided by the clinical study. Patients should realize what will need to be covered by themselves or their insurance policies.
- *Patients will have unlimited access to study personnel*: Patients may be very needy and demanding. In fact, some patients participate in clinical studies for the social interactions and attention.

In general, lowering a potential subject's expectations is preferable to raising them. Patients who are not happy with a study are more likely to withdraw, which may cost you valuable time and effort.

It is not necessarily a bad thing to increase the number of *patient refusers* (i.e., those who refuse to enroll in the clinical study). While it may be tempting to enroll patients as quickly as possible, losing subjects later in the study is much more costly and problematic than losing them before enrollment. Therefore, the screening process should aim to convert future patient discontinuers and dropouts (i.e., patients who decide to withdraw from the study) into patient refusers. Of course, the screening process should not dissuade appropriate patients, who would have completed the trial, from participating.

13.5 PATIENT ATTRITION

13.5.1 Patient Dropouts

Once patients are enrolled, keeping them involved in a trial is not a trivial matter. A *patient dropout* is a subject who chooses to withdraw from the study. The patient may formally drop out of the study, inform the investigator that he or she no longer wishes to participate, or simply disappear. Depending on the study design, deaths may be considered either dropouts or achievement of a specific study endpoint.

There are many reasons why a patient may drop out of a study. Some common ones include:

- *Other opportunities*: A subject may find a more desirable or interesting competing clinical study.

- *Job conflicts*: The study may be causing time demands or side effects that interfere with a patient's ability to work.
- *Personal issues*: Patients may need more time to focus on marital or family issues. Clinical studies demand a patient's time and effort, stressing his or her personal relationships. Remember that many patients in a clinical study have serious diseases that may already be causing some relationships to teeter. Spouses may feel jealous that patients are spending so much time with study personnel. Family members or friends may convince the patient to withdraw.
- *Psychological issues*: Depression, anxiety, paranoia, and psychological and psychiatric issues can manifest during the trial. These can either influence the patients to cease participation or be so debilitating that the patient cannot continue.
- *Relocation*: Patients may move far away from any of the study sites.
- *Dislike of study personnel*: Conflicts with study personnel may occur. Patients may perceive biases or stereotypes. Differing personalities and styles may be the source of problems. Some patients may voice their complaints before dropping out. Others may quietly endure problems before suddenly withdrawing.
- *Adverse and/or Side effects*: Patients may drop out when treatment side effects are either too frequent or too severe.
- *Lack of treatment effect*: Patients may become frustrated when their conditions do not improve or even worsen. Even when their conditions improve, they may be expecting more. If their conditions are debilitating or life-threatening, such concerns are very serious. You should consider discontinuing such patients before they drop out so that you can arrange appropriate care.
- *Disease improvement*: On the other hand, significant improvement in a patient's condition (whether or not the treatment was responsible) can convince the patient that he or she no longer needs the clinical study.
- *Study requirements*: Patients may find study requirements to be too onerous or insulting. Excessive paperwork, time demands, painful or irritating tests and treatments, and intrusive questions can all be issues.
- *Rumors*: News that an alternative treatment is more effective, that the clinical study treatment is harmful, or that the clinical study has problems can motivate patients to withdraw. Some patients are hungry for information (especially when the study is blinded) and will take every rumor and piece of information seriously without verifying the source.
- *Loss of motivation*: Patients may simply decide that they do not feel like participating in the study any more. In some cases, outside forces that motivated them to participate are no longer present (e.g., friends are no longer urging them, the clinical trial is no longer

popular or covered by the press, or they now have other things on their minds).

- *Peer pressure*: Hearing about other patient withdrawals may motivate a patient to follow the crowd. Even false rumors about patient dropouts can convince a patient to withdraw.
- *Financial constraints*: The patient may no longer have the financial means to participate in the study. The monetary compensation provided may not adequately offset travel costs and other medical and nonmedical expenses incurred by participating.

Regardless of the reason for the drop out, you should try to obtain the reason for each withdrawal. It is essential to determine if the drop out is in some way tied to study outcomes or endpoints. Anything related to treatment efficacy (e.g., withdrawal due to disease improvement or worsening) or safety (e.g., withdrawal due to side effects) will affect the analysis and interpretation of results. Even seemingly unrelated reasons may actually have efficacy and safety implications. For example, emotional or sexual side effects can cause marital problems, disease progression or side effects can inhibit job performance, and worsening conditions can lower a patient's tolerance for study requirements.

Ideally, all patient dropouts should participate in an exit interview and thorough examination. Getting the real reason for the drop out can be challenging. Patients may not want to be honest about their real problems and issues, especially ones that are potentially embarrassing or damaging. Patients may not want to offend you by denigrating your study personnel or treatments. They may be preparing for administrative or legal action against study personnel. Often, patients are not completely aware of the reason. They may experience and voice vague dissatisfaction but cannot pinpoint the source. Sometimes discussing the issues may convince the patient to remain in the study. However, never coerce a patient to continue. Participation must be out of his or her own free will.

13.5.2 Patient Discontinuers

Many times investigators decide to terminate patients from a study. Although these patients are often called dropouts, *Patient discontinuers* are enrolled patients who are removed from a clinical trial by the investigator. Common reasons for discontinuing patients include:

- *Noncompliant patients*: Some subjects may remain in a study but not comply with many study requirements. Distinguishing minor from serious noncompliance can be difficult. You have to decide if the noncompliant acts will jeopardize the integrity of the study.

- *Disruptive patients*: Patients may perform acts that threaten the operations of the study such as being verbally or physically abusive, finding and releasing private information, and stealing items. Whenever the safety or privacy of study personnel and other patients are at risk, you should consider terminating the perpetrating subject immediately.
- *Broken blind*: When subjects or research personnel are inadvertently unblinded, you need to determine if the subject can continue in the study. The decision depends on the answers to several questions. Who was unblinded? What are their roles in the study? How much and what kind of information was revealed? Did the unblinding affect the treatment administration or measurements? Is it possible to "re-blind" the subjects and study personnel (e.g., if only a few study personnel were unblinded, replacing them may be possible.) When the blind is broken, always assume the worst case scenarios until you can prove otherwise.
- *Clinical deterioration*: Worsening conditions may require immediate treatment outside the clinical study. Even if the study treatment has some effect, participation in a clinical study often prevents subjects from receiving optimal treatment. Be aware of harbingers of disease progression. Anticipating significant declines and taking action before it occurs is very important. Therefore, closely monitor patients for changes in symptoms and signs. Good clinical judgment is essential.
- *Safety concerns*: The treatment or the clinical study design and operations may be too risky for some patients. Very frequent or severe treatment side effects, diagnostic tests or other clinical study requirements that are too strenuous (e.g., a patient with severe lung problems running on a treadmill), and severe allergies are common reasons for discontinuing patients. Be aware that patients may mask or hide these problems for fear of appearing noncompliant, uncooperative, or weak. Also, they may not be aware of the risks.
- *Selection criteria violations*: During the course of the study, you may discover patients that no longer qualify (or should not have qualified in the first place) for the study. The testing and close observation in a clinical trial can be more stringent screening than the initial enrollment screening.
- *Ethical or legal conflicts/concerns*: Selection criteria should exclude patients for whom there may be ethical or legal problems for participating in the trial. However, selection criteria may not cover all possible situations or scenarios. For example, you may find that a patient has a grudge against the investigator or is prejudiced against someone or some entity involved in the study. The subject could even be "spying" on your clinical study.

Discontinuing a patient from a study is not easy. Patients may want to desperately remain in the study, especially if it is their only treatment option. Many patients become emotionally and socially attached to a clinical study (e.g., they are used to seeing the same people and place every week). Termination can seem like a personal insult or attack. Patients may feel like they failed or were fired. Following termination, patients could become depressed, anxious, angry, or disruptive. Some may seek administrative or legal action.

When you discontinue a patient, do not abandon him or her. Ensure that the patient has adequate follow-up care, especially if the patient's condition is deteriorating. Follow-up care should include medical treatment for the patient's condition and potential psychological treatment if necessary. Make sure that those providing follow-up care are fully aware of the patient's condition and the nature of the treatments they received. An exit interview and comprehensive examination should be part of the discontinuation process.

13.5.3 Patient Retention Strategies

As you can see, successfully recruiting patients is only part of the battle; retaining patients in a study is a challenge as well. In fact, retaining subjects in a clinical trial is similar to retaining employees in a company. The key is to create and promote an atmosphere that encourages patients to comply and remain in the trial.

- *Remember that the patients are volunteers*: None of the patients need to participate in the trial. Autocratic attitudes and rules will not work in a clinical study setting.
- *Clearly state expectations*: Ambiguous and ever-changing orders confuse, stress, and frustrate patients. Make sure that patients know what is expected of them before the clinical study commences. If changes are necessary, give patients adequate warning and understand that changes may disorient patients.
- *Understand that "one size does not fit all"*: Patients come in all sizes, shapes, and personalities. While standardization is important in clinical study protocols, patients have different ways on responding to their conditions and treatments physically and psychologically. They also have different ways of voicing dissatisfaction and complaints. You, your personnel, and your system should understand and be prepared to deal with this diversity.
- *Exhibit appropriate cultural and religious sensitivity*: Patients also will be from diverse cultures, socioeconomic backgrounds, professions, and religions. Communication barriers may exist, so translators should be available. All study personnel should be sensitive to different requirements, interpretations, and ways of expression. Understand that different people may have specific cultural and religious restrictions (e.g., some

religions do not permit certain activities after sundown or on Saturdays). Before enrolling patients in a study, make sure you clearly explain the requirements and check if the patients have any restrictions or requests.

- *Appropriate diversity among study personnel*: Patients are more likely to bond with study personnel with similar backgrounds. Your study personnel should incorporate enough diversity so that patients do not feel that it is one social group studying another.
- *Provide feedback and encouragement*: Like any humans, patients often crave feedback, particularly positive feedback. Appropriately reward their compliance with words of encouragement. Also, provide constructive suggestions when necessary. Patients cannot improve their performance if they do not know what they are doing is wrong.
- *Create an atmosphere and environment for patients to succeed*: Study schedules, facilities, and other arrangement should be conducive to patient compliance. Patients are more likely to miss visits if they have no available parking or the clinic is difficult to reach. If possible, avoid scheduling follow-up visits that conflict with patients' work schedules. Choose facilities that are comfortable and provide access to important comforts such as food, drink, and bathrooms. The more inviting the surroundings, the more likely patients will show up to their appointments.
- *Provide forums for feedback and complaints*: Give patients opportunities to voice their concerns. Silence or a lack of complaints does not mean the patient is satisfied. Actively request feedback. Ensure patients that they will be safe from retaliation if they do offer negative feedback.
- *Maintain fairness and equity*: Treat all patients with an equal amount of respect. Beware of prejudices and favoritism. Information can spread quickly, so that patients will quickly find out if they are being mistreated compared to other patients.
- *Avoid blaming the patient*: When a patient is being noncompliant, blaming the patient is easy. Instead examine the circumstances that may have led to the noncompliance. The patient may be facing hardships at home or at work. Perhaps the patient feel alienated. Your clinical trial operation may be to blame. Rather than criticize, find possible solutions.
- *Establish a rapport and build a social environment*: Patients are more likely to comply when they like the study personnel. Building a rapport with patients is important. To patients, part of the allure of a clinical study is having a whole team of people on which they may rely.
- *Provide multi-disciplinary support*: Patients should have access to experts and professionals that may handle a wide variety of problems including mental health professional, physical and occupational therapists, pharmacists, and social workers.

- *Realize that experience in one study will determine participation in future studies*: Patients who have a positive experience are more likely to enroll in future studies. This is particularly important if you plan extension or follow-up studies.

While all of these may seem daunting, remember that your study design and operations can go a long way to improving patient retention and compliance. The majority of patients want to comply and help your study succeed. Cooperation and commitment from your end will engender the same from their end. A little bit of investment can go a long way. Health care providers may not cooperate because they are suspicious of your study and feel obligated to protect their patients from becoming "experimental subjects." They may be concerned that their patients will be assigned to the control or placebo arm and not receive adequate treatment.

Chapter 14

Assessing Data Quality and Transforming Data

14.1 BACKGROUND

14.1.1 Importance of Data Quality and Format

Analyzing and interpreting clinical study data is like cooking. Before cooking, a good chef checks the quality of the ingredients (e.g., how fresh are the vegetables and fish, what is the grade of the meat) and then carefully converts the ingredients into usable forms (e.g., removes the bones from the fish, dices the vegetables, and tenderizes the meat). Without good quality ingredients, no chef (not even the Ming Tsai's and Wolfgang Puck's of the world) can prepare good quality dishes. Without properly preparing the ingredients, the dishes also will suffer.

Similarly, before you analyze and interpret clinical study data, verify the quality of the data and transform the data into forms that are readily analyzed and interpreted. Poor quality data can only yield poor quality results that can only generate very limited conclusions. Bad analysis can derail good quality data. But good analysis cannot rescue poor quality data. Data that is unreliable or improperly organized and categorized will not be amenable to proper analysis and interpretation.

Think of data as a photograph of the clinical study. Data should represent what actually occurred in the study. Data should be as clear and as complete as possible. Like photography, data quality has improved significantly over the past several decades. Like photography, the quality of data depends on multiple steps:

- Study design (analogous to the planning and execution of the photography shooting session, e.g., where the model stands, the lighting, and the setting).
- Choice and quality of measures (the film or camera hard drive).
- Quality of measurement devices (the camera).

- Experience, training, competence, and motivation of personnel taking and recording the measurements (camerapeople).
- Choice and quality of data capture, processing, and storage (film developing equipment, chemicals, and personnel or computer program and storage drive).
- Choice and quality of data analysis, tables, tests (photo album).

Pharmaceutical companies, medical device companies, research organizations, and academic researchers expend considerable time, money, and effort monitoring, assessing, and maintaining data quality. Many have separate committees for these tasks. However, despite careful planning and operations, data problems are inevitable. Nearly every study has missing data and errors. Even with top quality personnel and resources, unexpected events and random fluctuations may occur. By analogy, the best photographer photographing the best model with the best camera and the best film developing may produce some photographs that are out of focus, smudged, or poorly angled.

Data problems can be the product of isolated events or consistent operational problems. Therefore, assessing data quality can help improve your study design and operations. Without assessing data quality, serious study design problems can go unnoticed. Often, researchers will analyze and re-analyze poor quality data, blaming the analysis rather than questioning the process that generated the data.

14.1.2 Measures of Data Quality

Chapter 4 introduced the concepts of accuracy, precision, and validity in the context of measures. These terms also apply to assessing data quality. *Accuracy* applies not only to how well measurements correspond to the actual values of the phenomena being measured but also to how well the values of the numbers in the data set correspond to the measurements. (i.e. were the measurements accurately recorded?) In fact, whenever data is transcribed or transferred from one database to another, checking the accuracy of the new database is important (i.e., comparing the values in the first database with values in the second database). Therefore, double data entry (i.e., two independent people entering the same data twice and then checking if their entries are equivalent) is the standard practice. Accuracy is analogous to the degree to which you have the right ingredients for cooking. An inaccurate database is like having the wrong ingredients.

Precision in data and databases is somewhat different from precision in measurements. Precision, otherwise known as *resolution*, is the amount of discernible detail in data or a database. High resolution databases have significant details.

Consistency reflects the *internal validity* of the database. When values that are supposed to agree in a database in fact do agree, a database is consistent. The more discrepancies or contradictions, the less consistent a database is. There are different kinds of discrepancies or inconsistencies. *Temporal inconsistency* occurs when the timing of events is not possible. For example, even through Event 1 (e.g., hospitalization) causes Event 2 (e.g., hospital acquired infection), the database indicates that Event 1 occurs after Event 2. Another example would be a database that lists Event 1 and Event 2 as occuring at the same time, even though this would be impossible (e.g., a patient receives a colonoscopy, coronary angioplasty, and elective back surgery all on the same day). Thematic inconsistency is present when different fields that measure similar attributes, (i.e., have similar themes) do not agree (e.g., one field in the database states that a man has no congestive heart failure but another field lists that his cardiac ejection fraction is 17%).

You can evaluate consistency by building *redundancy* into your database. Redundancy is having the same or similar information for a given patient more than once in a database, i.e. different fields that measure the same phenomenon. (For example, a database may have the following fields: gender, last menstrual period, pelvic exam findings, and genetic karyotype.) An inconsistent database will exhibit discrepancies among redundant fields (e.g., *Gender:* Male; *Last menstrual period:* May 10; *Pelvic exam findings:* Strawberry cervix; *Genetic karyotype:* XY.) A man with a XY genotype should not have a menstrual period and a cervix). A consistent database is not necessarily accurate. Of course, the more redundancies, the more discrepancies you may have. Strategically building redundancies into the database can be a valuable tool for assessing data quality. However, currently most clinical studies are not yet sophisticated enough to consciously and regularly employ data redundancy (most redundancies are purely accidental). In general, the standard practice is to collect each piece of data only once but exert great effort (monitoring, double entry, and queries) to ensure that the data is accurate.

Database *completeness* is the degree to which all data are present in a database. An incomplete database has missing values. Later in this chapter, we will discuss causes of missing data. Redundancy in a database can help solve missing data problems. You can use redundant fields to fill in the missing data (e.g., if you have the following data: *Gender:* Missing, *Last menstrual period:* May 10, *Pelvic exam findings:* Strawberry cervix, and *Genetic karyotype:* Missing. You may guess that gender should be female and genetic karyotype should be XX). In our cooking analogy, completeness is similar to the presence of necessary ingredients. Incomplete dishes lack certain ingredients (e.g., sushi that lacks white rice; a cake without flour). Redundancy is like having different interchangeable ingredients (e.g., different types of flour) that may be used in place of each other in case one is missing.

Data *integrity* is the usability and soundness of the data. A databases' integrity depends on its validity and completeness. Invalid or incomplete data hurts a database's integrity. In our cooking analogy, data integrity is akin to the usability of the available set of food ingredients. Are they the right ingredients and are all of the necessary ingredients present? Are the ingredients damaged or incomplete (e.g., a sauce without all the right ingredients or mushrooms missing their caps).

Data is *reliable* if different investigators asking the same questions and doing the same kind of analysis on the data will arrive at the same conclusions. For this to happen, the data collection and entry has to be *consistent* (i.e., performed in the same way and format), *accurate*, and reasonably *precise* (e.g., recording the weight as greater than 100 pounds is less precise than recording it as 107 pounds). The collection and entry methods must also be *replicatable* (i.e., someone else would be able to perform the same procedures and get the same data). Standardizing all methods employed helps significantly. Extending our cooking analogy, ingredients are reliable if the same amounts prepared in the same way will generate the same taste and appearance. If a certain spice tastes very different every time it is used, the spice is not very reliable.

14.1.3 General Steps in Assessing Data Measures of Data Quality

In clinical trials, ensuring that the data set is accurate, reliable, and appropriate takes considerable time and effort. When a large quantity of data is collected in a clinical trial, missing or unreliable data, protocol violators, and contradictory data are inevitable. Therefore, you will have to make some difficult and critical decisions that may significantly affect study results and conclusions including:

- What are the acceptable thresholds (e.g., how much data can be missing before study results are jeopardized)?

- How will you manage missing or unreliable data?
- Which data set will you use for the primary analysis?

If possible, always avoid introducing bias into the study. Carefully reflect upon your decisions and how they may affect study results and interpretation. Remember that even though many statistical methods are intended for linear data, many biological phenomena are not linear.

Assessing data quality and transforming data involves several steps:

- Evaluate whether the study design was appropriate and the study was conducted rigorously.
- Check whether the assumptions underlying the study were accurate.
- Assess data completeness and decide how to handle missing data.
- Verify and validate data.
- Parse and transform data.

The following sections in this chapter discuss each of these steps in detail.

14.2 STUDY ASSUMPTIONS

14.2.1 Checking Study Assumptions

Assumptions are part of any study design. If you knew how everything would turn out and did not have to make any assumptions, there would be no need for a study. In fact, many times you do not realize that you are making assumptions...even in day-to-day life. For example, when you cross a one-way street in San Diego, you assume that cars will be coming from only one direction and will obey any red lights. Looking upward is not necessary because blimps or airplanes do not usually come down from the sky. Most likely no one has replaced the crosswalk with quicksand. These assumptions are based on prior experience. When the situation changes (e.g., you cross a street in an under-developed country located next to an unstable mountain), your assumptions and your plan of action change. Knowing when the situation changes is important.

Similarly, most clinical study design assumptions are based on prior experience and studies. Some assumptions are so prevalent and established that reviewing prior studies is not necessary. For example, you do not need to consult prior studies to know that injecting a small amount of saline into a patient's veins is safe, patient's heart rates usually increase when exercising, and certain races tend to have darker skin. Other assumptions are not as reasonable without supporting evidence, usually from prior similar studies. For each assumption, answer the following questions:

- *Do you need prior studies to support the assumption?* Ask yourself, would most people inside and outside your field know and agree with this assumption?

If yes then you probably do not need to support your assumption.

- *Did you look at a reasonable sample of prior studies?* Ideally a systematic review or meta-analysis of the literature provides the most complete answers. Realistically, reviewing every study is impractical. So at the very least, you should review the most important or most representative studies.
- *How applicable are prior studies to your study?* Answering this question can be very difficult since so many factors are involved. For example, do the prior studies have similar study population compositions to your study (e.g., a study on African Americans may not be applicable to Latinos)? Are the disease characteristics comparable (e.g., a more severe form of the disease will have a higher event rate than a less severe form)? Are the concomitant medications and co-morbid conditions similar (e.g., patients with heart disease and diabetes are not the same as patients with heart disease alone)?
- *How volatile is the assumption?* Does the parameter remain relatively constant or fluctuate significantly from study to study? For example, infectious disease transmission rates vary significantly by a patient's social contacts, immune status, environment, and disease severity. Therefore, prior studies may be very poor in predicting the transmission rates for your study.
- *How hard (i.e., objective) is the evidence behind the assumption?* Even if prior studies support an assumption, the prior studies may only provide anecdotal or subjective evidence. For example, no matter how many studies you do, you cannot generate objective evidence that certain races are more physically attractive than others. Physical attractiveness is subjective and significantly influenced by the prevailing culture and social norms.
- *How much time and what events have transpired since the prior studies?* Often, older studies become invalid after a certain period of time. Technological, environmental, cultural, and social changes can alter assumptions (e.g., patient diets are very different now vs. in the 1960s). Sometimes landmark events can dramatically alter the basis of some assumptions (e.g., new standard of care guidelines, significant changes in clinical practice, or scientific discoveries).

At the end of a study, re-checking all assumptions is important because:

- *It is impossible to ensure that all assumptions are accurate at the beginning of a study.* For example, you will not know if patients will be compliant with therapy until the study occurs.
- *Conditions change during the course of a study.* For example, patient's diseases may become more severe later in the study.
- *Some assumptions are based on other assumptions.* For example, you may assume that a percutaneous coronary

intervention will be performed competently if the operators are well trained, the patient reaches the catheterization laboratory in time, and the patient does not have a significant bleeding problem. The clinical study may demonstrate if the other assumptions hold.

- *Fundamental study design errors may not be apparent until the end of the study.* For example, the study may have allowed patient dropouts without capturing the reason for each dropout, i.e. whether it was due to adverse events, symptom resolution, lack of efficacy, etc.
- *Assumptions may affect how the analysis is performed.* For example, should you count each dropout as a failure, success, or something else.

Table 14.1 lists some common, important, but frequently overlooked assumptions to check. Think of assumptions that you did not consider when designing or starting the study. External factors also can skew the actual study to be different from the intended study. Many factors may make the enrolled study population quite different from the originally intended patient population, such as competing trials (e.g., a competing trial enrolling only Stage IV lung cancer patients, make your study to have disproportionately fewer Stage IV patients and disproportionately more Stage I–III patients) and weather and climate (e.g., bad weather can discourage certain patients from enrolling).

TABLE 14.1 Frequently Overlooked Study Assumptions to Check

Assumption	Description
Distribution of variables	Many assume either a normal or constant distribution for variables including the response variable
Background medications	Many assume that background medications stay the same (e.g., patients were allowed to receive rescue medications, and a new highly effective therapy was approved in the middle of the study, the original assumptions regarding the clinical course of the patients in the rescue group may need to be revisited)
Clinical event rate	Many assume a constant fixed event rate (e.g., two disease flares/month). In actuality, the event rate may fluctuate significantly or increase as the disease progresses
Patient population characteristics	Many often assume that the population is more homogeneous than it really is. The more population characteristics you know, the less homogeneous a population appears
Reproducible measurements	Many assume that measurements will not fluctuate as long as the clinical phenomenon being measured does not fluctuate
Causation/no causation (not "N")	Sometimes factors that do not seem to affect other things do in fact have an effect and vice versa (e.g., geography and nationality do influence patient response)
Measurements' effects on the outcome	It is impossible to make any measurement without the measurement affecting the results of the study. In some cases, this impact is profound, such as training effect of treadmill test. A patient's performance on the treadmill test often improves significantly on repeat test due to training effect
Placebo effect	
Experimental (Hawthorne) effects	Being part of an experiment can affect outcomes. For example, more MI patients receive aspirin and ACE inhibitors when they are in a clinical trial than when they are being treated outside a study, because clinicians tend to adhere more strictly to practice guidelines when they conduct a study than in general clinical practice
Constant hazard ratios	Some statistical tests assume that the drug or intervention will have a beneficial effect that is constant over time. For example, a drug may lower the risk of death by 25%. Sometimes these assumptions fail to hold. For example, all patients die at some point, so if your study lasts for a very long time, patients might start dying from other causes, making the hazard ratio change or even reverse
Certain mechanism of action or certain mechanisms of disease	As another example, if an assumption were that IL-6 levels were predictive of patients who were highly likely to have an event, and the alpha was allocated mostly to the subgroup with elevated IL-6 (let's say as an example, the high IL-6 group was allocated alpha of 0.04 and the overall group allocated 0.01), and data (external to the trial) has become available to rebut this assumption, then the analysis plan should be re-examined. Perhaps the alpha should be allocated in a different way
Biases	Potential biases can be overlooked
Influence of external factors	Be aware of any factors or events outside your study that have an impact on your study and data

14.2.2 Dealing with Invalid Assumptions

Invalid assumptions do not necessarily mean that you have to junk the data and study. Invalid assumptions are common. It is rare that a study will go completely as planned. For each invalid assumption, take the following steps:

- *Understand the nature of the invalid assumption and why it is invalid.*
- *Assess the magnitude of the assumption's effect.* Some invalid assumptions have very minor effects on the data and outcomes.
- *Determine whether the assumption is a fatal flaw in the study.* Occasionally an egregiously invalid assumption has such a significant impact on the outcomes that it renders the entire study invalid.
- *Determine what portions of the data are affected.* Sometimes an invalid assumption only affects part of the study (e.g., data before a major change in the study are unaffected).
- *Decide how to adjust the data set and statistical analysis plan.*

Remember, do not just view each invalid assumption in isolation. Sometimes two invalid assumptions will cancel each other out (e.g., patients took less medication than anticipated but were also lighter than expected) or magnify their impact (e.g., patients had more severe disease and were less compliant than anticipated).

Amending the Statistical Analysis Plan

When one or more of the assumptions turn out to be inaccurate, amend the statistical analysis plan and make sure you do this *prior* to unblinding the study. Otherwise, you will introduce bias (Figure 14.1). Changing the statistical analysis plan to fit the data can be like changing the way you play a poker game after you know the outcome.

Whenever you significantly change the study protocol, carefully assess and revise as necessary the original analysis plan. Even seemingly minor protocol changes can dramatically affect the data and the corresponding analyses (e.g., halfway through the study permitting the use of a previously excluded medication might affect the magnitude of effect, safety profile, or patient retention). The pre-change data may be quite different from the post-change data. Unfortunately, significant protocol changes during the study are sometimes unavoidable.

14.3 ASSESSING DATA COMPLETENESS

14.3.1 Missing Data

Missing data potentially can wreak havoc on a study. Missing data, of course, is missing information. This information may be irrelevant or essential for the study. (e.g., for a diabetic study, patient weights and blood sugar levels are likely essential, but patient occupations may or may not be important). If the amount is significant enough, missing data can harm the power of the study. Even small amounts of missing data can cause significant bias.

Missing data is the norm and not the exception. No study data is perfect. Rarely will a study data set be absolutely complete. In an ideal world, all data from a study would be complete, with no missing patients or missing values. All patients would have taken the assigned medication doses. No one would have dropped out from the study or died. But as we all know, real life is unpredictable. Expected and unexpected events occur. How to handle missing data is a complicated and potentially critical matter. It can have an enormous impact on the results of the study (e.g., in a mortality trial of 10,000 patients, with mortality of 5% [e.g., a thrombolytic trial], even 10 or 20 missing patients in one arm can easily change a positive study to a negative study).

The most common causes of missing data are:

- *Instrument failure*: Measurement instruments (e.g., imaging devices or blood pressure machines) can malfunction may not be available or replaceable.

Why you should amend the statistical analysis plan before unblinding the study

Here's an example:

- Unblind the study.
- *Analysis*: Discover that the difference in efficacy between active and control arms changes from the first part of the study to the second part.
- You then realize that a new drug was approved partway through the study.
- Realize that the patients who dropped out of the study after the approval of the new drug had better survival than the patients who dropped out before approval because they received the new drug.
- *Analysis plan*: Calls for including the dropout patients in the intent to treat overall survival analysis, and also calls for a one part proportional hazard model.
- *Poor practice*: Change the analysis plan *post-hoc* to amend the analysis either to exclude the dropouts or to change the model to a two part proportional hazard model (which to a degree mitigates the change in the survival of the dropout patients pre and post new drug approval).

FIGURE 14.1 Reasons to amend the statistical analysis plan before unblinding the study.

- *Noncompliance*: Subjects may refuse to participate in certain tests (e.g., avoiding tedious or painful tests) or answer certain questions (e.g., finding some questions to be offensive or too personal). They may intentionally or unintentionally miss appointments.
- *Failure to record data*: Study personnel can make mistakes. The more complicated the recording, the more likely recording problems will be.
- *Values out of measurement range*: Every measurement device or method has its range of potential values (e.g., lab assays cannot measure blood sugars above a certain level). Measurements that fall out of this measurable range will be listed as too low or too high to measure.
- *Measurements cannot be made*: Some situations prevent adequate measurements (e.g., patients may be too large to fit in the CT scan machine, unconscious so that they cannot answer a survey, or dehydrated so that they cannot produe a urine sample).
- *Ethical or legal barriers*: Obtaining certain types of data may be prohibited in certain patients (e.g., X-rays in pregnant patients or strenuous tests in the elderly).
- *Errors in storing or transferring data*: During the course of a study, data may go through many different hands and databases. Each step brings the chance that data is damaged or lost (e.g., computers may crash, case report form [CRF] pages be lost, or blackouts may occur). Privacy and data security considerations make data storage and transferring even more complicated.
- *Treatment discontinuations*: Treatment regimens may be too successful (e.g., enough positive efficacy data is generated) or unsuccessful (e.g., adverse effects) to complete.
- *Losses to follow-up*: Many situations can result in patient dropouts (e.g., patients move away).

Types of Missing Data

In 1976, Donald Rubin (who is currently John L. Loeb Professor of Statistics at Harvard University) proposed a taxonomy for describing missing data. Missing data can be categorized as missing completely at random, missing at random, or not missing at random.

When data is *missing completely at random (MCAR)*, the probability of a measurement being missing is entirely independent of its value or the value of other measurements. For example, since gender is fairly easy to determine and record, gender may in many studies be MCAR as long as there is no reason why women would be more or less likely to drop out from a study. MCAR data produces absolutely no bias and is the result of purely random events such as lost data or database malfunction. True MCAR data is rare since most events differentially affect certain values of data more than others.

When data is *missing at random (MAR)*, the probability of a measurement being missing is independent of its value, but dependent on the value of other types of measurements.

For example, high blood pressures are no more or less likely to be missing than low blood pressures. However, obese patients may be more likely to be missing blood pressures because their arm size exceeds the maximum for the blood pressure cuffs. MAR data is much more realistic and common than MCAR.

Not missing at random (NMAR) data creates the most bias, because the probability of a measurement missing depends on the value of the measurement. For example, older patients may be less likely to reveal their ages, wealthier patients may be less likely to reveal their salaries, or minorities may be more likely to drop out since they feel isolated or out of place. NMAR data creates significant bias. So to continue our examples, higher ages, higher salaries, or certain ethnic groups will have fewer observations in the database.

Determining whether missing data is MCAR, MAR, or NMAR is important but can be very difficult. You have to calculate the probabilities of different values of a measurement being missing (e.g., for ethnicity, Caucasians vs. African Americans vs. Latinos vs. Asian Americans) and the probabilities of different values when combined with other measurements (e.g., are wealthier Asian Americans more likely to be missing than wealthier Caucasians). As you can see, this can be a rather complex endeavor. Sensitivity analyses, (i.e., varying the values of a measurement and seeing how it affects the outcomes of interest) can be helpful.

14.3.2 Patient Dropouts

Dropouts rarely occur completely at random, that is, certain patients are more likely to drop out of a study. Patients may be more likely to drop out of a study if they experience:

- *Side effects from the treatment (including death).*
- *Progression of the disease (including death).* Patients may be anxious to switch to a proven medication or too ill to continue in the trial.
- *An inadequate response to the treatment.*
- *An excellent response to the treatment – so good that patient no longer felt the need for treatment.*

If the treatment group experiences one or more of any of the above causes than the placebo group, bias will result. Bias also will be present if any of the above is more likely in the placebo group than the treatment group.

Other causes of dropouts may either have random effects or cause bias:

- *New alternative treatments become available.* Patients from both treatment and placebo groups may leave the trial for better treatments.
- *Investigators decide to remove certain patients.* Investigators may find certain patient is noncompliant or otherwise inappropriate for the study.

- *Patients make significant lifestyle changes.* For example, move to another state, change jobs, or have children. Patients who feel that their therapy is working may make more effort to stay in the study.
- *The study is inconvenient.* For example, requiring too many visits, blood draws, or tests.

It can be difficult to predict which subpopulations may suffer more dropouts. As Table 14.2 illustrates, the same factor can make a patient more or less likely to drop out of a study.

Table 14.3 shows how having more dropouts among the less severe patients can bias the results. As you can see, the average patient disease severity worsens over time.

14.3.3 Dealing with Missing Data

Keep several things in mind when dealing with missing data:

- *Establish in advance how you will handle missing data before unblinding and analyzing the data (i.e., in the statistical plan)*: Defining and prescribing your methods in the statistical plan will prevent biases.
- *Make every effort to minimize bias*: If you need to determine how to deal with missing data after unblinding, an independent adjudication panel can review the data and determine a course of action. The adjudicators should be blind to both the patient assignment (i.e., which treatment groups they belong to) and trial results.

- *Any methods used and their results should be reproducible*: Someone else should be able to apply the same way of handling the missing data and arrive at the same results.
- *Make all efforts to minimize loss of information*: If the amount of missing data is substantial, simply discarding all missing data may result in too much wasted information. Choose a method that not only is valid and reliable but also will preserve as much information as possible.
- *Clearly document your methods*: Documentation should include all specific decisions and the rationale behind each decision. This should be part of the study report or an appendix to the study report.
- *To the best of your ability, determine and document the circumstances behind and cause of each missing value*: The circumstances and cause will help choose the most appropriate method of dealing with the missing data. This is especially true with patients who dropped out of the study. Knowing why each patient withdrew is extremely important (e.g., if the patient dropped out because a treatment was not working, you may have to consider subsequent missing values as treatment failure). Carefully design the CRFs to capture such information.
- *Study design can help minimize missing data*: The same circumstances may result in missing data in one type of study design but no missing data in another type of study design. For example, patients dropout of a study can result in missing data (i.e., you do not have measurements on the patient after he withdraws).

TABLE 14.2   Difficulty of Predicting Dropouts

Disease severity	Are more likely to drop out because…	Are less likely to drop out because…
Less severe disease	Have less to gain from staying in the clinical trial	Are healthier so can better comply with the trial requirements
More severe disease	Are hampered by poor health	Really need the treatment

TABLE 14.3   Example of How Dropouts Can Affect the Patient Population Over Time

	January	March	May	July
Patients with less severe disease (Score = 2)	50	45	40	30
Dropouts (less severe)	2	2	2	2
Patients with more severe disease (score = 10)	50	49	49	45
Dropouts (more severe)	10	10	10	10
Sum of severity scores	600	580	570	510
Total patients	100	94	89	75
Average disease severity score	6	6.17	6.40	6.80

However, before the study begins, you may specify that, whenever a patient withdraws due to lack of treatment effect or need for rescue medication, the patient has achieved an endpoint and completed the study. In such a case, no measurements will be needed after the patient withdraws.

- *Missing safety and efficacy data may require different methods*: We discuss this later in the chapter.

For each piece of missing data, determine its *ignorability* (i.e., whether the missing values affect the analysis and interpretation of the data). Missing values are ignorable if they do not affect the analysis and interpretation. The type of data, intervention, and condition studied determine ignorability. Missing efficacy or safety data is rarely ignorable. Other types of data may be ignorable depending on their nature and quantity. MCAR and MAR data are potentially ignorable, provided the percentage of missing data is relatively low. Any type of missing data is not ignorable if it constitutes a sizable proportion of the overall data set (e.g., missing half the data, even at random, can be devastating).

Sensitivity analyses also can help establish the ignorability of your missing data. Sensitivity analyses involve varying the missing variable along a range of different values (e.g., minimum to maximum) and ascertaining how this affects the results, analysis, or outcomes of the trial. If there is no effect, the missing values are potentially ignorable. The greater the effect, the less ignorable the missing values are. Sensitivity analyses also help determine how to handle missing values, as we will discuss later.

Several different possible methods can handle non-ignorable missing data.

Rational Substitution

Sometimes guessing the values of missing data is relatively simple and straightforward. (e.g., if a patient is currently a professional football player, you may assume that his functional status score will be the highest possible). Rational substitution requires making assumptions (e.g., you assume that a professional football player is physically fit enough to accomplish most activities of daily living). The more far-reaching the assumption required, the less appropriate it is to use rational substitution (e.g., it is too much to assume that the football player's physical exam will be completely normal).

Case Deletion

Complete Case Analysis

One option is to exclude all subjects with any missing data (i.e., incomplete cases) from your analysis. In other words, consider only subjects with a complete set of data (i.e., complete cases). This method (known as *complete case analysis* or *list-wise deletion*) may be appropriate if the number of complete cases is substantial and differences between complete and incomplete cases are minimal. Systematic differences between incomplete (e.g., more debilitated patients) and complete cases will introduce significant bias.

Available Case Analysis

Available case analysis is similar to complete case analysis, except that you only exclude subjects that have specific types of missing data. In other words, a subject does not have to have a complete set of data, just a minimum amount. For example, you may specify that a patient must have all blood pressure readings, echocardiogram results, and electrocardiogram results to be included in the analysis. Then available case analysis will include a subject missing all temperature readings and glucose levels but exclude a subject missing a single blood pressure reading. In general, the limitations of available case analysis are similar to those of complete case analysis. One of the challenges is determining the minimal level of data you will require.

Censoring

The biggest problem with case deletion is the great loss of information. Subjects with only a few missing values can still provide a large amount of potentially valuable information. To exclude all of the subject's data may be a tremendous waste, especially if subjects are hard to find.

Censoring is assuming that the patient does not exist during the time when his or her data is missing. For example, imagine that a study with 20 patients. During Time Periods 1 through 4, all data was complete. During Time Period 5, 2 patients were missing data. Censoring would view 20 patients as being present during Periods 1 through 4 but only 18 patients as being present in Period 5. In effect, censoring a patient reduces both the numerator and the denominator. This method is most common with survival analysis but can be part of any analysis that has a time component (e.g., in slope analysis, computing the slope without the missing data). Censoring is not possible with analysis such as number of hospitalizations that can happen multiple times. It would have to be something along the lines of "risk of hospitalization" at any given time.

There can be a variation on this – for instance, in the example above, patients who drop out due to an adverse event or lack of efficacy might be counted as having had a recurrence, while the patients who drop out for other reasons such as moving to another part of the country, might be censored.

Single Imputation

Imputation is finding a value to replace a missing or incorrect value. Imputation is akin to guessing or assuming. For example, the weather is usually warm and sunny in San Diego. If you failed to check the weather one day, you may assume or impute that it was warm and sunny. Depending on the situation, your assumption or imputation may be strong and justifiable or weak and haphazard. For example, pro tennis player Martina Hingis frequently played and almost always beat Anna Kournikova. If you missed one of their matches, you could safely assume or impute that Martina won. However, Martina did not always defeat Monica Seles. Imputing the result of their match would be far more difficult.

Single imputation is replacing each missing value with a single value (i.e., one value for every missing one). This replacement value is called an "impute" and can be the mean, median, mode, minimum, or maximum of the nonmissing values or any other derived value, whichever happens to make the most sense. Your choice depends on the situation, variable, intervention, and condition.

Single imputation is relatively simple and straightforward and may be reasonable when the fraction of missing data is small (e.g., less than 5%). It assumes that the missing values are known and exact. For example, say you have 100 women in a trial (ranging in height from 5-feet to 5-feet-8) and you are missing the heights for two women. Assuming that the two women are 5-feet-4 (your calculated median) would be single imputation.

However, single imputation can be problematic when there is significant variation in the variable of interest. Say your patient population includes a number of gymnasts, jockeys, football players, and basketball players (i.e., the subjects' heights vary widely). Would it be reasonable to replace every missing height with a median or mean of all the subjects' heights? This may lead to a gross overestimation of a jockey's height and a gross underestimation of a basketball player's height. Moreover, if the data is not MCAR then single imputation can exacerbate biases. For example, if only the female gymnasts' heights were missing and you replaced these missing values with the population's median height, all of the female gymnasts may be listed as much taller than they really are, biasing the data.

Use Simple Statistical Measures (e.g., Means or Medians)

Means or medians can effectively serve as imputed values if the patient population, conditions, and environment are not too variable and heterogeneous. The means or medians should be from the most similar and relevant portion of the observations. Depending on the situation, they may be means or medians of all nonmissing values for all patients, for similar patients, or for the same person in other time periods.

Using means or medians is potentially fraught with problems. They become more inaccurate as the percentage of missing values grow. Such simple statistical measures can be too simple for imputation, masking underlying variability.

Moreover, extreme measurements can greatly skew statistical measures such as means.

Treat as Failure/Worst Case

When imputing missing efficacy data, the simplest imputation method is to consider missing data as failures in the treatment arm and successes in the control arm. In other words, assume that your intervention does not have an effect whenever data is missing. This is easiest when the missing variable is dichotomous (i.e., has only two alternatives) in a landmark analysis (i.e., at a given point of time, which alternative did the subject experience?). For example, imagine that the endpoint with missing values is mortality at 6 months. Worst case analysis imputation would count all missing endpoint values as deaths in the active arm and as survivors in the control arm (Figure 14.2).

Such an imputation method may be difficult for nonlandmark analyses (e.g., survival or frequency analysis). What if the missing variable of interest is the frequency or rate of an event (e.g., number of atrial fibrillation episodes over 6 months)? What would be the worst case scenario? Would the patient have experienced a bad event (e.g., atrial fibrillation) every single week, every single day, or every single hour? You could select the highest rate of bad events among the patients with complete data. However, this assumes that the patients' missing data did not have the highest frequency or rate, which often is not a safe assumption since patients having the most problems may be most likely to be noncompliant or drop out of a study.

Such an imputation method may be difficult with variables that have multiple alternatives (e.g., chest pain level) or are continuous (e.g., length of time patient walked on a treadmill). For example, what is the maximum amount of time a patient can walk on a treadmill? How long do we assume a placebo patient (which would be considered a best-case scenario) walked on the treadmill? Do we assume that an active treatment patient (worse case) could not tolerate the treadmill at all?

When the missing value (e.g., dropout) rate is higher in the active arm than the placebo arm (which is usually the case), this imputation method is very conservative (i.e., stacked against the intervention). However, if missing value rate is higher in the placebo or control arm, this imputation method may be too permissive (i.e., favorable for the intervention).

Use Baseline Value

Some variables (e.g., blood pressure, heart rate, or laboratory values) are measured at the beginning of the study (baseline values) and may not change during the course of the study. If you have the baseline measurements and the condition is rather stable, it may be safe to assume that the measurements did not change (e.g., a patient who

Example:
A rheumatoid arthritis study has enrolled 50 patients into each of two arms (active treatment and placebo). The placebo group has 5 patients dropout of the study. The active group has 9 dropouts. The primary endpoint is the number of patients who experience an ACR20 response. A conservative imputation would assign "no response" to all patients who dropped out.

FIGURE 14.2 Example of worst case imputation.

TABLE 14.4   Example of Interpolation and Extrapolation

				Day					
	1	2	3	4	5	6	7	8	9
Interpolation	2	4	6	8	10	12	14	16	18
Extrapolation	3	6	9	12	15	18	21	24	27

The shaded boxes are the imputed values.

begins the study with an oxygen requirement of 2 L/min may require the same rate throughout a subsequent 6-week period). Using baseline values is problematic when the condition is not stable or the intervention is expected to affect the variables.

Last Observation Carried Forward

The last observation carried forward (LOCF) method of imputation uses the last recorded value before the missing value. So, for example, if the heart rate is 80 on Day 1, 82 on Day 2, and missing on Day 3, you may impute that the Day 3 heart rate is 82, i.e. the latest available measurement before the missing value. LOCF potentially can fill in all of the missing values after a patient drops out of a study (e.g., if the patient drops out Day 3 of a 20-day study, LOCF assumes that the heart rate for Days 4–20 is the Day 2 measurement or 82 beats/min). LOCF runs into problems when events occur between the last available measurement and subsequent missing values (e.g., patient suffered a heart attack in the evening of Day 2). LOCF also can be inaccurate when patients drop out of the study due to worsening of their conditions (e.g., a patient's heart condition gets worse so that his heart rate actually is supposed to steadily rise).

Conditional Mean Imputation

When a particular variable has missing values and is dependent on the values of other variables, you can build a regression model with that particular variable as the dependent variable. Complete observations can help estimate the regression coefficients for independent variables in the model. Then, the model can impute or predict the dependent variable's missing values based on the independent variables'

values. Probit or logit regression models are appropriate for binary variables. Poisson or other count regression models are appropriate for integer-valued variables. OLS or similar regression models are suitable continuous variables.

Interpolation and Extrapolation

Interpolation and extrapolation employ existing data values to develop a curve (i.e., regression analysis or curve fitting), which helps impute missing values. The curve may be a simple line (i.e., linear) or a more complicated curve. When the missing values are between existing data points, we call the process *interpolation*. When the missing values come after all the existing data points, we call the process *extrapolation* (see Table 14.4).

Variable Imputation

One of the most realistic, but potentially most difficult ways to impute missing values is variable imputation, i.e., to tailor each individual imputation to available data and circumstances. You look at the conditions surrounding and leading up to the missing value and then impute the value accordingly (e.g., counting patients who dropped out after treatment inefficacy as treatment failures, who dropped out after their symptoms resolved as treatment successes, who have worsening symptom scores before the missing value as treatment failures, and who have improving symptom scores as treatment successes). There are two general ways to employ variable imputation:

1. *Rule-based*: Establish a set of clear rules in advance. For example, whenever you see Situation X always impute using Procedure A.

2. *Blinded independent adjudication panel*: The panel can review the data and determine how to impute missing values.

Hot Deck Imputation

Hot deck imputation uses values from complete records of patients who are similar to the patient with missing data to impute the missing value. Let us illustrate with an analogy. Suppose we do not know how fast football player Dan Marino would run the 100-m dash. We could randomly choose one of the 100-m dash times of players similar to Dan Marino (e.g., quarterbacks who are similar height, weight, and age). As long as your sample is large enough, the more similar the players are to Dan Marino, the more likely the imputed time will be accurate.

Hot deck imputation works the same way with clinical trial data. The first step is to divide all the observations into different relevant groups. You may, for example, group everyone of the same gender, ethnicity, age, and socioeconomic status together (e.g., one group can be Latino men ages 40–50 with an annual income of $50,000–$75,000, a second group can be White women ages 30–40 with an annual income of $100,000–$125,000, etc). Then, for each missing value, randomly select a value from complete observations within the same group (which we will call the comparable group). For example, if the weight of a 35-year old White woman with an annual income of $110,000 is missing, randomly select a weight from among White women ages 30–40 with an annual income of $100,000–$125,000. The key is to narrow the characteristics so that the comparable group is similar enough to the patient with missing values but not so much that the comparable group has very few observations (e.g., having the comparison group be White woman ages 33–36 with an annual income of $109,000–$110,000 may be too specific). By choosing randomly from a comparable group, hot deck imputation, unlike single imputation, incorporates data variability.

Multiple Imputations

As we mentioned above single imputation replaces each missing value with a single value, generating a single full data set, i.e. a single *imputed data set*. Statistically analyzing this single imputed data set yields a single set of results. Single imputation assumes that each missing value is known exactly (e.g., the patient's height is 5-feet-5) and fails to account for any potential variability (e.g., the patient's height may be 5-feet-3, 5-feet-5, or 5-feet-7).

Multiple imputation overcomes this potential drawback of single imputation. This method incorporates uncertainty (e.g., you do not know exactly what a patient's height may be). Multiple imputation replaces each missing value with a set of possible values (multiple imputes). In multiple imputation, using different possible imputes for each missing value will generate multiple imputed data sets (e.g., in one imputed data set, Patient A's height is 5-feet-3; in a second imputed data set, Patient A's height is 5-feet-5; and in a third imputed data set, Patient A's height is 5-feet-7). Statistically analyzing each imputed data set separately yields multiple separate results (e.g., Data Set 1 results, Data Set 2 results, etc). You can then combine these different analysis results to produce one overall analysis.

Of course, the different possible imputes for each missing value should not be wild guesses. They should be educated predictions about what the missing value may be and the variability associated with that value. If a patient's weight is probably around 105 pounds, then you should not use 180 pounds and 85 pounds as possible values. Understanding the standard error, variances, and standard deviation for each variable is important.

14.3.4 Incomplete or Partial Data

What do you do when a certain measurement is either incomplete or only partially present (and neither completely missing nor complete)? This can occur in a composite endpoint (e.g., a patient answered all but 1 or 2 of the questions in a 10-question questionnaire). In some cases, you may be able to use some of the aforementioned imputation methods for missing values to "complete" or discard the incomplete data. There are also several additional options:

- *Treat the measurement as a percentage or fraction*: The simplest method is to calculate the fraction of the available data (e.g., consider a patient who answered 7 out of 8 questions correctly as having answered 8.75 questions correctly). Usually, you may assume that the portion of the measurement that is not available is consistent with the available portion.
- *Establish a cutoff or threshold*: Another method may introduce a cutoff or threshold, above which the data is considered missing (e.g., if greater than 15% of the values are missing in a composite endpoint then the incomplete data is missing data).
- *Establish rules*: You can design rules. Of course, all the caveats about imputing missing data apply to incomplete data – for example, if it is likely that the answer was left blank because the patients probably did not know the answer, then the answer might be best imputed as an incorrect response.

14.4 DATA VERIFICATION AND VALIDATION

14.4.1 Data Verification

Although many definitions of data verification exist, we define *data verification* here as checking whether the data set is complete and was collected and recorded by proper procedures. We discussed data completeness in the previous section. However, even though data is fully present, it may not be reliable or trustworthy. Data generation, recording, entry, or storage problems may have occurred. Taking the following steps is important:

- *Determining and reviewing the sources of the data*: This includes ensuring that all measurement instruments and personnel were reliable, the data came from the right locations and patients, and the data sources did not experience any importance changes during the study that may have corrupted the data.
- *Comparing the data collection, entry, and storage process with the study protocol and any other procedural guidelines*: Was everything done according to protocol? Were there any discrepancies? We discuss protocol deviations in Section 14.5.
- *Whenever data is entered or transferred, compare the original source with the new data set*: If data is transferred from Data Source 1 to a database, are the specific entries the same? Are there any discrepancies? Were there problems in data entry or transcription errors?

Analyzing all of the data may be too time- and resource-consuming. Depending on the situation, verifying random or selected samples of the data may suffice.

14.4.2 Data Validation

Many definitions of data validation exist. Here we define data validation as checking whether the data "makes sense" (we define validity in Chapter 4). This may include the following checks:

- *Presence check*: Are the necessary and relevant data fields present? Certain fields are almost always mandatory (e.g., the patient's age and gender). Certain conditions or interventions call for specific fields (e.g., when studying congestive heart failure you should have the patient's ejection fraction).
- *Range check*: Do values fall within the appropriate or pre-specified range? Are any numbers much higher or lower than expected or possible (e.g., a blood pressure measurement of 300/50 mmHg)? Are any values present that should not be present (e.g., if the possible options for a variable are "high," "medium," and "low," "very low," or "very high" should not be possible)?
- *Type check*: Do you see the right kind or type of data (e.g., age usually should be integers and not percentages or letters, cardiac ejection fraction usually should be percentages not letters or exponential numbers).
- *Format check*: Are the data in the appropriate formats? Are there numbers where there should be numbers and letters where there should be letters? Do the numerical values have the correct number of digits (e.g., zip codes

should be five digits)? Are decimal points in the right locations?
- *Spelling check*: When words are present, are they spelled correctly?
- *Length check*: Are the numbers of the appropriate length, i.e. have the correct number of digits (e.g., blood sugars should not have more than three digits)?
- *Internal consistency check*: When the same data is collected in different ways, do the values conflict with each other (e.g., is the date of a specific adverse event different in the CRF, adverse event form, and safety databases)? *Triangulation* means comparing measurements of the same phenomenon that were collected using different techniques.
- *Outliers check*: Are there any unusual values that seem out of line with the rest of the values (e.g., a patient weighs 70 kg on every visit except for one visit where his weight was recorded as 170 kg)?
- *Data behavior check*: Some data fields should closely correlate with other data fields (e.g., heart rate and temperature should rise and fall together; different measures of diabetic glycemic control should correspond with each other).
- *Data distribution (variability) check*: Are the values of the data assuming the expected distribution? In other words, are you seeing the appropriate variability in the data? For example it would be unusual for every patient to have the same respiration rate, weight, or height unless the study pre-specified that the values must be exact numbers. Data with too little or no variability suggests that the data may be erroneous or fabricated.
- *Intra-study comparisons*: Often, comparing data from one part of the study or study population with another is helpful. For example, data from the first 50% of the patients in the study should roughly match data from the second 50% of the study, unless there is logical reason why the two halves should be different.

Other data validation techniques may be helpful. Repeating measurements on a sample of the research subjects can confirm whether repeat measurements correspond with the data values (*respondent or subject validation*). You may look for and further explore any unusual or outlying data values (*deviant case or data analysis*). Unexpected or contradictory data values can be isolated cases or indicative of major general problems in data collection or entry.

14.5 PROTOCOL DEVIATIONS AND VIOLATIONS

14.5.1 Definitions and Causes

Often a study will not go completely as planned. There will be differences between the study protocol and how the study is actually conducted. We call these differences *protocol deviations*. When the investigators and relevant governing bodies (e.g., the sponsor approve a protocol deviation before initiating the study, it is called a *protocol waiver or exception*. The most common protocol waiver is allowing subjects who do not strictly meet the inclusion and exclusion criteria. When the protocol deviation is not approved by the relevant governing bodies, it is called a *protocol violation*. Protocol violations that affect the safety or efficacy of the intervention, the subject's rights, safety, or willingness to participate in the study, or the study's integrity or results are *major protocol violations*. Otherwise they are *minor protocol violations*.

Checking for protocol violations is essential but can be complicated, especially in large multi-national clinical trials. You must carefully compare the study protocol with the actual conduct of the study. This includes ensuring that patients were screened appropriately, patient visits occurred at the correct times, measurements were performed properly, and the intervention was administered correctly. Protocol violations may result in missing data (e.g., measurements that were supposed to be performed did not occur) or unreliable and unusable data (e.g., measurements for a patient who did not receive the correct dose of the drug may be inaccurate).

Many problems can cause protocol violations:

- *Poorly prepared study protocols*: The protocol instructions may be ambiguous or difficult to understand or follow (e.g., completing three blood draws, an electrocardiogram, a chest X-ray, and a survey within 30 min may be physically impossible).
- *Sloppy or poorly trained investigators*: Study personnel may not understand or have the training to execute the protocol.
- *Deliberately not following protocol instructions* (e.g., study personnel may want to cut corners or be opposed to performing certain tasks).
- *Communication, language, or cultural barriers*: Study personnel or subjects may not understand what is expected of them (e.g., instructions may be of a different language or study personnel may not communicate well).
- *Patient noncompliance*: Patients may accidentally or deliberately not follow directions.
- *Technical failures*: Equipment, computers, or laboratory assays can malfunction (e.g., radiology equipment breaks so that you must use an alternative test).
- *Prevailing conditions*: The environment can affect study conduct (e.g., a severe snowstorm can prevent subjects from making the required visits).
- *Limitations*: Study personnel and subjects may make every effort to follow instructions but cannot do so (e.g., subject is unable to walk so cannot complete a task).
- *Unforeseen events or accidents*: For example, a subject gets injured and cannot complete a task or an electrical blackout prevents the use of equipment or results in the loss of data.

- *Safety issues*: Sometimes following the protocol can actually endanger certain patients (e.g., the intervention causes unforeseen side effects or certain diagnostic tests or procedures prove to be harmful to patients with specific conditions).

14.5.2 Checking Protocol Compliance

A systematic approach to checking protocol compliance will help guarantee that no important aspects are overlooked. Careful and rigorous review of available records is paramount. The study must have adhered to Good Clinical Practices (GCP) and ethical standards. Some important steps in checking protocol compliance include the following.

Review Audit and Monitoring Records

As we discussed in earlier Chapter 12, throughout the study, active monitoring and periodic audits occur. Keeping and reviewing records from these activities will confirm the degree to which laws, rules, and procedures were followed (e.g., site visits ensure that the submitted data is accurate, complete, and match the patients' medical charts). Look for any GCP violations. Whenever discrepancies or unusual events occurred, you will have to decide whether and how they affected the data and results. Make sure you review documentation for any test samples or measurements (e.g., were the correct lab assays run or were the ultrasound examinations performed in the correct manner) and core laboratory quality checks. For any audits, make sure that the prespecified audit plan was followed and findings were addressed and completed. Compare monitoring reports with prespecified monitoring plans to ensure that the plan was followed. Confirm that any findings were addressed and "closed out." Of course, checking every single document and documentation is not necessary and often not feasible. You should examine enough documents to get a sense for how well the study was conducted.

Check Whether Patients Met the Selection Criteria

The next step is examining individual level data. Make sure that the patients enrolled in the study met the inclusion and exclusion criteria. Even slight violations in these criteria can significantly affect results. A significant number of selection criteria violations will invalidate the study. Selection criteria violations may be deliberate (e.g., investigators bending criteria to get certain patients into a study) or accidental. Deliberate violations may be allowable if the investigator receives a waiver and the waiver is fully documented. However, such violations may significantly damage the interpretability of the data.

Review the selection criteria and make sure that they were not vaguely worded or inadequate. Otherwise,

> *Warning*
>
> Some studies allow patients to be randomized before meeting all selection criteria and some of their eligibility assessments to occur at the end of the study [e.g., some "metastatic" cancer patients, who were initially enrolled on the basis of investigator assessment, turned out not to have metastasis after a more formal, rigorous assessment later in the study (*Journal of Clinical Oncology*, Vol 23, No 9 (March 20), 2005: pp. 2004–2011)]. In other words, some studies randomize patients before they have met all of the inclusion criteria. If at all possible, avoid such protocols. However, sometimes, such protocols may be unavoidable (e.g., in emergency treatments patients must be enrolled quickly before being fully assessed) and nearly always lead to data interpretation problems.

FIGURE 14.3 Enrolling patients before they meet all selection criteria.

inappropriate patients may have slipped into study. Check for any protocol amendments during the study that may have made previously eligible patients ineligible or previously ineligible patients eligible. This can make analysis difficult since the study population did not remain consistent throughout the study. Although usually you want to screen patients carefully before enrolling them in a study, sometimes you have to enroll patients before confirming that they meet all selection criteria. (Figure 14.3).

Check Intervention Compliance

It is extremely important to check whether each patient received the intervention in an appropriate manner. Did each patient receive the right dose? Did the doses occur according to schedule? Did the study personnel and patients follow the correct procedures when administering the intervention? Did the patient start and stop receiving the intervention at the appropriate times? Although intervention compliance is typically much better than in clinical practice, compliance in clinical trials is rarely 100%. Strategies to ensure compliance include the following:

- *Supervised intervention administration*: Some interventions are typically well-supervised (e.g., intravenous drug administration or surgical procedures). Others (e.g., patients taking pills at home) are most difficult or costly to supervise.
- *Tracer*: Several different inert, safe tracers are available to assess drug intake (e.g., fluorescein, riboflavin, or phenol red). Tracers usually can only determine recent drug intake.
- *Body fluid assays*: Many substances when administered to the body are detectable in different body fluids such as the blood, urine, saliva, or sweat. Assays may vary in sensitivity, specificity, and accuracy. Some assays can only detect the presence or absence of the substance. Some can detect different levels of the substance, which reflects the amount of substance the patient received. The pharmacokinetics and pharmacodynamics of the substance determine its appearance in different body fluids. It is usually difficult to find assays that can check placebo compliance.

- *Automatic recorders*: Some electronic devices can record the time an intervention is administered (e.g., electronic pill bottles that record the time the cap is opened).
- *Pill count*: Periodic counts of the number of pills a patient still has can help calculate the number of pills a patient has taken. Of course, patients may discard or lose pills, which will throw off the count.
- *Secondary effects*: Interventions may cause secondary effects (e.g., side effects) that can be tracked (e.g., some drugs will change urine color or hemodynamic parameters such as blood pressure). Detecting these changes is evidence that the patient is compliant.

Determine Whether the Intervention Actually Reached Its Target

Just because a patient received an intervention does not mean the intervention reached its ultimate destination. A patient may have taken a medication, but did that medication actually reach the bloodstream? Checking appropriate blood test results and pharmacokinetic measurements can provide the answer. Did the medication reach the target organ or tissue? Checking tissue samples may be helpful though usually impractical. A medical device may be inside a patient, but is it in the right location? Reviewing operative and available imaging reports can answer this question.

Check Whether Blinding was Appropriately Maintained Among Patients and Investigators

It can be helpful to double-check if patients were truly randomized and that patients and study personnel were truly unaware of what treatment each patient received. Make sure that one person kept the randomization code. Ask patients whether they can guess which treatment they received. Ask "blinder" study personnel if they can guess which patients received which treatments. If the patients and study personnel accurately guess the treatments, determine if such knowledge may have affected the results.

Check Comparability of the Different Study Groups

The populations in the different treatment arms should be relatively similar, with similar balances of major demographic and baseline characteristics. Check for any differences among the arms that may bias the study (e.g., different frequency of follow-up, different concomitant medications, or different compliance rates). Of course, perfect balances do not always occur, so make sure that any detected imbalances will not significantly affect the study results and interpretation. As we will discuss later in Chapter 15, sometimes statistical adjustments can compensate for imbalances, but they may be difficult and problematic to perform.

Check Comparability of Different Study Sites

Make sure that enrollment was well distributed among the different study sites. Determine if any sites had any unusual characteristics or situations. Ideally, each study site should have at least 4–5 patients and no more than 20% of all patients.

Check Subject Allocation (Usually Randomization) and Control Groups

Make sure that subjects were allocated in a reasonable manner to the different study groups. If randomization was used, did the study adhere to the right randomization procedure? Did the study maintain proper allocation concealment? Were the controls appropriate? Did the control groups follow protocol procedure?

Additional Checks

Some additional items to check include the following:

- Did follow-up visits and tests occur at appropriate times?
- Were tests interpreted using appropriate procedures?
- Did patients avoid prohibited medications?
- Did study personnel have the right qualifications?

14.6 DATA CLEANING

14.6.1 Data Screening (Error Detection)

Data cleaning is the process of correcting errors in the study database. *Dirty data* has many errors while *clean data* has relatively few errors. The line between clean and dirty data is very indistinct and arbitrary. In general, the more rigorous the study, the cleaner the data needs to be. We already

discussed some of the potential sources and types of errors. Some additional potential errors include the following:

- *Missing data proxies*: Sometimes people will enter a variable or number to serve as placeholder for missing data. Instead of leaving something blank, they will put "xxx" or "111" or some other series of letters or numbers. These can play havoc on data analysis.
- *Data transposition*: The process of entering or transferring data may accidentally shift blocks of data up or down several rows or left or right several columns.
- *Coding errors*: People may misread the coding key (which shows what codes are associated with what measurements) and enter incorrect codes or categories into a database.
- *Typing or transcription errors*: Spelling or typing mistakes are common.

Data cleaning is a two-part process. First, you have to find or detect errors (i.e., *error screening* or *detection*). Second, you have to correct or decide how to handle these errors (i.e., *data correction*).

The previous two sections addressed some of the error detection process. In general, your error detection arsenal consists of five major tools:

1. *Visual Inspection*: Simply looking at the data can catch many major errors. Row and column shifts may be fairly obvious. Improper data formats and obvious bizarre values may be very noticeable. Visual inspection is effective when the database is relatively small and fairly repetitive. Of course, the larger the database, the less effective visual inspection becomes. Even when the database is large, do not overlook visual inspection. Always, look at the data to make sure it makes sense.

2. *Data entry programs*: Some software programs will prevent the entry or existence of values that are inconsistent or erroneous. While some only work at the data entry stage, others can take existing databases and screen for errors using programmed algorithms.

3. *Descriptive statistics*: Checking some basic statistics (e.g., mean, median, minimum, maximum, standard deviation/variance, and mode) on each variable can go a long way. The minimum and maximum will identify significant outliers that may incorrect values. Strange or unusual values may skew or perturb any statistical measure but especially the mean, standard deviation, and variance. Consider some simple bivariate analyses (i.e., statistical tests that show the correlation between two different variables). If, for instance, height does not seem to correlate with weight, there may be a problem.

4. *Graphing*: Graphing the data may quickly identify errors. *Frequency histograms* of each variable will show significant outliers, strange distributions, and unusual skews in the data. If you expect a variable to have a normal distribution, any other distribution should raise concerns.

Scatterplots can show how one variable correlates with another variable.

5. *Sample scenarios and logic checks*: Think of different scenarios that should generate certain expected findings and run those scenarios in the data. For example, if you know that patients from a certain zip code should have lower income than those from another zip code, check to see whether the data supports this assumption. Be creative in designing and executing these "spot checks."

14.6.2 Data Correction

Some data errors are easily correctable. The correct spelling or number for a data entry error may be obvious. Shifting rows or columns back to their correct positions may be relatively straightforward. Going back to the original data source may remedy coding errors. When redundant data is available (i.e., the same values in different locations), checking the redundant source may help correct the error.

When data errors are more complicated, you may treat them as you would miss data. Many of the missing strategies and imputation techniques are at your disposal. The strategy and technique you choose depend on the situation. As with missing data approaches, the statistical analysis plan should pre-specify how to handle data errors before you even see the data. Otherwise significant biases could result.

14.7 DERIVING, CATEGORIZING, AND AGGREGATING DATA

14.7.1 Deriving Data

In addition to the raw primary data, data sets frequently include *derived data*. Derived data is generated from other data using calculations. For example, people usually do not directly measure the pulse pressure for a patient but instead, measure and record the patient's systolic blood pressure and diastolic blood pressure on the CRF. Subtracting the diastolic blood pressure from systolic blood pressure then generates the pulse pressure. The pulse pressure would be derived data. Derived data can come from raw primary data or other derived data.

There are many common examples of derived data:

- *Physiological parameters with multiple components*: For example, cardiac output is equal to stroke volume multiplied by heart rate.
- *Physical parameters with multiple dimensions*: For example, body mass index is a patient's weight (kg)/[height (m)]^2.
- *Clinical scoring systems*: For example, acute physiology and chronic health evaluation (APACHE) consists of many different variables reflecting chronic medical conditions as well as acute physiological parameters.

Preparing the data set may require making a number of different calculations to generate derived data. Carefully check the raw primary data and then the derived data when making these calculations. Sometimes the calculations will result in fractions that need to be either rounded up or down. Rounding should be consistent and comply with pre-specified rules (i.e., do not haphazardly round up and down different fractions). Since rounding can dramatically affect the data, a clear system or algorithm should be in place.

14.7.2 Aggregating and Categorizing Data

Preparation of the data set may also involve categorizing and aggregating data. This means combining data into analyzable groupings. By analogy, say you were determining which people in a certain vicinity you would consider dating. Having a list of detailed personality and physical descriptions may not be helpful without placing them into relevant categories. So descriptions such as "kicked several dogs while walking on the street," "yelled at the waiters and waitresses," and "threw trash at children" may fall under the category of "rude/mean behavior." Descriptions such as "helped your friend lift and move some items," "told you when you had some pudding on your face," and "remembered your birthday" may qualify for the category of "nice/considerate behavior." It would then be much easier to tabulate the incidences of "rude/mean behavior" and "nice/considerate behavior."

Data categories may be *pre-sprecified* or *emergent*. You establish pre-specified or preset categories before looking at the data. The study protocol and analysis plan should delineate the preset or pre-specified data categories. Pre-specifying efficacy categories prevents certain types of bias. Looking at efficacy data may lead you to establish categories that will unduly favor (or be biased against) the study intervention. For example, imagine that the study intervention caused mild improvement in most study patients but major improvement in only a few study patients. Using the categories "improved vs. did not improve" will lead to dramatically different conclusions from using the categories "major improvement vs. mild improvement vs. no improvement" should be pre-set or pre-specified. Pre-specifying categories is not always possible. For example, categorizing safety data often will require emergently establishing categories (i.e., after or while you look at the data). Some adverse events will be very usual or unpredictable and need new categories.

Categorizing data is important when data is similar but slightly different in ways that are not relevant to the analysis. Data on outcomes or events may be too detailed in description: For example, in some cases, the location of a myocardial infarction may not be relevant, so anterior myocardial infarctions and inferior myocardial infarctions can all fall into a "myocardial infarction" category. You

TABLE 14.5	How Narrow Categories can Cause a Loss of Signal				
Study group	Hematoma	Epistaxis	Stroke	Anemia	Any bleeding
Placebo	2.1%	1%	0.2%	6%	**8.6%**
Drug	2.9%	1.4%	.8%	8.2%	11.2%

may want to place synonymous terminology into a single category: For example, "heart attack" and "myocardial infarction" should be in the same category. The Medical Dictionary for Regulatory Activities can assist in establishing appropriate categories and map different terms into appropriate categories.

Be careful when placing (or *mapping* or *coding*) data into different categories. Inconsistent mapping or coding can significantly alter the perceived efficacy or safety of an intervention. For example, not placing anterior myocardial infarction into the myocardial infarction category would lead to underestimating the number of myocardial infarctions that occurred in the study population. As with all manipulations of the data, verify and validate your categorization methods.

The broadness vs. narrowness of the categories also can affect data analysis and interpretation. Categories should be narrow enough so that important differences between measurements or events are not lost. At the same time, they should not be so narrow that each category has too few incidences or events. When categories are too narrow, the analysis may miss certain associations. Table 14.5 illustrates an example. Here too specific categories (e.g., hematoma, epistaxis, stroke, and anemia which are all bleeding events) may prevent investigators from recognizing a drug that causes bleeding (i.e., too narrow categories leads to a loss of "signal").

Categorizing into Appropriate Time Scale

Frequently, data analysis will necessitate grouping the timing of events into large discrete time periods (e.g., months, half-years, or years). So when a study started in July 1, 2007 and an event occurred in August 25, 2007, this event occurred in the second month, during the first 3 months, or during the first year, depending on the length of the time periods you choose to use. Using very broad time periods (e.g., 6-month periods) to categorize the timing of events may clump together events that occurred very distantly from each other (e.g., an adverse event that occurred one day after drug administration may have very different implications from an adverse event that occurred 4 months after drug administration. However, both events could be lumped together in an "Adverse Events During First Six Months category"). In other words, the resolution of the categories is very important.

14.8 TRANSFORMING DATA

14.8.1 Types of Transformations

Let us return to our cooking analogy. Before using your ingredients, you may need to convert some of them into usable forms. Not all ingredients are immediately ready for cooking. For example, you may have to marinate the meat and mushrooms, wash and dice the vegetables, and clean the fish and poultry. The preparation method depends on the ingredient. Some methods are simple, while others are complex.

Transforming data is analogous to preparing and converting the ingredients. Data is not necessarily analyzable in its initial form. *Data transformation* is applying mathematical operations to the data to change its measurement scale so that the data is more amenable to statistical analyses.

Several situations may require data transformation:

- *The data is not linear*: Most statistical analyses assume that phenomena are linear, i.e. there is a constant relationship between two different variables. In other words, if one variable changes by a certain amount the other variable will always change by a fixed amount regardless of the initial values of the variables (e.g., increasing X by 1 will always increase Y by 2. So if X goes from 1 to 2, Y will go from 10 to 12. If X goes from 2 to 3, Y will go from 12 to 14.) Of course, this assumption of linearity frequently does not hold with biological phenomena.
- *The data does not have a normal distribution*: Many statistical analyses assume that data for a given variable is normally distributed. In other words, plotting the values of the variable in a histogram generates a normal curve. Of course, this is not always the case. While normal distributions are common, variables also can assume a wide variety of distributions. In addition to graphing the data and "eyeballing" it, running some statistical tests (e.g., checking skew and kurtosis or the Kolmogorov–Smirnov test) can determine normality.
- *Significant outliers are present*: Some values of a variable will be significantly higher or lower than the rest of the values. These so-called outliers may dramatically skew any statistical analyses.
- *Heteroscedasticity is present*: Homoscedasticity is an assumption that the variance remains constant or homogenous throughout different values of the variable. Many

statistical tests assume homoscedasticity. If the variance actually changes with higher or lower values of the variable, then heteroscedasticity is present.

Any of these situations may preclude the use of parametric statistical tests, unless you transform the data into usable forms (i.e., nonlinear data into linear data; other distributions into normal distributions; heteroscedastic data into homoscedastic data). Doing so is legitimate and relatively common. Depending on the situation, you may have to transform one or more variables. Common methods of transforming data so that statistical tests can be used include the following:

- *Log transform*: This involves taking the logarithms of the variable (e.g., $\log_b x$). The logarithm (to base b) of a number x (i.e., $\log_b(x)$) is the exponent y that satisfies $x = b^y$. In theory you could use any number for the base (i.e., b). If the base is 10, then the $\log_{10}$ of 1000 would be 3. If the base is the constant e (i.e., approximately 2.7182818), then $\log_e$ is also called the natural log. Log transforms convert exponential relationships into linear relationships. Log transforms can also remedy situations where the variance increases with the mean. When there are any numbers below 1.0 including negative numbers (you cannot take the logarithm of such numbers), you must vertically or horizontally translate (i.e., discussed below, add a constant value to all values of the variable) the variable so that all values are greater than 1.0. The most commonly used bases in log transformations are 10, 2, and e. Consider trying a range of bases before choosing one. Different bases are appropriate in different situations.
- *Reciprocal or inverse transformation*: This involves using the reciprocal ($1/x$) of the variable. Large numbers become small (e.g., 1000 becomes 0.001) and small numbers become large (e.g., 0.001 becomes 10,000). So remember that a reciprocal transformation reverses the order of the data. Multiplying all the values by -1 prior to the reciprocal transformation may be helpful (i.e., see vertical and horizontal reflection below, it reverses the order of the data before the reciprocal transformation which then reverses the order back to real order).
- *Square root transform*: This involves taking the square root of the variable ($\sqrt{x}$), i.e. every value that the variable assumes and can convert a Poisson distribution to a normal distribution. The square root transform has two major issues. Since you cannot take the square root of a negative number, when negative numbers are present, you must vertically or horizontally translate (i.e., see below, add a constant value to all values of the variable) the variable so that all values are greater than 0. Secondly, taking the square root of a number below 1.0 (which results in a number larger than the original number, e.g., $\sqrt{0.25}$ is 0.5) is quite different from taking the square root of a number above 1.0 (which results in a number smaller than the original number, e.g., $\sqrt{25}$ is 5). Therefore, avoid using the square root transform

when a variable has values both above and below 1.0, unless you first transform to data to be all above 1.0.
- *Arcsine (angular) transformation*: Taking arcsine x often helps with percentages and proportions.

Making data amenable to statistical analyses is not the only reason for data transformation. There are many other types of data transformations. As long as you apply a consistent mathematical formula to all values of a variable, you are transforming the variable and corresponding data. Additional situations where transformations may be useful include:

- *Systematic biases*: When biases occur that uniformly affect the data in a known manner (e.g., the measurement devices yielded measurements that were consistently lower by a specific amount), transforming the data may adjust for these biases.
- *Need for other transformations*: As we mentioned above, certain transformations are not possible until the data is adjusted (e.g., you cannot take logarithms of negative numbers).
- *Incompatible data format*: Sometimes data must be converted from one type of measurement to another (e.g., inches to centimeters, pounds to kilograms, or height and weight to body mass index).

Graphical transformations are basically data transformations that clearly alter the shape or location of a curve in specific ways. Like other data transformations, graphical transformations involve applying the same mathematical equation to every value of a given variable. Some common examples include the following:

- *Vertical translation*: This transformation involves adding a constant to the independent variable function [$y = f(x) + k$] after the function is calculated and has the effect of shifting the entire curve up (if the constant k is greater than 0) or down (if k is less than 0) along the y-axis. So if the function is $y = x^2$, $y = x^2 + 2$ would shift the curve two units up the y-axis.
- *Horizontal translation*: This transformation involves adding a constant to the independent variable [$y = f(x + k)$] before the function is calculated and has the effect of shifting the entire curve to the right (if the constant k is greater than 0) or left (if k is less than 0) along the x-axis. So if the function is $y = x^2$, $y = (x + 2)^2$ would shift the curve two units to the right on the x-axis.
- *Vertical and horizontal reflecting*: Reflection flips the curve about either the x-axis or y-axis. Multiplying the function by -1 [i.e., $y = -f(x)$] flips or reflects the curve about the x-axis. Multiplying the variable by -1 before calculating the function [i.e., $y = f(-x)$] flips or reflects the curve about the y-axis.
- *Vertical stretch or compression*: This transformation involves multiplying the function by a constant k [$y = kf(x)$] and has the effect of stretching the curve vertically by a factor of k if k is greater than 1 or compressing

or squeezing the curve vertically by a factor of k if the k is less than 1. So $y = (2x)^2$ would be 2 times as tall as $y = x^2$ and $y = (1/2)x^2$ would be half as tall as $y = x^2$.

- *Horizontal stretch or compression*: This transformation involves multiplying the variable by a constant k [$y = f(kx)$] before the function is calculated and has the effect of stretching the curve horizontally by a factor of k if k is greater than 1 or compressing or squeezing the curve horizontally by a factor of k if the k is less than 1. So $y = (2x)^2$ would be 2 times as wide as $y = x^2$ and $y = [(1/2)x]^2$ would be half as wide as $y = x^2$.

14.8.2 Using Transformations

When used properly, data transformations are very useful but when performed inappropriately, they can wreak havoc on data and results. Remember that logarithmic, square root, and reciprocal transformations alter the relative differences between different data points (e.g., the differences between the patient weight may appear less or more than they actually are). These transformations compress the distance between higher values more than the distance between lower values. Also, remember that reflections will reverse the order of the data points (e.g., the tallest patient will have the "lowest" height). Proper interpretation requires a proper understanding of how the transformations alter the data.

Before utilizing any transformations, closely examine the data. Decide what statistical analyses you will want to use for your study interpretation. Determine whether your data in its original form are amenable to these analyses. If they are not, determine what the data needs to look like to do the analyses. Choose the minimum number of transformations needed to convert the data into the proper form. Do not use transformations unless necessary.

Data transformation is an iterative process. You first graph the data to see if linearity, normality, and homoscedasticity are satisfied. If any of these conditions are not satisfied, then choose and apply a transform to the data and then check if the effect has been attained (e.g., the data becomes linear after the transformation). If it does not work, you may have to try a different transform.

Sometimes doing a series of different transformations is necessary. The order of the different transformations may be very important. Employing a horizontal translation and then a log transformation may be very different from employing a log transformation first and then a horizontal translation.

14.9 CHOOSING THE DATA SETS

14.9.1 Data Sets

So you have checked the quality of your study data, dealt with missing and erroneous values, calculated the derived data, and transformed the data into the appropriate format. The final step before data analysis is to choose what data to include in the analysis. The *data set* is what you get after you've gone through all the steps outlined in this chapter. The data set includes the data that will be used for the analysis, and more importantly, excludes data that you don't think is appropriate to include in your analysis.

Typically, you will need multiple different data sets: ones for efficacy, safety, and sensitivity analysis. The primary efficacy data set will be the one used to determine if the study intervention is effective. Secondary efficacy data sets serve to answer other additional questions about the intervention's effectiveness. The primary safety data set will be used to determine the safety of the intervention. You can perform sensitivity analyses on different data sets to see how results change under different assumptions and determine the robustness of any findings.

Different data sets are necessary for different analyses because some assumptions may not be appropriate for some analyses (e.g., you will sometimes exclude patients who had major protocol violations from the efficacy analysis data set but include them in the safety analysis data set).

In the end, you will want one data set that will be your primary efficacy analysis data set, and several other data sets for sensitivity and other analysis. The protocol usually specifies which patients and data to include in the primary analysis but sometimes judgment calls are necessary. The statistical analysis plan should specify exactly which subjects will be included in the primary analysis. You cannot choose one data set for the primary analysis, and then change your mind later because you do not agree with the results.

The data you choose depends on the type of analysis you will perform. There are two broad categories of analyses: per protocol and intention to treat (ITT). The difference between the two is patient adherence to protocol. Per protocol analysis only includes subjects who adhered to the study protocol and ignores data from subjects who violated protocol. By contrast, ITT analysis includes all subjects, regardless of whether they adhered to the study protocol. We discuss these analyses in detail in the following two sections.

14.9.2 Intention to Treat (ITT) Analyses

In an ITT analysis, the study treatment group includes *all patients who were assigned (usually randomized) to that study treatment group*, even those who dropped out or received incomplete or inaccurate doses of the treatment. Even patients who *never received a single dose* of the treatment belong in the study group. There is a saying to describe ITT: "analyze as randomized." So once patients are randomized, they are "stuck" in the analysis. Nothing that happens after randomization (e.g., noncompliance, protocol deviations, or dropping out) can exclude them being included in the analysis.

Initially, ITT analysis may not make sense for people not involved in clinical research (and even many people who are involved). Does this make sense? How can you use subjects who never received a study intervention to determine the effects of a study intervention? Isn't this akin to a theater critic including in her review of a show actors who were cut during the final round of auditions or football commentators talking about how players who were cut during training camp may affect a team's chances of winning a playoff game? Doesn't a patient have to experience a treatment from start-to-finish to qualify in the analysis?

However, a closer look reveals many reasons for and advantages of using ITT:

- *Determining thresholds for excluding subjects may be difficult*: When should patients be excluded from the analysis? How serious does the protocol deviation have to be? What may seem like a minor protocol deviation may in fact have major consequences. At the same time, major protocol violations may not be as significant as initially believed. Thresholds and tolerances for protocol deviations can be very subjective. ITT avoids such difficult decision making.
- *The causes of protocol deviations may be obscure and multi-factorial*: Why was the patient noncompliant with the study intervention? Did the investigator give the wrong directions? Were there significant side effects? Did the patient lack the socioeconomic means? All of these potential causes have different implications when it comes to measuring intervention efficacy. If you cannot accurately determine the cause of the deviation, isn't it easier to include all of the patients in the analysis?
- *Guarding against bias*: Since the reasons for protocol deviations and the criteria for excluding patients can be very subjective, ITT helps prevent bias. What if investigators consciously or unconsciously coerced certain patients to drop out of the study? What if patients in bad weather locations tended to withdraw from the study? What if certain study sites were rude and discourteous to patients, leading to patient noncompliance? What if certain socioeconomic groups were more likely to withdraw from the study?
- *Preserving information*: Excluding patients results in a loss of information. This loss can be significant if the patient completed most of the study appropriately. Loss of information can be devastating if the study population is small or a significant number of patients had protocol deviations.
- *Preserving efficacy and safety information*: Protocol deviations may be due to safety or efficacy issues. Patients may withdraw from a study if the side effects become intolerable, the intervention does not work, or the intervention cures them of their condition or symptoms. So in many ways, protocol deviations potentially are important efficacy and safety endpoints.
- *Maintaining balance achieved by randomization*: As we discussed in Chapter 5, randomization helps establish a balance of different characteristics (e.g., gender, age, and co-morbid conditions) among the different study arms. Excluding patients may disrupt this important balance and make the different study arms less comparable.
- *Clinical realism*: When a study intervention is used in real world clinical practice, protocol deviations will be very common. Patient treatment conditions and situation will be far from ideal. Many patients will miss treatments, get the wrong doses, and fail to follow-up appropriately. Excluding patients who violate protocol may be making the clinical study too pristine to be applicable to the real world.

ITT analysis is very common. Most primary efficacy data sets are chosen for ITT or modified ITT (which we will discuss later). In general, the Food and Drug Administration (FDA) will insist on a true ITT analysis for efficacy. In rare cases, they may agree to a modified ITT, as long as the modified ITT is pre-defined in advance. ITT is especially useful in any studies in which nonrandom dropouts are expected. So in open-label studies, patients will be able to obtain more information about the treatment and may even drop out before accepting the first dose. Even in a well-conducted blinded study, patients may drop out in a non-random manner (e.g., patients may require pre-medication with steroids and acetaminophen prior to receiving the active drug. This pre-medication may cause an adverse event and induce patients to drop out.).

Not everyone accepts the advantages of ITT. Some may argue that ITT introduces too much noise into the study, which may obscure the analysis and even hide potential intervention effects. If there are many dropouts and protocol deviations in the analysis, relatively few patients may exhibit an adequate improvement from the intervention. In other words, ITT analysis may be less sensitive at detecting an intervention effect. For this reason, ITT is generally not appropriate for safety analysis, which necessitates good sensitivity. An analogy would be judging a talent contest between two schools. Letting almost anyone participate from both sides may result in so many unqualified contestants who drown out the few highly talented individuals. This makes it difficult to determine which school has the most talented people.

Modified ITT

A modified ITT analysis includes all randomized patients that meet a specific minimum standard or simple set of criteria. The criteria should be simple, objective, and very straightforward. The criteria should not be related to the outcome (e.g., if you know that patients with lower socioeconomic status will be less likely to respond to your intervention, you cannot use socioeconomic status as a criterion). Using subjective criteria defeats the purpose of a

Should patients from sites with good clinical practice (GCP) violations be included in intention to treat (ITT) analysis?

This is an important and controversial issue? GCP violations are different from patient dropouts. In a way, a site with GCP violations is analogous to a site enrolling phantom patients or a site never even existing. For example, if very poor recordkeeping makes it impossible to determine whether the patients even received the drug, then censoring all the data from that site may be necessary.

FIGURE 14.4   GCP Violations and ITT.

modified ITT. The more common modified ITT will include all patients who received at least one dose of the study intervention (regardless of what happened to the patient after the initial dose). The study protocol should prespecify a modified ITT analysis and its criteria. Otherwise, selection bias can occur (e.g., if you find that a certain characteristic correlates with poor intervention response, you can later exclude patients with that characteristic from the analysis.) Another common modified ITT analysis excludes all patients who had major protocol violations (e.g., did not meet the study selection criteria). Usually the primary analysis should be an ITT analysis, but in some rare cases, a modified ITT may be appropriate. Modified ITT analyses are relatively common for secondary or exploratory analysis. Determining whether to include sites with protocol violations can be a challenge (Figure 14.4).

14.9.3 Per Protocol Analysis

Unlike ITT analysis, *per protocol analysis* only includes patients who successfully adhered to the protocol (i.e., no major protocol violations). In many cases, per protocol analysis may serve as the primary data analysis (FDA approval may be necessary). The major strength of per protocol analysis is the weakness of ITT analysis: it removes significant noise from study, noise that may prevent you from truly determining an intervention's effects. Conversely, we covered the major weaknesses of per protocol analysis when discussing the strengths of ITT analysis.

Understand that protocol stipulations are frequently subjective and arbitrary. Even a clearly written protocol leaves significant room for interpretation (e.g., missing how many doses constitutes a protocol violation). Prespecifying rules in the protocol is important. However, anticipating every possible peculiar situation is impossible (e.g., what if the tubing were to break while an intravenous drug was being administered? Did the patient get a full dose?) Moreover, some things that initially appeared to be protocol violations may not turn out to be violations.

Pseudo Per Protocol Analysis

Some apparent protocol violations are not necessarily true protocol violations. Study personnel may have strictly adhered to the study protocol but circumstances beyond their control occurred. For example, ambiguously written protocols, equivocal diagnoses, changing patient conditions, and emergent situations may cause problems even though patients and investigators were strictly adherent to the protocol. Pseudo per protocol analysis may allow some of these cases to be included in the analysis. While you should avoid such situations if possible, special deliberations can help arbitrate what data belongs in the data set.

Make decision about what to include in the data set on a study-by-study basis. Data included in the data set for one study may not be included in the data set for a very similar but different study. The situations and extenuating circumstances can be very complex. Some examples of common problems requiring such decision making include the following:

- *Incorrect treatment*: A randomization or site error can result in a subject receiving the wrong intervention (e.g., placebo instead of active medication). Before unblinding, decide how to treat such patients: For example, whether the patient should be considered a member of the study arm that he was originally assigned to (i.e., active treatment arm) or the study arm that most resembles what actually happened (i.e., placebo control arm).
- *Dosing errors*: Minor dosing errors (e.g., a few wrong doses, different dose escalation or de-escalation, or doses at the wrong times) may occur. Slight deviations may be acceptable. Well-written protocols will give acceptable ranges for dose deviations (e.g., the dose should be given once every 7 days plus or minus a day or two).
- *Other protocol violations*: Too many missed patient visits, patient visits outside the specified time window, broken blind, violated selection criteria, unauthorized medications or therapies, multiple admission to the same trial, and loss to follow-up are all common violations.

Chapter 15

Analysis of Data

15.1 DESCRIPTIVE STATISTICS

15.1.1 Description of a Single Variable

After we have assessed the quality of data, made appropriate imputations, and defined appropriate datasets, the next step is to analyze the data. By "analysis" we mean the process of describing and summarizing hundred or thousand pieces of data by calculating things like averages, standard deviations (SD), confidence intervals, *p*-values, etc.

This chapter will explore various statistical concepts and tests, but not to the extent that you will be able to perform the analysis without any expert help. In other words, the purpose of this chapter is to briefly explain the underpinning theory behind the statistical tests, point out the assumptions behind the tests, provide an understanding of how the results should be used, and describe the limitations.

The simplest statistical analysis is description of a single set of data such as "a set of height measurements" (each set is made up of multiple observations of the same variable, such as height measurements from 100 individuals). This is sometimes called *univariate analysis*. Its goal is to summarize the data.

As an example, rather than listing 1000 height measurements one by one, which would be tedious and difficult to review, univariate analysis allows you to say something like, "the mean height was 160 cm with SD of 15 cm." Mean, SD, and other similar calculations are called *summary statistics* and help us answer the question, "What does the data from height measurements look like?" Statistics of locations (e.g., mean, mode, and median) describe the "center" of the data, and statistics of dispersion (e.g., SD and variance) describe how the data is distributed.

Nominal/Categorical Variables

Depending on the type of variable being measured, different types of summary statistics can be generated. With nominal (also called categorical or discrete) variables, such as hair color, a simple *frequency distribution (histogram)* can be used to describe the data (Figure 15.1 and 15.2). In a frequency distribution, on the *x*-axis are the types of variables, such as hair color, and on the *y*-axis are the numbers of people who fall into that category.

Obviously, some summary statistics are not possible for some types of variables. It would be difficult, for example, to calculate the mean hair color. With nominal variables such as these, it is neither possible nor meaningful to calculate a mean, mode, median, or other summary statistic,

Hair color	Relative frequency (%)
Black	20
Blond(e)	10
Red	5
Brown	30

FIGURE 15.1 Relative frequency of hair color.

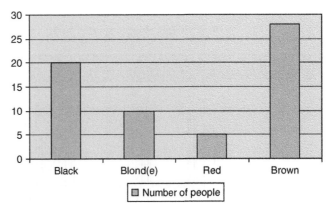

FIGURE 15.2 Frequency distribution (histogram) of hair color.

because the values such as "brown" and "red" cannot be added, subtracted, or otherwise manipulated.

Ordinal Variables

With an ordinal measure, you also use a frequency distribution but you would place the categories in an ascending format, as above. (Ordinal measures, if you recall, are measures that are not numerical but have some sort of rank relationship. In fact, they are sometimes called rank variables.) For example, in the chart above, the number of students in each type of school, there is a meaningful ordering, that is from lower grades to higher grades Figure 15.3.

There can be some summary statistic with ordinal variables. For example, mode and median would have some meaning.

Numeric Variables

With numeric measure (numerical measures, if you recall, are measures that have integers as values, that is there are no

fractions, no decimal points, and no negative numbers), one can also plot a histogram of patients' ages measured in years. The histogram might look like this if they are not grouped into intervals Figure 15.4.

Often, however, if you don't have a large number of data points, it may be difficult to get a true picture of the distribution. It is often useful to group values of measurements into intervals (e.g., 0–10, 11–20, etc.), to smooth out the histogram and get a better sense of the distribution. See below Figure 15.5.

As you can see, grouping often allows a better assessment of how the data is distributed. It smoothes out the random variations that can make interpretation difficult if individual level data is used. More data points there are, smaller the groups can be and still yield useful information. With very large number of samples, a group can be as small as individual integers.

The best way to summarize numeric variables in a variety of cases is to present median (where half the observations are higher and half are lower than the value), mode (the value that is the most frequent), and percentiles such as 25th and 75th percentile (where 25% of observations

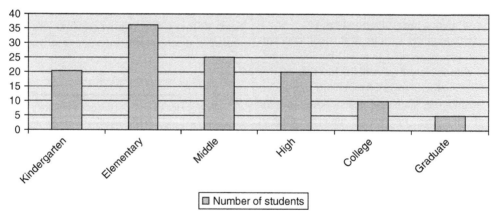

FIGURE 15.3 Histogram of educational levels.

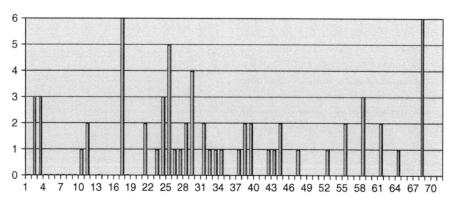

FIGURE 15.4 Histogram of patient ages.

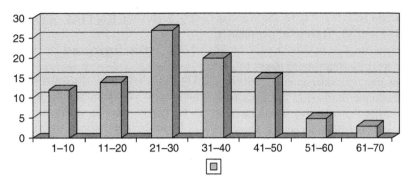

FIGURE 15.5 Histogram of patient ages, grouped into intervals.

lie below the value, whereas 75% of the observations lie above the value). This is because the shape of the curve for numeric variables is unpredictable and is often not normally shaped (bell shaped). Unless the shape of the curve is normal, mean and SD can be misleading because those statistics are based on normal distributions.

Of course, numeric variables can sometimes have a normal distribution and in these cases, mean and SD are useful.

Continuous Variables

Continuous variables are variables that can have infinite number of values, such as height (where height could be 160, 160.3, 161 cm, etc.), when probability distribution curves are used. These are curves where the area under a portion of the curve corresponds to the probability that a value will fall in the range. Though the curve may be of any shape, many things that can be measured with a continuous variable assume a bell-shaped curve, known as a normal distribution or a Gaussian distribution. We will discuss important characteristics of a bell-shaped curve later.

For continuous variables, mean and SD are most commonly used to summarize the data. As was discussed in Chapter 3, mean is the average value and SD is the square root of the variance. SD is a way of quantifying how "spread out" the data is. It is the square root of a closely related statistic called variance. Variance is the number you get if you take the difference between each observation and the mean, square the difference, and derive the average of the squares.

Of course, if the shape of the distribution for the variable is abnormal, then mean and SD may not be appropriate. Using these two summary statistics is predicated on a normal curve. With a normal curve, if you know where the center of the data is and how spread out it is (also known as dispersion), then you have a pretty good idea of how the dataset looks. However, if the data has multiple peaks, or if it is significantly skewed, other ways of describing the center of data (mode or median) or the spread of data (range or percentiles) may be more appropriate.

15.1.2 Comparison of Two or More Variables

As was discussed in Chapter 3, comparative analysis takes two or more sets of data and determines whether there is a relationship between or among them. For example, you might compare height and weight. Or you might compare the relationship among height, weight, and shoe size. Comparison between two sets of data is called bivariate analysis and comparison among three sets or more of data is called multivariate analysis.

A comparative analysis might show several things. It might show a correlation between the two groups. For example, with increasing dose of a drug, there might be increasing hours of sleep. It might alternatively show a difference between the groups. For example, it might show that a group receiving a drug has less anxiety than the placebo group. It might show equivalence or noninferiority (to be distinguished from lack of difference) between the groups. For example, a new anti-psychotic drug may be no worse than the standard anti-psychotic. It may also show that there is no relationship.

The simplest analysis is an analysis between two sets of categorical data. The comparison usually starts with a contingency table (also called cross-tabulations) such as the one below (Figure 15.6).

The correlation between the two variables (i.e., treatment and outcome in this case) can be calculated. The calculation is based on how uneven the distribution is across the diagonal cells and is called phi coefficient.

In addition, the relationship between the two categorical variables is often expressed in terms of the relative risk or odds ratio. The relative risk is the ratio of risk of an event in one group vs. another group. In the example above,

	Placebo	Drug
Died	21	41
Survived	16	83
Total	37	124

FIGURE 15.6 Contingency table.

the risk of dying on placebo is 21/37 = 0.57 and the risk of dying on drug is 41/124 = 0.33. Therefore, the relative risk of dying on placebo vs. drug is 0.57/0.33 or 1.72. If you are on placebo, you are 1.72 times more likely to die. The relative risk is rather easy to understand and for this reason, is often used in medicine. It also has the advantage of being independent of what the underlying rate is. The disadvantage is that it does not really address the absolute rate. If your risk of a deep vein thrombosis (DVT) is 1 in 10,000 and it doubles when you ride on a plane, the clinical significance is very different compared to risk of DVT going from 1 in 50 to 1 in 25, even though in both cases, the relative risk is 2.

The other disadvantage of the relative risk is that you get different results depending on which numerator you use. For example, the risk of *not* having a DVT changes from 9999/10,000 to 9998/10,000 in the above example of riding on a plane. This means that the relative risk of having a DVT is 2 if you ride on a plane, but the relative risk of *not* having a DVT is 0.9998. This is very counter-intuitive, and more importantly, it makes mathematical manipulation of the relative ratio very difficult because of the asymmetry.

Odds ratio is a somewhat less intuitive concept, so we'll go through it carefully. Let's start with the difference between risk and odds. Risk is the likelihood of something happening, such as "I have 25% chance of missing the next basket". The risk is 1 in 4. Odds are the likelihood of something happening vs. not happening. For example, "I have odds of 1:3 that I will miss the next basket".

Odds ratio is the ratio of the odds in one group vs. another group. In the above airplane example, the odds of dying on placebo are 21/16 = 1.31 and odds of dying on drug are 0.49. Therefore, the odds ratio of dying on placebo vs. drug is 1.31/0.49 or 2.67. The advantage of odds ratio is that no matter which denominator you use, it doesn't matter. The odds ratio of having a DVT is 1.002 and the odds ratio of not having a DVT is 1 divided by 2.002 or 0.4999. Therefore, odds ratio is often used in statistics because you can manipulate it mathematically much more easily.

The other common instance where odds ratio is used is for case control studies where the relative risk cannot be calculated. Case control studies are *retrospective* studies and once patients with and without an outcome are selected (e.g., 50 patients with DVT and 50 patients without DVT) and you look *backwards* in time to see how many had a particular risk factor. Since you choose how many patients with and without DVT are to be examine, the relative risk is meaningless (it changes depending on the whim of the investigator). Instead, you calculate the odds of patients with DVT having had the risk factor vs. the odds of patients without DVT having had the risk factor in order to derive the odds ratio.

When the rates of events are very low, the relative risk and odds ratio have very similar values, but when the rates are high, they yield very different values.

15.2 INFERENTIAL STATISTICS

15.2.1 Background

Once we have performed the descriptive analysis, the next step is to characterize and test the dataset to determine what results from the study can tell us about the population at large. In other words, the statistical tools are applied to the dataset and from this application, we try to guess what the broad population looks like.

If you recall, the patients in a study make up a "sample." In other words, they are a subgroup of the patient population at large (past, present, and future). The goal of a study is typically not only to describe what happened to the patient in the study but also to extrapolate the results to the patient population at large. The analysis on the sample is used to make some assertions about what the patient population at large might be like.

For example, the inferential analysis takes the data from the sample (e.g., 100 congestive heart failure [CHF] patients) and extrapolates the results to larger populations (such as 1 million CHF patients in the world). It asserts some conclusion about the broad population based on the data from the sample (the patients enrolled in the study that makes up a subset of the population).

The basic difference between the comparisons described in the earlier section and inferential analysis of the type is as follows:

- For descriptive statistics, correlations or other relationships are tabulated *for the datasets* themselves and are factual statements. For example, you might say, "in these 50 patients with poor night vision who were enrolled in the study, we found that those who ate carrots saw twice as well as those who did not."
- For inferential statistics, correlations or other relationships are assessed to determine whether they are convincing enough to draw some conclusions *about the patient population at large* that they are drawn from. For example, you might say, "based on the 50 patients in the study, we can conclude that if anyone, who has poor night vision, eats carrots will be able to see twice as well."

Obviously, that is a significant jump from the first statement to the second. Do we know the results weren't by chance? Do we know the patients who ate carrots didn't squint? Do we know the patients in the study weren't some subpopulation that is very different from the general population? There are many questions that must be addressed.

How do we go from the first statement to the second? We use inference, or statistical inductive reasoning. There are three major schools of inferential analysis: frequentist, Bayesian, and likelihood based. They share some common building blocks and tools but have fundamental differences in how they draw conclusions from data. We will focus on the frequentist methods in this chapter.

15.2.2 Inferring from a Single Sample: Standard Error and Confidence Interval

While most inferential analysis is applied to comparisons of two groups, it can be applied to a single group. In such analysis, the inferential analysis extrapolates from the sample data to extrapolate to the broader patient population. (Figure 15.7) This analysis is similar to descriptive analysis. This analysis includes, for example, confidence intervals. Confidence intervals, such as 95% confidence intervals, assert that in 95% of the cases, the mean of a population would fall within the set of values within the confidence interval.

Simply put, confidence interval tells you how "close" a value, such as the mean, derived from a sample is to the true mean of something. Confidence interval is the range of values that, if the study were to be repeated multiple times describes the proportion of the time that the confidence interval would include the true population value. For example, 95% confidence interval for mean blood pressure from a study would encompass the true population mean blood pressure in 95% of the cases. This is similar to saying that there is 95% chance that the true blood pressure is within the confidence interval. Although the true blood pressure may or may not be within the confidence interval, the likelihood that the confidence interval from a particular study encompasses the true value is 95%.

Confidence intervals can be used for a wide variety of values, including mean, hazard ratio, relative risk, and so on. It is an information-rich way of conveying the confidence of the value. As a rule of thumb, 1.96 times standard error (SE) defines the 95% confidence interval for a mean.

Also, most confidence intervals are two sided, meaning that the values lie between two numbers, but it can be a one-sided confidence interval, meaning that the true population value is below or above a certain value in X% of the samples taken.

	Single-Sample	Comparative/ Multi-Sample
Descriptive/Non-Inferential Describes the patients in the study	Mean, standard deviation, etc.	Mean of the difference
Inferential Asserts some conclusion Standard error about broader patient population based on study patient data		Confidence interval, *p*-value

FIGURE 15.7 Types of statistical analysis. Single-sample, non-inferential statistics are often just called "descriptive." Comparative, non-inferential statistics are often just called "comparative." Comparative, inferential statistics are often just called "inferential."

As an example, let's say you're trying to find out the average height of all the students in Springfield High School. There are 500 students in the school, so the most reliable way would be to line everyone up and measure everyone's height.

However, let's say there are some absentees on the day of measurement so you only measure 480 students. The average height you end up with is probably pretty close to the true average height. However, you wouldn't be surprised if you were slightly off.

Let's say, however, that you don't have much time, so you decide to randomly go into a few classes and measure 250 students. In that case, the average height you get is still probably close to the true value but you would be less confident. If you measured only 50 students, you would even be less confident.

How close is the average you get from a "sample" of 480, 250, or 50 students to the true value? The traditional way to quantify this is through a confidence interval. A confidence interval tells you how wide the margin of error is around the mean (or other statistic). For example, a 95% confidence interval for a mean of 170cm might be 165 to 175cm. Most people interpret this to mean that there is 95% chance that the true mean for the entire high school population is somewhere between 165 and 175cm. This is a reasonably accurate way of thinking about the confidence interval, although traditional statisticians (frequentists) will say that this is not a completely correct way to describe a confidence interval. In their way of thinking, probability only refers to likelihood of an event happening in the future. Since a confidence interval may or may not already include the true mean, their definition of a confidence interval is a bit more convoluted: it is the range of values such that if a large number of confidence intervals were calculated, the true mean would be included in the interval 95% of the time.

A more intuitive interval is the credible interval, which is a Bayesian concept similar to the confidence interval except it describes a range that has 95% (or other) probability of including the true value.

The most common type of the confidence interval is a 95% confidence interval but it can be any type (e.g., 80%, 99%, etc.). An 80% confidence interval would define the range with 80% chance (or confidence) of including the true mean; 99% would have 99% chance (or confidence) of including the true mean, etc. Obviously, 80% confidence interval would be narrower than 90% or 99% confidence interval.

A confidence interval is calculated by looking at how spread out your data is and how many data points you have. In the above example, a confidence interval should be narrower if you measure the height of 480 patients instead of 50. If all the measurements are very close to each other, the confidence interval will be narrow, and vice versa.

Confidence interval is a very good way to summarize the data, because it tells you what the likely true value is and how close you are to that true value. Therefore, it conveys much richer set of information than just the *p*-value.

330   SECTION V | Analysis of Results

In addition, confidence intervals can be used to test hypothesis and establish significance. You can calculate the difference between two samples. For example, difference in the average height from 50 patients from Springfield High School and 50 patients from Rockville High School. Let's say the average heights are 161 and 169 cm. The difference is 8 cm. If the 95% confidence interval around the difference does not include 0 (e.g., if it is 1–15 cm), then you can say that the difference is real, or statistically significant. If the confidence interval does include 0 (e.g., it is −2 to 18 cm), then you can say that the difference may not be real, because the possibility that the difference is due to chance has not been excluded.

One very important *caveat*: people often chart 95% confidence intervals for different samples and check to see if they overlap. It they do not overlap, that is taken to mean that the samples are statistically different, and if they do overlap, that is taken to mean that they are not statistically significant. This is wrong. Confidence intervals of 95% can overlap by as much as one-third (29%) but the samples may be statistically different at $p < 0.05$. One cannot compare confidence intervals from different samples. What you really should do is to calculate the difference between the samples and calculate the confidence interval around the difference.

Standard error (SE) is the other major statistic in simple inferential stat-istics. SE is a measure of how close the mean of the sample is likely to be compared to the mean of the population. Based on the SD, or the scatter around the mean of the study population (sample), one can estimate how close the study population mean is to the true mean for the population at large.

Important Point: Know the Difference Between SD and SE

SD and SE are often confused. SD tells you how "spread out" the data in a sample is. For example, you might have a group of patients whose average heart rate is 70. SD describes how much "deviation" you have from the average heart rate in that group of patients.

SE tells you how far averages you calculate from your dataset (from the sample) are likely to be from the true average for the entire population. In other words, SE tells you how far the average heart rate from above is likely to be from the average heart rate of all relevant patients in the world. It tells you how much "error" you will be risking if you think that the average heart rate from the group of patients is representative of the average heart rate from the entire universe of patients.

People often use SE incorrectly, by using error bars rather than using confidence intervals or SD in charts. This is often because SE is usually much smaller, since SE is SD divided by square root of the number of patients in the sample. You usually are interested in SD, which describes the sample population.

15.2.3 Comparing Across Samples

The more complicated, and more common, inferential analysis are based on comparing multiple samples (or arms), and attempt to assert a relationship between or among two or more patient populations based on the difference between or among two or more treatment groups in a study. The most common example in a clinical trial is hypothesis-testing for significance using the *p*-value between two groups. For example, primary efficacy endpoint of randomized controlled clinical trials is used to assert a causal relationship between some intervention and outcome between two groups.

As mentioned before, two or more samples can be compared and a correlation can be drawn across groups, or the groups contrasted. Each comparison can be characterized in terms of how likely or unlikely the correlation or the differences are. One way of characterizing the likelihood that the results are by chance is by *p*-values. The *p*-value indicates the probability of getting the results that are seen, purely by chance, if there are no differences between the groups. For example, let's say that a study is done in Crohn's disease patients, and the active group has a remission rate of 10% and the control group has a remission rate of 20% with a *p*-value of 0.01. This means that the likelihood of seeing results like this or more extreme (10% vs. 20%) is 1% unless the active and control groups were truly different.

It should be stressed that $p < 0.05$ is not synonymous with statistically significant. Significance is determined by both the *p*-value and prespecification of hypothesis (e.g., if you have multiple primary endpoints, the *p*-value required may need to be lower). Hypothesis-testing is usually based on *p*-values, but contrary to common assumptions, it is not always necessary. Hypothesis-testing can take multiple forms.

15.2.4 How to Generate a *p*-Value and Other Test Statistics

Depending on what kind of data, how many treatment arms, and the study design, there will be different ways of generating a *p*-value. The fundamental steps are:

1. Determine which set of variables will be used to compare the treatment arms (e.g., blood pressure, height, etc.).
2. Determine what the distribution of values would have been expected if there were no differences between the groups (in other words, if both samples had been drawn from the sample population and there were no real differences between them, just differences due to play of chance).
3. Use some way of summarizing the observed distribution so that it can be compared to what is expected. This can in theory be based on the shape of the distribution, mean value, or other similar parameters. The most common way of summarizing the difference is to derive a single value, such as *F*-value. This is a test variable, a number

that summarizes the likelihood of seeing the distribution that was seen in the study. In other words, it captures the essence of how "weird" the data is. In general, it is in the form:

$$\frac{\text{Values that are observed}}{\text{Values that are expected}}$$

4. Generate the *p*-value based on how unusual or unexpected the distribution is based on the value derived in 2.

Here is an example. Let's say we were measuring heart rates from two groups of patients. If the distribution looked like the one in Figure 15.8 you would probably think the two groups were different, because it would seem strange that they could be the same and yet by chance they would have a distribution like this. If someone were to tell you that these were from the same group of patients, you would think "that's strange." If, on the other hand, you saw something like this (Figure 15.9) then you would think they were probably drawn from the same population. Inferential statistics is just a mathematical way of capturing how "different" or "strange" the distribution is.

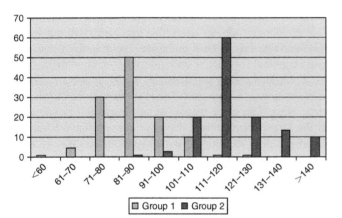

FIGURE 15.8   Heart rates.

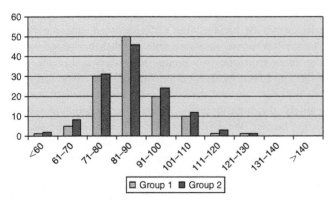

FIGURE 15.9   Heart rates.

We will discus many different types of statistical procedures in the following pages. The choice of test depends on the design of the study and types of variables. The key questions are:

- How many groups of patients are in the study?
- How many treatments did they receive?
- How many measurements did each patient get?
- What kinds of variables/measures were used?
- Are the data parametric in distribution?
- Are there same number of patients in each group?

15.2.5 Parametric vs. Nonparametric

In steps 3 and 4, there are two general ways of assessing the difference between the groups to see how "weird" the distribution is.

Parametric tests assume a normal distribution of values, or a "bell-shaped curve." For example, height is roughly a normal distribution in that if you were to graph height from a group of people, one would see a typical bell-shaped curve. This distribution is also called a Gaussian distribution.

Nonparametric tests are used in cases where parametric tests are not appropriate. Most nonparametric tests use some way of ranking the measurements and testing for weirdness of the distribution.

Typically, a parametric test has better ability to distinguish between the two arms. In other words, it is better at highlighting the weirdness of the distribution. Nonparametric tests are about 95% as powerful as parametric tests.

However, nonparametric tests are often necessary. Some common situations for nonparametric tests are when the distribution is not normal (the distribution is skewed), the distribution is not known, or the sample size is too small (<30) to assume a normal distribution. Also, if there are extreme values or values that are clearly "out of range," nonparametric tests should be used.

Sometimes it is not clear from the data whether the distribution is normal. If this is the case, previous studies using the variables can help distinguish between the two. The source of variability can also help. If numerous independent factors are affecting the variability, the distribution is more likely to be normal. You might think you could formally test to determine whether the distribution is normal, but unfortunately, these tests require large sample sizes, typically larger than required for the tests of significance being used. At large sample sizes, either of the parametric or the nonparametric tests work adequately.

Also, nonparametric tests are appropriate when the measure being used is not the one that lends itself to a normal distribution or where "distribution" has no meaning, such as color of eyes and Expanded Disability Status Scale (EDSS). In other words, nominal or ordinal measures in many cases require a nonparametric test.

15.2.6 Sidedness

In some cases, it may be possible to state in advance of the study that one is only interested if the one arm is better than the other, and not interested if the reverse is true. In that case, a one-sided tail could theoretically be used. For example, you might say that if the drug increases uric acid levels you are interested but if it lowers it you are not. However, in practice, this is rarely if ever done, because clinical trial results are almost always important regardless of the direction of benefit. Therefore, most tests are performed as a two-sided test – they look to see if either group has higher value than the other. For example, if a group received growth hormone and other group did not, the statistical test would be conducted. If either group had significantly higher growth rate, it would be considered to be a real difference.

15.2.7 Prespecification

The meaningfulness of the p-value is usually predicated on having a single primary endpoint prespecified in advance. Usually, the primary analysis is specified in the original protocol. In some cases, changes in the primary endpoint may be made, because of external factors: for example, another study shows that a different endpoint is superior or more sensitive. But these are rare. Sometimes internal factors such as excessive dropouts might force a change in the primary analysis plan. But these are also rare, and should always be changed before the unblinding of the data.

If the primary endpoint does not meet p-value of 0.05 or less, then the analysis cannot be subsequently changed to yield a "statistically significant" result. Any further generation of a p-value using other data or analysis results in a "nominal p-value" (the p-value that would have been, if it were a real p-value. This is purely hypothetical, kind of like the amount of money you would have won had you picked the right lottery numbers last week).

15.2.8 Types of Analysis

For the most part, the data you use for the analysis is the data you have – the dataset. In some cases, however, the dataset you have is incomplete. For example, you might want to know something about the 6-month response but you only have 6-month result from half the patients. Or you only have the 3- and 9-month results. In these cases, you can use various techniques to "fill in" or interpolate the missing values or "project out" or extrapolate. There are various statistical techniques for this. This can be useful, but the more missing values there are, great danger there is that the results will be incorrect. Similarly, you can model the results by building a mathematical representation of the results you see. This is commonly done with population PK analysis, but once again, at risk of being slightly off (or in some cases, significantly off).

15.2.9 Comparing Two or More Continuous Measures/Variables

The t-Test

The most common inferential question in clinical trials is: "Is there a difference in the clinical outcome I got from the patients in the placebo arm vs. the treated arm?" Commonly, the outcome is measured with a continuous measure, such as blood pressure. We will therefore explore this type of analysis first. This procedure cannot be used for variables that are not continuous. For example, if you are comparing hair color, this procedure will not work. The variable has to be a numerical, continuous value that can be added, subtracted, and otherwise manipulated.

First, let's clarify the question. Let's say we are testing a blood pressure medicine. The real question is, "Does the drug work?" In other words, we are interested in knowing if the blood pressure will decrease after we have administered the drug to patients with hypertension. We are also interested in whether the patients in the trial demonstrate a difference in the placebo and the drug arms, but only insofar as this will tell us whether patients with similar characteristics. So we are interested in extrapolating the results to patients with hypertension at large.

Statistically, what we are doing is trying to prove or disprove the null hypothesis, which says, "there is no real difference between the blood pressures seen in the two groups of patients: the differences are due purely to chance." What we do is we take the distribution of blood pressures from the two groups and see whether the distribution looks "weird." (For simplicity's sake, for now we will just use one set of blood pressure measurements, namely the measurements taken after administration of drug/placebo. We will later talk about taking the difference between two sets of measurements, such as pre- and post-drug blood pressures.) We do this mathematically by comparing two things: the difference in the means from the two arms vs. the expected value. By expected value, we mean what we would expect to see if there were no true differences between the two groups. In statistical terms we look at.

$$\frac{\text{Difference in the means}}{\text{Standard error of the difference in the means}}$$

Fortunately, you can calculate both of these from the values you obtain form the study. The top value is straightforward – you subtract the mean of one arm from the other. The bottom value can be calculated from the SD from the two arms – more spread out the data points, larger will be the value.

The above ratio is called t. The t is used to look up a p-value, usually from a standard table that reflects the likely distribution of t-values for normal distributions. If t is large – in other words, the means are very different from each other and you expect them to be very similar – you will end up with a small p-value. If t is small, you will end up with a large p-value.

We should keep in mind that this process is based on certain assumptions. For example, the table converting t- to p-value is based on an assumption that the distribution of data points has a normal distribution. The assumptions are:

- The population (not the sample, but the overall patient population) must have a normal distribution.
- The distribution of the population(s) must be similar in how spread out the data points are (have same variance).
- Each sample (the patients in each arm) must be independently and randomly drawn.

It is incumbent on you to notify the statistician if you suspect that any of the assumptions are violated, because you are in a much better position to know that. Violation of any of these assumptions can have a significant effect on the reliability of the statistical procedures we are discussing.

The F-Test (ANOVA)

When you have more than two arms, a similar analysis can be done. For example, let's say you have a group of patients who received placebo, a group who received angiotensin converting enzyme (ACE) inhibitors, and a group who received calcium channel blockers. You have three groups, and once again you compare the differences among the three means, one from each arm, against the value you would expect if the arms were equivalent. The null hypothesis would be "there is no difference in blood pressure among the three groups of patients: all are from the same population."

You compare the means as follows: first you calculate the variance of the population from the means. You can't subtract three or more means like you did with two, so you calculate how "different" they are by calculating from the means what the variance of the overall population would be, if in fact the null hypothesis were true and they were all drawn from the same population. It turns out that the SD of the means approximates the population variance.

Next, you calculate the variance of the population from the variance of each arm. It turns out if you take the mean variance from each arm – placebo, ACE inhibitor, and calcium channel blocker arms – it will approximate the population variance.

So you have two estimates of the population variance, both derived independently from the dataset. If the arms are all equivalent, the two estimates should match. If not, then they will be different. Therefore, the F is:

$$\frac{\text{Population variance calculated from the means}}{\text{Population variance calculated from average}}$$
$$\frac{\text{from the samples}}{\text{of sample variances}}$$

F should be close to 1 if the null hypothesis is true. You take the F and look up the p-value, once again from a table that is calculated based on a normal distribution, and you end up with a p-value.

Because this analysis uses the calculation of population variance to determine whether the groups are similar, it is called analysis of variance or ANOVA.

The assumptions required for F-test are similar to those for the t-test.

15.2.10 Analysis of Nominal Measures/Variables

z-Test

For nominal variables, we must use a different kind of analysis. Nominal variables, as you recall, are non-numeric variables such as hair color (black/brown/white) or survival (dead/alive).

You can't calculate a true "mean" for something like survival, because there is no such thing. "Dead" and "alive" don't even have numeric values. Instead what you use are rates or proportions. For example, if half the patients died and half survived, the proportion of patients surviving would be 0.5. We will use the proportion in the same way we used the mean to perform statistical tests. Similarly, although there is no true SD, you can calculate one that emulates it, for example by assigning 0 to death and 1 to survival. However, no matter whether you are looking at dead/alive, relapse/no relapse, etc., for any given proportion, this "SD" will be the same. In other words, if you know the proportion, you will know the SD. This is because when you only have two possible values (0 or 1); there is only one possible distribution of the values for a given proportion: if the proportion is 0.25, for example, one quarter of the values must be 1 and the rest must be 0. There is no other possible way to get 0.25.

So what you do is similar to the *t*-test. Namely you look at the following:

$$\frac{\text{Difference in the proportions from the arms}}{\text{Standard error of the difference in the proportions}}$$

Let's say you're comparing survival in patients who received a thrombolytic vs. those who didn't. You would calculate the numerator by subtracting the rate of survival of one arm from the other. You would calculate the denominator from the number of patients who survived or died in each group. This value is called *z*. As with *t*, you use *z* to look up the *p*-value.

You can only use *z*-test if there are at least five patients who died and five who lived. If there are fewer than these, the lookup table will be inaccurate. The lookup table is based on there being enough patients so that the distribution of proportions approximates a normal distribution. Otherwise you must use a special method, which is not covered in this book.

Other assumptions for the *z*-test include:

- There can be only two values, such as dead and alive. For nominal variable that has more than two values, such as hair color black/brown/red/blond, you must use the Chi-square test, which is described below.
- There can only be two samples or arms.
- The samples must be independent.
- Each patient in the sample must be selected independent of other patients.

Chi-Square Test

What about when there are more than two outcomes or more than two samples? There is another way to analyze nominal data by using the Chi-square test. This test relies on the contingency table. Let's go back to the contingency table (Figure 15.10).

If placebo and drug had no apparent impact on survival, then you would expect that 38.5% of the patients in each group would have died and 61.5% of the patients in each group would have survived.

The Chi-square test is based on calculating the following where *X* is chi:

$$X^2 = \text{Sum of } \frac{\left\{\begin{array}{l}(\text{Actual number in} \\ \text{the cell} - \text{expected} \\ \text{number in the cell})^2\end{array}\right\}}{\text{Expected number in the cell}} \text{ for each cell}$$

This number will be large if the actual numbers are very different from what's expected for many cells. Chi is used to calculate the *p*-value.

You can use this test for large contingency tables such as (Figure 15.11).

The Chi-square test cannot be used if there are cells with very small values. For example, for a 2 × 2 contingency table, the test cannot be used if there are any cells with values less than 5.

Fisher's Exact Test

Fisher's exact test is useful for contingency tables with very small sample sizes. For small tables, you can actually list all possible combinations of values for the cells and calculate the *p*-value. More extreme the distribution of the cells, smaller will be the *p*-value.

	Placebo	Drug	Total
Died	21	41	62 (38.5%)
Survived	16	83	99 (61.5%)

FIGURE 15.10 Contigency table.

	No event	Hospitalized	ER visit	Died
Placebo	13	43	80	22
Beta agonist	6	88	77	66
Leukotriene inhibitor	87	7	87	3
Steroid	223	32	232	22

FIGURE 15.11 Outcome in asthma patients.

15.2.11 Analysis of Ordinal Measures/Variables: Nonparametric Methods

Mann–Whitney Rank Sum Test: Comparing Two Nonparametric Samples

Many of the techniques described above require that the distribution curve be normal. The p-value calculations for the above tests are based on a normal distribution. For non-normal distributions and ordinal variables, rank test is used. Non-normal distributions are also called *nonparametric distributions* because you can't use simple parameters such as mean and SD to fully describe them. Therefore, the statistical tests we will now discuss are often called *nonparametric tests* or *nonparametric methods*.

As an example of a rank test, let's say that we are comparing multiple sclerosis patients as follows: we take each EDSS value and rank them from lowest to highest. The patient with the lowest EDSS score gets ranked as 1, the next lowest as 2, and so forth. Tied scores get the same rank, but you add together the ranks they would have had and average them. We can't just add and subtract EDSS scores because, as you recall, they are not linear – the difference between 2 and 3 is very different from 9 and 10.

Below is a table you would get if you had three placebo patients with EDSS scores of 2, 5, and 6 and you had three treated patients with scores of 1, 5, and 6 (Figure 15.12).

The rank score for placebo is $2 + 3 + 4 = 9$. The patient with the EDSS score of 2 had the second lowest score so she get 2 points, the next patient had the third lowest score so she gets 3, etc.

Now, to determine whether the rank score of 9 is "weird" or not, let's look at all the possible ways that the placebo patients could have had the ranks (Figure 15.13).[1]

Since in 6 out of the 10 possible combinations the rank score is 9 or less, 9 is not a very extreme or "weird" value. In fact, the p-value for rank score of 9 is 0.6, so the results are not statistically significant.

Of course, with larger samples, it is unwieldy to try to list all the possible combinations, so statisticians usually use formulas to calculate the p-value, as a shortcut. Nonetheless, the basic technique that we do, called Mann–Whitney rank sum test, is the same. You use this test when

you have two samples you are comparing, and the measurements are ordinal. You also use it for comparing two samples where the distribution is not normally shaped.

Kruskal–Wallis Test: Comparing More than Two Nonparametric Samples

When you have multiple samples, then what you do is similar to the analysis of variance. You start by ranking the patients as follows (Figure 15.14).

If there were no real differences between the groups, you would expect that the average rank in each group would be similar. Further apart the average ranks are, less likely it is that the arms have no differences. So, what you do is to calculate for each arm the difference between the observed average rank and the expected average rank, and then you square it to make it positive, and then you add the squares from each treatment group together (weighted for the differences in sizes of the groups). The expected

Combination of ranks for the placebo group					Sum of ranks
1	2	3			6
1	2		4		7
1	2			5	8
1	2			6	9
1		3	4		8
1		3		5	9
1		3		6	10
1			4	5	10
1			4	6	11
1				5 6	12

FIGURE 15.13 Sum of rank scores.

Placebo		Interferon		New drug	
EDSS score	Rank	EDSS score	Rank	EDSS score	Rank
2	3.5	1	1.5	1	1.5
5	6	3	5	10	9
6	7.5	6	7.5	2	3.5

FIGURE 15.14 Rank scores in multiple patient populations.

Placebo		Drug	
EDSS score	Rank	EDSS score	Rank
2	2	1	1
5	3	8	5
6	4	10	6

FIGURE 15.12 Ranking of EDSS scores.

---

[1] Derived from a similar example in Glantz, S.A. (2005). *Primer of Biostatistics*, 6th edn. McGraw-Hill, New York.

average rank is of course the rank you get from all the patients in the study – add up the ranks for everyone and divide by the number of patients. This should be the average rank for each treatment group if there are no differences between the groups. You then adjust this number based on the total number of patients in the study, and you get the Kruskal–Wallis test statistic. From this statistic, you can derive the *p*-value.

15.2.12 Survival Curves

The above described procedures work only when there are complete datasets, or datasets that are nearly complete. In other words, you must know the outcome for all or nearly all the patients (so that you can easily impute the missing values).

In many studies, though, you don't have access to the complete dataset. For example, in an oncology trial, with death as an endpoint, there may be patients who are still alive at the conclusion of a trial. Also, in many trials, there may be a significant number of patients who drop out. In the cases like this, we can use survival curve analysis. This analysis allows us to take patients with different lengths of follow-up and analyze them.

Survival curves are generally analyzed using two "functions." The first function is the probability of surviving until a certain time *t* and is called the survival function: $S(t)$. The second function is the probability of dying at a certain time *t* (if the patient is alive at that time, of course) and is called the hazard function: $h(t)$.

So what you do is to take the survival curve as follows (Figure 15.15).

The curve above is a common way to drawing the survival curves. On the *y*-axis is the proportion of patients who are still alive and the *x*-axis is the time, for example, the number of days from the start of the study. You can draw it one of two ways. The more common is the *Kaplan–Meier curve*, where each time a patient dies the survival is recalculated and reflected on the graph. That is shown above. The *actuarial method* uses fixed intervals such as days or months and calculates survival for each interval. *Life-table analysis* is a term used to refer to either of the methods.

At any given point in time, the rate of decrease (the slope) in one curve vs. the rate of decrease in the other curve is the hazard ratio.

The advantage of a survival analysis is that it allows *censoring*. During censoring, you remove the patient from *both* the numerator and denominator. In other words, if a study started with 100 patients in an arm, and let's say by month 3, 10 patients had died. The survival would be 90/100 or 0.9. Let's say that five patients drop out the following day. Then the survival would be 85/95 or 0.89 after you censor the patient.

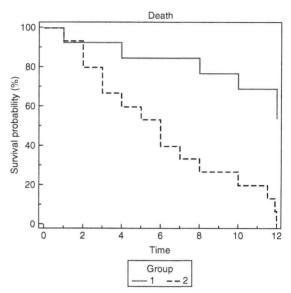

FIGURE 15.15   Survival curves.

You might censor someone who might have been lost to follow up or died of some cause unrelated to cancer, such as a car accident. You can also censor patients who did not die before the end of the study. You know, for example, that if a patient was in the study for 3 months before the study ended and he was alive the whole time, that he lived for at least 3 months but don't know how much longer. You can use the data up to 3 months, and then censor him after that point. For the Kaplan–Meier method, censoring is done when the dropout occurs, for the actuarial method, halfway through the time interval when the dropout occurs.

In theory, you can also censor if you don't know how long it's been since the patient had the initial event (e.g., you don't know the date of diagnosis and you are measuring survival from the date of diagnosis to death), which is called left censoring, but this is not typically done. You would typically just measure survival from time of study entry.

Of course, censoring is appropriate only if the dropouts occur for an unrelated reason. If the dropout is due to hospitalization or a severe adverse event, for example, it may be more appropriate to count the event as a death.

We should note that although we are talking about survival curves, you can use this technique for anything that happens once and only once per patient, such as time to cure, time to next relapse, etc. With sophisticated techniques, you can use survival curve analysis for event that happens multiple times as well, but this is highly dependent on assumptions regarding the relationship between the events so is not widely used.

There are several ways of analyzing survival curves. The first method is the Kaplan–Meier analysis which compares the number of deaths in each time period for the two arms. Each time period can be time between each death or a fixed time interval, such as 1 day or 1 month.

The second method is the Cox proportional hazard method (also called Cox regression), which is a regression analysis. With this technique, the difference between the two treatment groups is collapsed into one variable, the hazard ratio, and a regression (a mathematical model based on the variables) is performed. The regression will have the treatment group as a variable, and the output will often looks like this:

- Hazard ratio = 0.6
- 95% Confidence interval = (0.4, 0.9)

The hazard ratio is the hazard (or risk) of dying at any given point, if you're in one group compared to the other. For example, in an oncology trial, if on any given day, the patient in the control arm has 2% chance of dying and the patient in the drug arm has 1% risk of dying, then the hazard ratio would be 2. Of course, the hazard ratio should be 1 if there is no difference between the groups.

If the 95% confidence interval for the hazard ratio excludes 1, as in this case, then the difference between the two groups is probably real.

The advantage of the Cox method is that it allows the model to be adjusted for other covariates, such as imbalances in age, sex, etc. One problem with the Cox method though is that it assumes that the hazard ratio doesn't change over time. This is sometimes an inaccurate assumption. For example, in an oncology study with a long follow-up, where everyone dies sooner or later, this could be a problem. If the survival curves come together in the end then the Cox method will have poor ability to tell the difference between the two groups. As another example, let's say that a drug shortens the length of time one has a cold. For the first several days, the hazard ratio will be in favor of the drug, but after that, when almost all the patients on the drug have gotten better, and most of the placebo patients are still sick, then a greater proportion of the placebo patients will be recovering. So the hazard ratio turns in favor of the placebo group.

Also, if the survival curves cross, then these tests lose a great deal of power – clearly the hazard ratio does not stay constant over time in that instance.

If the hazard ratio does change over time, then there are more sophisticated versions of the test that change the hazard ratio partway through the study. However, it is often difficult to tell in advance when to change the hazard ratio, and it is inappropriate to fiddle with the test parameters like that *post hoc*, since you can change the *p*-value in your favor by doing that.

The third method is the log-rank test, which is essentially equivalent to the Mantel–Haenszel method. In this test, you are looking to see whether or not the difference in the patterns of survival/death is close to what you expect. To do this, you look at the number of patients in one group whenever someone dies and add up the difference between how many patients you expect to be alive vs. how many are actually alive. If the differences are large, then you will find that the *p*-value is low.

The assumptions for the log-rank test are:

- The two groups/arms are independent.
- The censoring patterns are not difference between the groups, and not related to prognosis.
- The hazards and hazard ratio do not change over time. However, the log-rank test is much more robust to changing hazard ratio than the Cox method.
- The events happened at the times specified.

Another way to compare the survival curves is the *Gehan's test*. In this test, you compare between each death in one group and each death in the other group. For each comparison, you assign 1, 0, or –1 depending on whether one event occurs before or after the other (or you can't tell, in which case you get a 0). Statisticians consider the Gehan's test to be weaker because a small number of early deaths can skew the results.

15.2.13 Paired Tests and Repeated Measures: When Same Patient Gets Multiple Measurements or Treatments

Paired or Unpaired Tests

The procedures thus far discussed are for cases where you are comparing one piece of data from each patient, such as one blood pressure reading. But what about cases where you have multiple pieces of data from each patient? For example, you might have one measurement before the patient receives his medication and one measurement after he receives it.

Of course, it is perfectly acceptable to just use the post-dose value, since in theory the average pre-dose values should be similar in each group. However, you can often get better statistical power by using the difference between the pre- and post-values from each patient. This is particularly true if the variability is very high *between* patients but lower when repeated in the same patient.

With these nested datasets, there are many different ways of comparing the data. For pre- and post-dose data, there are usually three ways to analyze the data as summarized below (the graph is modified from Spriet) (Figure 15.16).

If there is a relationship between the pre- and post-dose measurement – which is typically the case – then the most powerful (sensitive) way to analyze the data is to compare the means of the paired differences (paired differences are sometimes also called intra-patient difference). For example, if the walk distance is increased by 100% in every patient who is treated, and 10% in everyone else who is not treated, then the difference in the post-drug value minus pre-drug value should be calculated for each individual,

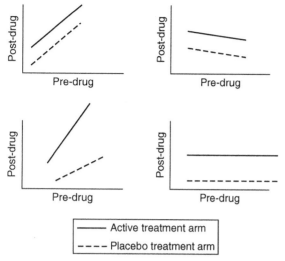

FUGURE 15.16   Pre and post-drug values for a nested dataset.

and then the mean of the intra-patient value be calculated for the placebo and the active groups.

If there is not a relationship between the pre- and post-dose measures, then paired comparisons will not improve the power for the analysis. This is the case with the bottom right graph – the baseline values have no impact on the post-treatment value.

When computing the differences, there are two options: absolute difference or relative (percent) difference. If the change in the values is proportional to pre-treatment values, as is the case with the bottom left graph above, then the percent change is more powerful. For example, if 10 cm tumor shrinks to 8 cm and 1 cm tumor shrinks to 0.8 cm, use the percent difference. Otherwise, the absolute value can be used. For example, if 20% ejection fraction increases to 25% and 40% ejection fraction increases to 45%, then use the absolute changes instead.

In a few cases, the changes are not proportional to the baseline value, but are not completely independent of the baseline value such as in top right hand graph. The slope is not 1, which means that even in the placebo group there is some change in response that is related to the baseline value. For example, in a waxing and waning disease, patients with the worst disease might naturally enter remission. In that case, what you want to do is subtract the natural variability that comes from the disease and the baseline condition. There is a statistical procedure that converts the data from looking like upper right hand graph in Figure 15.16 to the lower right hand graph, called analysis of covariance (ANCOVA).

Nested Datasets

There can certainly be more than two sets of data, and there might be sets of data that are nested. For example, there

might be four different dose groups in a study. Or there may be two sets of measurements in each of multiple treatment groups. The comparisons can be intra-patient, inter-patient, or both. For example, the pre- and post-drug depression scores might be compared to each other for every patient. This would be intra-patient comparison. Or the average height of two groups of patients may be compared. This would be inter-patient comparison. Or the mean depression score changes (post-drug score minus pre-drug score for each patient averaged over the group) may be compared between the placebo and active groups. The way the nested groups are analyzed, such as which groups are compared first, has important implications for the power of the analysis and the types of conclusions that can be drawn.

In general, the first way of nesting the patient (Figure 15.17), out of the two ways illustrated in the above tables (Figure 15.17 and 15.18) is preferred because the measurements for the same patient are not independent–that is, Figure values are normally more similar for multiple measures on the same patient than across patients.

Multiple Measurements

With multiple measurements, repeat measures analysis sometimes may be a wise way to analyze the data. For example, if a patient has 12 visits in the course of a study, then rather than just using the data from the final visit or first and the final visits only, repeated measures analysis allows all the data points to beused.

Patient 1	Patient 2	Patient 3
Pre-treatment	Pre-treatment	Pre-treatment
After one treatment	After one treatment	After one treatment
After two treatments	After two treatments	After two treatments

Compare within patients first, then across the patients

FIGURE 15.17   Nested groups.

Patient 1	Patient 2	Patient 3
Pre-treatment	Pre-treatment	Pre-treatment
After one treatment	After one treatment	After one treatment
After two treatments	After two treatments	After two treatments

Compare within same time points (across patients) first, then across the time points

FIGURE 15.18   Nested groups.

As was described in Chapter 7, repeat measures analyses can be very useful in diseases that wax and wane; but they may not be very powerful in diseases that progressively worsen. When diseases progressively worsen over time, the differences in measurements between the treatment and control group should become greater over time (i.e., if a drug aims to slow down the progression of heart failure, there should be a greater difference in cardiac function between treated and control patients later in the trial). Therefore, using only the first and last measurements may be more sensitive in detecting differences between the treated and control groups. Using a sports analogy, if one athlete is to start regularly lifting weights while another athlete does not, there may not be any difference in their game performance during the first year. However, after 4 years, the differences may be readily apparent.

A variation of repeated measures analysis is to look for a *sustained response* (i.e., does the intervention have the same response at multiple time points). In other words, the endpoint is dependent on a response being present at multiple different time points. An intervention having a positive effect at both weeks 5 and 10 is more convincing than having effects just at 5 or 10 weeks. This is especially helpful when there is a high placebo rate, that is the placebo appears to have a positive effect on a disease. For instance, if a Crohn's disease drug were effective, you would expect that patients who responded would have remission at both weeks 10 and 12, while those receiving placebo may have spurious measures that indicate remission sporadically but not on a sustained basis. Defining endpoints as disease remission at weeks 10 and 12 therefore decreases the rate of false remission in the placebo group. While this is a rather different sort of analysis compared to the tests described above, conceptually they are similar in that you take advantage of the expectation that values in the same patient is more likely to be similar.

Paired t-Test

The paired *t*-test is used when you have one group of patients who have both pre- and post-measurements. For example, let's say you have 40 patients who all take a weight reduction medication. Each patient has a weight measurement pre- and post-treatments. Rather than comparing the mean pre-dose value for the whole group against the mean post-dose value for the whole group, which would have fairly low statistical power (because you are only comparing two values), you can calculate the change in weight for each patient first (now you are looking at 40 differences). This gives you much better statistical power to tell if there is a difference, because if every patient loses exactly 2 pounds, it would be much easier to pick this up by looking at how much each patient has lost than looking at the average pre-treatment weight vs. the average

post-treatment weight. You could have half the people gaining 10 pounds and half the people losing 14 pounds and still end up with difference of 2 pounds (net loss) for the mean group weights:

$$\frac{\text{Mean change in weight}}{\text{Standard error of the difference in pre- and post-treatment weight}}$$

Ratio t-Test

In medicine, some drugs have an effect that is best expressed as a relative change rather than an absolute change. For example, a drug might shrink tumors by 50%. A 10-cm tumor might shrink to 5 cm and a 2-cm tumor might shrink to 1 cm. In that case, it would probably be appropriate to capture both shrinkages as 50% rather than one as 5-cm shrinkage and the other as 1-cm shrinkage.

Similarly, after one half-life, the drug concentration might decrease from 10 to 5 nM in one patient and from 2 to 1 nM in another patient. It would be misleading in this case to say that the drug is cleared faster in the first patient than the second patient.

When you expect a drug to have a relative effect, you will often want to compare the percentage change rather than the absolute change. You can use the ratio *t*-test to resolve this issue.

But the percent change or ratios are a bit difficult to compare directly because they are asymmetrical. When you double something, you increase it by 100%, but when you halve something you decrease it by 50%, not by 100%. When you triple something you increase it by 200%, but when you reduce it to a third, you decrease it by 67%, not by 200%.

In order to get around this issue, you use the logarithm of the ratio. This makes the percentages and ratios symmetrical. For example, increasing a value tenfold increases the log by 1 and decreasing it to one-tenth decreases log by 1.

Sometimes it will be difficult to decide whether an absolute change is clinically more meaningful than the relative change. Sometimes it is also difficult to tell whether a drug is going to have an absolute change or a relative change. Ultimately, the choice of which test to use comes down to a judgment call, based on clinical and statistical considerations, but it should be a decision based on sound understanding of the statistical implications.

Repeated Measures Analysis of Variance

Now, let's say you have a more complicated situation. In addition to measurements taken after treatment with the weight loss drug, the patients also obtain a weight measurement halfway through treatment. So you have three measurements per patient.

Baseline EDSS score	Post-drug EDSS score	Difference	Rank based on magnitude of the difference	Direction of difference	Signed rank
2	2	0	1	+	+1
5	3	−2	3	−	−3
5	1	4	5	+	+5
2	3	−1	2	−	−2
5	3	3	4	+	+4
2	10	−9	6	−	−6

FIGURE 15.19 Signed rank.

In this case, you use the repeated measures analysis of variance. This ANOVA is similar to the ANOVA from earlier, but the difference this time is that the measurements from the same person will tend to be similar to one another. So these measurements will not be "independent-" that is they will be influenced by the other measurements. The details of the analysis can be left to the statistician and his/her computer, but the general idea is the same as for the standard ANOVA – if the distribution appears weird, you reject the hypothesis.

Wilcoxon Signed Rank Sum Test

As you recall, the ANOVA is for continuous variables, such as height, blood pressure, etc. For nonparametric or ordinal variables, you will often use the Wilcoxon signed rank sum test. Let's return to the multiple sclerosis case. This time though, you not only have the measurements from the end of the study but also from baseline values.

You then add up the signed rank and obtain the *signed rank sum* Figure 15.19. If there is no effect, then the positive and negative differences should approximately cancel each other out because the changes would be random and in either direction. If there were an effect, then the signed rank sum would be very positive or very negative. You can list all possible combinations of possible ranks and based on how "weird" or "extreme" the signed rank sum you get is, you can calculate the *p*-value. Of course, for larger studies, your statistician will use formulas to calculate the *p*-value.

Friedman Test

For nonparametric situations, a rank test called the Friedman test can be used if a patient receives multiple treatments. In this case, the subject's response to each treatment is ranked against his/her response to other treatments. See below (Figure 15.20).

If all the drugs have a similar effect, then the distribution of the ranks should be random. If they have different effects, then the likelihood that one of them have different increases.

	Drug A	Drug B	Drug C
Patient 1	1	2	3
Patient 2	2	1	3
Patient 3	1	2	3
Patient 4	3	2	1
Patient 5	1	2	3
Patient 6	1	3	2

FIGURE 15.20 Ranking for Friedman test.

Testing for Trends

The repeated measures ANOVA and other methods discussed above are reasonable good ways of looking at repeated measures. They also are relatively flexible in that the measurements can be done with many different types of interventions. For example, the first measurement may be made at baseline, the second after drug 1, the third after drug 2, the fourth after drug 3, and so on. The drugs can be completely unrelated.

There is another way to analyze repeated measures, if the intervention is the same type. An example would be if the measurements are made at baseline, after 1 month of therapy with drug 1, after 2 months of therapy with drug 1, after 3 months of therapy with drug 1, and so on. The method relies on looking for a trend over time. Below is an example. Let's say a group of patients received a drug for osteoporosis and bone density was measured over time (Figure 15.21).

You can draw a *regression line* through the data points. A regression line is a line that best fits the data points. What does "best fit the data points" mean? Intuitively, it means that the line is as close as possible to as many data points as possible. Statistically, it means that if you are to take the distance between each data point and the line, square it, and add them all up, the line would minimize that total value. You square the value so that if the difference

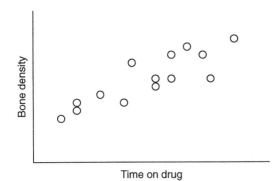

FIGURE 15.21 Bone density vs. time o drug.

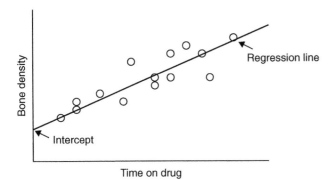

FIGURE 15.22 Regression line.

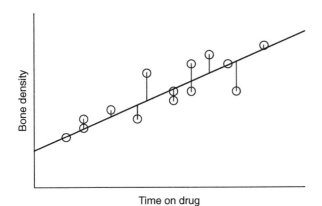

FIGURE 15.23 Least squared regression line.

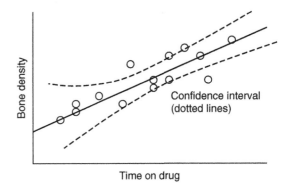

FIGURE 15.24 Confidence interval around regression line.

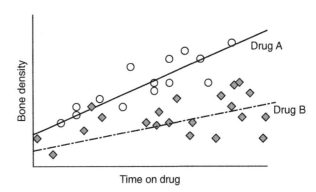

FIGURE 15.25 Comparison of regression lines.

values are to the true slope and intercept for all patients in the world (the entire population). This is analogous to the other values based on samples we've discussed before.

You can in fact do a lot of things with the regression line. You can in effect use it like you use the mean. For example, you can calculate the confidence intervals Figure 15.24.

You can also compare across two lines from two arms of a study (Figure 15.25).

There are three possible comparisons between two lines:

1. Comparison of the slopes.
2. Comparison of the intercepts.
3. Comparison of both the slopes and intercepts (a test for *coincidence*, that both lines are exactly the same).

The procedures for these comparisons are similar conceptually to the procedures for comparing other statistics like the means. The details won't be covered here, since it is best left to statisticians and their computers, but the broad outlines of how this is done is as follows.

First you calculate the regression line for all the patients, from both drug A and drug B groups. The null hypothesis would be that the drugs are no different, and if this is the case, all the patients can be treated as if they are form one group (Figure 15.26).

Next, calculate how good the "fit" is if you use two separate regression lines vs. using just the one for all patients.

is negative, it turns into a positive value. This method is called *least-squared regression*.

So you get the following (Figure 15.22)

And the least-squared regression is based on the distance as noted below with vertical lines (Figure 15.23).

Now we have a line that has *a slope* and *an intercept*. The slope and the intercept allow us to calculate the expected bone density for any time point. Of course, the regression line is the best-fit line for the group of patients (the sample) in the study, but not for the entire population of patients in the world eligible to receive the drug. There is the *SE* for both the slope and intercept, which quantifies how close the

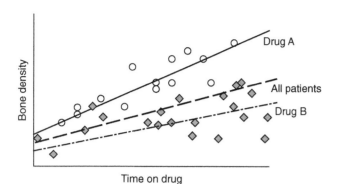

FIGURE 15.26 Null hypothesis line.

You do this by calculating the variability for each of the lines using the least-squared method outlined above. Of course, the fit will almost always be better from using two separate lines, but if the fit is *much* better then the p-value you will look up based on this procedure will be very small and you will conclude that the lines are different.

The above regression lines are based on the assumption that each data point can be a different patient. Through a more sophisticated mathematical manipulation, regression lines can be drawn even if there are multiple measurements per patient, and some of the data points are from the same patient. In fact, this can make the analysis much more powerful. This can then become a way to take repeated measurements from the same patient and test for differences between groups.

15.3 SELECTING TESTS AND CAVEATS

15.3.1 Choosing a Test

When do you use parametric vs. nonparametric tests? Choose the nonparametric test if

- the variables are clearly not normal/parametric/Gaussian;
- the variables are not continuous – such as ordinal or nominal measures;
- some values are extremely outliers that can't be measured, for example "glucose level is too high to be measured;"
- if you know from other studies that the variables are nonparametric.

On the other hand, parametric test is probably appropriate if

- there are many independent factors causing variability, since in that case the distribution will probably be Gaussian;
- the variables are known to be normal/parametric/Gaussian.

For large samples, it makes little difference which test you use. Both tests will do a good job. With small samples, the parametric test will yield overly low p-values for nonparametric samples, and vice versa.

When there is a choice of paired or unpaired tests, the paired test should almost always be used because they are more powerful, especially when measurements are matched (e.g., pre- and post-measurements, sibling measurements, etc.) (Figure 15.27).

Measurement type	Continuous, parametric	Nominal/ordinal/ nonparametric	Dichotomous (two possible outcomes)	Survival (time to event) (*not clear*)
Describe one group	Mean, SD	Median, percentiles	Proportion	Kaplan–Meier survival curve, median survival
Compare one group to a hypothetical value	One sample *t*-test	Wilcoxon test	Chi-squared or binominal test	
Compare two unpaired groups	Unpaired *t*-test	Mann–Whitney	Fisher's or Chi-squared	Log rank or Mantel–Haenszel
Compare two paired groups	Paired *t*-test	Wilcoxon	McNamara's	Conditional proportional hazards regression
Compare three or more unmatched groups	One way ANOVA	Kruskal–Wallis	Chi-squared	Cox proportional hazards regression
Compare three or more matched groups	Repeated-measured ANOVA	Friedman	Cochrane Q	Conditional proportional hazards regression
Quantify relationship between two variables	Pearson correlation	Spearman correlation	Contingency coefficients	
Predict value from another variable	Linear (or nonlinear) regression	Nonparametric regression	Simple logistic regression	Cox proportional hazards regression
Predict values from several measured or binominal variables	Multiple linear (or nonlinear) regression		Multiple logistic regression	Cox proportional hazards regression

Source: This table is derived from Mikulski, H. (1995). *Intuitive Statistics*. Oxford Press. New York.

FIGURE 15.27 Appropriate statistical tests for different types of analysis.

15.3.2 Assumptions

In the above sections, we have discussed many different types of tests for different situations. It is not critical to remember which test(s) to use in which situation, since you can always look that up. Neither is it critical to remember how the tests are performed, since a statistician and/or his/her computer will perform the tests.

What is critical, however, is to remember the assumptions behind the tests. The assumptions underpinning the statistical analyses must be accurate, or the tests will yield inaccurate results. You must understand and remember the assumptions because the clinician is responsible for alerting the statistician when the assumptions are incorrect. If an assumption is incorrect, the results of the analysis will be incorrect.

There is no way for a statistician to know, for example, that the blood pressure has a U-shaped curve in relation to survival – that a patient with systolic blood pressure (SBP) of 50 will have a poor prognosis; that a patient with SBP of 120 has a good prognosis; and that a patient with SBP of 300 has a poor prognosis. In the absence of input from a clinician, a statistician will likely assume a linear relationship.

As another example, there is no way for a statistician to know that you expect only a subgroup of patients to respond to a new therapy. If this happens, then the shape of the curve describing the response may become bimodal (two peaks): the responders and nonresponders. This causes two issues: the curve is no longer normal (parametric), which is a fundamental and important assumption in many of the tests; and the shape of the curves for the active and placebo groups are different which violates another critical assumption in many of the tests.

Fortunately, if the assumptions are violated, and this is recognized, then there is usually an alternate, more appropriate statistical test that can be used.

Below are some of the more important assumptions:

- For parametric tests, the population must be normally distributed. For many of the common tests (e.g., the *t*-test), the samples must be at least approximately normal in shape. For example, if you are examining ejection fraction, the distribution of ejection fraction values must form a bell-shaped curve. Sometimes this is an incorrect assumption. For example, you might have a subpopulation of patients with low ejection fraction due to a prior myocardial infarction (MI). You then have a bimodal distribution. Bimodal distribution in particular has a very negative impact on the tests, just like a very skewed distribution.
- For many parametric tests, the variance in the samples must be similar. The shape of the curve must be similar for both groups. This can be a problem, for example, if your drug widens or narrows the curve and the comparator group's curve does not change. For example, if you have a drug that lowers high glucose levels but does not cause hypoglycemia, and you are comparing against a drug that lowers glucose in every patient indiscriminately, you are likely to end up with a narrower glucose concentration curve with the first drug. For unequal variance, there are special tests that take into account the differences in variance.
- You must be using the right types of variables. For example, you must be using true continuous measures if you are using the tests designed for continuous variables, such as the *t*-test. For example, if EDSS is mistakenly thought to be a continuous measure, then the *t*-test may be performed on it. Any conclusions based on performing mathematical manipulation on EDSS dataset that assumes linearity and continuity will be at worst misleading and at best meaningless because 1 point change in EDSS means very different things depending on whether you are going from 1 to 2 or 5 to 6 or 9 to 10.
- As another example, Mini Mental State Examination (MMSE) is not a linear scale in studies of Alzheimer's disease. The decline in MMSE is not linear over time. Before standard mathematical manipulations can be done, the data should be transformed (basically stretched and deformed to make it linear). Alternatively, it can be treated as an ordinal variable. The choice can have a critical effect on the sample size and magnitude of effect that can be shown, as discussed below.
- Each sample is selected independently of other samples.
- Each sample must be randomly selected, without bias.
- For survival curves, the proportional hazard ratio stays constant. In other words, that the benefit of the drug stays consistent over time. This may be untrue, for example, if a new therapy is introduced partway through the trial, or if the patients who die quickly have different benefits from the drug compared to the others who die later.
- For some tests, your sample sizes may need to be large enough. If, for example, the sample size is less than 30, then the nonparametric analysis usually must be performed, rather than the standard statistical analyses. For Chi-square test, the expected number in each cell must be at least 5 or else the Fisher's exact test must be used. Fortunately, in most cases, statisticians will catch this, but if you are performing the statistical calculations yourself, then you should be aware of this pitfall.

15.3.3 Aggregate Data: Pro's and Con's

Any statistical analysis of a clinical trial is performed on aggregate data (collection of many pieces of data). It is necessary and sometimes important to analyze individual level data, especially when evaluating adverse events. This type of analysis is described later, but is usually the exception rather than the rule. Each statistical analysis relies on aggregate data, and the power of a clinical trial is the ability to aggregate data and draw conclusions from them. The aggregating data gives us power to manipulate the data and understand them in such ways that it would not be possible with individual data, but there are limitations.

One limitation is that some of the finer details of data are lost, no matter how good the analysis is. This is an inevitable trade-off, and an acceptable trade-off in most cases. However, in some cases, you don't merely lose the finer details. You might draw wrong conclusions because the aggregate data is misleading.

For example, using the mean is usually a good first-order look at the response. However, aggregate data can lead to wrong conclusions when the distribution of the data is atypical. This is discussed in detail in Chapter 7. For example, if the mean walking distance on a treadmill test increases by 30 seconds after a patient receives a drug, this is generally taken to be of clinical benefit. However, this assumes that most people have a similar response to the drug. If in fact some of the patients could walk 2 minutes longer but 25% of the patient walk 2 minutes shorter, this would be of very different clinical significance.

Conversely even if the mean doesn't change, the drug may be of use if a subgroup benefits. Let's say 25% of the patients do twice as well as before and the rest do somewhat worse and that it is possible to predict in advance or shortly after starting therapy which patients would be most likely to respond to drug treatment. This of course assumes that the negative effects are reversible (in the case of being able to tell early who the responders are going to be). For example, if after 1 week of starting the drug, it becomes clear which 25% of the patients are going to be able to walk longer, and the ones who are not responding can be taken off the drug and return to baseline immediately, the drug may be of benefit even if the mean does not change.

Limitations of Aggregate Data, Example

Three statisticians went hunting. One shot at a deer and missed 5 feet to the right. Another shot and missed 5 feet to the left. The third did a calculation, derived the average, and exclaimed, "We got him!"

On a related topic, if the drug has clear beneficial effect on one measure of disease (e.g., renal function in lupus patients), this may be a good signal that the drug is working. However, this assumes that the drug has a similar effect on all manifestations of the disease and the renal function is a surrogate for the disease as a whole. This is often the case, and it is possible that, for example, the drug actually worsens the hematological manifestation of the disease, while improving the renal function. In that case, capturing only one aspect of the disease would not accurately reflect the benefit of therapy.

Similarly, when a drug has an apparent beneficial effect over the short or the medium term, it is assumed that this is a good surrogate for its effect over the long term. In fact, it is rather rare that response over years is studied, even for chronic diseases. The benefit on rheumatoid arthritis over 6 months may be considered to predict benefit over many years. These types of assumptions may or may not be accurate.

The other instance where aggregate data can lead to wrong conclusions is when individual response curve is important in clinical use of the drug and the averaging of the aggregate data destroys that information.

In addition, the primary endpoint alone is rarely enough to provide enough data for assessing the total clinical benefit. It doesn't capture time to onset of action, rebound, durability of effect, consistency across subgroups, etc.

15.3.4 Confounding and Imbalances in Baseline Characteristics

Confounding is a very important aspect of data analysis. Confounders are factors, variables, or other characteristics that make the effect of an intervention appear higher or lower than it actually is.

A classic example is carrying matches and lung cancer, which was discussed in Chapter 1.

> An extensive study is undertaken to determine if carrying matches causes lung cancer. It is found that a strong correlation exists between the two. Match carriers are at an extremely high risk of developing lung caner. Of course, this conclusion is wrong, because the smoking is a confounding factor. People who carry matches tend to be smokers, and therefore smoking confounds the results of the study and causes the conclusions to be stronger than it really is.

Of course, one could ask whether the exact reverse might be true: it appears that smoking causes lung cancer but could it be that carrying of matches is the real cause and the smoking is a confounder? How can we tell which is which? The answer is that in and of itself, there is no way to distinguish a confounder from the true cause, unless a randomized study is performed. This is indeed an alternative definition of a confounder – something that cannot be distinguished from a true cause.

The classic requirements of a confounding factor are:

1. It is a risk factor for the outcome (disease, endpoint, etc.).
2. It is correlated (positively or negatively) with the intervention (or exposure).
3. It is not an intermediate in the pathway between the intervention and outcome (or in some definitions, be downstream of the intervention).

For example, rash would not be a confounder in a study of epidermal growth factor receptor (EGFR) antagonist for cancer, because EGFR antagonists cause rashes.

If the results of the study were adjusted for rash, it would be inappropriate because that would cancel out the true effect of the drug.

In an mycordial infarction (MI) study, the location of the infarct would be a confounder for percutaneous transluminal coronary angioplasty to reduce mortality, since inferior infarct patients have better outcome.

Confounding is an irascible problem in observational studies. It is impossible to ferret out all potential confounders or to distinguish confounders from true causes. The purpose of a randomized study is to neutralize the effect of confounding. While in a rare instances, just by chance, there can be confounding due to imbalances in baseline characteristics, but in general, the results of a randomized study do not need to be adjusted for imbalances in baseline characteristics. For example, even if it's known that age is a strong predictor of death after an MI, the results in general are not adjusted for difference in the age of patients randomized into the active and the placebo groups. Randomization should balance the patient populations in the two groups such that they are relatively equal.

Also, if certain baseline characteristics are known to be predictors of response, then the patients should be stratified at randomization. Moreover, adjustment for covariates will adjust for known (but not unknown) confounders, whereas randomization should do both. Adjusting statistically for the known confounders will introduce bias into the analysis, and probably does not add much in most instances.

However, in some cases, where the confounders are well characterized, and if prespecified, it is reasonable to adjust for confounders. In fact, even the Food and Drug Administration (FDA) has sometimes agreed to such adjustments even in primary analysis (e.g., the pivotal study for tenecteplase).

15.3.5 Interactions

In addition to confounders, there is a related but different phenomenon called interactions. Interactions are similar to confounding in that they can lead to misleading results, but they are fundamentally different in many significant ways. Perhaps the most important difference is that you can eliminate confounding by randomization, but you cannot eliminate interactions through randomization.

Interactions occur when a factor that may not in and of itself be a risk factor, but changes the strength of a risk factor. Drug interactions are common examples of interactions. Terfenadine and ketoconazole by themselves do not cause QT prolongation but together they do because ketoconazole inhibits metabolism of Terfenadine. Quantitative interaction occurs when the direction of change is consistent but the magnitude is different. Qualitative interaction means that the treatment effect goes in opposite directions.

While confounding involves two risk factors having an additive (or in few cases a subtractive) effect on the outcome, interactions generally have synergistic effects. In other words, interactions often occur in situations where both factors A and B must be present to exert an effect. An example would be smoking and inhaling on lung cancer. Inhaling is an interaction for smoking with respect to lung cancer. Both smoking and inhaling must be present to result in lung cancer. Smoking in and of itself would not cause lung cancer if the person never inhaled, and inhaling without smoking does not cause lung cancer.

In randomized trials, interactions often manifest themselves as subgroups that may or may not gain benefits. For example, a drug might have a beneficial effect on the blood pressure for the patients as a whole in the study, but on a subgroup analysis, it might turn out that the patients with high aldosterone levels do not benefit. This would be an interaction.

Interactions are important to identify because they can exist even in randomized clinical trials, and they allows identification of patients who gain more or less benefits than the group as a whole.

15.4 SLICING AND ANALYZING DATA IN VARIOUS PERMUTATIONS

15.4.1 Primary Endpoint and Multiple Comparisons

Conventional Primary Endpoint

The analysis of the primary endpoint is generally straightforward. If designed properly, the clinical trial should be geared toward the primary endpoint, and the question of whether the primary endpoint is met should be simple. The prespecified analysis is performed to derive the p-value of the primary endpoint comparing the two or more arms. If the p-value is less than 0.05, then:

1. The null hypothesis is rejected.
2. The primary endpoint is met.
3. Causation between intervention (treatment) and outcome is established.

Of the three criteria, the third one is the most important: establishment of a causal link.

However, there are several other types of analyses that typically done in addition to the primary endpoint analysis. These are outlined in the following sections.

It is important to emphasize again that the primary endpoint must be prespecified. It cannot be changed once the results are unblinded, due to the reasons outlined earlier in the book – that is a single, prespecified primary endpoint with alpha of 0.05 is the accepted test to establish causality in clinical trials. There are only a few exceptions or variations to this fundamental rule, which are explained in this section.

Multiple Comparison and Other Ways of Splitting the Alpha

As was previously mentioned, you cannot have multiple primary endpoints unless you either:

1. split the alpha or
2. arrange the testing hierarchically, or
3. do both.

We will discuss splitting of alpha in this section. Let's revisit what alpha is: it is the maximal probability of Type I error. Type I error, if you recall, is the mistake of rejecting the null hypothesis when it is actually true: that is, deciding that a treatment is better than placebo when it actually is not. Alpha is conventionally set at 0.05 or less in clinical trials.

Usually, the entire 0.05 is allocated to the primary endpoint, and there is usually only one primary endpoint. However, this does not necessarily need to be the case. Alpha splitting means that you take 0.05, which is the standard alpha, and allocate it across several different primary endpoints. One of the more common ways to do this is with multiple comparisons: looking at the same endpoint across many groups. For example, one might have a three-arm trial (placebo, low dose, and high dose) and allocate p (or alpha) of 0.025 to comparison between placebo and low dose and p of 0.025 to comparison between placebo and high dose. This results in two primary endpoints without violating the conventions for Type I error because $0.025 + 0.025 = 0.05$.

It is important to note that, in this case, the p-values must be less than 0.025 in order to be able to declare the comparison to be statistically significant. If, for example, the first comparison between the placebo and low dose groups yielded a p-value of 0.03, then this would not be statistically significant. If at the same time, the comparison between the placebo and high dose groups yielded a p-value of 0.01, then this comparison would be statistically significant.

This section is mostly concerned with multiple comparisons across multiple treatment groups. We should keep in mind that you can split the alpha across different endpoints as well. For example, even if you only have two arms (active and placebo groups), you might assign alpha of 0.04 for one endpoint such as survival and 0.01 for another endpoint such as reduction in hospitalization. You can also split the alpha among subgroups, such as 0.04 for everyone in the study and 0.01 for the subgroup with the most severe disease. For these types of alpha splitting, we advise that a conservative route of simply dividing the alpha be taken. Some of the more sophisticated techniques outlined below can be used in these types of alpha splitting, but the statistics can become quite complicated quickly.

As an additional point, the techniques for defining confidence intervals with the various methods of allocating the alpha are not well developed, and can present a problem in interpreting the results beyond just the simple question of "is there a statistically significant difference?" Confidence intervals are important in understanding the robustness of the result and precision of the estimates of the difference.

Bonferroni Correction

The simplest way to allow multiple comparisons is Bonterroni method. This means just take p of 0.05 and divide it by the number of tests to be performed. So in the above example, since there are three t-tests, the p-value needed for statistical significance is 0.05 divided by 3. Then, you can perform the t-test.

Bonferroni correction tends to be conservative. If you have more than a handful of t-tests, you will tend to under-call significance. The more comparison you do, the worse it will be. That's because it doesn't account for double counting – if you already have had a false positive result, you don't make things worse by having additional false results.

The reason why Bonferroni is conservative is as follows. If you perform pairwise tests such as the t-test on two arms of a study, they only take into account information from the two arms and ignore that there are other arms. Now, if you recall, the t-test compares the observed variability in the two samples vs. total variability in all the samples. In fact, you have information from more than two arms that will give you a better idea of what the total variability or the "spread" of values should be, but you are not using them in the pairwise tests. You are calculating the numerator and denominator from just two arms when in fact you could use information from all the arms for the denominator. This is why simple Bonferroni correction is more conservative (less likely to detect a real difference) than the other tests.

Also, there is some information carryover. If you compare arm 1 with arm 2, and then compare arm 2 with arm 3, you will have some information about arm 1 vs. arm 3. Tests like the t-test do not take this into consideration.

You can make the tests little less conservative by modifying the t-test so that it uses information from all the arms to estimate the expected "spread" of the values rather than just from the two arms being compared, but this will only help slightly. This is because the t-test is designed for comparing groups from studies with only two arms.

Why Bonferroni is Overly Conservative: By the Numbers

The risk of Type I error when you have three comparisons is as follows. If you just use 0.05 as the cutoff for significance, then with each comparison, you have 95% chance that you will not draw a false conclusion. So the probability you will not draws a false positive conclusion is $0.95 \times 0.95 \times 0.95$, which is 0.86. The probability that you will have one or more false positives is 0.14. The Bonferroni method calculates this probability as $0.05 \times 3 = 0.15$. So the values are relatively close.

The risk of Type I error for 10 comparisons is as follows. The likelihood you will not draw a false positive conclusion is $(0.95)^{10}$, which is 0.60. The Bonferroni method calculates this probability as $0.05 \times 10 = 0.5$. So the difference is much larger.

Holm Correction

The Holm *t*-test is less conservative than the Bonferroni *t*-test and is relatively easy to use. You start by ordering the *p*-values from each comparison you want to do, from smallest to largest. You sequentially test each comparison, except instead of using 0.05 divided by the number of comparisons as in the Bonferroni correction, you use 0.05 divided by (number of comparisons – number of comparisons you have already performed). So for the first comparison in the example above, you use 0.05/3, but if that's significant, you then use 0.05/2 followed by 0.05/1. You keep on going until you get a result that is not significant. As you can see, this is less conservative than the Bonferroni *t*-test.

Multiple Primary Endpoints Must All Be Met

One way of avoiding adjustment for multiple primary endpoints is to specify that all the primary endpoints must be met. One example is Alzheimer's disease studies where generally both an objective measure such as ADAS-COG and a general measure of cognition must both achieve statistical significance at $p < 0.05$ in order to declare the study to be positive. In other words, if only one of the primary endpoints is met, then the results are negative. This avoids the issue of multiple comparisons, since one is not cherry picking the best results out of multiple endpoints.

However, this is generally a poor solution to the multiple comparisons problem, because it greatly increases the chance of a Type II error. Unless the study is powered to control Type II error for both endpoints, which often would require enormously large trials, the risk of false negative is extremely high. To achieve $p < 0.05$ on two endpoints is a very high bar. One mitigating factor in many of these studies with multiple primary endpoints is that the endpoints are often collinear. If one endpoint shows a difference, there is usually a high chance that the other will be correlated. This will reduce the likelihood of Type II error.

Multiple primary endpoints are used sometimes because there is no single, general measure that can fully capture the disease outcome in that indication or field. Eventually, however, as the study of that indication becomes more sophisticated, and as the clinical trial medicine advances in that particular field, better instruments for measuring outcome are usually developed, such as composite measures.

The other instance where multiple primary endpoints must all be met is in multiple arm trials where the clinical utility of the drug or the regulatory approvability of the drug requires that multiple endpoints be met. For example, in a three-arm study with placebo, positive control, and experimental drug, the regulatory requirement for approval may be that both of the following endpoints must be met at the 0.05 significance level:

- Investigational drug is superior to placebo.
- Investigational drug is noninferior to the positive control.

Or, with a combination drug, the requirement may be that the combination drug shows superiority to each of the component drugs at significance of 0.05.

Other Methods

The other way of performing multiple comparisons is the use of the Tukey test mentioned above or the Student–Newman–Keuls (SNK) test. The SNK test is very similar to the Tukey test, except the former is less conservative. The SNK test is derived from the Tukey test except that while the Tukey test uses the number of groups in the whole study to compute the *p*-value table, the SNK test only uses the groups being compared.

Caveats

Please make sure that some other way of analyzing the data isn't more appropriate. For example, if the arms are placebo, 5 mg dose, and 10 mg dose, then a more powerful way of analyzing the data may be to test for a trend (e.g., placebo < 5 mg < 10 mg).

Or perhaps you are not interested in every pairwise comparison. You might have placebo, old drug, and new drug in the three different arms. You might only be interested in (1) placebo vs. new drug and (2) old drug vs. new drug, but not placebo vs. old drug. You don't have to split the alpha across three tests then. Or, in the above example, you only want to know if your drug has an effect or not, and you think both the 5 and 10 mg doses will work. Then you can pool the 5 and 10 mg groups or use the Dunnett's test, which is a way of comparing many groups and one group.

Hierarchical Testing

The other way of having more than one primary endpoint is by the use of hierarchical testing (sometimes referred to as contingent primary endpoint) (Figure 15.28). In this case, you start with a conventional primary endpoint such as the

---

| Primary endpoint 1: Experimental drug is noninferior to the standard of care ($p < 0.05$) |

If first test is met, then go onto the second primary endpoint

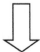

| Primary endpoint 2: Experimental drug is superior to the standard of care ($p < 0.05$) |

FIGURE 15.28 Hierarchial testing.

difference in survival between the placebo and active groups. If there is a statistically significant difference ($p < 0.05$) in the first hierarchical endpoint, then you can test the second hierarchical endpoint, such as the difference in hospital days between the active and placebo groups. If the p-value is less than 0.05 for the second hierarchical endpoint, then you can claim a causal relationship between the intervention and endpoint. You can continue your analyses with as many hierarchical endpoints as you wish, but you should be aware that lower down in the hierarchy one goes, greater the chance of a Type II error.

The key aspects of hierarchical endpoints are:

1. The p-value that you use for each of the primary endpoints, unlike with multiple comparisons, is 0.05.
2. In order to be able to get to the next endpoint in the hierarchy, the previous endpoint above it must have been achieved. This means that if the first hierarchical endpoint is not met, then all of the other endpoints fail. This is different from multiple comparisons where the endpoints are much more independent.
3. Each primary endpoint in the hierarchy established a causal relationship. This is different from simple secondary endpoints, since secondary endpoints do not establish causation. Secondary endpoints are exploratory.

One very typical use of hierarchical testing is for noninferiority studies. For example, if the study shows the experimental arm to be noninferior to the standard of care arm, then superiority may be tested with p-value of 0.05.

If the first test is negative, the second test cannot be performed. This is intuitive for the noninferiority. Obviously, it is not possible for a drug to be equivalent if it is inferior. It is less intuitive for subgroups – obviously it is possible for a drug to be efficacious in a subgroup and not for the group as a whole. Even if the first primary endpoint for the entire study is not met, it is possible that the secondary primary endpoint for a subgroup could be met. For example, herceptin works only for breast cancer patients with HER2 overexpression. Why can't the second primary hypothesis be tested even if the first test fails? The reason for this is to avoid multiple comparisons that can lead to a spurious result. It is not that a drug may not work for a subgroup – it is that the trial cannot be used as evidence for that conclusion because it violates the goal of keeping Type I error below 5%.

Hierarchical testing and multiple comparisons can be combined (Figure 15.29). For example, the first hierarchical test can be for a difference between the active and placebo arms for the entire group and then the second hierarchical test can be split into 0.025 for males and 0.025 for females.

15.4.2 Sensitivity Analysis

Sensitivity analysis is performed with assumptions that differ from those used in the primary analysis. Sensitivity analysis addresses the questions such as "will the results of the study change if we use other assumptions?" and "how sure are we of the assumptions?" Sensitivity analysis is typically performed to check the robustness of the results. For instance, if a study yields a p-value of 0.02 for the primary analysis but there are quite a few dropouts, then a sensitivity analysis might be performed while counting all the dropouts as patients who fail therapy. If the p-value becomes 0.03 under this scenario, then the results are robust. If it becomes 0.2 then the results are not robust.

Sensitivity analysis can be performed for a host of reasons, including Good Clinical Practice (GCP) violations,

---

Primary endpoint 1: There is a

difference between active and

placebo groups in survival

($p < 0.05$)

If first test is met, then go onto the second primary endpoint

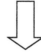

| Primary endpoint 2a: There is a difference between active and placebo groups in survival among females ($p < 0.025$) | Primary endpoint 2b: There is a difference between active and placebo groups in survival among males ($p < 0.025$) |

FIGURE 15.29   Hierarchial testing combined with multiple comarisons.

protocol violations, ambiguous/missing data, etc. Since imputations (see Chapter 14) for missing data can have a nontrivial effect on results of a study as well as the *p*-value, FDA will often request sensitivity analysis to ensure that the results of the test are robust with different imputations. For example, for dropouts, the FDA might ask for analysis that considers each dropout to be a failure (if there are more dropouts in the active group) or each dropout to be a treatment success (if there are more dropouts in the placebo group). In extreme cases, considering the dropouts in the active group to be failure and the dropouts in the placebo group to be success might be necessary.

15.4.3 Secondary Endpoints and Descriptive Analysis

The primary hypothesis in a clinical trial is a rather blunt one: for the group as a whole, does the drug work? While the soul of clinical trial medicine is to test a hypothesis, once it is proven, secondary and descriptive analyses become important and legitimate. These analyses add the color and detail that increase the utility of the study results.

Secondary endpoints, in a simplest definition, are all endpoints other than the primary endpoint. They might address a different measure, different subgroup, or different analytic method compared to the primary endpoint. Secondary endpoints, because they are not the primary endpoint, do not establish a firm causal link between the intervention and outcome in question.

Sometimes there are "tertiary endpoints" as well. Semantic differences aside, there are no formal differences between secondary and tertiary endpoints, other than the fact that investigators think that the tertiary endpoints have less clinical relevance than the secondary endpoints.

You can sometimes find both "primary efficacy endpoint" and "primary safety endpoint" in a trial. Statistically, there is usually only one true primary endpoint, and the efficacy is usually the one, unless the trial's main goal is to assess the safety or the trial is one of the rare studies that require both primary efficacy and safety endpoints to be met. The endpoint that drives the sample size should be the true primary endpoint.

For example, secondary endpoints and descriptive analysis may describe whether the benefit is evenly spread over the population such as the following:

- Who benefits? Who doesn't?
- Does the clinical benefit increase or decrease over time?
- Is the effect durable with continuous treatment, or after discontinuation?
- Does not the safety profile remain the same, improve, or deteriorate over time?

While analysis of secondary endpoints can be very helpful, they are often misused and overinterpreted. The greatest danger is multiple comparisons. Because there is no limit to the number of secondary endpoints, it is almost always possible to find "statistically significant" results for various secondary endpoints. If enough endpoints are examined, a spurious positive result can be found. Alternatively, an endpoint may suggest that the drug has a peculiarly poor efficacy on some endpoint when it actually doesn't, because when you do analysis on lots of different endpoints, it is always possible to identify some subgroup that appears to have an opposite outcome than the overall group.

One classic example of spurious findings due to multiple comparisons is the finding that patients who were Gemini or Libra had adverse effects from receiving aspirin in the ISIS-2 trial.[2]

The table below (Figure 15.30) illustrates the probability of at least one spurious statistically significant result ($p < 0.05$) given no true differences, if multiple subgroup analyses are performed:

The best way is to limit the number of secondary endpoints, and to prespecify them in the protocol. Prespecification both limits the number of analysis, and the type of analysis. Analyses that are not prespecified are most likely based on *post hoc* analysis that is constructed after the unblinding of the data. In other words, it is likely designed to be positive because the data is already unblended, and is often not a fair analysis.

Another alternative is to perform a global statistical test, before accepting any secondary endpoint. This is done by taking the whole set of proposed secondary analysis and performing a test for significance for the entire set. If the test results are $p < 0.05$, then the individual analyses are performed. This procedure is possible when the secondary analyses in question are all analogous and can be grouped together – for example, four different arms of a study can be tested to see if all four are equivalent with respect an

Number of tests	Probability
1	0.05
2	0.20
3	0.14
5	0.23
10	0.40
20	0.64

FIGURE 15.30 Probability of at least one spurious statistical result with multiple testing.

[2] ISIS-2 Collaborative Group Randomized trial of IV streptokinase, oral aspirin, both, or neither among 17, 187 cases of suspected acute myocardial infarction (1988). *Lancet*, **2**, 349–360.

endpoint, and if there is a difference, then each pair of arms can be analyzed separately.

Subgroup Analysis

Subgroup analysis is a type of secondary endpoint analysis based on taking a subset of patients in the study. It is an important analysis, and one that is particularly fraught with common misuses.

Baseline data collected in clinical trials are used for several different purposes. First, they are used to check that the randomization did indeed result in balanced groups across the treatment groups. Second, if there are significant imbalances, they can be used to adjust for the imbalances. Third, they can be used to examine whether the results are consistent across subgroups. Fourth, they can be used to examine the groups to determine whether there is a group that stands out and has a disproportionate effect compared to the rest of the study population.

Unfortunately, the fourth is often done when the overall study results are negative and there is extensive data mining to identify a subgroup that appears to have benefit. An example would be a study that the primary endpoint (e.g., FEV_1) is negative ($p = 0.15$), but the secondary endpoints (e.g., the number of exacerbations and mortality from asthma) is strongly significant ($p = 0.001$). **IF THE PRIMARY ENDPOINT IS NEGATIVE, EVEN STRONGLY POSITIVE SECONDARY ENDPOINTS SHOULD BE INTERPRETED WITH EXTREME CAUTION**. They are usually spurious.

The subgroup analysis is best used to determine whether there is a difference in response in the subgroup compared to the group at large, not whether there is a treatment effect in the subgroup or how the subgroup differs from another subgroup, unless the analysis is known to be well-powered. The way to do this is to perform an interaction test and see whether the subgroup exhibits a different effect than the overall study. This compares the results seen in the subgroup against the results seen in the overall study.

Subgroups can be defined in an infinite number of ways – essentially any characteristic that is different between patients such as age, sex, dose, etc. can be used. However, these, methods can all be grouped into three categories: baseline factors, treatment factors, and response factors. It is extremely important to distinguish among these three ways of dividing the population into subgroups because they have an enormous impact on the conclusions.

Baseline factors are factors that exist at the time of enrollment in the trial. Many of them are factors that are fixed such as sex, but some are not. These baseline factors are the most legitimate way of creating subgroups because they are unaffected by the treatment.

Some typical types of subgroups are:

- Demographics
  - Sex
  - Age
  - Geographic location
- By characteristics of the disease
  - Severity of disease
  - Disease subtypes (relapsing MS, progressive MS)
  - Length of disease
  - Refractoriness of the disease (steroid resistant, TNF inhibitor failures, etc.)
  - Frequency of relapses
  - Current flare (or absence of such)
- By prior medical treatments
  - Concomitant medications
  - Prior therapies
  - Prior failed therapies

The second type of factors is treatment factors. These are things that are done to the patients, either by the physician or because of the conduct of the study. These are factors that are normally beyond the control of the patients. They can affect outcome of the study, but should not be affected by the treatment in most cases. These are legitimate subgroups for many purposes, including sometimes inferring effect of treatment. For example, if patients who receive one manufacturing batch of the drug have a different outcome than the patients who receive another manufacturing batch, a reasonably strong conclusion regarding batches could be advanced. Some examples include:

- By study factors
  - Site of enrollment
  - Protocol violations
  - GCP violations
  - Number of doses
  - Manufacturing lots

The third and most dangerous type of factors is response factors. These are subgroups based on some effect that the drug has on the group, such as drug levels or pharmacodynamic measures. These are highly prone to confounding, and any conclusions drawn from them, such as correlation of a pharmacodynamic marker and outcome, should be interpreted with extreme caution. The interpretation of this type of subgroups will be further discussed in Chapter 16. Some of the response factors include the following:

- Pharmacokinetic
  - Drug levels
  - Metabolite levels
- Pharmacodynamic
  - Antibody titer
  - Integrin expression levels
  - IgE levels
- Clinical effects (that could be affected by treatment)
  - Presence of an adverse event (rash, nausea, etc.)
  - Dropouts
  - Number of missed doses (normally a treatment factor, but if compliance is affected by how well the drug works, can be a response factor as well)

– Response status (e.g., "average pain score among patients who responded")

The subgroups being examined should be prespecified at the beginning of the trial, and for important subgroups, they should have been stratified at randomization. Stratification allows for much stronger conclusions to be drawn, since the subgroups themselves are randomized.

Subendpoint Analysis

In some cases, composite endpoints are used as the primary endpoints. The issue in assessing the components of the primary composite endpoint (subendpoint analysis) is similar to that of the subgroup analysis in many ways. For example, the SF-36, a common measure of the quality of life (also called patient reported outcome) is composed of 36 different measures. The overall SF-36 can be a primary endpoint, and sometimes there is interest in examining each individual component separately.

As with subgroup analysis, if the overall SF-36 shows a significant difference, it is acceptable to examine the components separately. However, if the SF-36 does not show a significant difference, finding a difference in one or more of the components should not be interpreted to mean that there is indeed a difference.

With some composite endpoints, one of the components may be much more significant than another. For example, if the composite is death, ischemia, or revascularization, then it is important that death does not go in the opposite direction as the overall endpoint. Otherwise, even if there were a statistically significant benefit in the composite endpoint, the clinical benefit would be in doubt.

15.5 SPECIAL ANALYSIS

15.5.1 Crossover Study Analysis

In a crossover study, the first step in analysis is an interaction analysis to determine whether there is a difference between the two periods. If there is no difference, then the periods can be combined. Otherwise, only the first period can be used.

For example, let's consider a study where the first period group A receives placebo and group B receives active drug, and then in the second period group A receives active drug and group B receives placebo. The primary endpoint is reduction in the blood pressure. The first step is to determine whether the periods show an interaction. If there is not, then the group A period one data can be combined with group B period two and group A period two can be combined with group B period one.

15.5.2 Factorial Analysis

The first step in the factorial analysis is to look for interactions. If there is no interaction between the factors, the

Group PP	Group AP
Placebo anti-hypertensive	Active anti-hypertensive
Placebo anti-psoriatic	Placebo anti-psoriatic
Group PA	**Group AA**
Placebo anti-hypertensive	Active anti-hypertensive
Active anti-psoriatic	Active anti-psoriatic

FIGURE 15.31   Factorial design.

analysis is straightforward in that each factor is analyzed separately, ignoring the other factors.

If there is no interaction between the two treatments (if there is no synergy or dyssynergy between the anti-hypertensive and the anti-psoriatic), then for the analysis of the anti-hypertensive, PP + PA group would be compared to AP + AA group using standard analytic techniques, and for the anti-psoriatic, PP + AP group would be compared to PA + AA group (Fig. 15.31).

However, if there is an interaction, then the analysis must treat the study as a four-arm study, each group has to be compared against others, and the analysis can become quite complicated. What's more, the power of the study to detect a difference between the groups becomes much lower than anticipated, because the sample size decreases and the multiplicity comparisons may require smaller p-values to be met.

For example, a 2×2 factor study of ifosfamide and muramyl tripeptide where there was a strong interaction and the results were very difficult to interpret[3] (Figure 15.32):

Results (3-year event free survival rate).
  Neither drug: 71%
  Muramyl tripeptide: 68%
  Ifosfamide: 61%
  Ifosfamide and muramyl tripeptide: 78%

The addition of muramyl tripeptide alone seemed to have only little effect on survival, while ifosfamide seemed to decrease survival. However, adding both seemed to improve survival.

Study Groups	
Neither drug	Ifosfamide
Muramyl tripeptide	Ifosfamide and muramyl tripeptide

FIGURE 15.32   Factorial design.

---

[3] Meyers, P.A. *et al.* (2005). *Journal of Clinical Oncology*, **23**(9), 2004–2011.

15.5.3 Pharmacokinetics, Pharmacodynamics, and Dose Analyses

Analysis of pharmacokinetics (PK) and pharmacodynamics (PD) data is one area of clinical trial medicine that can be very different from the rest of the field. While most of clinical trial medicine relies on inferential reasoning (conclusions are based on statistical tests and *p*-values), much of PK and PD analyses are much more akin to traditional scientific endeavors using deductive reasoning. The output of PK and PD analyses are usually not conclusions of statistical difference among treatment groups but rather estimates of area under curve (AUC), half-life, etc. that are calculated rather than inferred. For example, in most PK studies, there is no placebo treatment arm against which the results are compared. It doesn't make much sense to compare AUC from the treatment and placebo groups.

There are exceptions of course. In some cases, PK and PD may be compared across groups of patients with renal impairment, hepatic impairment, or other changes in excretion. And in bioequivalence studies, the confidence intervals are compared between two treatment arms as discussed below.

Typically, the first step in PK analysis is to take the raw data and create a mathematical model from it. This is because PK is the science of change in drug levels across time. A single data point in and of itself does not give much information. The data points must be linked across time in order to yield useful information. The technique for linking the information across time is a model. A PK model is a mathematical equation that describes the relationship between drug levels and time. In many cases, there are other variables in the model such as age and renal clearance that also affect the relationship between drug levels and time.

Some of the methods in constructing a PK model have been addressed in Section 10.8.2 of Chapter 10. Briefly, the PK data is collected, a mathematical model that fits the data is constructed, and if possible, the model is validated by comparing the drug levels that the model predicts with additional data points that were not part of the dataset used to construct the model.

With a traditional PK dataset, where multiple samples are taken from each patient, the creation of the model is relatively straightforward. The specifics of model construction are beyond the scope of this book.

With a population PK approach, where multiple semi-random samples are taken from the patients in a sparse manner, the modeling is a bit more complicated because the missing data points need to be extrapolated. Therefore, the results of the modeling are more dependent on subjective or arbitrary assumptions. However, modern modeling techniques are very sophisticated, and take into account both variabilities across patients as well as within patients and are usually reliable. Also, this approach can be very helpful in that data from hundreds of patients can be collected, rather than from tens of patients as for traditional PK studies.

Other Analysis

In addition to the AUC, half-life, and other parameters, analysis of the PK and PD data should yield information about heterogeneity or homogeneity of the drug-PK response. For example, identification of subgroups that have different PK/PD effects is important. Factors that influence PK/PD parameters such as fed/fasting state, interactions with other drugs P450 metabolism should all be identified.

Characterization of the dose response curve with minimally effective and maximally tolerated doses being identified, is also important in many instances, although it is not always practicable to do so.

15.5.4 Bioequivalence

Bioequivalence studies are special type of studies where two drugs or two sets of formulation of the same drug are compared to show that they have nearly equal bioavailability and PK/PD parameters. These studies are often done for generic drugs or when a formulation of a drug is changed during development.

Typically, what is needed to demonstrate equivalence from regulatory viewpoint is to show that the experimental drug's PK profile falls within 20% of the reference drug. The 20% is an arbitrary number, but is satisfactory for the majority of drugs. In some cases, for drugs with a narrow therapeutic index such as warfarin, 20% may be too large.

Practically, what this means is that the upper limit of 95% confidence interval for the experimental drug must fall below 125% of the reference drug and the lower limit must fall above 80% of the reference drug. A value of 125% is used because the difference between 125 and 100 is 20% if one uses 125 as the denominator. Confidence interval is used because it is important that the drug is less than 20% different. If point estimate is used without confidence intervals, then a drug with very wide variability that on average is within 20% of the reference drug but quite often falls outside of that could be considered to be equivalent.

15.5.5 Equivalence and Noninferiority Studies

Interpretation of equivalence and noninferiority studies is based on the confidence intervals. The upper and lower ranges of confidence intervals must meet the prespecified criteria. The specific criteria are dependent on convention, the clinical study in question, and negotiation with the regulatory agency. Below are some examples:

- Bioequivalence studies require +/−20%.
- Noninferiority studies often require that experimental arm retains at least 50% of the benefit of the reference arm.
- Equivalence studies can require that the experimental arm retain at least 90% of the benefit of the reference arm.

15.5.6 Regression Discontinuity Analysis

As mentioned previously, patients can be assigned without randomization (Figure 15.33). One example is assignment of patients based on the intended outcome measure. For example, patients with severe lupus flare with glomerular filtration rate (GFR) below 30 can all be assigned to treatment and patients with GFR above 30 can be assigned to control. Regression discontinuity analysis can be used

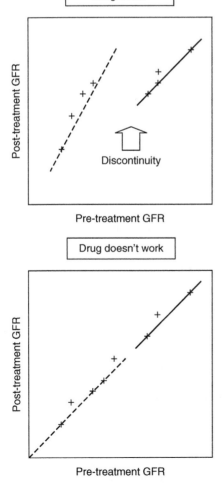

FIGURE 15.33 Regression discontinually analysis.

to analyze results of such randomization. By analyzing whether the regression line for the pre- and post-treatment values is discontinuous, it is possible to determine whether or not the drug is effective in the treated group. Counterintuitively, this type of analysis is not affected by regression to the mean or effect of the severity of the disease on outcome.

This analysis is based on modeling and has the inherent flaws of all modeling techniques.

15.6 ANALYSIS OF SAFETY DATA

15.6.1 Definition of Adverse Event

Let's start with the definition of an adverse event. The standard definition, which comes from "Reviewer Guidance: Conducting a Clinical Safety Review of a New Product Application and Preparing a Report on the Review," (http://www.fda.gov/CDER/GUIDANCE/3580fnl.htm) is as follows:

the term *adverse reaction* is used to refer to an undesirable effect, reasonably associated with the use of a drug that may occur as part of the pharmacological action of the drug or may be unpredictable in its occurrence. This term does not include all adverse events observed during use of a drug, only those for which there is some basis to believe there is a causal relationship between the drug and the occurrence of the adverse event. The term *adverse event* is used here to refer to any untoward medical event associated with the use of a drug in humans, whether or not it is considered drug-related. The phrases *serious adverse drug experience* and *serious adverse event* are used in this guidance to refer to any event occurring at any dose, whether or not considered drug-related, that results in any of the following outcomes:

- Death
- A life-threatening adverse experience
- Inpatient hospitalization or prolongation of existing hospitalization
- A persistent or significant disability/incapacity
- A congenital anomaly or birth defect.

Important medical events that may not result in death, life-threatening, or requiring hospitalization may be considered serious adverse drug events when, based on appropriate medical judgment, they may jeopardize the patient or subject who may require medical or surgical intervention to prevent one of the outcomes listed in this definition. Examples of such medical events include allergic bronchospasm requiring intensive treatment in an emergency room or at home, blood dyscrasias or convulsions that do not result in inpatient hospitalization, or the development of drug dependency or drug abuse. Documents developed by the International Conference on Harmonization (e.g., E2) add to serious events, which prolong hospitalization but do not include cancer and overdose.

Finally, the term *adverse dropout* is used in this guidance to refer to subjects who do not complete the study because of an adverse event, whether or not considered drug-related; adverse dropouts include subjects who receive the test drug, reference drugs, or placebo.

15.6.2 Limitations of Safety Analysis

As previously mentioned, most clinical studies are designed to test a hypothesis about an efficacy endpoint, not a safety endpoint. This presents several challenges.

First, this means that clinical trials are often not powered to detect safety events. For instance, a trial with 300 patients may be sufficiently large to detect whether a TNF inhibitor will improve signs and symptoms of rheumatoid arthritis, if the ACR20 response is 20% in the placebo arm and 70% in the active arm. However, it will not be sufficiently powered to detect a change in lymphoma rates if it is 0.5% in the placebo arm and 1% in the active arm.

Second, the safety endpoints are not defined in advance. There might only rarely be specific targeted adverse events clearly defined in advance, with clear pre-specifications on which will be considered to be an event, how the severity will be classified, and with clear provisions for consistent elicitation of the adverse event across various sites. This is usually the exception. Because it is extremely difficult to predict all possible adverse events, there is no way to prespecify in advance even if this is the goal of the study.

Furthermore, because adverse event endpoints are not generally predefined, they will generally not qualify for statistical hypothesis-testing. Therefore, most safety analyses will be exploratory. However, as will be discussed in the next chapter, the standard of proof for safety events is generally not statistical significance – even nonsignificant signals must often be considered seriously.

15.6.3 Goals of Safety Analysis

Similar to PK analysis, the goal of the safety analysis is not just to answer the question, "Do we see a safety problem," but rather to also answer:

- What kinds of events do we see?
- How severe are the events?
- How frequent are the events?
- How certain are we of the estimates of frequency and severity of the adverse events?
- Are they predictable, reversible; do they occur in certain subpopulations?
- How much power must we have to detect rare events, or even relatively common ones?

At the end of a clinical trial, or even at the end of a clinical development program, it will rarely be possible to have enough patients exposed to the drug to get a precise estimate of the safety of the drug. Therefore, safety analysis will usually last into the post-marketing period, long after the regulatory agency has approved the drug. Analysis of uncontrolled postmarketing data presents challenges associated with all uncontrolled data. Some of the issues with safety analysis of post-marketing data are as follows:

- Incomplete data – not all data will be collected, especially in the postmarketing setting.
- Unknown denominator – it is usually not possible to know for sure how many patients have been treated.
- No comparator – it is not possible to determine exactly what the comparator group should be, and how to adjust for the differences in demographic and disease characteristics.

Most analyses of safety are descriptive with certain limitations mentioned earlier. Nonetheless, it is possible to generate nominal p-values and confidence intervals for safety data across groups of patients and treatments, and these can be useful in interpretation of the data.

15.6.4 Classification of Adverse Events

Conventionally, adverse events can be divided into two types, Type A and Type B. Type A adverse events are due to a result of pharmacological action of the drug and are more predictable, common, and dose-dependent. Rash with EGFR inhibitors would be an example of Type A adverse events. Type B adverse events are idiosyncratic, not dose-dependent, and rare.[4] Examples of Type B adverse events are granulocytopenia seen with many drugs or progressive multifocal leukoencephalopathy (PML) seen with Tysabri.

Categorizations of Adverse Events

As previously mentioned, safety endpoints are not prespecified. Because of this, one of the most important aspects of analyzing safety data is to decide how to categorize the safety events. Safety signals can be missed if they are not categorized appropriately. To put it another way, safety signals may not be evident unless they are categorized into appropriate buckets.

Categorizing into Appropriate Disease Categories

In many cases, an adverse event can be considered to be in one of several groups. For example, urticaria can be a dermatological event or an allergic event. As another example, PML may be considered to be an infection or as a neurological disease.

In an effort to introduce standards into how adverse events are categorized, several dictionaries have been

---

[4] Rawlins, M.D., Thomson, J.W. (1981). Pathogenesis of adverse reactions. In Davis, D.M. (ed.), *Textbook of Adverse Drug Reactions*. Oxford University Press, Oxford.

developed by various organizations, including the World Health Organization. The dictionaries allow adverse events to be mapped or translated into standard terms, which allows analysis, display, and communication of the adverse events in a more standardized fashion.

At present, the dominant dictionary is the Medical Dictionary for Regulatory Activities (MedDRA) developed by the International Conference on Harmonization. Adverse event reporting to regulatory agencies must now be in the MedDRA format. Below is an example of MedDRA codes Figure 15.34.

Treatment Emergent vs. Nontreatment Emergent

Treatment emergent means that the adverse event does not exist at baseline, but occurs during treatment. In most cases, determination of treatment emergent vs. treatment not emergent is straightforward, but in several cases, it can be open to interpretation. Some examples are as follows:

- Patient had joint pain in one hand at beginning of study and it becomes more painful.
- Patient had joint pain in one hand at beginning of the study and it spreads to the other hand.
- Patient had joint pain at beginning of the study. It resolves during the study, and then recurs late in the study.
- Patient had joint pain on screening, the pain resolves by randomization, and then recurs during the study.

The best course of action is to predefine how these types of events will be handled, and be consistent in how they are categorized.

Counting the Number of Events

Once again, in most cases, it is not difficult to count the number of adverse events, but there are instances where it is open to interpretation, such as the following:

- Patient develops pain in one hand during the study, and while it is resolving, develops pain in the other hand.
- Patient suffers an MI requiring a hospitalization, and while in the hospital, has an arrhythmia and reinfarcts.
- Patient has an asthma exacerbation requiring steroid use, and before he finishes the steroid taper, contracts an upper respiratory infection and has a second exacerbation requiring steroids.

Once again, the key is to be consistent in how the events are counted.

Categorizing into Appropriate Scale

If the categories are too broad or too narrow, a signal may be lost. For example, a drug that causes bleeding may not be recognized as such if the hematoma, epistaxis, stroke, and anemia are not categorized together because within each group, the signal may not be evident but becomes evident when grouped together (Figure 15.35).

Categorizing into Appropriate Time Scale

Some safety events might occur only at certain periods of time. For example, an EGFR antagonist might cause

Adverse events category	AE/supra-ordinate term	MedDRA preferred term	MedDRA code
Allergy/immunology	Allergic reaction/hypersensitivity (including drug fever)	Hypersensitivity NOS	10020755
Allergy/immunology	Allergic rhinitis (including sneezing, nasal stuffiness, postnasal drip)	Rhinitis allergic NOS	10039087
Allergy/immunology	Allergy/immunology – other (Specify, __)	Not available	90004000
Allergy/immunology	Autoimmune reaction	Autoimmune disorder NOS	10003815
Allergy/immunology	Serum sickness	Serum sickness	10040400
Allergy/immunology	Vasculitis	Vasculitis NOS	10047128
Auditory/ear	Auditory/ear–other (Specify, __)	Not available	90004002
Auditory/ear	Hearing: patients with/without baseline audiogram and enrolled in a monitoring program	Hearing disability	10053491
Auditory/ear	Hearing: patients without baseline audiogram and not enrolled in a monitoring program	Hearing impaired	10019245

FIGURE 15.34 Example of MedDRA codes.

	Hematoma (%)	Epistaxis (%)	Stroke (%)	Anemia (%)	Any (%)
Placebo	2.1	1	0.2	6	8.6
Drug	2.9	1.4	0.8	8.2	11.2

FIGURE 15.35 Safety signal by grouping.

pulmonary adverse events only at the beginning of treatment. If the adverse event rates are examined only at 6 and 12 months or over the study as a whole, the signal might be missed.

Classification of Severity

We have already discussed the difference between serious adverse events and nonserious adverse events. These are regulatory classifications used for the purpose of reporting adverse events to regulatory authorities.

In addition, the most common way of grading the severity of adverse events is the National Cancer Institute's Common Terminology Criteria for Adverse Events (CTCAE). This is a system of grading the severity of adverse events from 1 to 5, originally developed for oncology trials. It is fairly comprehensive and is often used for non-oncology trials, especially in the evaluation of laboratory abnormalities. It is reproduced in Appendix D.

Relatedness

Adverse events collected in a clinical trial are graded on relatedness by the investigator and by the sponsor. They are classified into:

- Not related
- Unlikely to be related
- Possibly related
- Probably related
- Definitely related

Expectedness

Adverse events that are noted in the Investigators Brochure or in the package inserts are considered to be expected. Others are considered to be unexpected.

15.6.5 Descriptive Analysis of Safety Data

As previously described, the safety data analysis is descriptive, aims at ascertaining the adequacy of the dataset and collection/classification methodology. In general, the analysis proceeds in the following order.

First, the size of the database, the adequacy of exposure, and the methodology of data collection are assessed.

This is followed by assessment of deaths. The number of deaths, the causality of deaths, and the methodology of including or excluding the deaths in the database are assessed.

In particular, the impact of dropouts or patients lost to follow-up should be assessed. Both the crude mortality, as well as the exposure-adjusted mortality should be assessed. The exposure (the number of patients and duration of exposure) for the patients on active therapy usually is much greater than placebo, if the data from uncontrolled studies and open-label follow-up studies are included. Because of this, two sets of analysis should be done: one with only the placebo controlled data and one with the totality of all the patients (Figure 15.36).

Typically, every death narrative should be examined individually.

This should be followed by assessment of serious adverse events. The assessment of these events conducted in a manner similar to the assessment of deaths, but in addition, sequelae such as whether the event resolved and if so after how long, whether there was permanent disability or death, etc. should be examined.

This should be followed by assessment of dropouts, including the pattern of dropouts, the reason for the dropouts, and the proportion of dropouts across the various arms (Figure 15.37).

This should be followed by adverse events of interest. For example, for immunosuppressive drugs, infections should be examined closely. For thrombolytics, bleeding

	Number of deaths	Number of patients	Crude mortality	Patient-years of exposure	Mortality per 100 patient-years
Placebo					
Active					

FIGURE 15.36   Format of safety listing: death.

	Total dropout (%)	Adverse event (%)	Lost to follow-up (%)	Lack of efficacy (%)	Other (%)
Placebo	N	N	N	N	N
Active	N	N	N	N	N

FIGURE 15.37   Sample of disposition listing.

Placebo				Active		
	Shift normal to low (%)	Normal (including high to normal and low to normal) (%)	Shift normal to high (%)	Shift normal to low (%)	Normal (including high to normal and low to normal) (%)	Shift normal to high (%)
Albumin	N	N	N	N	N	N
Alk Pho	N	N	N	N	N	N
Etc.	N	N	N	N	N	N

FIGURE 15.38   Sample shift table.

	Placebo baseline	Placebo mean change	Active baseline	Active mean change
Albumin	Value	%	Value	%
Alk Phos	Value	%	Value	%
Etc.	Value	%	Value	%

FIGURE 15.39   Sample laboratory listing.

should be examined. Other targeted adverse events should also be assessed.

Next, the most common adverse events should be examined. In particular, those events that could be a harbinger for related but more serious events (e.g., gum bleeding and stroke) should be assessed carefully.

Next, the laboratory parameters should be assessed. Laboratory values can come from a core laboratory where all the samples are processed at the same laboratory with the same normal ranges and reproducible values. In other cases, the laboratory samples are processed at local laboratories where the range of normal values will differ slightly from the site to the site. In the latter case, the normal ranges need to be programmed into the database for each site.

The analysis of the laboratory is traditionally done with shift tables (Figure 15.38).

In some cases, analyzing the patients who have two or more simultaneous changes, such as bilirubin and SGPT, may be useful in identifying potential issues. In other cases, displaying the cumulative incidence of abnormal laboratory values may be helpful.

In addition to the shift tables, the changes in mean and median values from baseline to post-treatment values should be examined (Figure 15.39). This can reveal a trend, such as an increase in blood sugars or a decrease in the renal clearance that may be significant on its own, or portend potential problems that may affect some patients that experience an extreme case of the phenomenon. Below is a sample table. Mean change can be expressed as percent change, often based on the greatest change for each patient.

Some Common Adverse Events

Below is a list of some of the more common adverse events and classes of drugs often associated with them:[5]

- Hepatotoxicity (NSAIDs, thiazolidinedione PPAR gamma agonists)
- Pancreatic toxicity
- QT prolongation (any anti-arrhythmic, anti-psychotic, anti-histamine, fluoroquinolone)
- Vasodilator effects, such as hypotension (alpha blockers) or edema (dihydropyridine calcium channel blockers)
- Withdrawal effects (beta blockers, central alpha agonists, SSRI's, narcotics)
- Orthostatic hypotension (any anti-hypertensive, anti-psychotics)
- Hypertension (any sympathomimetic or phosphodiesterase inhibitor)
- Tachycardia
- Neutropenia (drugs related to ticlopidine, procainamide, clozapine)
- Bleeding (drugs inhibiting any aspect of clotting or platelet function, NSAID's)
- Aplastic anemia
- Increased coagulation times
- Muscle injury (any HMG CoA reductase inhibitor [statin] or other lipid-lowering drug)
- Sedation (any psychotropic drug)
- CNS stimulation

---

[5] http://www.fda.gov/CDER/GUIDANCE/3580fnl.htm.

- Anti-cholinergic activity
- Allergic reactions
- Sexual dysfunction (any anti-depressant, sedating drug)
- Elevated intraocular pressure
- Cataracts
- Retinopathy
- Worsening glucose tolerance/diabetes (diuretics, atypical anti-psychotics)
- Pro-arrhythmic effects and increased mortality (most non-beta blocker anti-rrhythmics)
- Increased CHF and SD mortality (any inotrope, some negative inotropes such as calcium channel blockers)
- Nephropathy (NSAIDs)

Analysis of Individual Level Data

One instance where individual level data is very important is adverse events. Sometimes it is important to go through all the details of an individual adverse event report and narrative to understand all the possibilities regarding the pathogenesis of the event and the magnitude of it. This is partially because the threshold for taking action on a safety issue is much lower than for efficacy. For example, if two out of four patients develop a very severe infection in response to a drug, then it might be sufficient to justify warning physicians about the drug. If two out of three patients have an unusually good efficacy this would not typically suffice to trigger a recommendation regarding efficacy.

15.7 INTERIM ANALYSIS

Interim analysis discussed in this section concerns classical interim analysis, usually performed to test for futility, safety, and/or efficacy. Interim analysis performed as part of a group sequential design, Bayesian study design, and adaptive/flexible study designs are discussed in another chapter.

Classical interim analyses are performed by an independent statistician who should be a person other than the regular study statistician, and who should not communicate the results to the sponsor or any of the personnel involved in conducting the trial. The results should go only to the independent data monitoring board, unless the interim analysis is being performed for administrative reasons such as initiating another study on basis of the interim results.

There are several analytic techniques for performing interim analysis (Figure 15.40). The most conventional way is to have a predetermined number of interim analyses and prespecified timing for them. This is called *Repeated Significance Tests*. It essentially means that part of the alpha is spent (or allocated) to the interim analysis, so that at the end of the study, the combined alpha of the interim analysis plus the final analysis do not exceed 0.05. The three most commonly used techniques are Pocock, Haybittle/Peto, and O'Brien/Fleming. The differences among the three

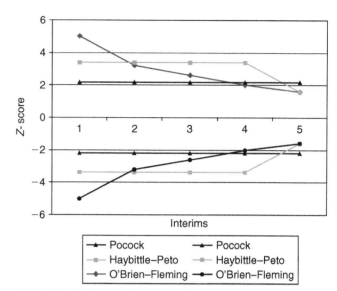

FIGURE 15.40　Statistical boundaries for interim analysis.

techniques mostly concern how much of the alpha is spent and when.

With the O'Brien/Fleming method, the statistical penalty (hit) is not as great at the beginning of the study. In other words, at the early interim analysis, the results have to be extremely compelling in order to trigger termination of the study. With each subsequent analysis, the boundaries become lower and lower.

A more flexible methodology is that of Lans/Demets which allows flexible timing and number of analysis, called alpha-spending function. This is usually not used in classical interim analysis. The most flexible approach is that by Wald, called Boundaries Approach, which allows for selection between two alternative hypotheses on the basis of the interim looks. This is not typically used in classical interim analysis either.

15.8 ADJUSTING FOR COVARIATES

Whenever there are imbalances in the baseline demographics between the treatment groups, or in the treatment factors such as trial site, there is a possibility that covariates might have biased the results. It is then possible to adjust for the potential bias by adjusting the results to take into account the imbalances. This is typically done by adding covariates to the model being used to test for statistical significance. Many of the statistical techniques, such as ANCOVA or Cox regression, will allow for adjustments, although not all will.

There is quite a bit of controversy regarding whether it is better to either minimize bias by stratification during randomization or correct the bias by adjusting the results after the fact. Our personal preference is to stratify as much as possible, because adjustment of the results can in and of itself introduce biases.

One of the most common adjustments is for imbalances in baseline characteristics. For example, age might be a strong predictor of outcome in many types of diseases. If the placebo arm enrolled patients with an average age of 60 and active arm enrolled patients with an average age of 65, then there might be a bias in the results purely due to the difference in age.

Adjustment for baseline imbalances is very controversial. In fact, the European Medicine Agency (EMEA) "Points to Consider on Adjustment for Baseline Covariates" flatly rejects it. In theory, proper randomization should make it unnecessary to adjust for baseline covariate. However, in fact, there is often an imbalance, because if sufficient numbers of baseline characteristics are collected, there is likely to be one or more imbalances.

On the other hand, if adjustments will be made, there are certain items that should normally be included in the model. Any variable considered to be important enough stratify on should be included. For diseases with baseline severity that can influence the outcome measures, such as such as Psoriasis Area and Severity Index scores for psoriasis or pulmonary function test values, baseline severity should be included in the model. If there are strong prognostic factors identified in the past from previous studies that should be included in the model as well.

In any case, it is extremely important to prespecify the covariates at the beginning of the study and at the latest before unblinding of the study. Covariates should *not* be selected after the unblinding. Also, response variables such as PK or compliance that can be affected by the intervention or treatment should not be included in the model.

As a general rule, it is very rare that adjustment for covariates changes the outcome of a study materially. We usually recommend avoiding adjustments and instead relying on thoughtful stratification.

Chapter 16

Data Interpretation and Conclusions

16.1 INTERPRETING DATA

16.1.1 Overview

After the data has been cleaned and the analysis completed, the data must then be interpreted. Interpretation is the process of taking the data and asking the question, "So what do these results mean?" Interpretation proceeds in two steps. The first step is study interpretation, or the process of figuring out what the results tell us about the drug's effectiveness within the trial. The second is external extrapolation, or the process of taking the study results and extrapolating them to the patient population at large, to patients who were not entered in the trial. It is the process of reaching conclusions about how the therapy should or should not be used for patients in clinical practice. If you recall, the process of clinical trial design proceeds as follows:

General medical question → Study hypothesis and study design → Study execution → Data

The process of clinical data interpretation recapitulates the process in reverse:

Data → Data analysis → Study interpretation → External extrapolation

We will discuss the last two steps in this chapter.

Study interpretation is the process of taking the data and the various statistical outputs from data analysis (discussed in the Chapter 15) and asking the question, "Does the data refute the null hypothesis?" It is the process of determining whether the intervention had a causal effect on outcome: in other words, whether the primary endpoint was met. If the intervention can be shown to have a causal effect on outcome, the study is said to have achieved *internal validity*. In addition, interpretation involves determining answers to secondary endpoints, and gleaning additional information about the results of the study.

After establishing internal validity, the next step is to draw conclusions, or to extrapolate the results of the study to the patient population at large. As was stated previously, clinical trial medicine is not a branch of aesthetics; it is a practical endeavor with the final outcome being change in clinical practice. Ultimately, the goal of a clinical trial is to be able to generalize the results of the study to the patient population as whole. The patients in a clinical trial are a subset (sample) of the patient population as a whole. The results of the study must be applicable to the patient population at large. If they are applicable, then the study is said to have *external validity*.

To put it another way, if the study shows that the intervention had an effect on the primary endpoint, among the *sample* of patients in the study, it has internal validity. If the study design, conduct, and results are such that the results can be extrapolated to the *population* from which the sample has been drawn, then the study is said to have external validity.

The processes of study interpretations and external extrapolation are highly dependent on the quality of the preceding steps. Faulty study design, sloppy execution, erroneous data analysis can all have a highly detrimental effect on the last steps. No matter how well the preceding steps are performed, however, there will always be flaws in those steps. Therefore, part of data interpretation to recognize and flag those flaws and to determine what impact they have on the interpretations and conclusions, as well as to determine whether there are ways to correct or ameliorate the flaws.

In addition, there are often ancillary questions that are part of data interpretation. These include questions such as, "If the study was negative, why was it negative?" and, "What does the data tell us about the next study to conduct?"

Steps in Interpretation

In general, study interpretation proceeds as follows.

First, descriptive assessment is performed. Typically, demographic data such as type of disease, length of disease, race, sex, age, etc. are assessed. Baseline characteristics are examined to understand the types of patients who were enrolled, and to assess whether there are notable differences in the characteristics of the patients who were randomized into the different arms. However, it is not appropriate to test demographic differences for statistical significance, since this is largely meaningless. The differences in demographics, if randomization was performed correctly, are due to chance, unless the randomization was not correctly done, so no matter how small the *p*-value, the *p*-value means nothing.

There are some descriptive assessments that can make an enormous difference in the interpretation of the study. One of them is assessment of protocol adherence. You want to make sure, for example, that the patients had the disease of the type and severity that the study was designed for. You want to make sure that the diagnosis was correct, that the appropriate tests and imaging was done as per-protocol, so that you can assure yourself and others that the appropriate patients were enrolled. Enrolling the appropriate patients is not a straightforward proposition. In many studies, many investigators enroll patients who are not eligible, or who do not have documentation that they have the disease. Making sure that the patients meet the inclusion and exclusion criteria is a critical part of study interpretation.

You also want to make sure that the patients received the drug, and received the drug at the right doses at the right times. You also should check that the assessments of drug effect, especially the primary endpoint assessments, were conducted at the right times. You should also check that the appropriate validation and calibrations were performed on the instruments, and that the study personnel were trained and certified appropriately. In short, you should verify that the patients were the appropriate patients; that they were treated and assessed properly; and that there is appropriate documentation to that effect.

Finally, you should verify that the appropriate laws and regulations were followed. For example, it is extremely important to verify that informed consents were obtained properly, for it would be unethical to use the data otherwise.

Efficacy is assessed next. The following sections explore this in detail, but briefly,

1. The *p*-value is assessed.
2. The threats to internal validity is assessed to determine if there are factors that will invalidate the *p*–value.
3. Secondary endpoints are assessed.
4. Exploratory endpoints and descriptive data is assessed.

Effectiveness, or external validity, is assessed next. This is an assessment of whether and how relevant the results are to the patient population at large.

Safety is assessed next. Finally, risk/benefit is assessed.

16.1.2 Testing Robustness

As a general rule, it is good practice to "pressure-test" the results of the study for robustness. Certainly, regulatory agencies such as Food and Drug Administration (FDA) will typically perform these pressure-tests. These tests examine the data to detect for anomalies that might suggest underlying problems with the design, conduct, or interpretation of the study.

One of the most important assessments is to examine missing data and missing patients and to determine whether there is a pattern in the missing data; whether the quantity of the data is so large that it threatens the validity of the study; and so on. Another typical assessment is to examine thoroughly the baseline demographics to determine whether there are baseline imbalances. There will always be some imbalances, but it is rare that it is significant enough to affect results. What you will be looking for are signs that randomization was performed incorrectly or in a biased fashion.

Subgroup analysis is also often performed, to determine whether there are certain groups of patients to whom the study results may not be applicable, or whether there might be a problem with the study. The subgroups typically include those with certain sex, age, geography, and sites, but may also include patients who were enrolled in the first half of the study vs. in the second half, or with one manufacturing lot of the drug vs. another, and so on.

Although this type of pressure testing is in essence a fishing expedition, the insights gained from it can uncover significant real issues.

16.1.3 Validation

If the endpoints in the study are not well established and well validated, they must be validated in the study. One of the first steps in interpretation of the results should be examination of the validation data to insure that the measures are reliable, reproducible, and valid.

16.2 THREATS TO INTERNAL VALIDITY IN WELL-CONTROLLED STUDIES

16.2.1 Avoiding Inappropriate Use of *p*-Value

At first glance, assessment of internal validity might appear simple:

> Look at the *p*-value. If it is less than 0.05, then the study is positive and internal validity has been achieved. Otherwise, it has not.

In an ideal world, for a randomized prospective controlled trial, the primary efficacy analysis would indeed be straightforward. Good study design will have insured that the endpoint is clear. Conduct of the trial will have been such that the data is reliable. Patients would have been enrolled appropriately. Compliance to the protocol has been good. In such a case, it is simply a matter of determining whether the study met its primary endpoint.

Certainly, it is tempting to close the book once the p-value is calculated and it is less than 0.05, and declare victory. After all, if the p-value is not less than 0.05, we always close the book and declare defeat. Unfortunately, things are never quite that simple. There are many instances where the p-value <0.05 does not translate into a positive study. There are many instances when the study, study conduct, or external factors conspire to turn even a "significant p-value" into a negative result.

The first common mistake is multiple comparisons. Please remember that there can be *only one primary endpoint* (except in specific instances where hierarchical testing is used or the alpha is divided), and *it must be declared in advance.* You cannot take a host of endpoints at the end of a study, perform statistical tests on them, and select the one that looks the best. This prohibition sounds simple but in practice, many people fail to follow it. Here is a typical example:

A study in COPD patients is performed, with hospitalizations as the primary endpoint. Unfortunately, clinical practice guidelines for COPD change in the middle of the study, and the number of hospitalizations is much lower than expected. The study therefore becomes underpowered, and while there is 25% reduction in hospitalization, the p-value is 0.08. However, it turns out that the mortality in the treated group is markedly lower than the placebo group, with 70% reduction in the mortality rate and p-value of 0.002. Not only that, but also in the patients who received the full course of the drug, the reduction in mortality is 90% and the p-value is 0.00001.

There is only one acceptable interpretation of the above example: the study results are negative. Full stop. The issue is that if you look hard enough, you can find endpoints with p-values of 0.05 or less in any failed study. You cannot scrounge for favorable endpoint and thereby rescue a failed study. The p-value has meaning only for the primary endpoint. Unfortunately, it would not be uncommon for the investigator with results like the above would declare that the drug has an effect.

Don't confuse nominal p-values with p-values. The p-values can be calculated for any comparison, but unless they are for the pre-specified primary endpoint they are *nominal p-values.* (The only exceptions are for special hierarchical or split alpha that is discussed earlier in the book and see below as well.) Nominal p-values cannot lead to causal conclusions. Any p-value that has not been pre-specified is a nominal p-value. It is a common mistake to perform multiple comparisons, and multiple *ad hoc* analyses, and to make the mistake of assuming a relationship when the correlation is by chance. This is particularly the case when the relationship makes intuitive sense, and the human tendency is to look for causality in those cases.

For studies with hierarchical primary endpoints (contingent primary endpoints), the first primary endpoint must be positive before the others can be tested. If the first endpoint is negative, all subsequent primary endpoints are, by definition, negative. If the second endpoint is negative, all subsequent primary endpoints are negative, and so on. For studies that have allocated alpha to multiple primary endpoints, the p-value for the endpoint meet the reduced alpha value assigned to it. For example, if a study allocates alpha of 0.01 to mortality and 0.04 to relapse rate, then mortality difference that yields a p-value of 0.02 would not be significant even though it is smaller than 0.05.

In a study with a traditional single primary endpoint, that endpoint must achieve a p-value of 0.05 less before other endpoints are tested. If the primary endpoint is met, then the secondary and tertiary endpoints can be tested in a meaningful way.

The other common misconception about p-values is that smaller the p-value, greater the magnitude of the treatment effect. This is erroneous. Here is an example:

Two companies are neck and neck in racing to develop a therapy for a congenital storage disease. Their drugs are nearly identical, but when the two companies announce their Phase II results nearly simultaneously, the results appear quite different.

- The first company announces a successful study with p = 0.0001.
- The second announces a successful study with p = 0.04.

What happened? Did the second company make a mistake in their trial design? Is the first company's drug more likely to work?

No, the drugs worked similarly, and to a similar magnitude in the two studies. However, the first company's studies had 300 patients, the second had 80. The p-values reflect two things: how well the drug works and how large the sample size is.

Impressive p-values don't necessarily mean that a drug works better, if the studies are not equivalent in design and size.

In other words, smaller p-values can come from either the drug working very well or from having a large number of patients in the study. You should not confuse the two.

Finally, remember when not to rely on p-values. It is appropriate to require p-value of less than 0.05 when the objective is to establish efficacy for a new therapy. It is not appropriate to require a p-value of 0.05 when assessing safety signals. The bar for safety should be much lower. Even a p-value of 0.5 may be meaningful if the consequences of risk are great enough. For example, if you are studying a drug for asthma, and there is an imbalance in the rate of heart attacks, you should take the signal very seriously even if the p-value is not even close to 0.05. You are weighing a non-life saving benefit against a life-threatening adverse event. The two are not equivalent. Waiting until *p*-value becomes significant may result in tremendous, irreparable harm being done. You wouldn't wait until there was 95% chance of a fire before taking out fire insurance, and nor should you wait until you're 95% sure there is a safety issue before taking action.

Inappropriate Interpretation of Negative p-Values

Nearly as bad as overinterpretation is underinterpretation. Absence of proof is not proof of absence. A negative study does not prove that the drug does not work. If a drug does not work, it may produce a negative study result, but there are other reasons for why a study may be negative. A study can be negative for the following reasons.

- Drug doesn't work.
- Study design is faulty. It used wrong dosing, wrong patient population, etc.
- The study is underpowered.
- You had Random bad luck.

Wrong study designs can often torpedo a study. For example, inhaled nasal steroids take several days to take effect. If the endpoint is to measure 10 minutes after administration, the drug will not show an effect even if it is effective. Many studies are underpowered for primary endpoint, and almost all are underpowered for some secondary endpoints, especially safety endpoints. A negative result in an underpowered study is not proof that the drug does not work with regard to that endpoint. It merely says that the study failed to *prove* the drug works. Whether drug does not work or whether it works but just did not work well enough to yield a positive result in the study cannot be determined.

Finally, even if the study is well powered, no study can be 100% powered. A study that is 80% powered will, by random bad luck, yield a negative result 20% of the time, even if the drug works. A study that is 90% powered will yield false negative results in 10% of the cases from random bad luck.

16.2.2 Flawed Study Design

Another common major threat to internal validity is flawed study design. If the study design is flawed from the beginning, it is almost impossible to achieve internal validity. There are infinite ways to design an uninterpretable study, but below are some of the most common.

One of the most common mistakes comes from selecting an inappropriate endpoint. Some of the pitfalls have been covered in Chapter 7 earlier chapter, such as selecting *an unvalidated surrogate*, picking the *wrong time point*, selecting *an endpoint that is nor responsive to the intervention*. One mistake that is subtle but devastating is selecting

an endpoint that is subject to *competing risk*, sometimes called *survivor bias*.

Competing Risk and Survivor Bias

Survivor bias is a very common misinterpretation. For example, if one were examining the rate of Congestive heart failure (CHF) after a myocardial infarction (MI), the patients who received tPA would have a higher rate than patients who received placebo. This is because patients who would have otherwise died without tPA survived after receiving tPA, but survived with compromised ejection fraction. In other words, the number of patients with CHF was increasing because the number of patients who died was decreasing and instead was becoming CHF patients.

Here is an analogy. In World War II, a plan was hatched to reinforce Allied bombers to reduce the percentage of bombers that were shot down on each mission. The engineers carefully mapped the location of bullet holes in the fuselages of bombers that returned to the base after missions and reinforced the areas where the bullet holes were found.

This unfortunately had no effect on the loss rate. It turned out that the most important parts of the bombers were the areas where no bullet holes were ever found. Those were the areas in which if bullets hit bombers, they would be crippled and would never make back to the base. In designing endpoints in clinical trials, it is important not to forget patients who die or dropout for other reasons. If you look only at patients who remain alive, or remain on the study, or in other ways "make it back to base," you may set the study up to be biased.

Here is an example.

A new drug is being developed for primary pulmonary hypertension patients. It is expected to slow the progression of disease, lowering deaths, and hospitalization.

Hospitalization is more common than death, so in order to increase the power of the study, hospitalization is selected as the primary endpoint.

But contrary to expectation, hospitalization is increased rather than decreased in the treated group.

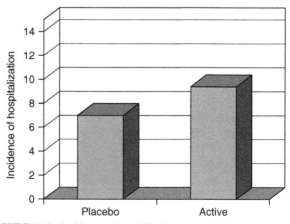

FIGURE 16.1   Incidence of hospitalization.

However, death plus CHF was decreased in the active group.

Of course, this is because the drug was very effective in preventing deaths and the patients who would have died on placebo survived on active drug, but with increased rate of hospitalization.

A related error occurs when you use composite endpoints that combine competing risk. For example, death/CHF endpoint might not show a difference between placebo and tPA arms in the above example even though there is a benefit, because the number of patients who die may decrease in the tPA group while the number of patients with CHF may increase. Clinically, surviving with CHF is a much better outcome than dying, and therefore it is not appropriate to combine the two in such a case. However, if both components of the endpoint move in a similar direction, or if the composite endpoint would move in the same direction, it might be appropriate.

Of course, in some cases, a composite outcome may be appropriate even if there is competing risk. For example, death/vegetative state after a stroke may be an appropriate endpoint because unlike CHF and death, death and vegetative state may be nearly equally bad so that converting a patient who would have died into a survivor in a vegetative state may not be clinically meaningful.

Inappropriate Study Procedures

Inappropriate study procedures can also confound a study and can negate study results. For example, let's say you were conducting a study of three doses of a new oral hypoglycemic. The frequency of the hypoglycemias is titrated by blood glucose measurements performed four times a day. The primary endpoint is MI rates across the dose groups.

This is a poor study design, because by titrating the drug frequency to the blood glucose level, the doses are confounded. There will be more doses given in the low dose group and fewer for the high dose group. If the low dose group receives 1 mg three times a day and the high dose group receives 3 mg once a day, one would not expect much of a dose response, for example. A better design would be to make frequency of dosing the endpoint, or alternatively would have called for fixed dose frequency across the dose groups. Alternatively, the design could have called for three groups with three difference target blood glucose levels and titration parameters.

Bias and Confounding

The *p*-value is also meaningless if there are significant biases. For example, if the patients are able to guess what drug there are on because of side effects, there might be a pronounced placebo effect. This would make it likely that the *p*-value would be low, but not because of the true effect of the drug but rather because of placebo effect. Of course, this would invalidate the results of the study.

This type of risk is particularly high for studies with subjective endpoints, such as in Crohn's disease or pain studies, where placebo effect can be pronounced. The likelihood of placebo effect affecting the results is much lower with objective endpoints such as death or changes in hemoglobin levels.

Anything that can affect the outcome can be a source of bias if it is present in different amounts in the two arms. For example, concomitant drugs can easily affect outcome. This can introduce bias if its use is different in the different arms. For example, if nonsteroidal anti-inflammatory drug (NSAID) use decreases in an arthritis study in the active group because the drug is working, this will introduce a bias. Therefore, the dose of concomitant medications should be held constant or prohibited in the trial. Potential confounders such as these should be examined carefully during analysis and interpretation of the study, since it can invalidate the results. Potential sources of bias include:

- Use of excluded medications
- Site differences
- Differential treatments by physicians
- Seasonal changes
- Observation bias
- Reporting bias, sometimes due to AE collected at different frequencies
- Time effect

16.2.3 Study Exe\cution Issues

Poor Study Execution

Poor execution can render results invalid for a variety of reasons. For example, if the protocol was not followed, or there were multiple violations, the results will be suspect. If the patients received only half the drug doses, or were misdosed

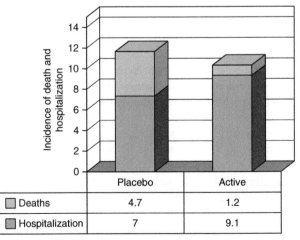

	Placebo	Active
Deaths	4.7	1.2
Hospitalization	7	9.1

FIGURE 16.2 Incidence of death and hospitalization.

or if the randomization was performed incorrectly of if there was fraud at some of the sites then the results may be invalid.

One of the most critical factors in study execution is enrollment of appropriate patients. If the inclusion and exclusion criteria are not tightly written, you may end up with patient populations that are not your intended population. If protocol waivers are frequently granted – which is of course poor practice – then many of the patients may be different from the intended population and also from one another. Heterogeneous population can be a significant problem in study interpretation.

Even when the protocol is well drafted, it is not uncommon to end up with patients who are not members of the intended patient population particularly if there is a strong incentive for the investigators or patients to bend the inclusion and exclusion criteria. For example, if the disease is a severe disease with no other therapeutic alternatives and there is widespread expectation that the drug will work, investigators may "misdiagnose" the patients with the diagnosis that better fits the inclusion criteria, or patients might claim to have symptoms that they really don't have.

Other potential issues with study execution include issues mentioned earlier in the book, such as instrumentation failure or lack of validation. For example, if the instruments used in the study were not properly calibrated, this could introduce a significant bias. Similarly, if the primary endpoint depends on a specific blood test such as a FACS analysis, and the shipping method was not validated for temperature, transit time, and other factors that might affect the test results, then even a result may be suspect. Or if the endpoint is ejection fraction, and the echocardiography technique and quantification algorithm are not standardized, there may be significant variation across the sites. This may render the results invalid.

Also, it is unfortunately not uncommon that blinding is broken either inadvertently or on purpose in the course of the study. Interactive voice response system (IVRS) errors are unfortunately not rare either, and this can be devastating to the study. Labeling errors and misdosing errors are also seen in many studies. Instrument errors or errors in labeling and shipping of laboratory samples is also seen in many studies.

Artifacts

Sometimes there are artifacts that negate the study results. Below is an example:

> You conduct a study comparing drug vs. placebo in patients with panic attacks. The primary endpoint is the number of panic attack episodes. At the end of the study, you find much to your delight that the placebo group had 89 episodes and active group had 67, with a p-value of 0.03. You get ready to publish the results, but then notice something disturbing. The patients,

after randomization, underwent 1 month of washout during which they were weaned from their previous drugs. After the washout period, they were started on placebo or active drug. During the washout period, when neither group was receiving therapy, the placebo group experienced 39 episodes and the active group 15 episodes. That means that during the 5 months when the groups were receiving their intended therapies, the number of panic episodes were 50 and 51.

Clearly, in this case, the study is negative, even though the p-value is less than 0.05. A drug cannot cause improvement before it is administered.

In other cases, you might find similar artifacts. For example, you might find that there is a difference between two arms in a survival study. But when you examine the survival curve, they start to diverge during the run-in period when no drug is being given and converge during treatment.

In other cases, study procedures may inadvertently cause a bias. For example, in cancer studies using progression free survival, the timing of the study visits and CT scans has a very important impact on time to event. Progression, or growth of the tumor, is generally detected at the time of the CT scan. If the CT scans are performed every week, the progressions will be detected earlier in many patients than if they are done every 3 months. If the randomization and schedule visits are such that patients in the placebo arm happens to have earlier visit schedule (even by a few days) than the patients in the treated arm. Then the placebo patients will tend to show fewer days to progressions even if the active drug has no effect on survival. Below is an illustration.

> Breast cancer patients are randomized into placebo and active treatments. All patients are to undergo CT scans every 3 months ± 1 month in order to look for progression, because progression free survival is the primary endpoint. It just happens that the placebo patients are scheduled, by chance, to return at average of 2.5 months, 5.5 months, 8.5 months, etc. while the active patients are scheduled to return at average of 3.5 months, 6.5 months, 9.5 months, etc. The placebo patients are found to progress, on average, 1 month earlier than the active patients.

Finally, you should make sure that placebo was truly inactive. In some cases, placebo or supposedly inactive component of the placebo formulation may have a beneficial deleterious effect on the study endpoints. For example, if you are testing cyclosporin for cystic fibrosis, and you have propylene glycol in your placebo solution, this may introduce an artifact since propylene glycol may exacerbate cystic fibrosis. The results may look better for the active arm simply because placebo made the patients fare worse. Or, if the physical act of injection into the eye improves age-related macular degeneration, then placebo injections may be as active as the drug injection.

External Events

Sometimes, external events, such as new drug being introduced, can have an impact on the trial. Below is an example.

A study of lung cancer is being conducted. Patients are treated with the drug X or placebo until they have progression (increase in the size of the tumor) and then they are discontinued from treatment. After progression, they are permitted to receive other therapies. Halfway through the study, a new drug is approved for lung cancer. The availability of the drug does two things. First, it increases the dropout rate. Second, it increases the survival of the patients who progress and are switched to the therapy. As a result, the drug X, which actually worsens survival compared to placebo, shows improvement in overall survival because so many patients treated with drug X dropout quickly and are switched to the newly approved drug.

Leaving aside the wisdom of allowing switching of drug before the primary endpoint has been met, external factors such as these can clearly influence the study.

16.2.4 Erroneous Statistical Analysis

Wrong Statistical Test

The second common mistake with p-values is erroneous analysis. It is not uncommon for investigators to simply use the wrong statistical test on the data. This can lead to p-values that are inappropriately too high or too low.

A common misuse of statistical tests is inappropriate use of tests designed to compare two groups, such as the t-test, on studies that have three or more groups. Rather than using a test like ANOVA that are appropriate for three or more group comparisons, some people will do two-way comparisons multiple times instead. In other words, they perform multiple pairwise comparisons. (Please note that pairwise comparisons are different from paired tests. Pairwise means you are comparing two groups, paired means you are matching multiple measurements for each patient.)

Here is an example.

A study of wound healing is performed with three arms: placebo (P), vascular endothelial growth factor (VEGF), and hyperbaric therapy (HT). The result come in and the following t-tests are performed with the following p-values.

TABLE 16.1 Multiple paired t-tests

Test	p-value
P vs. VEGF	0.02
P vs. HT	0.03
VEGF vs. HT	0.13

Therefore, the conclusion is that VEGF has a statistically significant effect and that HT has a statistically significant effect. However, this is wrong, as you probably already guessed, because there are three groups. If you do a two-way test for each pair of groups, you in effect have three primary endpoints being tested. You cannot use cutoff of 0.05 three times in three primary hypotheses. You have to use a set of cutoffs that insures that there is no more than 5% chance of generating a false positive. Therefore, the p-value that is required for significance is much smaller, such as 0.05 divided by 3, which is 0.017.

More importantly, comparing two groups at a time is inappropriate way to analyze this data. The first question that should be asked is, "Are all three groups the same, or are there one or more groups that are different?" This way of asking gives us more statistical power, and starts with the most basic question first. The first test that should be performed is the ANOVA. The results are as follows.

Because we only have one primary endpoint, the p-value required for significance is 0.05, which this easily meets. Now, once it is established that the three groups are not all equivalent, then one is still left with the question which is the group that is different.

One way of establishing which group is different is the Tukey test, which compares the means of the groups, starting with the highest vs. lowest mean and working its way through the groups. It is similar to the t-test but a rather complicated model is used to generate the table that renders the p-value from the test statistic, and the testing is performed in a sequential manner. Alternatively, you can perform multiple comparisons properly, as outlined below.

Some other common statistical mistakes include:

- Using two sample unpaired t-test for paired data.
- Using paired t-test for unpaired data.
- Using t-test on sets of observations from two individuals.

Contingency tables show the distribution of data, number of patients or events. Not all 2×2 tables are contingency tables. Contingency tables show mutually exclusive outcomes. All numbers in a contingency table are integers. Don't use contingency table methods on fraction, duration, percent changes, etc. since none of them are counts of events.

Wrong Assumptions

Another common erroneous use of statistical tests is use of tests when the assumptions required for the test to be valid are not applicable to the study.

All statistical tests are based on assumptions. These include assumptions of linearity, assumptions of minimal

TABLE 16.2 ANOVA Test

Test	p-value
P vs. VEGF vs. HT	0.004

sample size, and so on. Unless a statistician is alerted when the assumptions are violated, they may not make appropriate adjustments to the methods. An example would be using a parametric test when the samples are not parametric. Another would be to use a standard test such as a t-test when there are only a few patients in the sample. Another would be to assume equal variance when the variances are not equal. Another would be to treat noncontinuous measurements such as EDSS as if it were a continuous measure. Another would be to add and subtract scales or variables as if they were numbers when they are not true numbers.

Another would be to ignore biological nonlinearity, such as with blood pressure, and use tests that rely on linearity assumptions. Most biological phenomena are roughly linear, but at the extremes of measurements, many lose the linearity. For example, blood pressure has a U-shaped curve with relation to cardiovascular outcome in MI patients. Very low pressure is a poor prognostic indicator, as is very high blood pressure. Unless a statistician is alerted to this fact, he is liable to apply methods designed only for linear relationships to the blood pressure data, with resultant misleading conclusions. As another example, hazard function is usually assumed to be constant over time but this is not always the case. For example, for cardiovascular bypass surgeries, the mortality rate is the highest right after surgery, and then rises again a few days after surgery.

Another would be to ignore biological collinear relationships. Many biological processes are interlinked, and colinearity is a very common phenomenon. Most statistical tests, however, assume absence of colinearity. For example, it would be inappropriate to perform an analysis of atrial fibrillation paroxysm frequency without correcting for number of episodes that occur in the same patients, since one paroxysmal episode often increases the likelihood of a repeat episode. If you assume that each episode is independent, you are likely to end up with an inaccurately low p-value, since a handful of patients having multiple episodes might skew the data.

In some cases, it will not be known at the beginning of a study whether the assumptions will hold. For example, Cox proportional hazards test assumes constant hazard ratio for the course of the study. At the end of the study, it may be that the hazard ratio was not constant. Perhaps the drug took sometime to exert an effect so the curves did not start separating until sometime had passed. A well-written statistical analysis plan would plan for this and arrange for the assumptions to be tested before the analysis is performed, but unfortunately, sometimes this is not the case.

Also, be careful of very large or small samples sizes. Everything will be significant in large samples, and small studies have low power and violate assumption of some statistical tests.

Misinterpretation of Statistics

Sometimes there is frank misunderstanding of the statistical results. For example, people often chart 95% confidence intervals for different samples and look to see if they overlap. It they do not overlap, that is taken to mean that the samples are statistically different, and if they do, that is taken to mean that they are not. This is false; 95% confidence intervals can overlap by as much as almost a third (29%) and the samples may be statistically different at $p < 0.05$. One cannot compare confidence intervals from different samples. What you really should do is to calculate the difference between the samples and calculate the confidence interval around the difference.

Inappropriate Imputation

Another very common mistake is to utilize inappropriate imputation. For example, if multiple patients dropout of a study because they are feeling so good that they are no longer motivated to continue in the study as a result of receiving the drug, imputing all missing patients as failures would lead to misleading results. Imputation may be required for patients who, though they did not dropout, must be excluded from analysis, because they did not meet the inclusion/exclusion criteria, did not receive the drug, received a prohibited drug, or for other reasons.

All studies will have some missing data. Imputation techniques were discussed in an earlier Chapter 14. During interpretation of the data and analysis, careful attention should be paid to how the imputations were performed and how the imputations are affecting the results. Careful sensitivity analysis will help assess the impact of dropouts and imputation.

In some cases, imputation is not even performed. The patients are merely censored, or a "*completer*" or "*responder analysis*" is performed. Anytime that you perform the primary analysis on a population other than the full complement of patients who were randomized, you are performing a subgroup analysis. This is fraught with risks, and is described in detail in the next section.

16.3 BEYOND THE PRIMARY ENDPOINT

16.3.1 Background

The above section describes the threats to internal validity with well-controlled trials, and particularly with respect to primary analysis. These studies, when they are well designed, have the advantage of eliminating many of the biases and confounding seen with nonrandomized, poorly controlled studies.

There are many instances, however, when you will need to or want to perform studies or analysis that are not well-controlled or subject to potential additional biases. This is for two reasons. First, it is sometimes not possible or practicable to perform a study in an ideal fashion. Whether it is for economic reasons, ethical reasons, or for logistic reasons, it may be necessary to perform an uncontrolled study or otherwise conduct a study that is less than ideal.

Second, the primary endpoint and the *p*-value alone do not yield much information. Statistical significance does not automatically mean clinically significant.

Often, you will want to perform additional analysis to understand not just whether the drug has an effect on the endpoint or not but also how well it works, whether there are subgroups that respond in a different fashion, whether there is an interaction with demographic or other factors, and so on. You will rely on secondary analysis for this sort of data. In many cases, the secondary endpoint will have been pre-specified, but in many cases they will not have been.

Now, an important *caveat* is that though secondary and exploratory analyses are very informative and important, you should note that they are far more prone to biases and confounding. Performing these types of analysis properly is much greater challenge than performing primary analysis properly.

16.2.2 Adding More Meat Around Primary Endpoint

A *p*-value in and of itself tells you whether there was a significant effect on the outcome, but does not tell you how large the magnitude of the outcome was. In clinical practice, you want to know not only just whether the drug impacts outcome but also how much difference it makes. A drug that reduces cholesterol by 1% is very different from the one that reduces it by 50%.

For this reason, point estimates and confidence intervals are often used to describe the effect of the intervention on the primary (and other) endpoints. Point estimate is the best guess regarding how much effect the treatment has, or what the value of the parameter being estimated is. Confidence interval describes how confident you are about the point estimate; 95% confidence is typically used, and it is a measure that describes the values in between which you would expect the true value to lie in 95% of the cases.

Point estimate plus confidence interval is often preferred over a *p*-value because the point estimate is an indication of how much effect there is, while the confidence interval is an indication how strong (statistically) the likelihood of difference is. The first is driven by the effect of the drug while the second is driven by the size of the study. This is in contrast to the *p*-value, which collapses the two (how well the drug works and how large the study is) into one value.

You can display a confidence interval for each arm or for the difference. For example, in a study comparing rug vs. placebo for blood pressure control, you might display the results as the following. The confidence intervals are in the parenthesis.

Placebo: 130 mmHg (120, 140)
Drug: 120 mmHg (115,125)

In this case, the confidence interval for the blood pressure in the placebo patients is between 120 and 140 mmHg.

Or you might display the results as a difference of ratio as follows:

Drug/Placebo: 1.1 (1.05, 1.2)

When you're looking at ratios, such as the number above, if the confidence interval does not include 1, it generally means that the results are significant.

In general, when you are performing subgroup analysis or analysis of nonrandomized data, you can look for the following factors to add additional credence to your analysis.

- Replication in another independent study.
- Presence of a dose–response relationship.
- Reproducibility of the observation in independent samples within the study, such as within individual sites.
- Availability of a biological explanation.

16.3.3 Aggregate Data Can Sometimes Be Misleading

Another reason why the primary endpoint, by itself, is an inadequate way of describing the study results is that aggregate data has limitations.

The basis for clinical research is the ability to aggregate data. Aggregate data is very helpful in most instances, and allows us to process complicated data sets in a manageable manner. So sometimes when individual data are aggregated, the information is simpler, easier to understand, and captures most of the properties. It is easier to say that mean blood pressure decreased by 10 mmHg rather than to state: "in Patient 1, the blood pressure decreased from 130 to 115 mmHg, in Patient 2, it decreased from 120 to 110 mmHg, in Patient 3 it increased from 110 to 118 mmHg …."

In other cases, it does not. It is important to realize sometimes that aggregate data can reflect individual data poorly. Adding five small lumps of clay gives you one large lump of clay but adding five small eggs together does not give you one large egg. It gives you five small eggs in a pile. Another analogy would be corporations. Corporations are aggregations of people that act as one person, and can do many things that a person can do, and in some cases better than a person. It can own property, it can enter contracts, and it can sue and be sued. However, a corporation is not a person and cannot do certain things a person can do, such as go to high school, get pregnant, or run for president. In the same way, you can add, subtract, and otherwise do many mathematical and statistical manipulations of summary statistics (such as means and standard deviations) but not all of them.

Similarly, aggregate data cannot capture some of the properties of individual data. An example would be a study of omalizumab in asthma. The treated group showed decreased hospitalization rate. It also showed decreased steroid use. It would seem that one could then claim that the drug lowers steroid use without increasing steroid use. However, that would be an erroneous conclusion. Even though the drug reduces hospitalizations and steroid use, it may or may not reduce hospitalizations and steroid use in the same individuals. It is possible, for example, that in 50% of the patients, hospitalization rate dropped by 90% and steroid use remained the same; while in 50% of the patients, hospitalization rate increased by 25% and steroid use decreased. That would mean that in patients who reduced steroid use, the risk of hospitalization increased.

The intellectual illusion here occurs because individuals are not the same as the group. Individuals within the group may move in opposite direction as the group mean.

The other example is the group vs. individual pharmacokinetic (PK) curve shown earlier. An individual's response curve may be much steeper than the group response curve. Assuming that the group response curve is same as the individuals' would be very dangerous in some cases.

So, when interpreting the results of a study, it is important to examine individual level data and subgroup level data.

16.3.4 Threats to Internal Validity in Nonclassical Study Designs

When there is no concurrent control arm, there may be bias from time effects. For example, treatment protocols might change overtime. Or seasonal changes may influence the results, as in an allergy study. These threats to validity come from factors external to the study.

Subjects themselves may change, due to progression or disease, aging, or other factors. This is called maturation.

Tolerance, conditioning, or training effects may be seen when a patient undergoes repeated testing. For example, patients may memorize eye charts if the same eye chart is used repeatedly.

Investigator bias can also become a significant factor in nonclassical studies.

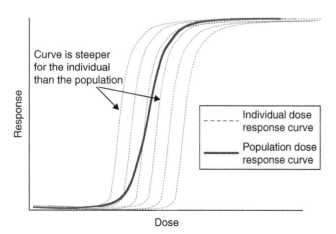

FIGURE 16.3   Individual and group PK response curves.

16.3.5 Statistical Flukes and Optical Illusions

Primate brains are not hardwired to process aggregate data properly. There is natural tendency to use heuristic processing, which is good for anecdotal data encountered in everyday life, but this can lead to wrong conclusions when processing statistical information. This section describes some of the more common errors.

Regression to the Mean

Regression to the mean is a counterintuitive concept to many people. It is fortunately not a major problem in causing false positive results in randomized studies, but in nonrandomized studies or analysis, especially subgroup analysis, it can be a major problem. It is also a major problem in estimating sample size of studies, and can reduce power of studies.

Regression to the mean can occur with any variable or event that fluctuates over time. Here is an example.

> Let's take a hundred die. You roll them, and find that there are 15 die that rolled to a six and 15 that rolled to a one. You take the first group and call them "the sickest population" and take the second group and call them "the healthiest population." You then re-roll each group of die. Will you get higher numbers in the first group and lower numbers in the second group? Of course not. They will tend to yield mean values of about 3.5. They will "regress to the mean" of 3.5.

Similarly, if you take a group of patients and select ones that have highest and lowest values of something, you will often find that when you re-measure them, the highest group will yield lower scores than before and the lowest group will yield higher scores than before. For example, if you take a group of people who have normal blood pressure, and measure them, you will likely find people who have high and low pressure readings just by chance. On re-measuring, they will regress to the mean.

Of course, if the group is heterogeneous – for example, you take a group of people some of whom have hypertension and some of whom do not – then you will find persistent differences in the readings, although you will find the differences will decrease on the second measurement due to slight regression to the mean.

The take-away is: never compare subgroup in one arm against the entire group from the other arm. Stratification by severity at time of randomization can protect against regression to the mean.

Regression to the mean is often seen across studies as well. Often, a Phase II study will yield spectacular results, and the subsequent Phase III will be less impressive. Given the number of Phase II studies that are conducted and given that only a subset proceed into Phase III, it would be expected that in general, Phase III results would be less impressive than Phase II.

A promising drug for patients with angina is being developed. Unfortunately, it fails to meet the primary endpoint (symptom severity) in the Phase II study.

But, preclinical data suggests that only the more severe patients would benefit because the drug affects receptors that are most upregulated in severe disease.

So, a subgroup analysis is performed on the 50% most severe patients.

The results look good, so the drug is advanced into Phase III for the more severe patients and it fails.

The lesson is as follows. In a waxing and waning diseases, all patients will have good periods and bad. Taking only the patients who are having worse than usual days will result in patients appearing to improve on repeat measurement.

Let's go back to the data and look at it again in a different way. In the Phase II study, even the placebo patients appear to improve with treatment (with placebo) if only the severe patients are considered. This is clearly an example of regression to the mean.

Proportions

One concept that can be hard to grasp is the concept of proportions. Most people are used to comparing things in terms of relative size or value. For example, you might say that one shoe costs twice as much as another. Or you might say that one person is 10% taller than another.

However, when you are comparing proportions, you have to be very careful. By proportions, we mean things that are expressed as percentages or fractions. They include things like percentage of patients who die, percentage of visits that are missing, fraction of patients who dropped out, and so forth. With proportions, there are always two ways to look at the numbers, and you have to be careful that you look at it from both angles. Below is an illustration.

- A company claims that its new drug reduces morality by 90%.
- Another drug is supposed to reduce mortality by 9%.
- Yet another claims to reduce mortality from 10% to 1%.
- Another company says that survival is increased from 90% to 99%.

All of these claims are equivalent. The difference between 1% and 10% is the same as the difference between 90% and 99%.

- 1% mortality = 99% survival
- 10% mortality = 90% survival

The difference between 0% and 90% is comparable to the difference between 90% and 99%.

- 10% to 100% is 10-fold difference
- 1% to 10% is 10-fold difference

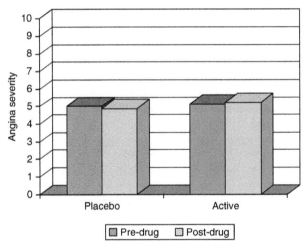

FIGURE 16.4 Angina severity.

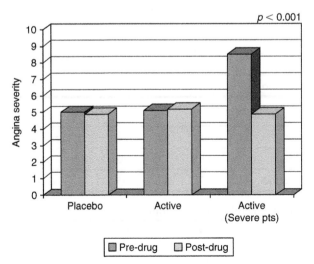

FIGURE 16.5 Angina severity in severe subgroup.

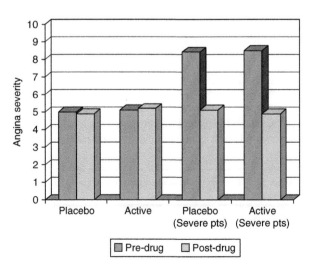

FIGURE 16.6 Angina severity in severe subgroup receiving placebo.

You should remember to distinguish between *absolute difference, relative difference*, and *odds ratio*. Absolute difference is the mathematical difference when one subtract one number from another: $100\% - 90\% = 10\%$. Relative difference is the difference in relation to the baseline value: $25\% - 20\% = 5\%$ $5\%/25\% = 20\%$. Odds ratio is the relative odds:

$$\frac{24\%/75\%}{20\%/80\%} = 1.33$$

Subgroup Reversals

You should also remember that statistics is not absolute. There will be some variability in results, and sometimes this will look contrary to expectations. People tend to underestimate the likelihood of these statistical flukes. Here is an example.

> A new drug is being developed for wound healing. The Phase II results are convincing, with 30% wound healing in placebo and 63% in active group ($p = 0.002$). However, one of the sites displays a worrisome effect. Therefore, there were 60% wound healing in placebo and only 25% in active. An investigation is launched to determine what happened at the site, whether the randomization codes were mixed up, etc.

This investigation is unwarranted. With enough sites, one or more sites will show reversal of effect, just by chance. The table below shows the probability of at least one site showing reversal of effect (alpha of 0.05, 80% power).

Nonreproducible Studies

Similarly, if you repeat the same study enough times, even a drug that works well will yield a negative result. After all, most studies are powered at 80% or 90% power. That means that for each study, there is 20% or 10% chance that the study will be negative even if the drug works. If you conduct four studies that are powered at 80%, then you will have only $0.8 \times 0.8 \times 0.8 \times 0.8 = 0.41$ or 41% chance that all the studies will be positive, even if the drug works.

Simpson's Paradox

The next three topics, Simpson's Paradox, Combining Groups, and Will Rogers Phenomenon are all statistical flukes introduced when disparate groups are combined or interact.

TABLE 16.3 Probability of at least one center showing treatment reversal

Number of centers	1	2	3	4	5	6	7	8
Probability of treatment	.003	.05	.15	.29	.43	.56	.67	.75

Simpson's Paradox is a relatively common, and very counterintuitive phenomenon that is often encountered when subgroups are examined, or when two groups are combined. In cases where the paradox is seen, analysis of the two smaller groups appears to show an effect from the therapy, but the effect disappears when the two groups are combined. For example, drug X seems to improve survival in women and in men when examined separately, but appears not to when both men and women are combined into one group. Below is an example.

> Men with a particular type of cancer who are treated with drug have higher survival rate. Women who are treated with drug have higher survival rate. However, when both men and women are combined, those who are treated with placebo have a higher survival rate.

The reason this happens is that though drug improves survival in men and women, men have overall survival rate that is higher than women, and most men received placebo while most women received drug. This violates the independence assumption that is required before groups can be combined together for analysis, because the groups are very different from each other.

Simpson's Paradox occurs when the direction of an association between two variables is reversed when a third variable is controlled. In this case, the first two variables are drug/placebo and alive/dead. The third variable is men/women.

Here is a real life example that might be easier to understand.

> University of California, Berkeley, was sued in the 70s for bias against women applying to graduate school. Below are the admission figures for fall 1973. It shows that there is a statistically significant difference in the admission rate between men and women.

TABLE 16.4 Simpson's Paradox

Men

	Died	Lived	Survival rate
Drug	6	81	93%
Placebo	36	234	87%

Women

	Died	Lived	Survival rate
Drug	71	192	73%
Placebo	35	55	69%

Both men and women combined

	Died	Lived	Survival rate
Drug	77	273	78%
Placebo	61	289	83%

But, Berkeley's (successful) defense is as follows. When broken down by individual departments, most departments were actually admitting more women than men.

It was found that no department was significantly biased against women; in fact, most departments had a small bias against men.

The explanation is that women applied to the more competitive departments that had lower admission rates.

Here is a graphical explanation of Simpson's Paradox. The dark grey is one subgroup, and the correlation goes in one direction. The light grey is another group, and the correlation goes in the same direction. The two groups are not similar to one another. If both groups are combined, the overall correlation, identified by a dotted line, goes in the opposite direction.

Combining Groups

This brings us to a related phenomenon. Don't combine two populations in a correlation analysis. If you have different groups, and you do a correlation analysis on them there might appear to be a difference when there is none. In the below graph, you can see that although there is no real correlation between two variables (food and tendency to fetch sticks), a spurious correlation emerges when two disparate groups are combined in the analysis.

There is no correlation between food intake and the tendency to fetch sticks. Dogs like to fetch stick and eat more than cats. But, when you graph dogs and cats on the same graph, it appears that by feeding your animal more, you can make it want to fetch sticks more.

Will Rogers Phenomenon

With appropriate apologies in advance to Californians (of which one of the authors is one), the Will Rogers Phenomenon is called such because of the quip form Will Rogers:

> *When the Okies left Oklahoma and moved to California, they raised the average intelligence level in both states.*

This paradox occurs when the mean value of a phenomenon is different in two groups, and some patients are transferred between two groups. Below is an example.

Over many years, survival for a certain type of colon tumors has been very stable. Patients with metastatic tumors had median survival of 12 months, and patients with non-metastatic tumors had median survival of 20 months. However, a recently conducted nonrandomized single arm study with drug Z showed very promising results: metastatic median survival of 14 months and non-metastatic median survival of 48 months. Ecstatic investigators conduct another, randomized study. The results unfortunately are negative.

The explanation is as follows. A better analysis technique for tumors allowed investigators to scan for and detect small metastasis. Therefore, many patients who would previously have been considered to be non-metastatic were now considered to be metastatic. These patients

TABLE 16.5 Simpson's Paradox: Berkeley admissions		
	Number of applicants	% Admitted
Men	8442	44%
Women	4321	35%

TABLE 16.6 Berkeley admissions by department				
Department	Men		Women	
	# Applicants	% Admitted	# Applicants	% Admitted
A	825	62%	108	82%
B	560	63%	25	68%
C	325	37%	593	34%
D	417	33%	375	35%
E	191	28%	393	24%
F	272	6%	341	7%

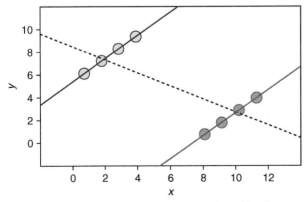

(Public domain image, from http://en.wikipedia. org/wiki/Image: Simpson%27s_paradox_continuous.svg)

FIGURE 16.7 Graphic illustration of Simpson's Paradox.

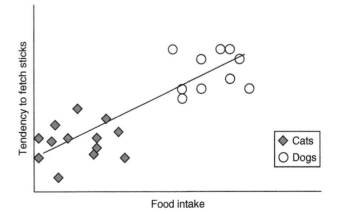

FIGURE 16.8 Spurious correlation between food intake and stick-chasing behavior in dogs and cats.

had median survival of 18 months. Adding them to the metastatic group increased median survival in that group. Subtracting them from the non-metastatic group increased median survival in that group.

16.2.6 Subgroup and Subtemporal Analysis

Proper and Improper Uses of Subgroup Analysis

Subgroup analysis can be very useful and important if used properly. It can help define those patients who benefit the most, and can identify patient who do not benefit or are at higher risk of safety events. No drug affects all patients in a homogeneous manner, and there can be significant variations across different populations, particularly populations with different sex, age, weight, and genetic profiles. There might be subgroups that benefit more than the main group, or a subgroup that respond poorly compared to the other groups. This topic is covered in the Chapter 7 and 9, but it is worth reminding ourselves that subgroup analysis is important, though risky, part of analyzing the data. It is important because the subgroup differences might be important in using the drug as effectively and safely as possible.

However, you should remember that subgroup analysis is appropriate when the primary efficacy endpoint has been achieved, and you want to examine the drug's efficacy across the subpopulations in a more granular fashion. Subgroups analysis is *inappropriate* when the primary efficacy endpoint has been missed, and you want to examine the drug's efficacy across the subpopulations in order to find a subgroup for whom the drug work. The former is data mining; the latter is data dredging.

As mentioned before, the subgroup analysis is best used to determine whether there is a difference in response in the subgroup compared to the group at large, not whether there is a treatment effect in the subgroup or how the subgroup differs from another subgroup.

You cannot take a study that is negative overall, and rescue it by finding a subpopulation in which it works. You can certainly generate a hypothesis based on that type of data dredging, but you cannot take another shot at establishing internal validity after your first attempt fails. Subgroup analyses are particularly perilous when the overall result is negative, and one of the subgroups appear to have tremendous benefit.

In describing the subgroup analysis, it should be noted how many subgroups were included in the analysis – if 4 out of 5 subgroups show a difference, that is very different from 4 out of 100.

Even when the subgroup analysis is appropriate, it is still risky because many biases and confounders can creep into a subgroup analysis. By definition, when you perform a subgroup analysis, you are analyzing a patient population that is different from the one that was randomized. Whenever you do this, you can introduce all the biases associated with nonrandomized studies.

Subgroups Defined by Baseline Characteristics

There are many ways to divide the population into subgroups, but broadly speaking, these methods fall into either of two categories: by characteristics that exist at the beginning of the study and by characteristics that change in the course of the study. Of the two, the former is much more legitimate than the latter.

Characteristics that exist at the beginning of the study, which we will call *independent factors*, such as sex, age, disease type/severity, geography, sites, etc. are much less subject to bias because they are unaffected by treatment. On the other hand, characteristics that can change in the course of the study, or *dependent factors*, such as PK/PD, dropouts, response, number of doses missed, etc. are highly subject to bias, and is very dangerous to use to define subgroups.

The strongest, most robust subgroup analyses are those performed on stratified groups. For example, if patients with anterior MI are stratified from patients with nonanterior MI (randomized in separate blocks), the subgroup analysis are much more powerful. The subgroups have been prespecified, and the randomization is balanced across the subgroup.

There are some standard subgroups that are almost always examined, such as demographic factors (gender, age, race, age, weight, demographics, etc.). You should keep in mind that p-values for these comparisons are nominal p-values. Subgroups are rarely adequately powered to show statistical differences, so in many cases you will not find that the subgroups achieve significance. For example, if the p-value for survival is 0.01 for the overall group but 0.2 for the males, that does not mean that the drug has no effect in males – it may just be a function of smaller sample size in that subgroup.

In fact, if you do enough subgroup analysis, you will find some subgroups where the therapeutic effect is opposite that of the overall group. In almost all cases, these should be ignored, except for hypothesis generation, unless there is a pre-specified, biologically plausible reason for anticipating such a difference. Of course, in such cases, the study ought to have been powered to see such a difference or those patients should have been stratified to separate strata and excluded from primary analysis.

Using Dependent Variable to Subgroup

Defining subgroups by a dependent variable is problematic, as a general rule.

One kind of subgroup analysis is particularly vulnerable to bias: when a subgroup is used as the basis for the primary analysis. This occurs not infrequently because many studies are plagued with dropouts and protocol violators. So instead of performing a true intent-to-treat analysis, a "modified" intent-to-treat analysis is performed. This might be a per-protocol analysis, a completer analysis, or some other permutation. All of these are subgroup analysis, and as such, are subject to the drawbacks of subgroup analysis. Anytime you analyze a patient population that is different from the one that was randomized, you can introduce a bias. This is "the curse of the subgroup analysis," where many investigators have, to their detriment, been led astray by analyzing a subgroup.

Completer analysis includes only patients who completed the study. Responder analysis includes only patients who responded to the drug. *Pharmacodynamic responder analysis* is the practice of including only patients who had a biological response to the drug in the analysis. One example would be to include only patients who raised antibodies against a vaccine in the analysis. *Pharmacokinetic responder analysis* is similar, except only patients who had adequate levels of drug absorbed are included in the analysis. *Per-protocol analysis* includes only patients who did not have protocol violations, or who did not have major protocol violations in the analysis.

Completer Analysis

Here is an example of a completer analysis:

A new steroid cream is being developed for atopic dermatitis. The initial results are not statistically significant. However, there were quite a few dropouts and therefore an analysis only of the patients who dropped out is performed. This analysis is very encouraging, and on the basis of that, a large Phase III study is undertaken.

The Phase III is negative.

What happened is that the steroid actually worsened the symptoms, and worsened it the most in the patients with the most severe disease. As a result, most of the most severe patients in the active arm dropped out, making the average disease severity look better in the active arm. Looking at subgroup that remained in the study, lasted through titration, or was available for long-term analysis will almost always introduce bias. They will always be the best responders. But they may also enrich for patients who are the most motivated, who have the best support systems, or otherwise have characteristics that will result in a different response than the overall patient population.

Responder Analysis

Here is an example of responder analysis.

A promising new therapy for arthritis is being developed. It appears to be highly effective in some patients. Unfortunately, it causes severe itching in some patients that can lead to discontinuation. A Phase II is conducted, and as expected, dropouts are significant (about 30%). The results are therefore analyzed looking only at patients who completed the study (completers).

The results among those patients who tolerated the drug and completed the study look promising, though statistical significance is not reached.

Now, someone on the team recalls that comparing average scores (continuous endpoint) rather than looking just at success/failure (dichotomous endpoint) can increase the power of the study. Also, the biology of the drug suggests that it will only work in some patients. Therefore, the average pain score among those who reported pain relief is examined (responder analysis). In the responder population, the results are overwhelmingly positive. In other words, it looks like the drug only works in some patients but in those where it works, it works astonishingly well.

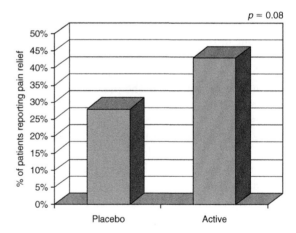

FIGURE 16.10 Nonsignificant pain relief.

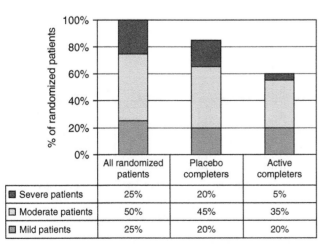

	All randomized patients	Placebo completers	Active completers
■ Severe patients	25%	20%	5%
□ Moderate patients	50%	45%	35%
▨ Mild patients	25%	20%	20%

FIGURE 16.9 Completer analysis.

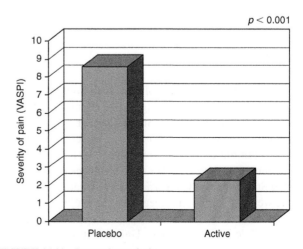

FIGURE 16.11 Responder analysis.

The drug is advanced into Phase III. It fails to show a benefit in Phase III.

Clearly, the issue is that it did not in fact work tremendously well in patients in whom it worked. Whenever you just look at responders, you will likely find that the responders look much better than the overall population. While this can sometimes be a true representation of drug's effect – some drugs do work only for some patients – it is more often an artifact, because you are systematically excluding patients who did poorly.

This sort of responder analysis should be distinguished from a subgroup analysis where the patients are segregated on basis of a baseline characteristic, such as HER2 positive breast cancer patients before treatment with Herceptin. While still subject to some issues, this sort of analysis is much more reliable than an analysis that depends on some variable, such as response or PK, that occurs after the drug is given.

Now, to continue the responder analysis example:

Let's say that as with the atopic dermatitis example, many of the most severe patients dropped out. The arthritis drug caused intense pruritus in the patients with the worst arthritis. The patients with the worst arthritis dropped out.

The numerator is similar between the groups, but denominators change, because more patients drop out in the active group. The sicker patients are the ones who tend to dropout. The healthier patients are the ones most likely to improve spontaneously. Among the responders in the placebo, some patients are from the severe group, who had higher pain scores to start with. Among the responders in the active group, almost none are in the severe group because they nearly all dropped out. The pain scores from the severe group skew the mean score in the placebo group.

	Placebo	Active
Responder	27	26
Completer	82	61
Response rate	33%	43%

An analogy might be as follows. Using only responders to gauge the efficacy of a drug is like trying to determine whether Chile or the United States is richer by using average income of Mercedes owners in each country. A very small proportion of the people in Chile own a Mercedes but their average income is higher than Mercedes owners in the United States since in Chile 5% of the population owns 90% of the wealth. That doesn't mean that the average Chilean is richer than an average American, nor does it mean that the GNP of Chile is higher than the United States.

Subgroups Defined by PK, PD, or Biomarker

PK and PD measurement and biomarkers are extremely useful tools. In particular, they can help design studies and can serve as surrogates for endpoints, dramatically reducing timeline for drug development. For example, a common biomarker/PD marker is viral load. Drugs that reduce viral loads well in hepatitis or AIDS tend to turn out to be drugs that work well.

Similarly, baseline biomarkers or genetic/RNA/proteomic baseline markers can be very useful. One example is HER2: high levels predict response to Herceptin.

However, biomarkers or PK/PD that change in the course of therapy cannot be used to legitimately subgroup patients. It is fine to use them to subgroup the patients if the purpose is to generate a hypothesis or for purely exploratory analysis, but conclusions based on such subgroups are subject to potentially severe bias.

PK/PD Subgroup Analysis

One extremely common type of analysis is an analysis correlating PK or PD subgroups with outcome. These types of analysis should only be used as an exploratory analysis. You certainly cannot use them to "save" the results of a failed trial. For example, you can't say, well only 10% of the patients had a titer, and those patients did very well, so the drug does work – see, those patients who had high titers.

Here is an example.

A promising drug for gastroenteritis is being developed. The study misses primary endpoint of diarrheal symptom severity, but there does seem to be some effect at the higher dose.

One of the formulation experts thinks that the drug may not have been absorbed well in these patients with diarrhea. Obviously, if drug is not absorbed, then it can't be expected to work. So, the hypothesis is that perhaps patients who absorbed the drug did well.

So a new analysis is performed. Patients are divided into three groups based on the drug levels

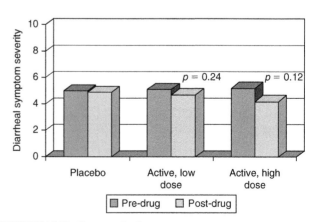

FIGURE 16.12 Response by dose groups.

in plasma. There is a profound decrease in symptom score in patients who absorbed the drug best.

The drug is advanced into large Phase III study with high dose, and the study is negative.

The explanation is that the patients who had the best prognosis had less severe form of gastroenteritis, and as a result, they were able to absorb drug better. So, they absorbed drug better because they were in a subgroup with better prognosis, not the other way around. Using any variable that changes during the course of the study (PK, PD, etc.) can lead to erroneous, confounded conclusions.

Similar analysis is often performed with vaccines – such as when only the patients who raise antibodies after vaccination is included in the analysis. These are similarly subject to bias. The legitimate way to design and analyze studies such as these is to randomize patients into groups, with each group being titrated a target PK/PD. In other words, Group 1 would be titrated serum drug level of 1 mcg/ml, Group 2 to 5 mcg/ml, and Group 3 to 10 mcg/ml, etc.

Subtemporal Analysis

Subtemporal analysis is analyzing data only from one period of a study. It is somewhat different from subgroup analysis, in that all patients may be analyzed but only data from a limited time period is used for the analysis, rather than from the entire study.

Below is an example.

A drug was being developed for Crohn's disease. In first stage, patients with active CD flares were randomized to either placebo or drug. The results were positive, with drug inducing remission in a significantly higher number of patients than placebo. The second stage enrolled only patients who had achieved remission, and was designed to assess the durability of remission. Therefore, patients were re-randomized to either placebo or drug.

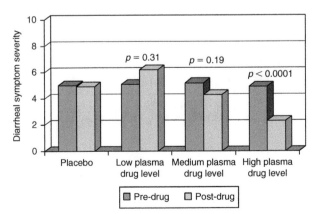

FIGURE 16.13 Response by plasma levels of the drug.

A subtemporal analysis was performed on the patients from the point of re-randomization to loss of remission. The patients who were re-randomized to the drug had a much longer remission than those who were re-randomized to placebo.

This analysis is flawed, because if the drug caused a rebound effect, such that patients who were initially on the drug and then were placed on placebo had rebound, then the drug would seem to prolong the durability of remission when in fact it was no better than placebo in maintaining remission. In fact, this is what happened. The patients who went into remission on placebo and stayed on placebo did much better than patients who went into remission on drug and were then re-randomized to placebo. In other words, the drug was not statistically better when comparing patients who were on placebo the entire way through and patients who were on drug all the way through. However, by taking data only from re-randomization, and making the baseline remission, the subtemporal analysis failed to take into account the randomization data from the first randomization and yielded misleading results.

In any study where there is risk of carry-over, you must be careful not to perform a subtemporal analysis that ignores the previous treatment.

Be very cautious with subgroup analysis. Use intent-to-treat analysis whenever possible. If subgroup analysis is important, use baseline variables, not variables that can change during the course of the study, or stratify at randomization by the baseline variable.

16.4 OTHER TYPES OF DATA ANALYSIS

16.4.1 Interpreting Survival Data

Survival data is often presented as a Kaplan-Meier curve, with a hazard ratio. Hazard ratio is a bit nonintuitive – it means the risk of dying at a certain time for one arm vs. the other. If the ratio is 1 that means that the risks are the same. If it is greater than 1, then the risk is higher, and vice versa. The drug is usually the denominator, so 1.5 means for example, that the risk of dying is higher on the drug by about 50%.

Clinical benefit is more easily understood in other ways. For example, median survival is a more intuitive term. It is the point at which half the patients die.

If one is trying to look at the average survival gain, it is expressed in life-years and is the area between the two curves.

Depending on the shape of the survival curve, it makes more sense to express the results in one way vs. another. For the below graph, it might be more meaningful to talk about median survival or average survival gain because the survival curves converge at the end. The drug appears to increase the median survival but not the maximum survival.

In the below graph, where the disease progresses much more slowly, it might make more sense to talk about survival at 12 months. In fact, the median survival for the active group has not been reached yet.

16.4.2 Oncology Data Analysis

The current endpoints used for oncology studies include Response Evaluation Criteria in Solid Tumors (RECIST) criteria, progression, progression free survival, time to progression, and survival. In Phase I and Phase II studies, RECIST is often used. This is a crude method of measuring linear dimensions of tumors and using it as a surrogate for response to the drug. The results are expressed as one of the following.

- CR (complete response) = disappearance of all target lesions
- PR (partial response) = 30% decrease in the sum of the longest diameter of target lesions
- PD (progressive disease) = 20% increase in the sum of the longest diameter of target lesions
- SD (stable disease) = small changes that do not meet above criteria

While RECIST is of some use with traditional cytotoxic agents, it suffers from several flaws. One is that some of the newer agents do not shrink tumors. Two is that RECIST often does not correlate with clinical benefit. Three is that it only measures macroscopic tumors, and does not measure microscopic metastasis. Four is that by collapsing tumor response into four categories, it reduces the amount of data available for interpretation.

Waterfall plots is one way to address the last of these issues. It is a way of plotting the tumor size across the entire spectrum of response and gives a much richer view of the results.

RECIST is a crude measure, which means that if you see a signal (tumor shrinkage) then the drug probably has activity. If you don't, however, it does not necessarily mean that the drug does not have activity.

The issues with many oncology studies are that many of them are uncontrolled and are in combination with other drugs. This makes it difficult to assess the results because it is not clear what the responses would have been with the concomitant drugs alone, and what the baseline rate would have been. The problem is exacerbated by the fact that in any given type of cancer, survival tends to be very different depending on their staging, performance scores, etc. This makes it difficult to assess what the response rate would have been without the drug if there is no control arm.

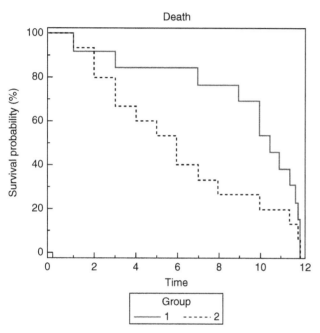

FIGURE 16.14   Converging survival curves.

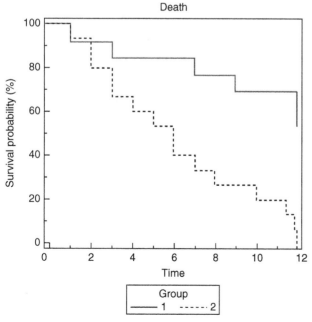

FIGURE 16.15   Diverging survival curves.

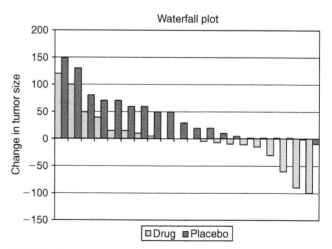

FIGURE 16.16   Frequency of arrhythmias and duodenal ulcers.

Time to progression is also fraught with difficulties. First, the definition of progression must be well defined so that there is consistency across investigators and treatment groups. Since many oncology studies are unblinded, there is an incentive for investigators to proclaim progression earlier in placebo patients, especially if they can then roll over onto active therapy. Also, as previously noted progression is generally detected via regularly scheduled imaging studies. The scheduling and frequency of the imaging can influence the rate at which progression is detected.

Using survival as the endpoint is ideal. Mortality is objective, and it is readily ascertainable. Unfortunately, this can increase the length of the study, sometimes unacceptably so. Also, you should be careful and determine whether patients rolled over into an active therapy either within the study or outside it after progression, because that can influence mortality.

16.4.3 Cluster randomized study analysis

Cluster randomized studies, if you recall, are studies in which the randomization is not at the patient level but at a higher level, such as by hospital, by geography, or other variable. Cluster study analysis is a bit more complicated than a typical analysis because the unit of analysis is often not the unit that was used to randomize. For example, if the randomization was at the hospital level, such that some hospitals were assigned to placebo and others to active drug, you are interested in not just whether changing the therapies at the hospital level affects outcome but also whether each individual patient is treated with the drug the outcome would be affected.

It is important to pre-specify what the primary endpoint is – whether it is at the cluster level or at the individual patient level. You cannot test both at the p-value of 0.05 level.

There is higher risk of bias in cluster randomization because the investigators and in some cases the patients might know which treatment the cluster has been assigned. For example, if one hospital has been assigned to thrombolysis for MI patients and another to percutanerous transluminal coronary angioplasty (PTCA), then there might be a bias on the part of patients or referring physicians to direct some patients one way or another.

Patients in a cluster are often correlated with respect to outcome. Because of the intra-cluster correlation, the statistical analysis must adjust for this when performing the statistical tests.

16.4.4 Equivalence and Noninferiority Study Analysis

The design of equivalence studies has been discussed earlier in the book extensively in Chapters 3 and 7. When interpreting the results of an equivalence of noninferiority studies, it is important to keep in mind that if the study is not well designed, there is an incentive to conducting a sloppy study. Sloppy studies tend to muddle the results and tend to make the results look similar across the treatment groups. In a standard study, there is therefore an incentive to conduct the study in a rigorous manner, but in an equivalence study, the incentive is the opposite.

Because of this, the equivalence studies are designed around confidence intervals rather than point estimates. Sloppy studies will tend to make the point estimates converge, but will also increase the size of the confidence interval. Therefore, a well-designed equivalence study will test for the confidence intervals to fall within a certain boundary, with respect to the confidence interval for the comparative group.

The above is also applicable for noninferiority studies.

If the primary analysis is noninferiority, and the analysis is positive, then a test for equivalence or for superiority may be performed without a statistical penalty. In other words, if you prove that the therapy is noninferior to the comparator therapy, then you can test for equivalence or for superiority (at p-value of 0.05). This is in effect to hierarchical testing, and an instance where hierarchical testing is usually appropriate.

16.4.5 Interpretation of PK, PD, and Dosing Data

We have already discussed one of the most common pitfalls in analysis of PK/PD data, namely the temptation to correlate PK and PD values to outcome when the study was not designed to titrated patients to a pre-specified PK or PD values.

The end goal of PK/PD studies is to determine a safe and effective dose. The other goal, if possible, is to establish a dose–response curve, including minimally effective dose and maximally tolerated dose. Ideally, PK and PD studies will allow you to select the dose with the highest efficacy and lowest toxicity. And ideally, you will have enough data to clearly define minimally effective dose, highest tolerated dose, and the dose–response curves across a range of patients. Unfortunately, time and resource constraints require some compromises.

For some indications with very severe unmet medical need, such as oncology, it is often necessary to proceed with the highest tolerated dose because you will typically want the highest dose possible. For diseases with severe unmet medical needs where speed is the essence, such as for AIDS in the early days of the epidemic, it may be necessary to proceed quickly as soon as an acceptable dose has been identified, rather than waiting to identify the optimal dose.

There are some common misinterpretations with respect to dosing and PK/PD. In general, investigators tend to always underestimate toxicity in Phase I and Phase II for each dose. This is because limited number of patients have been treated, and it is nearly axiomatic that once additional patients have been treated additional safety issues will arise.

Also, in dose escalation studies, there is a tendency to ascribe efficacy to higher doses. In other words, if a drug is effective at 10 mg dose, a dose escalation study that tests 0.1 mg followed by 1 mg, 5 mg, 10 mg, 20 mg, 40 mg, etc. will typically find that 20 mg or 40 mg is the effective dose. You generally will overshoot the actual effective dose. Often, this is due to the fact that there are so few patients in each dose group. So a drug that will improve outcome in say 30% of the patients often will not show efficacy at the effective dose just because there hasn't been enough patient tested. In some cases this phenomenon can also occur because there can be spontaneous improvements in disease over time.

On the other hand, some drugs take a long time to exert effect, and there may be a cumulative dose effect. These effects can artificially make lower doses appear less effective than they really are. It should be very carefully ascertained that there has been enough time to assess the effect of the drug with enough time. In forced titration studies where same patient is titrated upward, it is important to be cognizant of the potential confounding due to delayed response. It is not unusual to be led astray in this type of study. For example, if a patient receives 0.1 mg followed by 1 mg, 5 mg, 10 mg, 20 mg, 40 mg, and the effect is seen at 20 mg, the true effective dose may be 30 mg, but there is carry-over effect from the earlier doses.

In optional titration studies, or titration to an endpoint, only the poor responders may be titrated to higher dose. This may result a false U-shaped curve. This can occur because at low doses, there are no responses because the drug dose is too low. And at high doses, there are no responses because only the highly refractory patients are titrated to very high doses. The less refractory patients have already responded to the medium doses.

For pharmacodynamic endpoints, it is important to be very rigorous about drawing conclusion linking the pharmacodynamic results to clinical outcome. Below is an example where clearing of bacteria is the pharmacodynamic endpoint.

A trial is conducted for sepsis. 80% of the patients in the active and 20% of the patients in the placebo arm had blood cultures clear of bacteria, and 70% of the active and 10% of the placebo patients survived.

It is tempting to conclude that the drug is effective for sepsis and furthermore that the drug acts by clearing bacteria. However, this is premature to conclude unless more analysis is performed.

TABLE 6.9 Clearance of bacteremia

	Cleared bacteremia	Did not clear bacteremia	Total
Survived	110	28	140
Died	50	12	60
Total	160	40	200

For example, what if only 15% of the active patients cleared bacteremia before clinical recovery and the 80% clearance rate was after the primary endpoint of 30 day mortality?

What if the bacteremia was assessed before the mortality but the patients who cleared were not the same patients who survived?

What if it turns out that though the difference in the 30 day mortality is pronounced, the 90 day survival were 5% in both arms?

16.4.6 Immunogenicity Data

In interpreting immunogenicity (anti-drug antibodies) data, you should remember that there are no universally accepted standards for defining a positive immunogenicity test. The cutoff values for a "positive" results varies from one organization to the next. If the cutoff is very low, then there will be high rates of positive results, including false positive results. Even patients who have never been exposed to the drug may test positive. If the cutoff is very high, then even patients with immune responses may test negative.

In addition, some of the current immunogenicity tests suffer from a major flaw in that if there is drug in the plasma, it will interfere with the assay and the results will be negative even in the presence of antibodies.

If there are antibodies to the drug in the patient, the next questions are whether they are persistent and whether they are neutralizing. Some antibodies persist over months to years, while others are much more fleeting. The antibodies with the greatest clinical impact are those that cause anaphylaxis. These are rare. The antibodies with the second greatest impact are those that neutralize the drug, especially if they cross react with endogenous proteins. Antibodies that are not neutralizing, and antibodies that chaperone the drug (increasing the half-life) generally are much less worrisome.

16.4.7 Pharmacogenomic Analysis and Related Analysis

Interpretation of pharmacogenomic data is still evolving. With the advent of single nucleotide polymorphism (SNP) maps, ultra-rapid sequencing, and high density gene chips, the greatest challenge in pharmacogenomics is sorting through a mass of data and determining which correlations are real and which are spurious. The most convincing way of establishing pharmacogenomic correlation is via a biological rationale that is specified *a priori*. For example, if you suspect in advance that the drug will be affected by P_{450} enzyme expression, and you find that is the case, a causal relationship may be established much more easily than if you sift through thousands of pharmacogenomic markers and find one that has high correlation with outcome. In the latter, the exercise would be helpful for establishing a hypothesis, but should only be considered for that purpose.

Because classic pharmacogenomic analysis relies on independent factors, namely the DNA sequence, it is not subject to the issues seen with PK/PD or other dependent factors. Most drugs will not change the DNA sequence of the patients.

However, proteomics, epigenetic analysis, RNA expression analysis, and other similar analysis may be influenced by drugs, and the analysis of such data must be performed with all the usual *caveats* pertaining to dependent factor subgrouping in mind.

16.4.8 Instrumental Variable

Instrument variable is one way of establishing causality in the absence of randomization. It is useful when you have two variable that are correlated but you don't know which is the cause and which is the effect. For example, you might find that in a group of patients with arthritis, visits to the physician are correlated with NSAID use. You are not sure if they visit the physicians because of gastric bleeding due to the NSAID use, or whether NSAID use increases because the physicians prescribe them when the patients come in for a visit. Therefore, you might select an instrumental variable, which is a variable that is correlated with one of the two original variables but could not be caused by the other variable. In this case, it might be insurance coverage for physician visits. Insurance is correlated to the number of physician visits, but NSAID use would not typically increase insurance coverage. If there is a correlation between insurance coverage and NSAID use, then the second hypothesis is probably correct.

16.5 INTERPRETATION OF SAFETY DATA

16.5.1 Challenges

Adverse events occur in all clinical trials. The adverse events might stem from a host of causes, including the following.

- Due to the drug
- Due to the disease
- Due to concomitant medications
- (Discovered) due to ascertainment
- Due to combination of the above

The goal of safety interpretation is to determine the causation of the adverse event, frequency of the event, and sequelae of the event.

There are four major challenges in interpretation of safety data. The first is that most studies are not adequately powered to detect safety events that would be of interest. Safety events that occur at low rates are often clinically

meaningful. This means that absence of safety signal in a study does not mean that the safety profile is acceptable.

The second is that p-value of 0.05 is not an acceptable target for safety events. You should not wait until you reach p-value of 0.05 before taking action on potential safety issues.

The third is that it is impossible to define all potential safety issues in advance. Safety events must be captured and categorized as they occur in most cases. This means that safety endpoints cannot, ahead of time, be categorized neatly like efficacy endpoints.

The fourth is that with some safety events, it is difficult to determine whether the incidence is increased or just represents the underlying background rate.

By nature, safety data interpretation is exploratory. Hypothesis testing is not possible except in few instances where the study is designed as a safety study, has randomized groups including a comparator, and is adequately powered. Despite the warning in the above sections about subgroup analysis and multiple analyses, safety interpretation relies on just such techniques.

The techniques to assist interpretation of nonrandomized data, such as utilizing previously generated data external to the study, assessing dose response, assessing internal consistency of patterns, should all be utilized in the interpretation of safety data.

16.5.2 Heuristics

Common Adverse Events

Much of safety interpretation depends on heuristics and Bayesian interpretation. One of the most common heuristics depends on commonly seen adverse events.

With small molecules, there are some stereotypic adverse events: hematological, hepatic, renal, dermatological, and pro-arrhythmic adverse events. All small molecules should be assessed carefully for these common adverse events, including neutropenia, thrombocytopenia, liver failure, renal failure, rash, and *Torsades de Pointes*.

With large molecules (proteins) these types of adverse events are rare, because biologics tend to only have adverse events that are extensions of their biological effect. For example, thrombolytics cause intracranial hemorrhage. Natalizumab causes viral infections (PML). There are a few exceptions, such as Trastuzumab and cardiotoxicity, but they are rare. One common adverse associated with biologics though is immunotoxicity and all biologics should be assessed carefully for immunotoxicity.

Preclinical Toxicology and Biology

Adverse events seen in preclinical toxicology studies often provide a clue regarding potential adverse events in the clinic. Adverse events that mimic and seen in toxicology studies should be taken seriously and examined closely.

Also, of course, biological relevance should play a strong role in interpretation of the adverse event. If it is plausible that the drug could cause the adverse event – for example, an antibiotic and *C. difficile* – then the likelihood of causation is higher.

Cytochrome P_{450} studies often are highly reliable in predicting metabolism issues or drug–drug interactions.

Class Effects

If a certain type of adverse event is known to be associated with a class of drugs, such as myopathy with statins, then it is highly likely that the new drug in that class will share the adverse event.

The chemical structure of the compound may also be a clue to the types of adverse events it might cause. Certain chemical moieties are associated with higher incidence of bone marrow suppression, liver failure, and other adverse events.

Dose Response and Overdose, and Time Effect

An adverse event that is real may exhibit a dose response. In particular, patients who overdose on the drug may exhibit adverse events that might be less obvious in other patients. Some drugs cause cumulative effects, and a time response may be observed: the adverse event may manifest only after the drug has been administered long term.

Relationship of the adverse events to frequency and timing of visits and dosing should be examined. This can increase or decrease the incidence of adverse events – in general, more frequent the visit, higher the rate of adverse events if the adverse event is real. There may also be a stereotypical timing relationship between visits/doses and adverse event.

If re-challenge is possible and ethical, it can provide very strong evidence that the adverse event is real and related to the drug.

Harbinger Events

Some adverse events are harbingers of more serious adverse events. For example, elevated liver function tests often presage more serious hepatic adverse events. Prolonged QT interval may presage risk for life-threatening arrhythmias.

Unmasking

The adverse event may be unmasked only under certain circumstances or in particularly vulnerable populations, such as patients such as elderly or pregnant who are particularly at risk. Or it may only be seen in some patients, or only with concomitant medications like terfenadine and erythromycin.

General Pattern

Adverse events should be examined in context of other adverse events. In addition to dose response and harbinger events, the frequency of the adverse events and overall timing and distribution pattern should be examined carefully to detect any possible pattern.

Expectedness

Investigator assessment of expectedness is on the basis of limited data. He usually doesn't have access to the overall safety database so he's at a significant disadvantage because he cannot see a potential pattern in the adverse events. Sponsor assessment of expectedness is somewhat better, but expectedness on an individual adverse event level is often misleading.

Expected Baseline Rate

If the adverse event is exceedingly rare, such as PML, causation can be relatively readily assigned. However, often the baseline rate is not as rare, and in many cases, it is not clear what the baseline rate is. Nonetheless, comparison to expected rate is often useful in understanding the adverse event pattern.

Relationship to Prompting

Adverse events that are elicited tend to be noisier (more spurious signals), because patients tend to recall more events. However, they are also more sensitive, and tend to be more consistent. If elicitation will be used, then you might want to pre-define certain adverse events are targeted adverse events, with specific definitions. This will make the data much more robust and amenable to analysis.

Ascertainment Bias

Ascertainment bias is not uncommon, especially with elicitation or mandated regular screening. Detection of squamous cell cancer, for example, is often increased due to ascertainment bias.

Dropouts

Dropouts should be examined carefully, because dropouts are often due to adverse events.

Other Explanations

If there are other plausible explanations for the adverse event, such as a concomitant medication that is known to cause the adverse event, then it makes less likely that the adverse event is due to the drug being studied, although you must be careful not to rule out a potential causal link merely on basis of alternative explanations.

16.5.3 Descriptive Analysis

Unlike efficacy results, safety events should be examined as individual events as well as in aggregate. Community acquired pneumonia that resolves after 10 days course of penicillin on an outpatient basis is different from one that requires hospitalization and prolonged IV antibiotics to resolve.

All deaths should be examined closely on an individual level. Serious adverse events should be treated similarly. Line listing of each patient and his or her adverse event profile should be reviewed, though in less detail than the deaths or serious events.

You should pay close attention to precipitating factors, mitigating factors, risk factors (including demographics, concomitant medications, etc.). If risk factors or precipitating factors can be identified, it may be possible to avoid the adverse event or exclude patients at highest risk from receiving the medication. Ideally, a single risk factor that is identifiable would be very helpful to patients and physicians. In some cases, you might need to come up with a composite risk score instrument that predicts the adverse event.

There are some stereotypical patterns of adverse events. Some events are acute, and occur at the beginning of therapy and do not recur. Others occur at beginning of therapy and continue. Yet others only occur after extended period of exposure or upon re-exposure. It is helpful to characterize the adverse events as much as possible so that prognostic information can be given to patients and physicians.

16.5.4 Consequence Analysis

In addition to the quantity of adverse events, the sequelae of adverse events are important. Did it result in death? Was it reversible or did it result in irreversible morbidity or death? You should pay careful attention to the severity of the adverse event, duration, resolution (or lack thereof), treatments required. Short-lived, reversible adverse events that can be managed with an intervention warrant a very different level of concern than catastrophic, irreversible adverse events.

16.5.5 Assessing Rare Safety Events

Rare adverse events, such as PML or pulmonary hemosiderosis, if they occur, are relatively easy to link to drug. Even one case of an event such as these would raise a very high index of suspicion that there is a causal relationship.

The difficulty with rare adverse events is most acute when the event does not occur. Most studies have very low power to detect rare adverse events. In general, if no specific adverse event is detected in a trial, then the upper bound-ary of the 95% confidence interval is 3/size of the study. For example, if no scleroderma is seen in a trial of 3000 patients, the upper boundary of the 95% confidence interval for scleroderma is 1 in 1000. Since many rare adverse events occur at a rate less than 1 in 10,000, you would have to conduct studies with tens of thousands of patients to rule out adverse events in that range of frequency.

There are a few ways, though, to increase the detection sensitivity. One is to study the drug in patients at high risk, if it is feasible and ethical to do so. For example, incidence of PML is high in transplant patients, so if a drug does not cause PML in that setting, it is less likely that it will cause it in a non-immunocompromised setting.

The other, mentioned already, is to look for harbinger signs, such as nuisance bleeding, LFT abnormalities, and increased common viral infections. They may presage intracranial hemorrhages, hepatic failure, or opportunistic infections.

16.5.6 Assessing Common Adverse Events

Common adverse events are difficult to assess, because causality is difficult to establish. If the population being studied already has an incidence of the adverse event – patients who received Cox-2 inhibitors who also had risk of MIs – or the disease itself might cause the adverse event – such as post-MI patients who are already at risk of arrhythmias and received anti-arrhythmic drugs – causation is particularly difficult to establish.

The conventional way to establish that the drug is causing the adverse event is to demonstrate that it is increasing the rate of the events. This is not always easy. In fact, passive collection of adverse events in uncontrolled studies can usually only detect common adverse events if the rate increases by 10-fold or more. Even a randomized study can generally detect about 2-fold increase. Of course, you should not wait until the p-value reaches less than 0.05 before taking action, but nonetheless, it is often hard to detect a signal in such instances.

The other way to detect common adverse events is to look at the circumstances around adverse event. For example, if patients tend to experience a headache 30 minutes after administration of a drug, and it happens consistently, it may be possible to detect that as a drug-related adverse event.

Also, special manifestations of the adverse event may turn it into an uncommon adverse event. For example, tuberculosis is a common adverse event, but disseminated tuberculosis is not. Disseminated TB should be considered to be a signal in most trials because spontaneous occurrence of it is very rare.

It is sometime helpful to perform an epidemiological assessment of external data, such as a data registry from a large health care provider, to generate comparisons but unless the numbers are very large and the differences between the database and the study profound, it is difficult to come to a definitive conclusion.

Below are regulatory definitions of frequency of various types of adverse events.

16.5.7 Effect of Lumping and Splitting

As mentioned above, categorization of safety events can have a profound impact on whether you can detect a signal or not. Here is an example.

A promising drug for refractory seizures is being developed. Unfortunately, it appears to have two drawbacks. First is the potential to cause arrhythmias. Second is

the potential to cause duodenal ulcers. Therefore, the Phase III safety data is carefully examined to assess potential signal in those two categories.

Fortunately, neither concern seems to have been justified, as no signal is apparent.

Unfortunately, if the net for arrhythmias is cast more widely to include not just the term, "arrhythmia" but also "sudden death," "palpitations," "syncope," (which can be other presentations of arrhythmia) then a signal becomes apparent.

Unless the safety events are categorized appropriately, it is easy to miss a signal.

Similarly, the fact that the drug causes acute duodenal ulcers may be completely missed. In this graph, you only see a signal for the duodenal ulcer if you "zoom" to the right level. If the adverse events are split into nausea, bloody stools, ulcers, anemia, etc. the number of events in each category is too low to generate a signal. On the other

TABLE 16.10 Regulatory terminology for frequency of adverse events

Very common	>= 10%
Common (frequent)	>=1% to <10%
Uncommon (infrequent)	>0.1% to <1%
Rare	>0.01% to <0.1%
Very rare	<0.01%

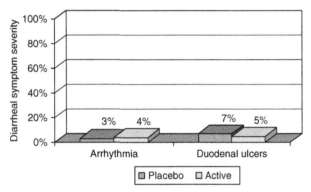

FIGURE 16.17   Frequency of arrhythmias and duodenal ulcers.

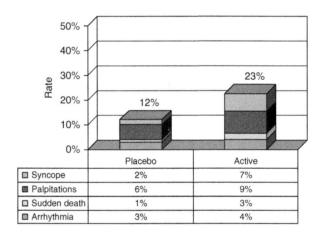

	Placebo	Active
Syncope	2%	7%
Palpitations	6%	9%
Sudden death	1%	3%
Arrhythmia	3%	4%

FIGURE 16.18   Cumulative frequency of arrhythmia related events.

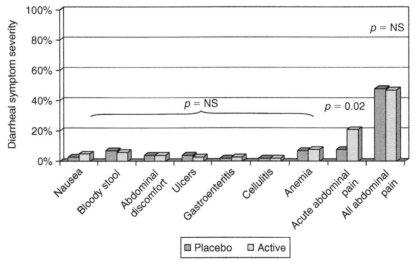

FIGURE 16.19   Cumulative frequency of abdominal pain events.

hand, if all abdominal pain is examined, then pain caused by a host of other factors swamps the signal. Only when acute abdominal pain is examined does the signal become apparent.

In most cases, it is necessary to survey the safety data at several levels of categorization and several different ways of categorization in order to be sure that you are not missing a signal.

16.5.8 Specific Safety Adverse Events

Liver Toxicity

Liver toxicity is one of the most common major adverse events. The Liver is the site of metabolism of many drugs, and small molecules often tend to exert a toxic effect on the liver. Elevated LFT's can predict liver toxicity in some cases, but unfortunately, there are currently no reliable tests for predicting catastrophic hepatic failure.

Hy's Law identifies several portents of liver failure:

1. An increased rate of transaminase elevations (3x ULN, 5x ULN, 10x ULN, etc.).
2. No evidence of obstruction (elevated AP).
3. Even a very small number of cases (one or two) of transaminase elevation accompanied by a rise in bilirubin to 2x ULN.

QT Prolongation

QT prolongation is a surrogate for *Torsade* de Points, a potential fatal arrhythmia. QT prolongation, however, is not a completely reliable surrogate, since many drugs that cause QT prolongation do not cause life-threatening arrhythmias. The FDA requires most drugs to undergo formal testing to assess QT prolongation and arrhythmic potential.

Neutropenia

Bone marrow suppression is a recognized potential side effect of small molecules. It is often caused by an immune response to the drug that also attacks hematopoetic cells. Neutropenia can be a result, but thrombocytopenia or pancytopenia may also occur. These reactions tend to be idiosyncratic (nondose related).

Drug–Drug Interaction

Drug–drug interaction can be caused by a host of factors, including direct chemical reaction, interaction through P_{450} up- or down-regulation, competition for binding to albumin, and so on. It can sometimes be predicted. Most clinical programs should assess potential for drug–drug interaction with other drugs that are expected to be used frequently.

Food–drug interaction may also occur, and should be assessed as well.

Addictive Potential and Withdrawal Effects

Some drugs have the potential to be habit-forming. Drugs that have high risk of this such as opiods and sleeping drugs should be assessed for this potential. Some drugs upregulate or downregulate homeostatic systems in the body and withdrawal could be harmful if performed abruptly. Benzodiazepines and certain anti depressants are examples of this. It is important to characterize such properties.

Tolerance

Other drugs cause tolerance. The effects wear off after continuous exposure, such as nitrates. Part of safety evaluation should include assessing for tolerance.

Rebound

Some drugs can cause rebound. The disease may return worse than it was at the beginning of treatment. Rebound assessment should also be part of safety assessment.

Assessing Laboratory Data

The goal of laboratory data assessment is to distinguish true signals from random noise, and to correlate the signals to potentially clinically significant phenomena.

The laboratory data assessment and interpretation proceeds in several steps. First, you should assess the overall pattern of changes in laboratory parameters. This can be performed by examining the mean values, then by examining the shift tables and similar display (scatterplots, box plots, cumulative distribution displays, and tables). It takes a pronounced effect to change the mean value substantially, so shift tables tend to be more informative. Then, outlier values should be examined. The shift tables tend to have the highest yield, followed by outliers.

Then, individuals who exhibit very large changes in one or more laboratory values should be examined. If the laboratory value changes are concurrent with or precede an adverse event, then this should be noted.

There are several challenges in sifting real signals from noise. First, there is regression to the mean or to outliers. If the study inclusion criteria call for patients whose hematocrit is below 35, then there will likely be some regression to the mean and some patients will appear to increase their hematocrit just from regression to the mean. Or, if the inclusion criteria call for hematocrit between 40 and 41, the distribution will spread out back to a normal curve on repeat measurement because even if the true value is 40 or 41, natural variation in measurement will re-establish a Gaussian distribution.

Also, there will always be outliers, from chance. Remember that approximately 5% of the values will lie outside 2 standard deviations from normal values. More frequently you measure the laboratory values, more outliers you will detect.

"Normal values" and cutoffs for flagging outliers have a critical impact on laboratory value analysis. If a central lab is used, then this issue is less critical, but these criteria should be carefully assessed, and if necessary, sensitivity analysis using different values should be performed.

In a controlled study, comparisons therefore should be made to the control group's laboratory values. This can help distinguish artifact from real signal.

Once a signal is detected, and once you believe that the signal is real, as opposed to random noise, you should characterize the signal. Does it tend to occur in certain subgroups? Does it occur at certain doses of the drug? Does it occur at certain times? Does it reverse when the drug is discontinued? Does it stop even if the patients continue on the drug? Does it get worse if the patients continue on the drug? Is it followed by clinical sequelae?

16.6 BROADENING THE CONCLUSIONS

16.6.1 External Validity

The objective of a clinical trial is to deliver results that can be used to improve patient care. In the final step of interpretation, the conclusions from the study are extrapolated to the patient population at large and beyond the narrow hypothesis being tested. In this step, external validity is asserted.

However, most studies are conducted on a sample of patients. In every case, the sample differs from the overall patient population in some respect, either intentionally or inadvertently. The study procedures and patient care should be as similar to clinical practice as possible but these too can never be identical to clinical care. Endpoints used in the study should capture as much of the disease burden and impact as possible but they, by necessity, must be a distillation of the full spectrum of disease burden.

Therefore, at the end of a study, you must examine the results along with the study design and study conduct and determine how the results can be applied to the patient population at large. This is a tall order. The conclusions must be based on reliable and high quality data. The analysis must be free from fallacies or technical mistakes. The results must be convincing and robust to sensitivity analysis, and the confidence intervals must be acceptable. The results must be relevant to clinical endpoints. The endpoint must be broad enough to encompass or represent the main aspects of a disease. The risk–benefit ratio must be acceptable. The patient population,

the way the study was conducted, and the way that the patients received care must be similar enough to the patient population at large so that the results will be generalizable.

This dichotomy between the trial results and real life is sometimes described as "Efficacy vs. Effectiveness." *Efficacy* is whether a drug in a rather artificial situation of a clinical trial, particularly a blinded randomized clinical trial (RCT), shows clinical effect. *Effectiveness* is whether it has clinically meaning effect in the practice setting.

For example, a study might show that a drug increases cardiac output in CHF patients. Ultimately, though, the question being answered is: Is the treatment doing more good than harm, and how much, for how long, and for which patients? The conclusions have to take into account considerations such as,

- How much was the increase in cardiac output?
- What was the safety profile?
- Did all patients experience cardiac output augmentations or just a definable subset?
- How certain is it that increasing cardiac output will result in clinical improvement?
- How robust is the data? What do the sensitivity analysis show?
- How narrow was the inclusion/exclusion criteria?
- How closely did concomitant medications and treatment pattern mimic real clinical practice?

16.6.2 Examine the Patient Population

The first step in assessing external validity is to compare the patients in the study, both intended and actually enrolled, against the intended patient population. The goal of a trial is to enroll a broad range of patients, with the hypothesis that the patients are homogeneous and that they will have a homogeneous response. Results of a study are only directly applicable for the group of patients with the severity and type of disease, time course, concomitant medications, stage of disease, and dosing. They may be indirectly applicable to patients who are not exactly analogous.

You should ask,

- Do the inclusion criteria reflect the target population?
- Do the exclusion criteria bias the results, making them inapplicable to certain portions of the population?
- Were all clinically important clinical criteria considered?

For example, if the study enrolled only patients in the VA system, most subjects will be male. This might make extrapolation to female patients problematic. It is typical that inclusion and exclusion criteria exclude patients who are old, who have multiple concurrent medical problems, and who are complicated. It is inevitable that the study population will be a narrower, better defined population than the overall patient population, but you should confirm that the criteria were not unacceptably narrow.

You should also look at the demographics of the patients who were actually enrolled and determine whether they reflect the intended patient population. For example, if the study was intended to study all multiple sclerosis patients, but ended up enrolling mostly RRMS, then the results may not be completely applicable to PPMS.

16.6.3 Inappropriate Endpoint

The importance of selecting an appropriate endpoint is discussed in Chapter 7, but in order for the study to have external validity, the endpoint must be clinically relevant. For example, if the drug is intended for treatment of rhinorrhea, the endpoint should be at several days, not at 12 months. If the drug is intended for treatment of lung cancer, it should focus on endpoints such as survival, not joint pain.

Surrogate

The greatest difficulty with external validity in clinical trials continues to be nonvalidated surrogate endpoints. Many investigators and clinicians, because they operate day to day in the world of surrogates such as X-rays, echocardiograms, and CT scans, often overestimate the value of surrogates. You should remember that surrogates in clinical trials should be interpreted with great caution. Below is a classic example of a surrogate gone wrong.

> Many patients die of sudden death secondary to arrhythmias after an MI. It is well established that the patients with the greatest number of premature ventricular contractions (PVCs) are at the highest risk of death. In the past, several drugs were developed to prevent PVCs, and they were believed to be effective in preventing life-threatening arrhythmias.
>
> Cardiac Arrhythmia Suppression Trial (CAST) was a study of anti-arrhythmic drugs designed to demonstrate that the drugs lowered mortality post-MI. It was initiated amidst controversy, because many physicians thought it was unethical to randomize patients to placebo.
>
> Unfortunately, the drugs did not prevent the arrhythmias, but rather caused to increase them and in fact increased the incidence of sudden death. CAST was terminated early by the Data Safety Monitoring Boards (DSMB).

Surrogates are often used in clinical trials and the results of the studies are then extrapolated to influence clinical practice. As this example shows, the surrogates can be misleading. Below is another example.

> There is overwhelming data proving that in CHF patients, higher the level of TNF, more likely they are to die. Because of this a large study was conducted to reduce mortality by administering TNF inhibitor.

> The study conclusively showed that blocking TNF increased, rather than decreased, mortality.

Biomarkers that are correlated with a disease can sometimes be a good surrogate if they are in the causal pathway, and a good drug target if they are in the causal pathway between the drug action and clinical outcome. However, they are more often an epiphenomenona and therefore not in the causal pathway, or are caused by the disease, rather than causing the disease. In some cases, as with TNF, they may be a protective counterregulatory response to the disease.

Therefore, correlation with diseases or disease outcome in and of themselves does not mean that it can serve as proxy for the clinical outcome. A surrogate can be helpful if used correctly, but they must be validated first.

16.6.4 Relative vs. Absolute Difference

Another important concept is the concept of relative vs. absolute difference. If a drug reduces the rate of exacerbations from 40% to 30%, the relative reduction is 25% and the absolute is 10%. Depending on clinical circumstances, one or the other might be more appropriate. It is important to weigh both, and to be clear when one is being used vs. another.

In some studies, the results may be impressive in terms of relative difference but not in terms of absolute difference. For example, a drug might decrease the incidence of deep vein thrombosis (DVT) after flying on an airplane. The relative difference might be impressive: 75% reduction. However, since the rate is very low to begin with, the absolute reduction might be miniscule and clinically insignificant: 1 in 50,000 to 1 in 200,000.

16.6.5 Practicability Considerations

Clinical trials are often conducted in highly controlled circumstances with well-trained personnel and adequate support personnel to make even difficult or cumbersome procedures practicable. Unfortunately, in clinical practice, some therapies that are workable in clinical trials turn out to be impractical.

For example, an oral drug that is administered five times per day may be acceptable (barely) in a clinical trial, but would be almost impossible to prescribe in clinical practice. So would a subcutaneous drug that is injected three times per day. Similarly, a drug that requires 20 minutes of preparation would probably be too cumbersome to be acceptable as a self-administered therapy for a non-life-threatening disease.

Sometimes concomitant procedures can make the drug impracticable. For example, a drug that requires multiple blood tests before and after each dose of the drug makes the drug unacceptable in some indications.

Of course, the severity of the disease, the efficacy of the drug, and availability of alternate therapies will all influence the acceptability and practicability of the drug. Nonetheless, external validity cannot be achieved if the procedures and administration techniques used in the clinical trial cannot be feasibly transferred to the real life clinical setting.

16.6.6 Risk–Benefit Analysis and Generalizability

The primary endpoint of a trial is often expressed in a dichotomous fashion: positive or negative. Either the trial met its endpoint or it did not. However, the ultimate utility of a trial depends on a host of factors, including the risk–benefit ratio. Did the magnitude of the benefit outweigh the magnitude of the side effects? More broadly, did the magnitude of the benefit outweigh the cost, inconvenience, known side effects and the potential unknown (as of yet) side effects?

In order to make this determination, several factors go into play.

First, you should determine how much benefit was observed. This is *not* the same as *p*-value. It is possible to achieve very small *p*-values with a trivial clinical benefit if the sample size is large enough. For example, an increase in walk distance of 10 m may have a *p*-value of 0.01 with a sample size of 100, and the same increase might have a *p*-value of 0.00001 with a sample size of 5000.

Second, was the benefit seen in everyone or was there a subgroup that benefited the most? Is it possible to predict who will benefit? Does the benefit accumulate over time? Is there tachyphlaxis? Is there rebound?

In other words, you should determine how much benefit there is, and how it is distributed among the patients. You should also determine if there are ways to maximize the magnitude of the benefit.

Next, you should examine the safety profile. What were the adverse events that were observed? Is it possible to determine who is at risk of the harm? Is it possible to detect the adverse event early, and perhaps early enough to treat it?

Just as with efficacy, you should determine how many safety issues there are, and how they are distributed among the patients. You should also determine if there are ways to minimize the impact of the adverse events.

However, one aspect of safety makes the risk–benefit assessment asymmetrical. While efficacy is often fairly well defined from the clinical study, risk is almost always incompletely defined. This is because most studies are not large enough to characterize the safety profile well. Just as no drug is 100% safe, no clinical study or program will completely characterize the safety profile. Therefore, when assessing the risk–benefit, you must be cognizant that you are weighing the known benefits against both known and as-yet unknown risks.

16.6.7 Conclusions

As you are drawing the final conclusions, you should keep in mind some of the classical mistakes that many people make. Some of the mistakes arise from the inherent design of the study. For example, confirmation bias is the tendency to look for confirmatory evidence, and not for evidence to disprove one's assumptions; and it tends to be common – cognitively, humans tend look for data to confirm their prior beliefs and ignore the ones that tend to refute it. This is often true in clinical trials. It may be noted that a headache seems to develop in patients who have had coffee with the drug. One of the first things that researchers would do would be to determine whether stopping the coffee would decrease the incidence of headaches. They look for confirmation. What they do not do is to stop the sugar, or start patients on coffee. They tend not to conduct the experiment that would refute the hypothesis.

A mistake that arises from rescue bias is the tendency to find faults in the study to invalidate it if the results are not as expected – for example, finding that the patient population selected is not representative, or that the blinding was inadequate.

Auxiliary hypothesis bias is similar to rescue bias, but rather than invalidating the results of the study, this is the tendency to try to limit the generalizability of the study – that had the wrong dose been used, or the follow-up been longer, had the patients been younger, etc. Mechanism bias is similar – it is related to what happens with multiple comparisons – and refers to the natural human tendency to accept even a spurious results if it makes sense.

Well-controlled randomized clinical trials (RCT) have been a major advance over traditional, anecdotal sources of medical knowledge. These trials harness the power of aggregate data, and leverage the ability of randomization to minimize bias. The results of well-controlled RCT's have revolutionized medicine and the reliability of medical evidence. However, there are many potential traps and fallacies in designing, executing, and analyzing clinical trials. When improperly done, wrong results and conclusions can follow, and the consequent damage can be amplified by the respect that clinical trials are accorded today. This makes it especially important that extreme rigor is applied to all stages of these clinical trials.

FDA Internal Compliance Manuals

7. FDA *Compliance Program 7348.811*: *Bioresearch Monitoring*: *Clinical Investigators*

OCTOBER 1, 1997

7348.811 CHAPTER 48 – BIORESEARCH MONITORING

CLINICAL INVESTIGATORS OCTOBER 1, 1997 SEPTEMBER 30, 2000

PART I: BACKGROUND

Since the Investigational New Drug Regulations went into effect in 1963, *the Food and Drug Administration (FDA)* has exercised oversight of the conduct of studies with regulated products. The Bioresearch Monitoring Program was established in 1977 by a task force, *that* included representatives from the drug, biologic, devices, veterinary *drug*, and food areas. *Compliance programs (CP) were developed *to provide uniform guidance and specific instruction for* inspections of clinical investigators (CP 7348.811), sponsors (CP 7348.810), biopharmaceutic laboratories (CP 73 48.001) now known as *in vivo* bioequivalence, institutional review boards (CP 7348.809), and *nonclinical* laboratories (CP 7348.808).

New regulations dealing with obligations of clinical investigators, sponsors, and monitors (21 CFR Parts 312, 314, 511, and 514) were published on March 19, 1987, and became effective on June 17, 1987. Regulations *for clinical investigations of devices* (21 CFR Part 812) became effective on January 18, 1980.*

Guidance documents for the monitoring of clinical investigations were published in January 1988 and May 1997, ICH Good Clinical Practice: Consolidated Guideline (for human drugs and biologics); and Good Target Animal Study Practices: Clinical Investigators and Monitors (for veterinary drugs).*

PART II: IMPLEMENTATION

Objective

*The purpose of the bioresearch monitoring program is to assure the quality integrity of data submitted to FDA to demonstrate the safety and efficacy of regulated products, and to determine that human rights and the welfare of human and animal research subjects are adequately protected.

The objective of this program is to obtain compliance of clinical investigators with the regulations and to assess through audit procedures whether records substantiate data submitted to FDA.*

Program Management Instructions

1. Coverage
   All assignments for inspections will issue from Headquarters.
   a. Clinical investigators
      Individuals within and outside the United States working under an application for research, or marketing permit. Areas to be covered include food additives, drugs, biologics, devices, and animal drugs (including animal food additives).

      Foreign inspections of clinical investigators are assigned when the studies covered provide data critical to product approval regardless of whether the studies are conducted under an FDA application for research.
   b. Sponsor/investigators
      This group consists of individuals who initiate and also conduct the study. Assignments covering this group will be relatively few in number. Most assignments of these investigators will come from the Center for Biologics Evaluation and Research.

Other Requirements

1. All Headquarters and Field units are encouraged to recommend to the appropriate Center any investigator *that* they believe needs to be inspected. All recommendations should include the following:
   a. the name and address of the clinical investigator;
   b. the name of the test article(s) being investigated, the application for research, or marketing permit number(s); and
   c. the basis for recommendation.
   The Field should notify the Center contact when a previously uninspected *Institutional Review Board (IRB)* or an IRB not inspected within 5 years is identified during the course of a clinical investigator inspection.
2. The assignment memo *should* specify a due date *and the headquarters address where the EIR should be sent*. The reasons for expediting any assignment, including outstanding assignments, *should* be provided. To expedite inspections, Center personnel *may* contact the Director of the appropriate District Investigations Branch *to* request an FDA investigator *be assigned* to perform the inspection. The *designated investigator should contact* the Center contact person as soon as possible for a briefing on the background of the planned inspection and to make arrangements *for* participation by headquarters personnel. When the Center and the District agree upon arrangements, the Center will issue a confirmatory assignment, that is *electronic mail*, fax, mail, to the District.
3. Pre-inspection contact with the Center
   The District will resolve any questions it has on the assignment with the appropriate Center program contact.
   During the course of the inspection, additional communications will often occur between the District and the Center. This is encouraged to ensure the rapid and efficient completion of the inspection and the report preparation.
4. Inspection feedback
   Any suggestions from the field for improvement in this program should be forwarded to the Division of Compliance Policy (DCP, HFC-230) with a copy to the Division of * Emergency and Investigational Operations* (DEIO, HFC-130)*.
5. Inspection teams – Field/Headquarters
   a. Team leader
      The field investigator will serve as team leader and is fully responsible for the conduct of the inspection in accordance with Investigations Operations Manual (IOM) section 502.4.
   b. Headquarters participants
      Headquarters personnel will serve in a scientific advisory capacity to the team leader and will participate in the inspection by:
      1. identifying specific studies to be covered by the inspection team and providing information

pertinent to the scheduled inspection directly from the involved Center(s);
2. attending pre-inspection conferences;
3. participating in the on-site inspection; and
4. aiding as necessary in preparation of the establishment inspection report and the FDA 483 as required.

Any difficulties involving headquarters participation in the inspection should be discussed with district management and, if not resolved, immediately referred to DCP (HFC-230).

PART III: INSPECTIONAL

Inspections will involve a comparison of the practices and procedures of the clinical investigator with the commitments made in the applicable regulations as described in this part of the program.

Many inspections will include a comparison of the data submitted to the sponsor with supporting data in the clinical investigator's files. This will always be the case in human drugs and biologics inspections. Original records should be examined and may include office records, hospital records, laboratory reports, records of consultations, etc.

Inspectional Operations: General Instructions

1. The nature of these inspections makes unannounced visits to the clinical investigator impractical. Appointments to inspect should, therefore, be made by telephone, unless otherwise instructed in special cases by the Center. To facilitate the inspection of a clinical investigator at a Veterans Administration (VA) facility, the FDA investigator should also contact the Medical Center Director. For military installations, the Chief of Professional Services should be the initial contact.
   The FDA investigator should, however, keep the time span between initial contact and actual inspection as short as possible. What appears to be undue delay *(such as more than 10 working days without sufficient justification)* of the inspection on the part of the clinical investigator shall be reported immediately to the Center.
2. If during the inspection, access to records or copying of records is refused for any reason, the FDA investigator should call the supervisor and report the refusal so that the assigning Center can be advised promptly by telephone. The same procedure should be followed when it becomes evident that delays instituted by the inspected are such that they constitute a de facto refusal. IOM Section 514 provides additional guidance.
   If actions by the *person being inspected* take the form of a partial refusal of inspection of documents or

areas to which FDA is entitled under the law, call attention to 301(e) and (f) and 505(k)(2) of the FD&C Act, and if the refusal persists, proceed with the inspection and then telephone your supervisor. The assigning Center should be contacted for instructions.

If a course of action to deal with a refusal cannot be resolved expeditiously by the Center or the Office of Regional Operations (ORO), DCP should be advised by the assigning Center.

3. If deviations from the regulations *that might affect data validity, endanger test subject health or welfare,* are encountered during an inspection, call the Center contact so that a determination can be made as to whether the inspection should be expanded to be more intensive or to include other studies or target groups. The appropriate Center will provide guidance on initiating an in depth audit inspection; however, the FDA investigator should continue the inspection.

4. For efficiency, a concurrent inspection may be indicated for a previously uninspected IRB or an IRB, which has not been inspected within the past 5 years. If such an IRB is found during the course of a clinical investigator inspection, contact the assigning Center for guidance and assignment. See CP 7348.809 for the IRB contact for each Center.

5. Issue a Form FDA 483, Inspectional Observations, at the conclusion of the inspection when deviations from regulations are observed. Deviations from guidance documents do not warrant inclusion on the FDA 483; however, they should be discussed with management and documented in the EIR.

Inspection Procedures

This part identifies the nature of the information that must be obtained during each inspection to determine if the clinical investigator is meeting obligations under appropriate regulations. This outline provides only the minimal scope of the inspection and each FDA investigator should extend the inspection as the facts evolve. The inspections conducted should be sufficient in scope to determine the clinical investigator's practices for each point identified. The FDA investigator should *not* attempt to scientifically evaluate the data or protocols maintained by the clinical investigator; however, relevant documents should be reviewed, as appropriate. Evaluation of the scientific merit of the study is done by the FDA scientific reviewers receiving the application. Full narrative reporting of any deviations from existing regulations is required, and deviations must be documented sufficiently to form the basis of a legal or administrative action. For example, any records containing data not comparable with data submitted to FDA should be copied and documented as to what caused the discrepancy. Title 18 violations may require extensive documentation.

Discuss the situation with your supervisor and the appropriate Center prior to embarking on this type of coverage.

Each inspection *must* include a list of all studies performed by the clinical investigator including those for government agencies and for commercial sponsors. This is needed in case a problem is found in an inspected study which requires reevaluation of claims in other agency documents or which requires notification of another government agency.

Authority and Administration

1. Determine how (e.g., telephone, memo, etc.) the monitor explained to the clinical investigator the status of the test article, nature of the protocol, and the obligations of a clinical investigator.
2. Determine whether authority for the conduct of the various aspects of the study was delegated properly so that the investigator retained control and knowledge of the study.
3. Determine if and why the investigator discontinued the study before completion.
4. List the name and address of the facility performing laboratory tests.

If any laboratory testing was performed in the investigator's own facility, determine whether that facility is equipped to perform each test specified.

List name(s) of individuals performing such tests and indicate their position.

Protocol

1. *Obtain copies of the protocol and all IRB approvals and modifications (including dates) to the protocol. Unavailability should be reported and documented. If a copy of the protocol and IRB approvals and modifications is sent with the assignment background material, they should be compared to the protocol and approvals at the site. If they are identical, duplicate copies do not need to be obtained, but the documents sent with the assignment should be returned with the EIR. The narrative should note that the protocol and IRB approvals and modifications were identical.*
2. Did the protocol remain unchanged with respect to:
   a. subject selection *(i.e., inclusion and exclusion criteria)*,
   b. number of subjects,
   c. frequency of subject observations,
   d. dosage,
   e. route of administration,
   f. frequency of dosage,
   g. blinding procedures,
   h. other (specify)?

3. Determine whether all changes to the protocol were:
   a. documented by *an approved amendment*,
   b. dated,
   c. maintained with the protocol,
   d. *approved by the IRB and reported to the sponsor before implementation*, and except where necessary, to eliminate apparent immediate hazard to human subjects.

Note: *Deviations from* protocol are not changes in the protocol.

Subjects' Records

1. Describe the investigator's *source documents* in terms of their organization, condition, completeness, and legibility.
2. Determine whether there is adequate documentation to assure that all audited subjects did exist and were alive and available for the duration of their stated participation in the study.
3. Compare the *source documents* in the clinical investigator's records with the case report forms completed for the sponsor. Determine whether clinical laboratory testing (including EKGs, X-rays, eye exams, etc.), as noted in the case report forms, was documented by the presence of completed laboratory records among the *source documents*.

   Determine whether *all* adverse *experiences* were reported in the case report forms. Determine whether they were regarded as caused by or associated with the test article and if they were previously anticipated (*specificity and* severity) in any written information regarding the test article.

   Concomitant therapy and/or intercurrent illnesses might interfere with the evaluation of the effect of the test article. Were concomitant therapy and/or intercurrent illnesses included in the case report forms? Determine whether the number and type of subjects entered into the study were confined to the protocol limitations.

   Determine whether the existence of the condition for which the test article was being studied is documented by notation made prior to the initiation of the study or by a compatible history.
4. Determine whether each record contains:
   a. observations, information, and data on the condition of the subject at the time the subject entered into the clinical study;
   b. records of exposure of the subject to the test article;
   c. observations and data on the condition of the subject throughout participation in the investigation including results of lab tests, development of unrelated illness, and other factors which might alter the effects of the test article; and

d. the identity of all persons and locations obtaining raw data or involved in the collection or analysis of such data.
5. Determine whether the clinical investigator reported all dropouts, and the reasons therefore, to the sponsor.

Other Study Records

Review information *in* the clinical investigator's records *that* will be helpful in assessing any under-reporting of adverse *experiences* by the sponsor to the agency. The Centers will send you the following information obtained from the sponsor with the assignment (currently not routine for CVM):

1. the total number of subjects entered into the study,
2. the total number of dropouts from the study (identified by subject number),
3. the number of assessable subjects and the number of inassessable subjects (the latter identified by subject number), and
4. *the adverse experiences, including deaths (with subject number and a description of the adverse experience or cause of death).*

The data supplied by the sponsor to the agency should be compared to the information submitted by the clinical investigator to the sponsor from the clinical investigator's files. For the adverse reactions and deaths use the clinical investigator's correspondence files as it is not practical to search through each case report form. Document any discrepancies found.

Consent of Human Subjects

1. Obtain a copy of the consent form *that was* used.
2. Determine whether written informed consent was obtained from subjects prior to their entry into the study. *A representative sample of consent forms should be reviewed for compliance with 21 CFR 50. If any problems are found the sample should be expanded to determine the extent of the problem.* If oral consent was obtained, *determine if it conformed to 21 CFR 50.

Institutional Review Board (IRB)

1. Identify the name, address, and chairperson of the IRB for the study.
2. Determine whether the investigator maintains copies of all reports submitted to the IRB and reports of all actions by the IRB. Determine the nature and frequency of periodic reports submitted to the IRB.

   Determine whether the investigator submitted a report *to the IRB* of all deaths, adverse experiences and unanticipated problems involving risk to human subjects [21 CFR 312.66].*

3. Did the investigator submit to and obtain IRB approval of the following before subjects were allowed to participate in the investigation?
   a. protocol
   b. modifications to the protocol
   c. report of prior investigations
   d. materials to obtain human subject consent
   e. media ads for patient/subject recruitment

4. Did the investigator disseminate any promotional material or otherwise represent that the test article is safe and effective for the purpose for which it is under investigation? Were these*promotional materials* submitted to the IRB for review *and approval before use?*

Sponsor

1. Did the investigator provide a copy of the IRB approved consent form to the sponsor?
2. Determine if periodic reports were submitted to the sponsor.
*3. *Determine if and how the investigator submitted a report of all deaths and adverse reactions to the sponsor.
4. Determine whether all intercurrent illness and/or concomitant therapy were reported to the sponsor.
*5. *Determine whether all case report forms on subjects were submitted to the sponsor shortly after completion.
*6. *Determine whether all dropouts, and the reasons therefore, were reported to the sponsor.
*7. *Did the sponsor monitor the progress of the study to assure that investigator obligations were fulfilled? Briefly describe the method (on-site visit, telephone, contract research organization, etc.) and frequency of monitoring. Do the study records include a log of on-site monitoring visits and telephone contact?

Test Article Accountability

1. Determine whether unqualified or unauthorized persons administered or dispensed the test article.
   What names are listed on the FDA-1571 (for Sponsor–Investigator) *and* FDA-1572? Obtain a copy of all FDA-1572s.
   If copies of the FDA-1572s were sent with the assignment background material, they should be compared to the FDA-1572s at the site. If they are identical, duplicate copies do not need to be obtained, but the FDA-1572s sent with the assignment should be returned with the EIR. The narrative should note that the FDA-1572s sent with the assignment and examined at the site, were identical.

2. Determine accountability procedures for test article; verify the following:
   a. receipt date(s) and quantity;
   b. dates and quantity dispensed, identification *numbers of subjects*;
   c. whether distribution of the test article was limited to those *subjects* under the investigator's *or subinvestigators* direct supervision;
   d. whether the quantity, frequency, duration, and route of administration of the test article, as reported to the sponsor, was generally corroborated by raw data notations;
   e. date(s) and quantity returned to sponsor or alternate disposition, authorization for alternate disposition, and the actual disposition;
   f. Compare test article usage with amount shipped and returned. If available, inspect unused supplies and verify that blinding, identity, lot number, and package and labeling agree with other study records describing the test article.

3. Inspect storage area.
   Determine whether the test article was stored under appropriate conditions.
   *Determine whether the test article is a controlled substance and whether it is securely locked in a substantially constructed enclosure.
   Determine who had access to the controlled substance.*

4. What is the date the last subject completed the study? Were test articles returned when either:
   a. the investigator discontinued or completed his/her participation;
   b. the sponsor discontinued or terminated the investigation; or
   c. the FDA terminated the investigation?
   If none of the above, determine whether alternate disposition of the test article exposed humans or food-producing animals to *risks from the test article(s)?*

Records Retention

1. Determine who maintains custody of the required records and the means by which prompt access can be assured.
   Determine whether the investigator notified the sponsor in writing regarding the custody of required records, if the investigator does not retain them.

2. Determine whether the records are retained for the specified time as follows:
   a. Two years following the date on which the test article is approved by FDA for marketing for the purposes which were the subject of the clinical investigation; or
   b. Two years following the date on which the entire clinical investigation (not just the investigator's part in it) is terminated or discontinued by the sponsor.

(For some studies selected as the basis of the inspection, the above time periods are not applicable.)

*Electronic Records and Signatures

*FDA published the Electronic Records; Electronic Signatures; Final Rule (21 CFR 11) on March 20, 1997. The rule became effective on August 20, 1997. Records in electronic form that are created, modified, maintained, archived, retrieved, or transmitted under any records requirement set forth in agency regulations must comply with 21 CFR 11. The following questions are provided to aid evaluation electronic records and electronic signatures:

1. What is the source of the hardware and software?
2. Who was responsible for installation and training?
3. Was the same hardware and software used throughout the duration of the study?
4. Was there any maintenance, including upgrading, conducted on the systems?
5. Were there any problems experienced during the course of the study?
6. What is the source of data entered into the computer?
   a. Direct (no paper)?
   b. Case report form?
   c. Office record?
   d. Other?
7. Who enters data? When?
8. Who has access to the computer? Security procedures?
9. How are data previously entered changed? By whom? Is an audit trail produced?
10. How are data submitted to the sponsor (i.e., modem, network, fax, hard disk, floppy disk, electronic transfer, mail, messenger, picked up)?
11. If the *sponsor* discovers errors, omissions, etc., in the data received, what contacts are made with the investigator? How are corrections effected, and how are they documented?
12. Does the clinical investigator retain a copy of the electronic data submitted to the sponsor?*

Animal Clinical Studies

The regulations for investigational new animal drugs, 21 CFR 511.1, do not contain all the provisions of the human drug regulations. There is no requirement that forms 1571 or 1572 be used. The sponsor must submit a Notice of Claimed Investigational Exemption per 21 CFR 511.1(b)(4)(i), (ii), (iii), (iv), and (v). There is no requirement that an approved protocol be used, or even that a protocol be submitted to CVM. For these reasons, inspections of animal clinical trials are extremely important as a

means of interim review. CVM assignments will include, when available, the Notice of Drug Shipment, the version of the protocol provided to CVM by the sponsor for the study(ies) to be conducted, and a checklist or list of questions provided by the reviewer to focus the direction of the inspection on critical attributes of the study(ies). *The investigator should contact the assigning office prior to initiating the inspection and maintain communication during and after the inspection.*

*CVMs guidance document "Good Target Animal Study Practices: Clinical Investigators and Monitors" was issued in May 1997. The guidance document supersedes the January 1988 "Guidance for Monitoring of Clinical Investigations" as it relates to clinical studies of new animal drugs and replaces CVM's 1992 guidance document "Conduct of Clinical Investigations: Responsibilities of Clinical Investigators and Monitors for Investigational New Animal Drug Studies." The guidance document offers focus to field investigators as to what study procedures CVM considers acceptable. This guidance document is listed in the reference section of this program. When CVM issues an assignment, a copy of the guidance document will be included and may be given to the clinical investigator at the exit discussion. Deviations from this guidance document should not be recorded on the FDA Form 483, but may be discussed at the exit interview:

1. Examine the facilities if possible, including requirements of animal quarters, segregation of animals, and method of identification. If appropriate, take photographs of the research facilities for inclusion in the EIR.
2. Report on the condition of the animals and adequacy of husbandry practices.
3. Report the method of identification in trials using food-producing animals.
4. Compare the protocol submitted to the CVM by the sponsor with the copy of the protocol used by the clinical investigator. Note any differences and document any deviations from either protocol in the EIR.
5. Collect a copy of the clinical investigator's final report.

6. Determine if multiple versions of data exist and which data are source data. Document discrepancies between versions, that is paper and electronic media.

7. Determine whether scientific measurements are made on individual animals or on groups, that is herds, pens, or flocks. Determine whether the investigator maintains records on these groups.

8. Determine the number of animals by age, weight, sex, and breed. Compare to the protocol and report any discrepancies.

9. Determine whether this is the only study each test animal has participated in within a 30-day period prior to initiation or after completion of the study.

10. Document the history of the test animals including any prior treatments or vaccinations.

11. Determine the actual inclusion/exclusion procedure that was done compared to the procedures noted in the protocol and describe any differences.

12. Document any other drugs, vaccines, or pesticides used on the animals during the study.

13. Determine the scope and extent of the blinding procedures employed in the study and document any practices that may have compromised the blinding procedures.

14. Determine whether the medicated feed is mixed on premises. (If not, report name and address of the mill utilized.)

15. Review the drug mixing procedures for animal feeds.

16. Determine the method used to identify each lot of drug or medicated feed, and the number of samples and types of assays run on the finished feed to verify dosage level. *If available for sampling, check with the assigning office on the need to collect a sample.*

17. If the investigation involves food-producing animals, determine whether the investigator observed the time periods (withdrawal, withholding, or discard periods) required for authorization to use edible products from such animals.

18. Determine if there is any evidence of unreported adverse reactions, toxic symptoms, or other observations in the investigator's notes. Include observed symptoms, clinical pathology, and diagnostic procedures.

19. Account for all the animals and drugs that were authorized for the study. Collect documentation of animals lost from a study and those that are removed from or added to the study. Examine necropsy and disposal reports for all animals lost during the trial and determine the method of disposal of animal wastes and carcasses.

20. Determine whether the investigator informed the owner(s) of each subject that the test article is being used for research purposes and whether owner consent was documented. (Current regulations do not require written consent.)

Device Studies

The regulations for investigational devices are found in 21 CFR 812. They do not contain all the provisions of the drug regulations. There is no requirement that Forms 1571 or 1572 be used but there is a requirement for a signed investigator agreement.

1. Determine whether the clinical investigator has used the test articles under the emergency use provisions. If so, determine if the clinical investigator has adequately complied with the guidance documents for emergency use.

2. Determine if the clinical investigator is involved in any nonsignificant risk studies and if so, provide a list of these studies and ascertain if they are being conducted in compliance with regulations (must have nonsignificant determination by IRB and IRB approval).

3. Determine if the clinical investigator has been involved in any use of a custom device; if so, determine compliance with 21 CFR 812 regulations.

4. Determine if the clinical investigator has been involved in any studies using humanitarian devices as provided by 21 CFR Part 814. A humanitarian use device (HUD) is a device that is intended to benefit subjects by treating or diagnosing a disease or condition that affects or is manifested in fewer than 4000 individuals in the United States annually. Determine whether IRB approval was properly obtained.

Report Format

*Reports covering inspections of clinical investigators should be prepared in accordance with IOM Section 590.

When significant violations of the FD&C Act or other Federal statutes are suspected, OAI reports must contain full narratives and accompanying documentation to support the inspectional findings. If obtaining all documentation will unduly delay the submission of the report to the Center, prepare and submit the report to the Center and then continue the investigation after consultation with the assigning Center to obtain necessary documentation. (See also Part V.)

The assigning Center may request a full EIR narrative in the assignment memorandum.

Abbreviated establishment inspection reports (EIR) may be prepared in a "Summary of Findings Report" format as described below for all non-violative inspections (NAI). For VAI inspections, abbreviated reports must contain sufficient narrative and accompanying documentation to support the inspectional findings. The abbreviated report must contain information about prior inspectional history, where the study was conducted, the responsibilities and functions of the primary personnel involved, and a definitive statement about what documents were examined, for example "I was provided in the inspection package 10 case report forms. I attempted to compare them with corresponding hospital charts. All were available. No discrepancies were found. Signed consent forms were present in each chart."

Note: An abbreviated report does not mean that an abbreviated inspection can be conducted. All inspections conducted under this compliance program shall be complete and full data audit inspections. The specific headings appearing under Part III "Inspection Procedures" should be fully addressed during the data audit inspection.

Abbreviated Report Format

Note: The following statement should precede the abbreviated EIR: This is an abbreviated report of a full Clinical Investigator/Data Audit Inspection.

The following items must be included in an abbreviated report:

1. Reason for inspection:
 - Identify the headquarters unit that initiated and/or issued the assignment.
 - State the purpose of the inspection.
2. What was covered:
 - Identify the clinical study, protocol number, sponsor, NDA/PMA/PLA/ANDA, etc.
 - Location of study.
3. Administrative procedures:
 - Report the name, title, and authority of the person to whom credentials were shown and FDA-482 Notice of Inspection was issued.
 - Persons interviewed.
 - Who accompanied you during EI?
 - Who provided relevant information?
 - Identify the IRB.
 - Prior inspectional history.
4. Individual responsibilities:
 - Identify study personnel and summarize their responsibilities relative to the clinical study.
 - Statement about who obtained informed consent and how it was obtained.
 - Identify by whom the trial was monitored, and when, etc.
5. Inspectional findings:
 - Statement about comparison of data recorded on the case report forms or tables supplied by the Center with the clinical investigators source documents.

- State what records were covered, that is patient charts, hospital records, lab slips, etc.
- Number of files and case report forms reviewed are of the total study population.
- Statement that test article accountability records were or were not sufficient.
- Discussion of 483 observations, reference the exhibits/documentation collected.
- State whether there was evidence of under reporting of adverse experiences/events.
- Statement about protocol adherence.
6. Discussion with management:
   - Discussion of 483 observations and non-483 observations.
   - Clinical investigators response to observations.*

Sample Collection

Routine collection of samples from clinical investigators is not contemplated. If samples are desired or appropriate, specific instructions will be issued by the Center (see item 16, Animal Clinical Studies). If there is a noticeable difference (such as color, size, shape, dosage form, route of administration, etc.) between the test article and the placebo or control, collect investigational samples (1 package) of each.

PART IV: ANALYTICAL

Sample analysis will not normally be required of the field laboratories.

PART V: REGULATORY/ADMINISTRATIVE STRATEGY

1. Each *Establishment Inspection Report* and the exhibits will be forwarded directly to the appropriate Center. All letters will be issued from the appropriate Center. *The EIRs should be sent by overnight express or certified mail, but never by interoffice mail. Exhibits should be banded, bound, or secured.*

   Copies of inspection reports, which contain findings of such a serious nature that they raise the possibility of one or more violations of the FD&C Act or other federal statutes should also be forwarded to the District Compliance Branch. Based on this review, the District Compliance Branch may issue investigation assignments for the development of the case. These intentions will be communicated promptly to the Center for consultation and concurrence prior to issuance of such investigational assignments.

2. Centers will coordinate their regulatory/administrative efforts when more than one Center is involved. The Associate Commissioner for Regulatory Affairs will resolve all regulatory policy disagreements between Centers prior to action.

3. *District EIR Classification Authority*

   The District Investigations Branch is encouraged to review and initially classify inspection reports generated under this compliance program, including those containing data audits. The final classification decision will be made by the Center and communicated to the District as described below.

4. *Center EIR Classification Authority*

   The Center has the *final* classification authority for all bioresearch monitoring inspection reports.

   Instances may arise when Center review results in a reclassification of an EIR reviewed and classified by the District. The Center will provide to the appropriate District copies of all final classifications including any reasons for changes.

5. *EIR Classifications*

   The following guidance is to be used in conjunction with the instructions in FMD-86 for District and Center classification of EIRs generated under this compliance program:

   a. NAI – No objectionable conditions or practices were found during the inspection *(or the objectionable conditions found do not justify further regulatory action).*

   b. VAI – Objectionable conditions or practices were found, *but the District is not prepared to take or recommend any administrative or regulatory action.*.

   c. OAI – *Regulatory and/or Administrative actions will be recommended.*

Follow-up Actions

1. All District follow-up action, including reinspection, will usually be done *in response to an assignment from headquarters*. On occasion, district compliance branches may initiate case development activities and may issue investigative assignments whenever review of the inspection report raises the possibility of severe violation of the FD&C Act or other Federal statute. This intention *should* be *prior to initiation of these

activities* communicated to the affected Center and to *DCP* (HFC-230).

2. The regulatory/administrative actions that can be used under this compliance program are not mutually exclusive. Follow-up of an OAI inspection may involve the use of one or more of the following:

   a. Issuance of a Warning Letter.

   b. Informing the sponsor that the study is not acceptable in support of claims of *safety or* efficacy in an application for research or marketing permit.

   c. Sponsor inspection (may be concurrent with other action including termination of the IND according to 21 CFR 312.44, or the INAD according to 21 CFR 511.1, or the IDE according to 21 CFR 812.30).

   d. Initiation of disqualification procedures or entry into a consent agreement with the clinical investigator under 21 CFR 312.70, 21 CFR 511.1, *or 21 CFR 812.119.*

      Disqualification of the investigator may be simultaneously considered along with a recommendation for criminal prosecution.

   e. Initiation of stock recovery by sponsor. (See *Regulatory Procedures Manual* Part 5, 5-00-10).

   f. Seizure of test articles if not exempted by regulation.

   g. Injunction.

   h. Prosecution under the FD&C Act, for example, 301(e) or Title 18, for example, Sec. 2, 371, 1001, or 1341.

3. If, following the inspection, the District has communication (written or oral) with the firm concerning the inspection, Headquarters should be kept advised of any such communications. Similarly, if the Headquarters unit has communication (including any written correspondence) with the firm following the inspection, including any judicial/administrative action, the District will be advised of such communication and will be provided a copy of memorandum of contact.

   Districts are encouraged to consult with the appropriate Center compliance or regulatory management unit contact prior to recommending action.

PART VI: REFERENCES AND PROGRAM CONTACTS

References

1. 21 CFR *Part 11 Electronic Records; Electronic Signatures*

   Part 50 Protection of Human Subjects

   Part 56 Institutional Review Boards

   Part 312 Investigational New Drug Application

   Part 314 Applications for FDA Approval to Market a New Drug or an Antibiotic Drug

   Part 361 Prescription Drugs for Human Use Generally Recognized as Safe and Effective and Not Misbranded: Drugs Used in Research

   Part 511 New Animal Drugs For Investigational Use

   Part 514 New Animal Drug Applications, Sections 514.1, 514.8, 514.111

   Part 571 Food Additive Petitions

   Part 812 Investigational Device Exemptions

   Part 814 Premarket Approval of Medical devices (Section 100 – Humanitarian Use Devices)

2. 45 CFR Part 46 Protection of Human Subjects (NIH Requirements)

3. FD&C Act Secs. 301(e), 501(i), 505(i), 507(d), 510(b), (e), and (i), 512(j), 520(g)

4. Specific Forms

   a. Form FDA-1571, Investigational New Drug Application, 21 CFR 312.40

   b. Form FDA-1572, Statement of Investigator, 21 CFR 312.53(c)

   c. Notice of Claimed Investigational Exemption for a New Animal Drug, 21 CFR 511.1(b)(4)

5. CVM guidance document, May 1997, "Good Target Animal Study Practices: Clinical Investigators and Monitors"

6. Guide for Detecting Fraud in Bioresearch Monitoring Inspections, April 1993.

Program Contacts

When technical questions arise on a specific assignment, or when additional information or guidance is required, contact the assigning Center. Operational questions should be addressed to ORO (HFC-132).

Specific Contacts

Office of the Associate Commissioner for Regulatory Affairs

*James F. McCormack, Ph.D.
Bioresearch Monitoring Program Coordinator
Division of Compliance Policy (HFC-230)
Telephone: 301-827-0425, Fax: 301-827-0482*

Thaddeus Sze, Ph.D.
Bioresearch Program Monitor
Division of Emergency and Investigational Operations (HFC-132)
Telephone: 301-827-5649, FAX: 301-443-6919

Center for Drug Evaluation and Research (CDER)

Bette Barton, Ph.D., M.D.
Chief, Clinical Investigations Branch (HFD-344)
Telephone: 301-594-1032, Fax: 301-594-1204
(or specific contact person named in the assignment)

Center for Biologics Evaluation and Research (CBER)
Patricia Holobaugh
Bioresearch Monitoring Team (HFM-650)
Telephone: 301-827-6221, Fax: 301-594-1944
(or specific contact person named in the assignment)

Center for Veterinary Medicine (CVM)

Dorothy Pocurull
Bioresearch Monitoring Program Staff (HFV-234)
Telephone: 301-594-1785, Fax: 301-594-1812

Center for Devices and Radiological Health (CDRH)

Robert K. Fish
Division of Bioresearch Monitoring (HFZ-312)
Telephone: 301-594-4723, Fax: 301-594-4731

Center for Food Safety and Applied Nutrition (CFSAN)

John J. Welsh, Ph.D.
Division of Product Policy (HFS-207)
Telephone: 202-418-3057, Fax: 202-418-3126

PART VII: HEADQUARTERS RESPONSIBILITIES

After review of EIRs containing findings of a serious nature the Centers will initiate necessary action with notification to the Division of Compliance Policy.

Potential regulatory/administrative approaches are discussed in Part V.

The Center will inform the field via copies of letters or reviewer's memo of the Center classification. Optionally a special memo may be generated. * HFC-130 and HFC-230 should receive copies of correspondence from all OAI classifications and when the final classification differs from the initial classification.*

Copies of all correspondence generated by this program should be supplied to the field.

a. *Division of Compliance Policy/ORA*
Coordinates policy issues.
Is the liaison with other Federal Agencies with whom FDA has Memoranda of Agreement or Memoranda of Understanding concerning this program.
Notifies interested governmental third parties whenever a regulatory action is effected against a clinical investigator.
b. *Center*
Identifies studies to be audited, and develops the inspection assignment package. Assignments issue directly from the Center to the field.
Reviews all EIRs, makes final classifications of EIRs and initiates and follows up on all regulatory action*s*. Reviews and approves prosecution recommendations made by the field.
Supplies to the field copies of all correspondence between the inspected and FDA.

c. *Office of Regional Operations (ORO) – Division of *Emergency and Investigational Operations (DEIO) and Division of Field Science**
1. DEIO:
Provides inspection quality assurance, training of field personnel, and operational guidance.
Maintains liaison with Centers and Field Offices and resolves operational questions.
Coordinates and schedules joint Center and multi-District inspections.
2. DFS:
Assigns laboratories for sample analysis and responds to method inquiries.

8. FDA *Compliance Manual: Bioresearch Monitoring Sponsors, Contract Research Organizations and Monitors*

Program 7348.810
CHAPTER 48 – BIORESEARCH MONITORING SPONSORS, CONTRACT RESEARCH ORGANIZATIONS AND MONITORS
Date of Issuance: February 21, 2001
Guidance for FDA Staff

This document is intended to provide guidance. It represents the Agency's current thinking on this topic. It does not create or confer any rights for or on any person and does not operate to bind Food and Drug Administration (FDA) or the public. An alternative approach may be used if such approach satisfies the requirements of the applicable statute and regulations.

Implementation Date: February 21, 2001
Completion Date: Continuing

PART I: BACKGROUND

This compliance program is one of four agency-wide Bioresearch Monitoring Compliance Programs. Regulations that govern the proper conduct of clinical studies establish specific responsibilities of sponsors for ensuring (1) the proper conduct of clinical studies for submission to the Food and Drug Administration (FDA) and (2) the protection of the rights and welfare of subjects of clinical studies. The specific regulations are found in 21 CFR 312 (CBER and CDER), 21 CFR 812 (CDRH), and 21 CFR 511.1(b) (CVM). The specific responsibilities of sponsors of clinical studies include obligations to:

1. Obtain agency approval, where necessary, before studies begin.
2. Manufacture and label investigational products appropriately.

3. Initiate, withhold, or discontinue clinical trials as required.
4. Refrain from commercialization of investigational products.
5. Control the distribution and return of investigational products.
6. Select qualified investigators to conduct studies.
7. Disseminate appropriate information to investigators.
8. Select qualified persons to monitor the conduct of studies.
9. Adequately monitor clinical investigations.
10. Evaluate and report adverse experiences.
11. Maintain adequate records of studies.
12. Submit progress reports and the final results of studies.

Sponsors may transfer responsibility for any or all of these obligations to Contract Research Organizations (CROs). (*Note*: The medical device regulations (21 CFR 812) do not define or delineate responsibilities for CROs.) Under the regulations such transfers of responsibility are permitted by written agreement. Responsibilities that are not specified in a written agreement are not transferred. When operating under such agreements, the CROs are subject to the same regulatory actions as sponsors for any failure to perform any of the obligations assumed.

Monitors are employed by sponsors or CROs to review the conduct of clinical studies to assure that clinical investigators abide by their obligations for the proper conduct of clinical trials.

A sponsor–investigator is an individual who both initiates and conducts an investigation, and under whose immediate direction the investigational article is administered, dispensed, or implanted. The requirements applicable to a sponsor–investigator include both those applicable to an investigator and a sponsor. See CP 7348.811 for Clinical Investigators.

PART II: IMPLEMENTATION

A. Objective

The FFDCA requires the submission of reports of clinical investigations that have been conducted to show whether an investigational product is safe and effective for its intended use. Inspections under this program will be conducted to determine:

1. How sponsors assure the validity of data submitted to them by clinical investigators.
2. The adherence of sponsors, CROs, and monitors to applicable regulations.

B. Program Management Instructions

1. Coverage
   a. Sponsors
      This group consists of those individuals, organizations, or corporations that initiate clinical investigations and have been so identified by FDA through receipt of an investigational exemption, or application for research or marketing permit for an article. A sponsor is defined in the regulations at 21 CFR 312.3, 510.3(k), and 812.3(n).
   b. Contract Research Organizations
      This group consists of those organizations or corporations which have entered into a contractual agreement with a sponsor to perform one or more of the obligations of a sponsor (e.g., design of protocol, selection of investigators and study monitors, evaluation of reports, and preparation of materials to be submitted to FDA). In accord with 21 CFR 312.52 and 511.1(f), responsibility as well as authority may be transferred and thus the CRO becomes a regulated entity. (*Note*: The medical device regulations (21 CFR 812) do not contain provisions for CROs.)
   c. Monitors
      This group consists of those individuals who are selected by either a sponsor or CRO to oversee the clinical investigation. The monitor may be an employee of the sponsor or CRO, or a consultant.
2. Procedure
   a. Inspection Teams
      In certain instances inspections will be conducted with Center personnel participating as team members.
      1. A field investigator will serve as team leader and is responsible for the cooperative conduct of the inspection. Responsibilities of the team leader are explained in the Investigations Operations Manual (IOM) 502.4.
      2. Center personnel will serve as scientific or technical support to the team leader and shall participate in the inspection by:
         a. Attending pre-inspection conferences when and if scheduled.
         b. Participating in the entire on-site inspection as permitted by agency priorities.
         c. Providing support, as agreed upon with the team leader, in the preparation of specific sections of the inspection report where the Center participant's expertise is especially useful.
      Any difficulties among participants in the inspection should be discussed with District management and, if not resolved, immediately referred to the HFC-130 contact for this program.

b. Specific
1. If a sponsor has contracted out all or part of their responsibilities, notify the Center contact of this fact and continue the inspection. The Center will decide whether to follow up with an inspection at the CRO or monitor and issue any additional assignments.
2. Whether a sponsor or CRO monitor is used, a monitor inspection will cover monitor's obligations for overseeing the investigation as instructed in Part III.

PART III: INSPECTIONAL

• General Instructions

1. All inspections of sponsors, CROs, and monitors are to be conducted *without* prior notification unless otherwise instructed by the assigning Center.
2. Each inspection will consist of a comparison of the practices and procedures of sponsors, CROs, and monitors to the commitments made in the application for investigational exemption (including 510(k)), and applicable regulations and guidelines as instructed by the report formats in the attachments. Use the firm's copy of the application to compare with actual practices.

   Devices only: Requests for inspections from CDRH normally involve Significant Risk (SR) devices that require full compliance with the Investigational Device Exemption (IDE) requirements. In addition to covering the identified SR device, the investigator should determine whether the sponsor/monitor is involved in clinical investigations of Nonsignificant Risk (NSR) devices, which require compliance with the abbreviated IDE requirements of 21 CFR 812.5, 812.7, 812.46, 812.140(b)(4) and (5), 812.150(b)(1) through (3) and (5) through (10). When appropriate, the investigator should choose at least one (1), but no more than three (3), NSR device investigations to determine the level of compliance with the abbreviated requirements.

   Determine whether the sponsor/monitor is involved in any clinical studies involving the humanitarian use of a device described in 21 CFR Part 814 Subpart H. Determine whether the sponsor has submitted any Humanitarian Device Applications Exemptions. Review distribution records for humanitarian use devices at the sponsor site to ensure compliance with exemption criterion (<4000 patients/year), proper accountability, confirmation of institutional review board (IRB) approval prior to

distribution, and prompt notification to CDRH's Office of Device Evaluation of the withdrawal of approval by an IRB.
3. If significant violative practices are encountered, the assigning Center should be notified and will provide guidance on continuing the inspection.
4. If access to records or copying records is refused, or if actions by the inspected party take the form of a partial refusal, call attention to 301(e) and 505(k)(2) of the Act. If this does not resolve the issue, proceed with the inspection and at the earliest opportunity notify the Bioresearch Monitoring Program Coordinator (HFC-230) and the contact for the assigning Center. IOM Section 514 provides general guidance on dealing with refusal to permit inspection.
5. Issue a Form FDA 483, Inspectional Observations, at the conclusion of the inspection when deviations from regulations are observed. *Deviations from guidance documents should not be listed on the FDA 483*. However, they should be discussed with management and *documented* in the EIR.

• Establishment Inspections

1. Organization and Personnel
   a. *Determine* the overall organization of the clinical research activities and monitoring of the selected studies.
   b. *Obtain* relevant organizational charts that document structure and responsibilities for all activities involving investigational products.
      1. *Identify* all departments, functions, and key individuals responsible for areas of sponsor activities such as protocol development, selection of investigators, statistical analysis, clinical supplies, monitoring, and quality assurance.
      2. *Determine* who has the authority to review and approve study reports and data listings.
      3. *Determine* who is responsible for final evaluations and decisions in the review of adverse experiences.
   c. *Obtain* a list of outside services and contractors (CROs, laboratories, IRBs) and *document* the services they provide and who is responsible for their selection and oversight.
      1. When a sponsor transfers responsibility for their obligations to a CRO:
         a. *Determine* if the transfer of responsibilities was submitted to the agency as required by 21 CFR 312.23(a)(1)(viii), 314.50(d)(5)(x), 511.1(b)(4)(vi), and 514.1(a)(8)(viii).
         b. *Document* any instance where transfer of responsibilities was not reported to the agency.

    c. *Obtain* a copy of any written agreement transferring responsibilities.

  2. If a CRO is contracted to collect adverse experience reports from clinical investigators, *determine* who at the sponsoring firm is responsible for obtaining these reports and submitting them to FDA.

    d. *Obtain* a list of all monitors (for the studies being inspected) along with their job descriptions and qualifications.

2. Selection and Monitoring of Clinical Investigators

  a. *Obtain* a list of all investigators and *determine* if there is a FDA-1572 (21 CFR 312.53(c)(I)) or a signed investigator agreement (21 CFR 812.20(b)(4) &(5)) for each clinical investigator identified.

  b. Regulations require that the sponsor select clinical investigators qualified by training and experience (21 CFR 312.53(a), 511.1(b)(7)(I), and 812.43(a)). *Determine* the sponsor's criteria for selecting clinical investigators.

  c. *Determine* if the sponsor provided the investigator all necessary information prior to initiation of the clinical trial. This may include clinical protocols or investigational plans, labeling, investigator brochures, previous study experience, etc.

  d. *Determine* if the sponsor identified any clinical investigators who did not comply with FDA regulations. Did the sponsor secure prompt compliance? *Obtain* evidence of prompt correction or termination by the sponsor.

  e. *Identify* any clinical investigators whose studies were terminated and the circumstances. *Review* monitoring reports for those clinical investigators and *determine* if those instances were promptly reported to FDA as required by 21 CFR 312.56(b) and 812.43(c)(3).

  f. Identify any noncompliant clinical investigator not brought into compliance and not terminated by the sponsor. *Determine* the reason they were not terminated.

3. Selection of Monitors

  a. *Review* the criteria for selecting monitors and determine if monitors meet those criteria.

  b. *Determine* how the sponsor allocates responsibilities when more than one individual is responsible for monitoring functions, for example a medical monitor may have the responsibility for medical aspects of the study (and may be a physician) while other monitors may assess regulatory compliance.

4. Monitoring Procedures and Activities

  a. Procedures

    1. *Review* the procedures, frequency, scope, and process the sponsor uses to monitor the progress of the clinical investigations. (Device regulations (21 CFR 812.25(e)) require written monitoring procedures as part of the investigational plan.)

    2. *Obtain* a copy of the sponsor's written procedures (SOPs and guidelines) for monitoring and *determine* if the procedures were followed for the selected study. In the absence of written procedures, conduct interviews of the monitors as feasible and *determine* how monitoring was conducted.

  b. Activities

    1. *Review* pre-trial and periodic site visit reports.

    2. *Determine* if the sponsor assured, through documentation, that the clinical investigation was conducted in accordance with protocols submitted to FDA.

    3. *Determine* if responsibilities of the clinical investigators were carried out according to the FDA regulatory requirements (21 CFR 312.60, 312.61, 312.62, 312.64, 312.66, 312.68, 812.46, 812.100, and 812.110).

  c. Review of Subject Records

    1. *Compare* individual subject records, supporting documents, and source documents with case report forms (CRFs) prepared by the clinical investigator for submission to the sponsor.

    2. *Determine* if, when, and by whom CRFs are verified against supporting documents (hospital records, office charts, laboratory reports, etc.) at the study site.

    3. *Determine* if all CRFs are verified. If a representative sample was selected, *determine* how the size and composition of the sample was selected.

    4. *Determine* if a form is used for data verification and *obtain* a copy. *Obtain* a copy of any written procedures (SOPs and guidelines) for data verification.

    5. *Determine* how the sponsor assures that IRB approval is obtained prior to the enrollment of subjects in the study.

    6. *Determine* how the sponsor assures that informed consent is obtained from all subjects in the study.

    7. *Determine* how the sponsor handles serious deviations from the approved protocol or FDA regulations. If serious deviations occurred, *obtain* evidence that the sponsor obtained prompt compliance or terminated the clinical investigator's participation in the investigation and reported it to FDA.

    8. *Determine* if the sponsor makes corrections to CRFs and if the sponsor obtains confirmation or verification from the clinical investigator.

    9. If sponsor-generated, site-specific data tabulations are provided by the assigning Center, *compare* the tabulations with CRFs and source documents.

d. Quality Assurance (QA)

Clinical trial quality assurance units (QAUs) are not required by regulation. However, many sponsors have clinical QAUs that perform independent audits/data verifications to determine compliance with clinical trial SOPs and FDA regulations. QAUs should be independent of, and separate from, routine monitoring or quality control functions.

Findings that are the product of a written program of QA will not be inspected without prior concurrence of the assigning FDA headquarters unit. Refer to Compliance Policy Guide 7151.02 for additional guidance in this matter.

1. *Determine* if the firm conducts QA inspections and audits.
2. *Determine* how the QAU is organized and operates.
3. *Obtain* a copy of any written procedures (SOPs and guidelines) for QA audits and operation of the QAU.
4. Describe the separation of functions between the QAU and monitoring of clinical trials.
5. Sponsors are required to submit a list of audited studies (21 CFR 314.50(d)(5)(xi)). If the assigning Center provides the list, *compare* the list with the sponsor's records.

5. Adverse Experience/Effects Reporting
   a. Regulations require that FDA be promptly notified of unanticipated adverse experiences/effects with the use of investigational articles.
      1. Drugs/biologics 312.32(c) and (d) – Telephone within 7 calendar days if fatal or life threatening; written reports within 15 calendar days if both serious and unexpected.
      2. Veterinary drugs 511.1(b)(8)(ii) – Promptly investigate and report any findings associated with use of the new animal drug that may suggest significant hazards.
      3. Devices 812.150(b)(1) – Within 10 working days of unanticipated adverse device effects.
   b. *Determine* if adverse experiences reported from clinical sites were relayed to FDA as required by regulation.
   c. *Determine* the sponsor's method or system for tracking adverse reactions and for relaying information of adverse experiences to participating investigators.
   d. *Obtain* copies of any notification to investigators relating to adverse experiences.

6. Data Collection and Handling
   a. Study Tabulations
      1. Sponsors are required to submit in an NDA/PMA analyses of all clinical studies pertinent to the proposed drug/device use (21 CFR 314.50(d)(5)(ii-iv) and 814.20(b)(3)).

         a. *Obtain* a list of all clinical studies contained in the application(s) referenced in the inspection assignment.
         b. *Identify* any studies not included in the NDA/PMA and *document* the reason they were not included.
   b. Investigator Tabulations
      1. Sponsors are required to obtain from each clinical investigator a signed agreement (form FDA 1572 for human drugs and biologics and an investigator agreement for devices) prior to initiation of the clinical trial (21 CFR 312.60 and 812.43 (a)).
         a. *Review* all signed agreements submitted to the associated IND/IDE.
         b. *Identify* any clinical investigators with signed agreements not included in the NDA/PMA and document the reason they were not included.
   c. Data Tabulations
      1. FDA regulations require that sponsors submit data tabulations on each subject in each clinical trial in an NDA/PMA (21 CFR 314.50(f)(1) and 814.20(b)(6)(ii)).
         a. *Determine* if the number of subjects in the studies performed under an IND/IDE is the same as the number reported in the NDA/PMA.
            ● *Determine* the number of subjects listed in each of the clinical trials and compare the number of subjects in the tabulations to the corresponding CRFs submitted to the sponsor.
            ● *Document* any subjects not included in the NDA/PMA and the reason they were not included.
         b. Data Collection and Handling Procedures
            1. *Review* the sponsor's written procedures (SOPs and guidelines) to assure the integrity of safety and efficacy data collected from clinical investigators (domestic and international).
            2. *Verify* that the procedures were followed and *document* any deviations.
      2. Record Retention
         a. Refer to 21 CFR 312.57, 511.1(b)(7)(ii), and 812.140(d).
      3. Automated Entry of Clinical Data
         In August 1997, the Agency's regulation on electronic signatures and electronic record-keeping became effective. The regulation, at 21 CFR Part 11, describes the technical and procedural requirements that must be met if a firm chooses to maintain records electronically and/or use electronic signatures. Part 11 works in conjunction with other FDA

regulations and laws that require recordkeeping. Those regulations and laws (predicate rules) establish requirements for record content, signing, and retention.

Certain older electronic systems may not have been in full compliance with Part 11 by August 1997 and modification to these so called "legacy systems" may take more time. Part 11 does not grandfather legacy systems and FDA expects that firms using legacy systems are taking steps to achieve full compliance with Part 11.

If a firm is keeping electronic records or using electronic signatures, *determine* if they are in compliance with 21 CFR Part 11. *Determine* the depth of part 11 coverage on a case by case basis, in light of initial findings and program resources. At a minimum, ensure that: (1) the firm has prepared a corrective action plan for achieving full compliance with part 11 requirements, and is making progress toward completing that plan in a timely manner; (2) accurate and complete electronic and human readable copies of electronic records, suitable for review, are made available; and (3) employees are held accountable and responsible for actions taken under their electronic signatures. If initial findings indicate the firm's electronic records and/or electronic signatures may not be trustworthy and reliable, or when electronic recordkeeping systems inhibit meaningful FDA inspection, a more detailed evaluation may be warranted. Districts should consult with center compliance officers and the Office of Enforcement (HFC-240) in assessing the need for and potential in depth review of, more detailed part 11 coverage. When substantial and significant part 11 deviations exist, FDA will not accept use of electronic records and electronic signatures to meet the requirements of the applicable predicate rule. See Compliance Policy Guide (CPG), Sec. 160.850.

The following are basic questions to be evaluated during an inspection of electronic recordkeeping practices and the use of electronic signatures by sponsors, CROs, and monitors.

Primary raw data collection should be *reviewed* to *determine* when changes were made and by whom. Concentrate on any original data entries and changes that can be made by anyone other than the clinical investigator.

a. Software
   0. Who designed and developed the software?
   1. Can it be modified, or has it been modified? If so, by whom?
   2. If the clinical investigator can modify it, how would the sponsor be aware of any changes?
   3. Has the software been validated? Who validated the software? What was the process used to validate the software? How was the validation process documented?
   4. Are error logs maintained (for errors in software and systems) and do they identify corrections made?

b. Data Collection
   0. Who is authorized to access the system and enter data or change data?
   1. Are original data entered directly into an electronic record at the time of collection or are data transcribed from paper records into an electronic record?
   2. Is there an audit trail to record:
      a. changes to electronic records,
      b. who made the change, and
      c. when the change was made?
   3. Are there edit checks and data logic checks for acceptable ranges of values?
   4. How are the data transmitted from the clinical investigator to the sponsor or CRO?

c. Computerized System Security
   0. How is system access managed, for example access privileges, authorization/deauthorization procedures, physical access controls? Are there records describing the names of authorized personnel, their titles, and a description of their access privileges?
   1. What methods are used to access computerized systems, for example identification code/password combinations, tokens, biometric signatures, electronic signatures, digital signatures?
   2. How are the data secured in case of disasters, for example power failure? Are there contingency plans and backup files?
   3. Are there controls in place to prevent, detect, and mitigate effects of computer viruses on study data and software?
   4. Are controls in place to prevent data from being altered, browsed, queried, or reported via external software applications that do not enter through the protective system software?

d. Procedures
   Are there written procedures for software validation, data collection, and computerized system security?

4. Test Article
    a. Integrity
        0. Describe the procedures the sponsor uses to ensure the integrity of the test article from manufacturing to receipt by the clinical investigator:
            a. *Determine* if the test article met required release specifications by review of the Certificate of Analysis.
            b. *Determine* where the test article was stored and if the conditions of storage were appropriate.
            c. *Determine* how the sponsor verifies article integrity during shipment to the clinical investigator.
        1. *Determine* if test article was properly labeled (See 312.6, 511.1(b)(1), and 812.5).
        2. *Determine* if the test article was recalled, withdrawn, or returned.
    b. Accountability
        0. *Determine* whether the sponsor maintains accounting records for use of the test article including:
            a. Names and addresses of clinical investigators receiving test articles (report names and addresses). See 312.57, 511.1(b)(3), and 812.140(b)(2).
            b. Shipment date(s), quantity, batch or code mark, or other identification number for test article shipped. See regulations above.
            c. Final disposition of the test article. See 312.59, 511.1(b)(7)(ii), and 812.140(b)(2).
            d. Final disposition of food-producing animals treated with the test article (511.1(b)(5)).

            A detailed audit should be performed when serious violations are suspected.
        1. *Determine* whether the sponsor's records are sufficient to reconcile test article usage (compare the amount shipped to the investigators to the amount used and returned or disposed of).
        2. *Determine* whether all unused or reusable supplies of the test article were returned to the sponsor when either the investigator(s) discontinued or completed participation in the clinical investigation, or the investigation was terminated.
        3. If the test article was not returned to the sponsor, *describe* the method of disposition and *determine* if adequate records were maintained.

4. *Determine* how the sponsor controls and monitors the use of devices that are not single-use products, such as lithotripters or excimer lasers.
5. *Determine* if the sponsor is charging for the test article and document the fees charged.

5. Sample Collection
    a. Samples may be obtained at the direction of the assigning Center.
    b. During the inspection, if collection appears warranted, contact the assigning Center for further instructions.

6. Establishment Inspection Reports (EIRs)
    Information contained in EIRs may be used in support of approval or denial of a pre-marketing application. The EIR must document all findings that could significantly impact the decision-making process.
    a. Full Reporting
        0. A full report will be prepared and submitted in the following situations:
            a. The initial inspection of a firm.
            b. All inspections that may result in an OAI classification.
            c. Any assignment specifically requesting a full report.
        1. The EIR should contain the headings described in IOM 593.3, in addition to the headings outlined in Part III, B. The report must always include sufficient information and documentation to support the recommended classification.
    b. Abbreviated Reporting
        0. An abbreviated report may be submitted in all but the above situations. An abbreviated report does not mean that an abbreviated inspection can be conducted. Abbreviated reports must contain sufficient narrative and accompanying documentation to support the inspectional findings. The specific headings appearing under Part III "Inspection Procedures" should be fully addressed during the inspection. The EIR should be clearly identified as an abbreviated report.
        1. The report should include all the headings described in IOM Section 593.1 and include:
            a. Reason for inspection.
            b. Prior inspectional history.
            c. Updated history of business.
            d. Administrative procedures.
            e. Persons interviewed and individual responsibilities.
            f. Areas covered during the inspection.
            g. Discussion with management.

PART IV: ANALYTICAL

If sample analysis is required at a field laboratory, contact Division of Field Science (DFS) at 301-443-7103.

PART V: REGULATORY/ADMINISTRATIVE STRATEGY

A. District EIR Classification Authority

The District is encouraged to review and initially classify EIRs under this compliance program.

B. Center EIR Classification Authority

The Center has the *final* classification authority for all Bioresearch Monitoring Program inspection reports. The Center will provide to the District copies of all final classifications, including any reason for changes from the initial classification.

C. EIR Classifications

The following guidance is to be used in conjunction with the instructions in FMD-86 for initial District and Center classification of EIRs generated under this compliance program:

1. NAI – No objectionable conditions or practices were found during an inspection (or the objectionable conditions found do not justify further regulatory action).
2. VAI – Objectionable conditions or practices were found, but the agency is not prepared to take or recommend any administrative or regulatory action.
3. OAI – Regulatory and/or administrative actions will be recommended.

D. Regulatory/administrative follow-up will be in accordance with 21 CFR 312, 511, and 812. FDA can invoke other legal sanctions under the FFDCA or Title 18 of the United States Code where appropriate.

E. The following are available to address violations of regulations:
   1. Warning and Untitled Letters
   2. Re-inspection
   3. Termination of an exemption (IND, IDE, INAD)
   4. Refusal to approve or license
   5. Withdrawal of approval (PMA, NDA, NADA)
   6. Determination of not substantially equivalent or recission of a 510(k) for devices
   7. Implementation of the Application Integrity Policy
   8. Initiation of stock recovery – see Regulatory Procedures Manual Part 5, 5-00-10
   9. Seizure of test articles
   10. Injunction
   11. Prosecution under the FFDCA and other Federal statutes, that is 18 U.S.C. 2, 371, 1001, and 1341.
   12. Referral of pertinent matters with headquarters' concurrence to other Federal, state, and local agencies for such action as that agency deems appropriate.

PART VI: REFERENCES AND CONTACTS

• References

1. FFDCA – Sections 501(i), 505(i), and 505(k)(2).
2. Regulations in 21 CFR Parts 11, 50, 56, 312, 314, 511, 514, 809, 812, and 814.
3. Specific Forms
   a. FDA Form 1571 – Investigational New Drug Application (See 21 CFR 312.40).
   b. FDA Form 1572 – Statement of Investigator (See 21 CFR 312.53(c)).
   c. Notice of claimed investigational exemption for a new animal drug (See 21 CFR 511.1(b)(4)).
4. ICH Good Clinical Practice Consolidated Guideline, May 1997.
5. Guideline for the Monitoring of Clinical Investigations, January 1988.
6. Good Target Animal Study Practices: Clinical Investigators and Monitors, May 1997.

• Program Contacts

When technical questions arise on a specific assignment, or when additional information or guidance is required, contact the assigning Center. Operational questions should be addressed to HFC-130.

1. Office of the Associate Commissioner for Regulatory Affairs
   a. Office of Enforcement, Division of Compliance Policy: Dr. James F. McCormack, HFC-230, 301-827-0425, Fax 301-827-0482.
   b. Office of Regional Operations, Division of Emergency and Investigational Operations: Dr. Thaddeus Sze, HFC-130, 301-827-5649, Fax 301-443-6919.
2. Center for Drug Evaluation and Research (CDER), Division of Scientific Investigations:
   a. Good Clinical Practice Branch I – Dr. John Martin, HFD-46, 301-594-1032, Fax 301-827-5290.
   b. Good Clinical Practice Branch II – Dr. Antoine El Hage, HFD-47, 301-594-1032, Fax 301-827-5290.
3. Center for Biologics Evaluation and Research (CBER)

   Division of Inspections and Surveillance – Mr. Joseph Salewski, HFM- 664, 301-827-6221, Fax 301-827-6748.

4. Center for Veterinary Medicine (CVM)

   Bioresearch Monitoring Staff: Ms. Dorothy Pocurull, HFV-234, 301-827-6664, Fax 301-827-1498.

5. Center for Devices and Radiological Health (CDRH)

   Division of Bioresearch Monitoring: Ms. Barbara Crowl, HFZ-311, 301-594-4720, Fax 301-594-4731.

6. Center for Food Safety and Applied Nutrition (CFSAN) Division of Product Policy: Dr. John Welsh, HFS-207, 202-418-3057, Fax 202-418-3126.

PART VII: HEADQUARTER'S RESPONSIBILITIES

A. Office of Regulatory Affairs
   1. Division of Compliance Policy
      a. Coordinates compliance policy and guidance development.
      b. Coordinates responses to inquiries regarding agency interpretation of regulations and policy.
      c. Serves as the liaison with other Federal agencies and foreign governments with whom FDA has Memoranda of Agreement or Memoranda of Understanding.
      d. Resolves issues involving compliance or enforcement policy.
      e. Advises and concurs with Centers on recommended administrative and regulatory actions.
      f. Coordinates modifications and future issuance of this compliance program.

   2. Division of Emergency and Investigational Operations
      a. Provides inspection quality assurance, training of field personnel, and operational guidance.
      b. Maintains liaison with Centers and Field Offices and resolves operational questions.
      c. Coordinates and schedules joint Center and multi-District inspections.
   3. Division of Field Science
      a. Assigns laboratories for sample analysis and responds to method inquiries (DFS).

B. Centers
   1. Identify the sponsors or CROs to be inspected (including applications for investigational exemptions, and applications for research or marketing permits to be covered), and forward inspection assignments and background data, for example protocols, correspondence, and reviewers' concerns, to the field.
   2. Review and make final classifications of EIRs. Conduct follow-up regulatory/administrative actions. Provide the field copies of all correspondence between the sponsor or CRO and FDA. Provide technical guidance and support to the field as needed.

Form Approved: OMB No. 0910-0291, Expires: 10/31/08
See OMB statement on reverse.

U.S. Department of Health and Human Services
Food and Drug Administration

For use by user-facilities,
importers, distributors and manufacturers
for MANDATORY reporting

Mfr Report #

UF/Importer Report #

MEDWATCH

FORM FDA 3500A (10/05)

Page _____ of _____

FDA Use Only

PLEASE TYPE OR USE BLACK INK

A. PATIENT INFORMATION

1. Patient Identifier	2. Age at Time of Event:		3. Sex	4. Weight
	or _____		☐ Female	_____ lbs
	Date of Birth:		☐ Male	or _____ kgs
In confidence				

B. ADVERSE EVENT OR PRODUCT PROBLEM

1. ☐ **Adverse Event**   and/or   ☐ **Product Problem** (e.g., defects/malfunctions)

2. **Outcomes Attributed to Adverse Event**
   (Check all that apply)

   ☐ Death: _____   ☐ Disability or Permanent Damage
   _____(mm/dd/yyyy)_____
   ☐ Life–Threatening   ☐ Congenital Anomaly/Birth Defect
   ☐ Hospitalization – Initial or Prolonged   ☐ Other Serious (Important Medical Events)
   ☐ Required Intervention to Prevent Permanent Impairment/Damage (Devices)

3. Date of Event (mm/dd/yyyy)	4. Date of This Report (mm/dd/yyyy)

5. **Describe Event or Problem**

6. **Relevant Tests/Laboratory Data, Including Dates**

7. **Other Relevant History, Including Pre-existing Medical Conditions** (e.g., allergies, race, pregnancy, smoking and alcohol use, hepatic/renal dysfunction, etc.)

C. SUSPECT PRODUCT(S)

1. **Name** (Give labeled strength & mfr/labeler)

   #1
   #2

2. **Dose, Frequency & Route Used**	3. **Therapy Dates** (If unknown, give duration) from/to (or best estimate)
#1	#1
#2	#2

4. **Diagnosis for Use** (Indication)	5. **Event Abated After Use Stopped or Dose Reduced?**
#1	#1 ☐ Yes ☐ No ☐ Doesn't Apply
#2	#2 ☐ Yes ☐ No ☐ Doesn't Apply

6. **Lot #**	7. **Exp. Date**	8. **Event Reappeared After Reintroduction?**
#1	#1	#1 ☐ Yes ☐ No ☐ Doesn't Apply
#2	#2	
9. **NDC# or Unique ID**		#2 ☐ Yes ☐ No ☐ Doesn't Apply

10. **Concomitant Medical Products and Therapy Dates** (Exclude treatment of event)

D. SUSPECT MEDICAL DEVICE

1. **Brand Name**

2. **Common Device Name**

3. **Manufacturer Name, City and State**

4. **Model #**	**Lot #**	5. **Operator of Device**
		☐ Health Professional
Catalog #	**Expiration Date** (mm/dd/yyyy)	☐ Lay User/Patient
Serial #	**Other #**	☐ Other: _____

6. **If Implanted, Give Date** (mm/dd/yyyy)	7. **If Explanted, Give Date** (mm/dd/yyyy)

8. **Is this a Single-Use Device that was Re-processed and Re-used on a Patient?**
   ☐ Yes   ☐ No

9. **If Yes to Item No. 8, Enter Name and Address of Re-processor**

10. **Device Available for Evaluation?** (Do not send to FDA)
    ☐ Yes   ☐ No   ☐ Returned to Manufacturer on: _____ (mm/dd/yyyy)

11. **Concomitant Medical Products and Therapy Dates** (Exclude treatment of event)

E. INITIAL REPORTER

1. **Name and Address**	**Phone #**

2. **Health Professional?**	3. **Occupation**	4. **Initial Reporter Also Sent Report to FDA**
☐ Yes ☐ No		☐ Yes ☐ No ☐ Unk.

Submission of a report does not constitute an admission that medical personnel, user facility, importer, distributor, manufacturer or product caused or contributed to the event.

409

MEDWATCH

FORM FDA 3500A (10/05) *(continued)* Page ____ of ____

FDA USE ONLY

F. FOR USE BY USER FACILITY/IMPORTER *(Devices Only)*

1. Check One
- [ ] User Facility
- [ ] Importer

2. UF/Importer Report Number

3. User Facility or Importer Name/Address

4. Contact Person

5. Phone Number

6. Date User Facility or Importer Became Aware of Event *(mm/dd/yyyy)*

7. Type of Report
- [ ] Initial
- [ ] Follow-Up #

8. Date of This Report *(mm/dd/yyyy)*

9. Approximate Age of Device

10. Event Problem Codes *(Refer to coding manual)*

Patient Code ____ - ____ - ____

Device Code ____ - ____ - ____

11. Report Sent to FDA?
- [ ] Yes _____ *(mm/dd/yyyy)*
- [ ] No

12. Location Where Event Occurred
- [ ] Hospital
- [ ] Home
- [ ] Nursing Home
- [ ] Outpatient Treatment Facility
- [ ] Outpatient Diagnostic Facility
- [ ] Ambulatory Surgical Facility
- [ ] Other: _____ *(Specify)*

13. Report Sent to Manufacturer?
- [ ] Yes _____ *(mm/dd/yyyy)*
- [ ] No

14. Manufacturer Name/Address

G. ALL MANUFACTURERS

1. Contact Office – Name/Address *(and Manufacturing Site for Devices)*

2. Phone Number

3. Report Source *(Check all that apply)*
- [ ] Foreign
- [ ] Study
- [ ] Literature
- [ ] Consumer
- [ ] Health Professional
- [ ] User Facility
- [ ] Company Representative
- [ ] Distributor
- [ ] Other:

4. Date Received by Manufacturer *(mm/dd/yyyy)*

5.
(A)NDA # _____
IND # _____
STN # _____
PMA/ 510(k) # _____
Combination Product [ ] Yes
Pre-1938 [ ] Yes
OTC Product [ ] Yes

6. If IND, Give Protocol #

7. Type of Report *(Check all that apply)*
- [ ] 5-day
- [ ] 7-day
- [ ] 10-day
- [ ] 15-day
- [ ] 30-day
- [ ] Periodic
- [ ] Initial
- [ ] Follow-Up # ____

9. Manufacturer Report Number

8. Adverse Event Term(s)

H. DEVICE MANUFACTURERS ONLY

1. Type of Reportable Event
- [ ] Death
- [ ] Serious Injury
- [ ] Malfunction
- [ ] Other:

2. If Follow-up, What Type?
- [ ] Correction
- [ ] Additional Information
- [ ] Response to FDA Request
- [ ] Device Evaluation

3. Device Evaluated by Manufacturer?
- [ ] Not Returned to Manufacturer
- [ ] Yes [ ] Evaluation Summary Attached
- [ ] No *(Attach page to explain why not)* or provide code:

4. Device Manufacture Date *(mm/yyyy)*

5. Labeled for Single Use?
- [ ] Yes
- [ ] No

6. Evaluation Codes *(Refer to coding manual)*

Method ____ - ____ - ____ - ____

Results ____ - ____ - ____ - ____

Conclusions ____ - ____ - ____

7. If Remedial Action Initiated, Check Type
- [ ] Recall
- [ ] Repair
- [ ] Replace
- [ ] Relabeling
- [ ] Notification
- [ ] Inspection
- [ ] Patient Monitoring
- [ ] Modification/ Adjustment
- [ ] Other: _____

8. Usage of Device
- [ ] Initial Use of Device
- [ ] Reuse
- [ ] Unknown

9. If Action Reported to FDA Under 21 USC 360i(f), List Correction/ Removal Reporting Number:

10. [ ] **Additional Manufacturer Narrative** and / or **11.** [ ] **Corrected Data**

The public reporting burden for this collection of information has been estimated to average 66 minutes per response, including the time for reviewing instructions, searching existing data sources, gathering and maintaining the data needed, and completing and reviewing the collection of information. Send comments regarding this burden estimate or any other aspect of this collection of information, including suggestions for reducing this burden to:

Department of Health and Human Services
Food and Drug Administration - MedWatch
10903 New Hampshire Avenue
Building 22, Mail Stop 4447
Silver Spring, MD 20993-0002

Please DO NOT RETURN this form to this address.

OMB Statement:
"An agency may not conduct or sponsor, and a person is not required to respond to, a collection of information unless it displays a currently valid OMB control number."

Reviewer Guidance

Conducting a Clinical Safety Review of a New Product Application and Preparing a Report on the Review

U.S. Department of Health and Human Services
Food and Drug Administration
Center for Drug Evaluation and Research (CDER)

February 2005
Good Review Practices

Reviewer Guidance

Conducting a Clinical Safety Review of a New Product Application and Preparing a Report on the Review

Additional copies are available from:

Office of Training and Communication
Division of Drug Information, HFD-240
Center for Drug Evaluation and Research
Food and Drug Administration
5600 Fishers Lane
Rockville, MD 20857
(Tel) 301-827-4573
http://www.fda.gov/cder/guidance/index.htm

U.S. Department of Health and Human Services
Food and Drug Administration
Center for Drug Evaluation and Research (CDER)

February 2005
Good Review Practices

TABLE OF CONTENTS

I.   INTRODUCTION 415
II. GENERAL GUIDANCE ON THE CLINICAL SAFETY REVIEW 415
     A.   Introduction 415
     B.   Explanation of Terms..416
     C.   Overview of the Safety Review 416
     D.   Differences in Approach to Safety and Effectiveness Data...............................417
     E.   Identifying and Assembling Source Materials for the Safety Review 418
     F.   Identifying Major Concerns at the Outset 419
     G.   Auditing Source Materials...419
     H.   The Purpose of Individual Case Review/"Drug-Relatedness" 419
III. SPECIFIC GUIDANCE ON THE CONTENT OF THE SAFETY REVIEW......................420
     7.0 INTEGRATED REVIEW OF SAFETY 420
     7.1 Methods and Findings 420
         7.1.1 Deaths..421
         7.1.2 Other Serious Adverse Events...423
         7.1.3 Dropouts and Other Significant Adverse Events....................................423
                7.1.3.1 Overall Profile of Dropouts 424
                7.1.3.2 Adverse Events Associated with Dropouts 424
                7.1.3.3 Other Significant Adverse Events...425
         7.1.4 Other Search Strategies 425
         7.1.5 Common Adverse Events..425
                7.1.5.1 Applicant's Approach to Eliciting Adverse Events in the Development Program......................425
                7.1.5.2 Establishing Appropriate Adverse Event Categories and Preferred Terms...............................426
                7.1.5.3 of Common Adverse Events – Assessment of Various Databases 426
                7.1.5.4 Common Adverse Event Tables 427
                7.1.5.5 Identifying Common and Drug-Related Adverse Events...........427
                7.1.5.6 Additional Analyses and Explorations 428
         7.1.6 Less Common Adverse Events 428
         7.1.7 Laboratory Findings...429
                7.1.7.1 Overview of Laboratory Testing in the Development Program...429
                7.1.7.2 Selection of Studies/Analyses for Drug-Control Comparisons of Laboratory Values 429
                7.1.7.3 Standard Analyses and Explorations of Laboratory Data 429
                        7.1.7.3.1 Analyses Focused on Measures of Central Tendency...................430
                        7.1.7.3.2 Analyses Focused on Outliers or Shifts from Normal to Abnormal..............430
                        7.1.7.3.3 Marked Outliers and Dropouts for Laboratory Abnormalities 430
                7.1.7.4 Additional Analyses and Explorations 431
                7.1.7.5 Special Assessments: Hepatotoxicity, QTc, Others................431
         7.1.8 Vital Signs 431
                7.1.8.1 Extent of Vital Signs Testing in the Development Program.......431
                7.1.8.2 Selection of Studies and Analyses for Overall Drug-Control Comparisons 431
                7.1.8.3 Standard Analyses and Explorations of Vital Signs Data.........431
                        7.1.8.3.1 Analyses Focused on Measures of Central Tendency...................431
                        7.1.8.3.2 Analyses Focused on Outliers or Shifts from Normal to Abnormal..............431
                        7.1.8.3.3 Marked Outliers and Dropouts for Vital Signs Abnormalities.........431
                7.1.8.4 Additional Analyses and Explorations 431
         7.1.9 Electrocardiograms 431
                7.1.9.1 Extent of ECG Testing in the Development Program, Including Brief Review of
                         Preclinical Results 432
                7.1.9.2 Selection of Studies and Analyses for Overall Drug-Control Comparisons 432
                7.1.9.3 Standard Analyses and Explorations of ECG Data 432
                        7.1.9.3.1 Analyses Focused on Measures of Central Tendency...................432
                        7.1.9.3.2 Analyses Focused on Outliers or Shifts from Normal to Abnormal..............432

7.1.9.3.3 Marked Outliers and Dropouts for ECG Abnormalities 432
7.1.9.4 Additional Analyses and Explorations...432
7.1.10 Immunogenicity..432
7.1.11 Human Carcinogenicity 432
7.1.12 Special Safety Studies...432
7.1.13 Withdrawal Phenomena/Abuse Potential..432
7.1.14 Human Reproduction and Pregnancy Data..433
7.1.15 Assessment of Effect on Growth 433
7.1.16 Overdose Experience 433
7.1.17 Post-marketing Experience 433
7.2 Adequacy of Patient Exposure and Safety Assessments...434
7.2.1 Description of Primary Clinical Data Sources (Populations Exposed and Extent of Exposure) Used to Evaluate Safety...434
7.2.1.1 Study Type and Design/Patient Enumeration 434
7.2.1.2 Demographics 435
7.2.1.3 Extent of Exposure (Dose/Duration) 435
7.2.2 Description of Secondary Clinical Data Sources Used to Evaluate Safety 435
7.2.2.1 Other Studies...435
7.2.2.2 Postmarketing Experience 435
7.2.2.3 Literature...435
7.2.3 Adequacy of Overall Clinical Experience 436
7.2.4 Adequacy of Special Animal and/or In Vitro Testing..436
7.2.5 Adequacy of Routine Clinical Testing..436
7.2.6 Adequacy of Metabolic, Clearance, and Interaction Workup..436
7.2.7 Adequacy of Evaluation for Potential Adverse Reactions for Any New Drug and Particularly for Drugs in the Class Represented by New Drug; Recommendations for Further Study 437
7.2.8 Assessment of Quality and Completeness of Data..438
7.2.9 Additional Submissions, Including Safety Update 438
7.3 Summary of Selected Adverse Reactions, Important Limitations of Data, and Conclusions...........438
7.4 General Methodology 439
7.4.1 Pooling Data Across Studies to Estimate and Compare Incidence 439
7.4.1.1 Pooled Data vs. Individual Study Data..439
7.4.1.2 Combining Data...440
7.4.2 Explorations for Predictive Factors 440
7.4.2.1 Explorations for Dose Dependency for Adverse Findings 440
7.4.2.2 Explorations of Time-Dependency for Adverse Findings 441
7.4.2.3 Explorations for Drug–Demographic Interactions...441
7.4.2.4 Explorations for Drug–Disease Interactions..442
7.4.2.5 Explorations for Drug–Drug Interactions 442
7.4.3 Causality Determination 442
List of Tables...444

Reviewer Guidance[1]
Conducting a Clinical Safety Review of a New Product Application and Preparing a Report on the Review

> This guidance represents the Food and Drug Administration's (FDA's) current thinking on this topic. It does not create or confer any rights for or on any person and does not operate to bind FDA or the public. You can use an alternative approach if the approach satisfies the requirements of the applicable statutes and regulations. If you want to discuss an alternative approach, contact the FDA staff responsible for implementing this guidance. If you cannot identify the appropriate FDA staff, call the appropriate number listed on the title page of this guidance.

I INTRODUCTION

This good review practice (GRP) guidance is intended to assist reviewers conducting the clinical safety reviews as part of the New Drug Application (NDA) and Biologic License Application (BLA) review process, provide standardization and consistency in the format and content of safety reviews, and ensure that critical presentations and analyses will not be inadvertently omitted. The standardized structure also enables subsequent reviewers and other readers to readily locate specific safety information.

This guidance is an expansion of Section 7 of the clinical review template and is entirely compatible with that template. The structure of this guidance, as an annotated outline, is meant to correlate exactly with the section headings of the review template, providing the pertinent guidance under each heading. The guidance also provides, as attachments, illustrations of displays and graphs that have been used successfully in the past. These are not requirements, but examples, and reviewers can substitute for, or modify, them, or simply find them unnecessary in particular cases. It is expected that new attachments will be added as examples become available.

The commentary and suggestions under each section of the guidance, together with appended examples, provide

suggested analyses, methods of presentations, and discussion of special cases and potential difficulties. Some flexibility in implementing the guidance will be needed, as different types of applications and datasets may require modifications to the structure outlined in this guidance. If sections are omitted, the review should briefly explain the reason for the omission.

FDA's guidance documents, including this guidance, do not establish legally enforceable responsibilities. Instead, guidances describe the Agency's current thinking on a topic and should be viewed only as recommendations, unless specific regulatory or statutory requirements are cited. The use of the word *should* in Agency guidances means that something is suggested or recommended, but not required.

II GENERAL GUIDANCE ON THE CLINICAL SAFETY REVIEW

A Introduction

This GRP guidance provides an annotated outline of the safety component of a clinical review of an application (NDA, BLA) and guidance on how to conduct and organize the safety review.[2] It is usually most efficient and informative

---

[1] This guidance has been prepared by the Integrated Summary of Safety group, a subcommittee of Good Review Practices Track 8. The Track 8 Committee has been charged with developing a guidance for the clinical review of a marketing application under the Good Review Practices (GRP) initiative.

[2] It is recognized that no drug is safe in the sense of being entirely free of adverse effects. Reference in the Food, Drug and Cosmetic Act to the "safety" of a drug for the uses recommended in labeling has been interpreted as meaning that the benefits of a drug outweigh its risks for those uses. The safety review, however, is not a risk benefit analysis, but rather, is the part of the NDA review that assesses and describes the risks of the drug.

to include all the safety findings, whatever the source, in the safety section of the clinical review (i.e., apart from the description of individual studies in the efficacy review). In some cases, however, it may be more appropriate to discuss some or all aspects of safety as part of the discussion of individual efficacy studies and reference them in this section (e.g., studies with mortality outcomes, development programs in which most of the safety data come from one or two large multi-center studies, and when evaluation and review of safety data may be more convenient or informative study by study).

The safety review has two distinct components: (1) identification and assessment of the significance of the adverse events reported in clinical trials (controlled or uncontrolled) and (2) evaluation of the adequacy of the applicant's safety evaluation. This guidance describes an approach that integrates safety findings across all studies and other clinical experience. Consideration of the safety findings in individual studies, without a thoughtful integration of the overall safety experience, is not adequate for a safety review.[3]

Although much of the guidance in this document is directed primarily toward the clinical reviewer and toward the analysis of particular events, the evaluation of safety data also involves analyses of event rates, estimation of risk over time, exploration of possible subgroup differences, and identification of risk factors associated with serious events, all analyses that involve substantial knowledge of methods of validly quantifying risk and providing measures of uncertainty. Clinical reviewers should therefore collaborate with their biostatistical colleagues when necessary in the preparation of reviews and consider when it may be appropriate to conduct a joint statistical and clinical review for particularly important safety issues.

The conceptual framework of this guidance is similar to the framework used for advising manufacturers on submitting safety data in FDA's *Guideline for the Format and Content of the Clinical and Statistical Section for New Drug Applications* (Clinical/Statistical guidance)[4] as well as in the guidance *M4: The Common Technical Document for the Conduct of Human Clinical Trials for Pharmaceuticals – Efficacy*.

---

[3] It is important to distinguish between the concept of performing an integrated safety review and the separate question of whether or not to pool data across studies in the conduct of that review. For the purpose of this document, an integrated safety review refers to the principle of bringing together in one place in the review all data and analyses pertinent to a particular safety issue (e.g., liver toxicity). Whether one looks primarily at data from individual studies or at datasets resulting from pooling of certain studies to address a particular safety concern is not critical to the concept of an integrated review. Either approach, or both approaches, will usually be used by a reviewer in carrying out an integrated review.

[4] See http://www.fda.gov/cder/guidance/statnda.pdf.

B Explanation of Terms

Because several related terms are used in this guidance that could cause some confusion, the following explanations are intended as clarification.

For purposes of this guidance, the term *adverse reaction* is used to refer to an undesirable effect, reasonably associated with the use of a drug that may occur as part of the pharmacological action of the drug or may be unpredictable in its occurrence. This term does not include all adverse events observed during use of a drug, only those for which there is some basis to believe there is a causal relationship between the drug and the occurrence of the adverse event. The term *adverse event* is used here to refer to any untoward medical event associated with the use of a drug in humans, whether or not it is considered drug-related. The phrases *serious adverse drug experience* and *serious adverse event* are used in this guidance to refer to any event occurring at any dose, whether or not considered drug-related, that results in any of the following outcomes:

- Death
- A life-threatening adverse experience
- Inpatient hospitalization or prolongation of existing hospitalization
- A persistent or significant disability/incapacity
- A congenital anomaly or birth defect.

Important medical events that may not result in death, be life-threatening, or require hospitalization may be considered serious adverse drug events when, based on appropriate medical judgment, they may jeopardize the patient or subject and may require medical or surgical intervention to prevent one of the outcomes listed in this definition. Examples of such medical events include allergic bronchospasm requiring intensive treatment in an emergency room or at home, blood dyscrasias or convulsions that do not result in inpatient hospitalization, or the development of drug dependency or drug abuse. Documents developed by the International Conference on Harmonisation (e.g., E2) add to serious events those that prolong hospitalization but do not include cancer and overdose.

Finally, the term *adverse dropout* is used in this guidance to refer to subjects who did not complete the study because of an adverse event, whether or not considered drug-related; adverse dropouts include subjects who received the test drug, reference drugs, or placebo.

C Overview of the Safety Review

The safety review has four principal tasks:

1. To identify and closely examine serious adverse events that suggest, or could suggest, important problems with a drug – specifically, adverse reactions severe enough to

prevent its use altogether, to limit its use, or require special risk management efforts.

2. To identify and estimate the frequency of the common (usually nonserious) adverse events that are, or may be, causally related to the use of the drug.

3. To evaluate the adequacy of the data available to support the safety analysis and to identify the limitations of those data. At a minimum, this includes assessments of whether the extent of exposure at relevant doses is adequate.

4. To identify unresolved safety concerns that will need attention prior to approval or that should be assessed in the post-marketing period, including such concerns as the absence of data from high risk populations or potential interactions.

In addition, the safety review should:

- Identify factors that predict the occurrence of adverse reactions, including patient-related factors (e.g., age, gender, ethnicity, race, target illness, abnormalities of renal or hepatic function, co-morbid illnesses, genetic characteristics, such as metabolic status, environment) and drug-related factors (e.g., dose, plasma level, duration of exposure, concomitant medication).

- Identify, where possible, ways to avoid adverse reactions (dosing, monitoring) and ways to manage them when they occur.

- For a drug that is to be approved, provide a comprehensive evaluation of risk information adequate to support a factual and sufficient summary of the risk information in labeling.

D Differences in Approach to Safety and Effectiveness Data

Approaches to evaluation of the safety of a drug generally differ substantially from methods used to evaluate effectiveness. Most of the studies in Phases 2–3 of a drug development program are directed toward establishing effectiveness. In designing these trials, critical efficacy endpoints are identified in advance, sample sizes are estimated to permit an adequate assessment of effectiveness, and serious efforts are made, in planning interim looks at data or in controlling multiplicity, to preserve the Type 1 error (alpha error) for the main end point. It is also common to devote particular attention to examining critical endpoints by defining them with great care and, in many cases, by using blinded committees to adjudicate them. In contrast, with few exceptions, Phases 2–3 trials are not designed to test specified hypotheses about safety nor to measure or identify adverse reactions with any pre-specified level of sensitivity. The exceptions occur when a particular concern related to the drug or drug class has arisen and when there is a specific safety advantage being studied. In these cases, there will often be safety studies with primary safety endpoints that have all the features of hypothesis-testing, including blinding, control groups, and pre-specified statistical plans.

In the usual case, however, any apparent finding emerges from an assessment of dozens of potential endpoints (adverse events) of interest, making description of the statistical uncertainty of the finding using conventional significance levels very difficult. The approach taken is therefore best described as one of exploration and estimation of event rates, with particular attention to comparing results of individual studies and pooled data. It should be appreciated that *exploratory analyses* (e.g., subset analyses, to which a great caution is applied in a hypothesis-testing setting) are a critical and essential part of a safety evaluation. These analyses can, of course, lead to false conclusions, but need to be carried out nonetheless, with attention to consistency across studies and prior knowledge. The approach typically followed is to screen broadly for adverse events and to expect that this will reveal the common adverse reaction profile of a new drug and will detect some of the less common and more serious adverse reactions associated with drug use.

With respect to assessment of serious events, there are two distinct situations. First, there are the events readily recognized as consequences, or at least potential consequences, of the treatment (i.e., adverse reactions) because they would be unusual in the population under study. Second, and particularly critical, are serious events that are not so readily attributed to the drug because they can occur even without the drug, for example, because they are known to result from the underlying disease or are relatively common in the population being studied (e.g., heart attacks, strokes in an elderly population) and could therefore represent intercurrent illness. Adverse events that do not seem typical of what drugs do (i.e., that are not hematologic, hepatic, renal, dermatologic or pro-arrhythmic) can be especially difficult to attribute to a drug. The history of the relatively late recognition of the practolol syndrome (sclerosing peritonitis, oculomucocutaneous syndrome), retroperitoneal fibrosis with methylsergide (Sansert), pulmonary hypertension with aminorex and other appetite suppressants, thromboembolic disease with oral contraceptives, endometrial cancer with post-menopausal estrogens, suicidal ideation with interferons, and more recently, cardiac valvular disorders with fenfluramine, illustrates this problem. Perhaps most difficult of all is the situation where the adverse event is, or could be, a consequence of the disease being treated. Thus, it was extremely difficult to discover that many drugs for heart failure (beta agonists, phosphodiesterase inhibitor inotropes, and a vasodilator, flosequinan) caused increased rates of the same kinds of death seen with the underlying disease (i.e., due to progressive heart failure or arrhythmias), that anti-arrhythmics could provoke new arrhythmias, and that interferon could cause depression in patients with cancer or multiple sclerosis, conditions that are themselves associated with mood alteration. Distinguishing the effects of a drug on the immune or other impaired systems in patients with cancer or HIV infection can also be difficult. Many years ago, a last resort drug for rheumatoid arthritis (RA), azaribine (Triazure), was approved despite a number of arterial thrombi seen during development because those were thought to be more common in patients with RA (the drug was removed from the market shortly after approval, however, when unusual thrombotic events, e.g., thrombosis of a digital artery became apparent). Drugs for seizure disorders and schizophrenia can be difficult to assess with respect to causing sudden death because patients with the disorders they treat have a relatively high rate of this event. Usually, the only way to establish that these are adverse reactions is through controlled trials of significant size. Sometimes, the controlled trials to evaluate effectiveness will be large enough to address these issues, but sometimes, where there is a significant concern, special, large safety studies may be needed.

There is no simple answer to these difficult assessments, but this guidance, similar to section H of the Clinical/Statistical guideline (*Guideline for the Format and Content of the Clinical and Statistical Sections of New Drug Applications*)[5] and the guidance *M4 The CTD — Efficacy*, suggest an approach, namely, close examination of all patients who die or who leave a study prematurely because of any adverse event (whether or not thought drug-related),[6] with explicit consideration of the possibility that the event was drug-related (the "prepared mind" approach). With respect to discovering that a drug causes a modestly increased rate of serious events that are relatively common in the population, only large controlled trials can provide a satisfactory answer and the reviewer needs to consider whether such trials are needed. In some cases, there are reasonably well-established surrogate markers that can predict severe injury. For example, an increased rate of transaminase elevations accompanied by a small number of cases in which bilirubin elevation accompanies the transaminase elevation can predict the occurrence of more severe liver injuries in some patients, and visual field defects may portend irreversible peripheral vision loss. Similarly, substantial QT interval prolongation on the electrocardiogram (ECG) predicts the occurrence of Torsade de Pointes (TdP)-type ventricular tachycardia.

E Identifying and Assembling Source Materials for the Safety Review

Before beginning the safety review, the reviewer should identify and assemble (or locate electronically) all available materials for the review. These materials include the following:

- The applicant's Integrated Summary/Analysis of Safety (ISS).
- Adverse event tables in the NDA/BLA submission.[7]
- Case report forms (CRFs) for patients who experienced serious adverse events or who dropped out of a study because of an adverse event. The reviewer should request these CRFs if the applicant does not include them in the submission (although they are required under 21 CFR 314.50). If the number of cases is very large (e.g., for dropouts) and many of the events are similar, it may be reasonable to request only a sample of CRFs.[8] Note that, in some cases, dropouts attributed to other reasons will upon review be associated with an adverse event.
- Individual patient adverse reaction data listings, laboratory listings, and baseline listings, usually accessible electronically.[8]
- The applicant's narrative summaries of deaths, serious adverse events, and other events that resulted in dropouts.
- If available, displays of individual patient safety data over time for patients who experienced serious adverse events.
- The safety sections of the sponsor's proposed labeling.
- Common Technical Document (CTD) safety-related sections (module 2, sections 2.5.5, 2.7.4), which give an overview of the applicant's approach to the safety evaluation and a detailed summary of the safety data.
- Any other safety-related documents, such as discussions of related drugs, descriptions of use of adverse drug reactions (ADR) coding dictionaries to combine data across studies, specific studies of safety hypotheses.

---

[5] See http://www.fda.gov/cder/guidance/statnda.pdf.

[6] 21 CFR 314.50(f)(2) requires that CRFs be submitted for each patient who died during a clinical study or who did not complete the study because of an adverse event, whether believed to be drug-related or not. It should be clear from the application that the ISS and other safety reports include all adverse events that were seen during development, not just those judged by investigators or the applicant to have been potentially drug-related. This is also a useful point to make at a pre-NDA/BLA meeting.

[7] If the reviewer determines that adverse event tables provided by the applicant are accurate and fairly represent the data they purport to display, the tables may be included in the safety review as appendices. If applicant-generated tables are used, the review should identify the applicant as the source.

[8] The reviewer should be able to easily access individual patient information. The reviewer may want to clarify formatting and accessibility concerns at the pre-NDA meeting. For hardcopy submissions, an index that directs the reviewer to the exact location (volume and page number) of the CRF, the narrative summary, and the individual patient safety data display is essential (for sample index see Table 8.0.1). For electronic submissions, the PDF files should have sufficiently detailed *bookmarks* to offer easy navigation by the reviewer. For example, narratives should be bookmarked by patient ID number, not just by study treatment or treatment assignment.

F Identifying Major Concerns at the Outset

Although the review will assess the data submitted, it may be useful to identify at the outset particular concerns that will be explored because they are suggested by the pharmacology of the drug or by safety concerns with pharmacologically related drugs. Thus, the clearance pathway of a drug will suggest certain potential drug–drug interactions or certain effects of decreased renal or hepatic function. Similarly, the pharmacologic class, and prior experience, could lead to focus on particular laboratory or clinical abnormalities (e.g., muscle or liver abnormalities with HMGCoA reductase inhibitors, QT prolongation with fluoroquinolone antiinfectives, gastrointestinal, renal, and cardiovascular effects of nonsteroidol anti-inflammatory drugs, liver abnormalities with endothelin receptor antagonists, cognitive impairment with sedating drugs, sexual dysfunction with selective serotonin reuptake inhibitors). These concerns are considered further in Section 7.2.5.

G Auditing Source Materials

Although there are no established standards for auditing safety data in a submission, the review should describe efforts to assess consistency of the data provided (e.g., comparing information included in CRFs, case report tabulations, and narrative summaries for individual patients). For important adverse events, for example, it is generally important to consider not only the applicant's narrative description, but the associated CRF or hospital records and submitted laboratory, radiology, or pathology results.

H The Purpose of Individual Case Review/"Drug-Relatedness"

An important part of the safety review is reviewing individual cases of death, serious adverse events, adverse events leading to discontinuation (adverse dropouts), and discontinued patients who are lost to follow-up. One reason to review the details of individual cases is to determine whether the event was coded to the correct preferred term. The assessment of causality for specific adverse events in NDAs/BLAs is heavily dependent on comparisons of event rates between treatment groups, and the numerator of these rate calculations includes events coded to the same preferred term. A case might be incorrectly included in the numerator of a rate calculation if the event is incorrectly coded to a specific preferred term. Events may be incorrectly coded to preferred term by the applicant when they summarize the data or because an investigator used a verbatim term incorrectly when recording the event in the CRF. An example of incorrect coding would be if an investigator used the verbatim term *acute liver failure* for a case of increased ALT and the applicant coded the event to acute liver failure. One would not want to include such a case in the numerator of a risk calculation for acute liver failure. Similarly, a case could be incorrectly excluded from a numerator. Inconsistent coding (e.g., peripheral edema coded as "heart failure" for one patient, but "metabolic abnormality" for another) could result in an inappropriately low numerator.

A second reason to conduct individual case review of deaths, serious adverse events, and adverse events leading to discontinuation is to determine whether there is a likely explanation for the event other than the drug that is the subject of the application, such as another drug or concomitant illness (e.g., documented acetaminophen overdose in a case of acute liver failure would argue against attribution to the test drug; documented cholecystitis would argue against attribution of cholestasis to the test drug). If there is no likely alternative explanation for the event, the event must be considered at least possibly drug-related, and should be included in a rate calculation.

A third reason for individual case review of deaths, serious adverse events, and adverse events leading to discontinuation is to look for other reasons that might exclude the drug as a cause of the event. One example would be when an adverse event occurred during a placebo washout period before exposure to study drug occurred. Events that occur prior to exposure would not be included in the numerator of risk calculations. Events that begin long after discontinuation of the drug might also be considered unlikely to be drug-related, but care must be taken in excluding them, as there are examples of such late drug-caused reactions (e.g., FIAU (fialuridine, a nucleoside analog) where liver failure was seen well after the drug was stopped, probably because it induced mitochondrial DNA damage that became a problem only when mitochondria tried to replicate) and because some chronic reactions might not be detected immediately.

A fourth reason for individual case review of deaths, serious adverse events, and adverse events leading to discontinuation is to look for results of re-challenge. A potentially important source of information about causality is when an individual is re-challenged with drug, accidentally or deliberately. Recurrence with re-challenge is a potentially strong indicator of causality, but interpretation of the results of re-challenge is highly dependent on the natural course of the event being considered. For noncyclical events that are exceedingly rare in the background (e.g., acute liver failure, aplastic anemia) recurrence of the event upon re-challenge (i.e., positive re-challenge) provides strong evidence of causality. Positive re-challenges are less definitive for diagnoses/events that can occur in cyclical or recurrent fashion (e.g., worsening glucose control in a subject with diabetes mellitus), but close observation of the patient's whole course (i.e., both challenge periods and dechallenge periods) may be helpful. Re-challenges that do not result in recurrence of the event (i.e., negative re-challenge) suggest (but do not prove) that the drug did not cause the event.

One must consider such factors as whether it was possible for the event to recur, the dose of drug and duration of exposure at which the subject was re-challenged, and whether the length of observation following re-challenge was sufficient to allow recurrence of the event of interest.

It is important to distinguish the processes described above from the causality analyses of drug-related events often provided by investigators and applicants in NDA/BLA submissions. The analyses of drug-related adverse events presented by applicants are usually based on assessments made by investigators at the time of an event, are highly dependent on information about the side effect profile of the drug available at the time of the study (e.g., what is in the investigator's brochure), and are not informed by awareness of the entire safety database. These analyses are generally not expected to provide much useful information in assessing causality.

Assessment of the drug-relatedness of an adverse event is fundamentally different for relatively frequent and relatively rare events. For the former, a reviewer would compare the incidence of adverse events occurring in the study drug group to that in the placebo (or other control) group (in RCT). For rare events, the expected rate in a clinical trial database would be zero. Thus, if even a few cases (sometimes even a single case) of a rare life-threatening event occurred when none was expected, that would represent a serious safety problem for a drug product that does not provide unique efficacy or some other advantage over available treatments.

III SPECIFIC GUIDANCE ON THE CONTENT OF THE SAFETY REVIEW

The following sections bear the same names and numbers of the section of the clinical review template that contains the safety review (Section 7.0).

This guidance organizes the safety review into three main sections:

● Methods and Findings (Section 7.1)
This section contains 17 subsections. Overall, this section should describe the relevant data sources, the safety assessments that were carried out, and the major findings of the detailed safety review. Section 7.1 should use a systematic approach to describing available data. It should focus first on the serious and potentially serious reactions, the kind that can affect the approval decision or severely limit the use of the drug (see Subsections 7.1.1–7.1.4). Focus should then move to the more common reactions that rarely influence approval but are often critical to patient and physician acceptance of the drug. Section 7.1 should then consider less common events, laboratory findings, vital signs, ECGs, immunogenicity, human carcinogenicity, human reproductive

toxicity, withdrawal phenomena, abuse potential, and overdose (Subsections 7.1.5–7.1.17).
● Adequacy of Patient Exposure and Safety Assessments (Section 7.2)
This section should address the adequacy of exposure (e.g., overall patient numbers and numbers for specific demographic subsets, duration of exposure, the dose levels at which exposure took place,[9] the quality and completeness of safety evaluations, whether all necessary evaluations were conducted (e.g., animal tests, *in vitro* tests, long-term safety testing, specific assessments of ECG effects), and whether any additional safety assessments are needed (either pre- or post-approval). This section should also include a subsection on additional submissions of safety data, including safety update(s).
● Summary of Selected Drug-Related Adverse Events, Important Limitations of the Data, and Conclusions (Section 7.3)
This section should identify and briefly summarize the critical findings of the safety review, including the adverse events the reviewer considers to be important and drug-related and any important limitations of the safety database.

This guidance also discusses general analytical methods that may be useful for multiple aspects of the safety assessment in Section 7.4 (see page XX). This section discusses pooling of data, explorations for adverse reaction predictive factors, dose-dependency evaluations, time-dependency evaluations, duration of adverse reactions, drug–demographic interactions, drug–disease interactions, and drug–drug interactions.

The annotated outline of the review begins here.

7.0 INTEGRATED REVIEW OF SAFETY

7.1 METHODS AND FINDINGS

This section consists of 17 subsections (e.g., death, other serious adverse events, laboratory findings). Each of these

---

[9] The proportion of patients exposed to the dose range that is effective should be considered. A total exposure consistent with ICH recommendations (1500 total with 300–600 for 6 months and 100 for 1 year), may, on examination, reveal far fewer who received an effective dose (i.e., the dose that would be used). ICH E-1 ([The *Extent of Population Exposure to Assess Clinical Safety: For Drugs Intended for Long-Term Treatment of Non-Life-Threatening Conditions, March 1995* (http://www.fda.gov/cder/guidance/iche1a.pdf)]) is clear in its expectation that the 6-month and 1-year exposures should be at dosage levels intended for clinical use. Although it is silent with respect to the 1500 figure, exposure at lower doses would not be expected to be informative about the safety of the clinically useful dose.

subsections is organized somewhat differently, depending on the content. In presenting analyses in the safety review, it is important to clearly distinguish between the applicant's analyses and conclusions and those of the reviewer.

In discussing serious adverse events and dropouts (Sections 7.1.1–7.1.3), it is critical that the reviewer identify individual patients in a way that enables subsequent readers to readily access data and supporting information if needed (e.g., study #, investigator #, patient ID#).

7.1.1 Deaths

Identifying Deaths Relevant to the Safety Review

Deaths occurring during the following time periods or under the following conditions should be assessed:

- Deaths occurring during participation in any study, or during any other period of drug exposure.
- Deaths occurring after a patient leaves a study, or otherwise discontinues study drug, whether or not the patient completes the study to the nominal endpoint, if the death:
  - is the result of a process initiated during the study or other drug exposure,s regardless of when it actually occurs; or
  - occurs within a time period that might reflect drug toxicity for a patient leaving a study or otherwise discontinuing drug. For drugs with prompt action and relatively short elimination half-lives, 4 weeks is a reasonable time period. For drugs with particularly long elimination half-lives or drug classes with recognized potential to cause late occurring effects (e.g., nucleoside analogs, gene therapies, or cell transplants), deaths occurring at longer times after drug discontinuation should be evaluated.

The reviewer should consider all deaths that occurred in a drug's development program and any other reports of deaths from secondary sources (e.g., post-marketing or literature reports), without regard to investigator or applicant judgment about causality. It is also important to consider deaths on control treatments for comparison, even though they are obviously not related to the drug in the application. Individual deaths should be listed in a table (see Table 7.1.1.1), unless they are an effectiveness study outcome.

Applicants will provide line listings of all patients who died in studies, together with a brief narrative. (See *E3 Structure and Contents of Clinical Reports*, Section 12.3.[10] The narratives may also be placed in the Integrated Summary of Safety).

Distinguishing Expected from Unexpected Deaths

Certain causes of death are sufficiently unusual in the absence of drug therapy, even in large databases, that they would almost always be considered unexpected (e.g., aplastic anemia or acute hepatic necrosis) and deserve detailed individual discussion. Other fatal events occur at such frequency in the general population that they would be expected to occur in any large database absent drug therapy (e.g., fatal strokes and heart attacks), especially in the elderly.[11] In most cases, these events need to be examined for frequency but discussion of individual cases is not helpful. Expected deaths would include the following:

- Deaths in studies in which mortality is an endpoint and the cause of death is expected for the disease or condition.
- Deaths in studies in diseases where high mortality rates are expected and the cause of death is expected (e.g., cancers). Note, however, that early deaths in cancer studies are a concern as patients are usually selected for clinical trials because they were not expected to die soon.
- Coincidental deaths resulting from progression of underlying disease present at enrollment in a study (e.g., a patient who dies from progression of cancer or Alzheimer's disease or an acute myocardial infarction (AMI) attributed to underlying coronary artery disease present prior to study entry.
- Deaths from inter-current long-term illness. These include the wide variety of fatal events that can be seen in any population, especially a relatively elderly population, such as sudden death (presumably representing an arrhythmia), fatal infections, surgical emergencies, or intra-cranial hemorrhage).

Even though fatal events may be expected in a population, the reviewer should not without further consideration readily accept the conclusion that a fatal event is due to the underlying disease or an inter-current illness and not the drug. For each fatal event, the reviewer should specifically consider the possibility that the event represents an as yet unsuspected adverse reaction. Even if there is nothing about these deaths to suggest a drug cause, it is critical to assess whether the rate of these events is increased. The best way to do this, of course, is by comparison with a control group (a single trial or pooled), but if no control group is available, it may be of value to look at databases of other drugs used in the same population.

When distinguishing between unexpected and expected deaths, the reviewer should make clear the bases for the distinctions (e.g., early deaths in cancer patients are unexpected if the entered patients were chosen because they were not expected to die soon; hematologic deaths are unexpected in

---

[10] The International Conference on Harmonisation of Technical Requirements for Registration of Pharmaceuticals for Human Use (ICH) *E3 Structure and Contents of Clinical Study Reports.*

[11] Note that *unexpected* is used differently from its use in 21 CFR 312.32, where it refers to adverse events not identified in the investigator's brochure and therefore reportable in an IND Safety Report.

a post-infarction study). For unexpected deaths, the individual medical events associated with the death should be carefully evaluated and discussed in detail in the review. Expected deaths should be classified as to type of death, but it is usually not necessary to discuss in detail the individual medical events associated with those deaths. What is critical is to consider whether there is a suggestion that their rate is increased, the adequacy of the data to evaluate this, and the need to know more (e.g., because of experience with related drugs).

Pooling of Relevant Data

Before conducting any mortality analyses, the reviewer must consider the poolability of the data pertinent to deaths. If data are not poolable, analyses should be conducted for separate databases, then examined together. See Section 7.4.1 for discussion of pooling.

Overall Mortality Analysis

The review should include an analysis of overall mortality for all Phases 2 and 3 exposures across treatment groups as well as cause-specific mortality to the extent possible. The *fineness* of classification depends on the quality of data and the number of events (cardiovascular (broad) vs. AMI, sudden death, CHF (more specific)), recognizing that assessing cause-specific mortality is very difficult even in the best circumstances, such as a study in which there is an attempt to describe such endpoints prospectively.[12] Death from an AMI can be indistinguishable from death resulting from an arrhythmia, for example. Analyses should be corrected for differences in drug exposure using person-time in the denominator to calculate mortality rates.[13] If person-time exposure is not included in the submission (ideally, it should be requested at the pre-NDA/pre-BLA meeting), it should be requested as soon as the need is recognized. This correction can be done only for those deaths for which person-time data are available. It may be useful to present both crude mortality and mortality expressed in person-time in an appendix table (see Table 7.1.1.2 for sample display). Life table approaches may be helpful in cases when there are more than a few deaths, and when the direction of different studies varies significantly. Ideally, one would have mortality data from other databases for comparison (e.g., from other drugs in the same class).

Discussion of Applicant's Assessment of Deaths

The reviewer should describe and evaluate the applicant's assessment of deaths, including the following:

- The applicant's criteria for including deaths in the NDA/BLA (e.g., whether the criteria were reasonable, whether the criteria were met).

- The methods used by the applicant to detect and classify deaths.
- The applicant's method of analyzing overall mortality and cause-specific mortality.
- The applicant's judgments on the drug-relatedness of events associated with deaths.

Reviewer's Assessment of Deaths

The reviewer's assessment of deaths, reflecting both the applicant's and the reviewer's analyses, should include the following:

- Listing of information upon which reviewer assessment is based (e.g., CRFs, narrative summaries, consultant reports, autopsy reports).
- Tabular summary of deaths. Deaths should be summarized in an appendix table, as illustrated in Table 7.1.1.1. It may be useful to distinguish between those deaths for which exposure data are available and those for which such data are unavailable (e.g., for post-marketing deaths, exposure data may never be available). In the table and subsequent discussion, there should be a clear identifier so that subsequent reviewers can identify the particular patient.
- Analysis of overall mortality for Phases 2 and 3 drug exposures across treatment groups (see Table 7.1.1.2).
- Analysis of cause-specific mortality across treatment groups (this could use a table similar to Table 7.1.1.2).
- The reviewer's overall judgment about the drug-relatedness of medical events associated with death (i.e., which deaths were probably explained by factors other than the study drug (e.g., another drug, underlying illness, another illness common in the population) and which could not reasonably be explained by such factors). Differences from the applicant's evaluation should be noted and discussed.
- Further discussion of the individual events associated with death and believed to be potentially drug-related, either because they are increased in rate compared to control or because of the nature of the event (e.g., events typically drug-related, such as aplastic anemia or acute hepatic necrosis, or events that would not be expected in the population studied such as sclerosing abdominal or pulmonary conditions or rapidly progressive unexplained renal failure). Any uncertainty about drug-relatedness should lead to inclusion of the event. For each of these individual events, brief narratives should be included in the review or (if numerous) attached in an appendix.
- Other relevant analyses, such as analysis of dose response (administered dose, body weight and surface area adjusted dose, cumulative dose, schedule (including duration of infusion for IV drugs) analysis of mortality within critical subgroups (e.g., demographic, disease severity, excretory function, concomitant therapy), drug–demographic, drug–disease, and drug–drug interactions (see Section 7.4).

---

[12] Temple R., Pledger, G., The FDA's Critique of the Anturane Reinfarction Trial, *N Engl J Med* 303:1488–1492, 1980.

[13] Since placebo and active control patients can generally have had shorter durations of exposures than patients given the new drug, they may have had less opportunity for serious events to have occurred.

- When deaths occur in uncontrolled studies, best available estimates of mortality in the population studied, in the absence of the treatment (see Section 7.4.3).
- When deaths are relatively frequent, the reviewer should consider some of the approaches described for Common Adverse Events (see Section 7.1.5).

7.1.2 Other Serious Adverse Events

Identification of Nonfatal, Serious Adverse Events

The reviewer should identify, without regard to the applicant's causality judgment, all serious adverse events that occurred in the drug's development program or were reported from secondary sources (e.g., post-marketing or literature reports). Serious adverse events may, in addition to signs, symptoms, and diagnosable events, include changes in laboratory parameters, vital signs, ECG, or other parameters of sufficient magnitude to meet the regulatory definition of a serious adverse drug experience.[14]

Applicants generally provide a line listing of all patients in Phases 2 and 3 of the development program who had an event meeting FDA's criteria for a serious adverse event. For each such event, the applicant should also provide a brief narrative (see ICH *E3 Stsructure and Content of Clinical Study Reports*, section 12.3.2). Because the definition of serious is subject to some interpretation, the reviewer should make clear how the applicant created the list. For example, applicants may include events considered serious by investigators, even if they do not technically meet the FDA or ICH definition for a serious event. If such events are included, the inclusion parameters should be noted.

Discussion of Nonfatal Serious Adverse Events

This section of the review should contain the following:

- A brief description of data sources used in the review of individual cases (e.g., CRFs, applicant's narrative summaries, hospital records).
- The tabular summary of serious adverse events (see sample listing, Table 7.1.2.1)
- An analysis of overall rate of serious events and rate of specific serious events, for each treatment group in critical subgroups (e.g., demographic, disease severity, excretory function, concomitant therapy), and by dose. The median duration of exposure should be examined across treatment groups. If there is a substantial difference in exposure across treatment groups, incidence rates should be calculated using person-time exposure in the denominator, rather than number of patients in the denominator, similar to the presentation for deaths in Table 7.1.1.2.

- Reviewer's overall assessment of which serious adverse events were probably explained by factors other than the study drug (e.g., another drug, underlying illness, another illness common in the population) and which could not reasonably be explained by such factors including any pertinent information from *nonserious* events (e.g., seizures not leading to hospitalization, all syncope) that may be related to the serious event.
- Further discussion of each individual serious adverse event judged to be drug-related (i.e., each adverse reaction), as needed, including any relationship of the reaction to death. For each of these reactions, brief narratives should be included in the review or (if numerous) attached in an appendix.
- A discussion or listing of serious events considered unlikely to be drug-related (may be identified in the tabular summary, illustrated in Table 7.1.1.1).

If serious nonfatal adverse events are relatively frequent, the reviewer should consider some of the approaches described for Common Adverse Events (see Section 7.1.5).

7.1.3 Dropouts and Other Significant Adverse Events

FDA regulations require that the CRFs from patients who discontinue treatment in association with an adverse event (adverse dropout) be submitted with the application (21 CFR 314.50(f)(2)) and their analysis constitutes a critical part of the safety evaluation (see Section 7.1.3.2).

ICH *E3 (Guideline on Structure and Content of Clinical Study Reports)* defines a new category of *other significant adverse events*. It includes the following:

- Marked hematological or other lab abnormalities not meeting the definition of serious. This will need to be an individual judgment, probably depending on the drug (e.g., CPK elevation could have a different implication for a statin and a different drug).
- Any events that led to an adverse dropout or any other intervention such as dose reduction or significant additional concomitant therapy (an expansion of the *adverse dropout* concept that appears in 21 CFR 314.50(f)(2), and in the Clinical/Statistical guideline, *and M4: The CTD — Efficacy*).
- Potentially important abnormalities not meeting the above definition of serious and not leading to death or modification of therapy (e.g., a single seizure, syncopal episode, orthostatic symptoms).

If the applicant has included listings for other *significant adverse events* these may be described here, under a subsection separate from the discussion of dropouts (see Section 7.1.3.3). Alternatively, marked laboratory changes may be described under Laboratory Findings (Section 7.1.6).

---

[14] See 21 CFR 312.32(a); 314.80(a); 600.80(a).

7.1.3.1 *Overall Profile of Dropouts*

The review should contain an overall profile of dropouts from clinical trials. The profile should classify dropouts from the overall Phases 2 and 3 study pool by reason for dropping out (e.g., adverse event, treatment failure, lost to follow-up). Where there are clinically relevant differences in dropout rates for certain subsets (e.g., dropouts in placebo-controlled trials vs. dropouts in other studies; dropouts in certain demographic or disease-related subgroups), the profile should also classify dropouts for those subsets. The reviewer should explain the basis for selecting identified subsets and provide mutually exclusive tabulations in which individual patients are counted only once.[15] Ordinarily, the dropouts should be categorized in a table or tables appended to the safety review (see Table 7.1.3.1.1). It can be useful to display, graphically or in tables, the cumulative dropout rates for each treatment group within each study, especially for cause-specific reasons, when this information is available and to assess patient baseline risk factors that contribute to differential cumulative dropout patterns. When pooling data, consideration of dropout patterns over all studies may reveal information that is useful to the overall safety evaluation.

When classifying dropouts, the reviewer should carefully examine the reasons identified by the applicant for subjects dropping out. Heightened scrutiny is warranted for:

- Dropouts classified as administrative, lost to follow-up, or a similar term.
- Dropouts for which the applicant changed the investigator's determination of the reason for the drop out.

Discontinuations attributed to adverse events require submission of the corresponding CRF but CRFs may not be submitted for dropouts classified as administrative or lost to follow-up. If such CRFs are not available, the reviewer may need to request at least a sample of them to determine whether these dropouts may have occurred in association with an adverse event. Where dropouts are reclassified by an applicant (i.e., assigned a reason for dropping out other than the one given in the CRF), the review should indicate how and by whom such reclassifications were made and comment on the appropriateness of decisions.

Ordinarily, the reviewer should combine patients categorized as dropping out for inter-current illness and patients categorized as dropping out for ADR (if the applicant makes that distinction) under the general category of dropouts for adverse clinical events (CRFs should be provided for both of these categories). This categorization is neutral from the standpoint of causality judgment, recognizes the great difficulty in making distinctions between ADR and inter-current illness, and encourages the reviewer to consider the possibility that what seemed to be another illness or a consequence of the underlying illness was, in fact, an ADR.

The reviewer should examine the number and distribution of dropouts to identify potential problems with study conduct or analyses (e.g., a substantial number of dropouts due to *lost to follow-up* and sites with disproportionately high dropout rates should be a sign of concern). For example, early dropouts generally, and differential (drug group vs. placebo group) early dropouts in particular, often present difficulties in conducting and interpreting the effectiveness analysis and may suggest breakdown of blinding. The review should discuss any concerns about dropouts and the methods employed by the reviewer to address them.

7.1.3.2 *Adverse Events Associated with Dropouts*

The analysis of adverse events associated with dropouts is important for two distinct reasons. First, it identifies the type and frequency of adverse events that patients were unable to tolerate even in a clinical trial setting, where there is arguably more support for enduring adverse events than in a clinical practice setting. This provides important prescribing information that can contribute to dose selection, and in some cases, to choosing a method of titration. In most cases, there will be little doubt about which of these events are attributable to the drug because the events will be of relatively high frequency, even if withdrawals because of them are not, and the main issue will be their frequency and importance. It is usually not necessary to review these events case by case.

Second, and the reason CRFs for dropouts due to adverse events are provided automatically to reviewers, these adverse dropouts may provide a clue to unexpected, but important, adverse reactions (e.g., fibrosing intra-abdominal or pulmonary illnesses, progressive liver or kidney diseases, cardiac valve damage, neurological diseases, arteritis, thromboembolic diseases, all of which have been caused by drugs) that can easily be dismissed as inter-current illness. The frequency of these events is likely to be very low, and the review should contain an analysis of each such adverse event that resulted in withdrawal from the study, whether or not the event was attributed to the drug. The reviewer should avoid dismissing such events as inter-current illness and specifically consider the possibility that each dropout not due to a known effect of the drug might reflect an unexpected effect of the drug. The applicant will usually provide a line listing of adverse dropouts (Table 7.1.3.2.1) and this listing (which need not be attached to the review) can serve to identify events needing further scrutiny. Review of the CRFs can often provide critical insights. The reviewer should describe how she or he analyzed these events.

---

[15] *Mutually exclusive* refers to the reason for dropping out. Patients should be identified with only one of the reasons. However, patients may be represented in more than 1 column (treatment group) of a table (e.g., patients in a crossover study may have survived several treatment arms and then dropped out).

With respect to the more common adverse events leading to discontinuation of treatment, the review should present:

- The incidence of adverse events associated with dropouts. Ideally, incidence would be presented in a table or tables appended to the safety review with separate tables for subsets of the overall clinical data pool in which there were clinically meaningful differences in dropout incidence (Table 7.1.3.2.2). Tables displaying incidence of events should include each event that led to a dropout even if a single patient had more than one such event.
- Whether the event can reasonably be considered drug-related; this conclusion will be based on comparisons between treatment groups in controlled trials and can be informed by the overall rate of the adverse event (Section 7.1.5), and the known pharmacology of the drug.
- The dose response and time dependency of the dropouts and drug–demographic, drug–disease, and drug–drug interactions (see Section 7.4 General Methodology).

For the rarer events that could suggest an important adverse reaction, the critical review determination is whether any of these events suggest drug-induced injury. These events need to be considered individually, with narratives and reference to other databases as appropriate.

Where the review contains applicant-generated tables, it is important for the reviewer to determine and describe how the tables were created. A table may identify one or more adverse events as having caused a particular patient to withdraw, in which case it would represent the actual incidence of specific adverse events that led to dropout. This approach is preferred. Alternatively, a table may list the adverse events that a subject experienced at the time of dropout and not identify any event (or events) as causing the dropout. This approach does not provide the actual incidence of adverse events associated with dropouts and is of less value. The reviewer should make clear in the review which of these approaches was used, or whether an alternative approach was used.

7.1.3.3 *Other Significant Adverse Events*

If a submission separates out information on adverse events that led to dose reduction or significant additional concomitant therapy,[16] but not to discontinuation of treatment, those findings should be described using an approach similar to that proposed above for adverse dropouts.

7.1.4 Other Search Strategies

In addition to reviewing deaths, serious adverse events, and adverse events associated with dropouts, it may be useful

to construct algorithms involving combinations of clinical findings that may be a marker for a particular toxicity (e.g. serotonin syndrome, cough, chest congestion and shortness of breath that may constitute drug-related bronchospasm, or drug-induced Parkinsonism). When such algorithms are used, the algorithm and results of the search using the algorithm should be described in the review. Generally, and where possible, such searches should be done while the reviewer is blinded to treatment, as this will minimize bias when identifying cases.

It should be noted that the causal relation of a drug to uncommon serious adverse events may be supported by less serious events that are more common. For example, the likelihood that a drug caused a small number of cases of serious liver toxicity may be supported by a higher rate of transaminase elevation.

7.1.5 Common Adverse Events

This section of the review focuses on establishing the common adverse reaction profile for the drug and determining the content of the adverse reaction table (s) to be included in labeling. NDAs typically contain numerous tables and analyses of adverse event incidence (e.g., by study, by various pools of studies, and for the overall database). In general, what are included are *TESS*, treatment emergent signs and symptoms (i.e., signs and symptoms not present at baseline, or not present at the severity seen on treatment). To approach these data, the reviewer should generally go through the steps outlined in Sections 7.1.5.1–7.1.5.5.

7.1.5.1 *Applicant's Approach to Eliciting Adverse Events in the Development Program*

Adverse events can be elicited by open-ended questions or checklists with varying degrees of specification. Each approach has advantages and disadvantages, but results can differ greatly and may lead to marked differences in reported adverse event rates across studies (it would not usually be appropriate to pool results obtained using both methods). The reviewer should describe the applicant's method or methods of eliciting adverse event data in clinical trials, including whether checklists were used, the frequency with which patients were assessed, and whether the approaches differed among studies. Identification of signs (abnormal findings observed by a clinician) would seem to be less of a problem, as these are elicited by physical examination, but use of a physician exam checklist could lead to a different result from a more general requirement for physical exam. If different approaches were used (e.g., checklists in studies conducted in the United States, open-ended inquiries in European studies), the reviewer should consider and discuss in the review the effect, if any, on the adequacy of adverse event information collected.

---

[16] This is recommended in the ICH *E3* guidance.

7.1.5.2 Establishing Appropriate Adverse Event Categories and Preferred Terms

Although investigator adverse reaction terms are provided as part of study reports and are listed in case report tabulations, the integrated analysis of the ISS requires the applicant to use some way of grouping closely related events to obtain an overall rate for a category of events. This is accomplished by using a so-called *dictionary* of preferred terms, such as COSTART,[17] MedDRA,[18] the latter a more granular listing developed under the auspices of ICH. These *dictionaries* are in fact lists of preferred terms and leave (especially COSTART and other older dictionaries) considerable discretion to the classifier to choose the term that best reflects the verbatim term reported by the investigator. The categorization of such systems, however, may not capture, or can dilute, the true meaning of certain events. In addition, terms used in COSTART may not be informative (e.g., pain, tooth disorder). It is expected that as MedDRA becomes more widespread, this will no longer be such a problem. It is critical that the reviewer assess the appropriateness of the applicant's categories and the coding of adverse event verbatim terms to preferred terms and understand how the verbatim terms (including terms in languages other than English) were classified.

In assessing the applicant's coding of events, the reviewer should compare the applicant's preferred terms to the verbatim terms used by investigators and patients, focusing on the events leading to dropouts or other changes in treatment as well as to serious adverse events. The applicant will usually provide (ideally this will have been agreed to at the pre-NDA/BLA meeting, but if not, it should be sought early in the review) the following tables and listings for assistance with this assessment; they should be provided in a form the reviewer can manipulate, such as a SAS transport file, not just in PDF format:

- Adverse event tables in individual study reports based on investigator terms for events.
- A comprehensive line listing of all adverse events in Phases 2 and 3 studies with a column containing investigator terms coded under a preferred term (see Table 7.1.5.2.1. This table is for reference only; it would not be included in the review)
- Listing of preferred terms and the investigator and patient terms that were subsumed under the preferred term. This table is for reference only; it would not be included in the review, although parts of it might be).

The reviewer should consider the following:

- Whether terms are too narrow (*splitting*), resulting in an underestimation of the true incidence for a particular event or syndrome (e.g., somnolence, drowsiness, sedation, and sleepiness probably all refer to the same event).
- Whether the terms are too broad or over-inclusive (*lumping*), so that important events that should be examined separately are diluted by less important events (e.g., loss of consciousness and syncope subsumed under hypotensive events or hypotension).
- Whether terms used lack a commonly understood meaning (e.g., mouth disorder, tooth disorder, GI disorder) and, if so, whether the incidence of individual events subsumed under these terms should be expressed separately or mapped to a different preferred term.
- Whether terms exaggerate a finding (acute liver failure for a transaminase elevation) or minimize the importance of an event (hypotension for a syncope episode).
- Whether the coding of adverse events is similar across treatment groups.

In any of these cases, the reviewer (or the applicant at the request of the reviewer) may have to recalculate rates using alternative terms or different groups of terms.

Usually it will be impossible to evaluate all or even most adverse event terms in this much detail. However, certain preferred terms should always have the subsumed verbatim terms examined because they may conceal important events. For example, *accidental injury* often includes fractures and/or lacerations related to falls. The fall, itself, however, may not have been captured as an adverse event. Additionally, *edema* may sometimes include *facial edema*. Since facial edema often represents an allergic reaction, one would not want allergic events lumped together with peripheral edema events. In general, adverse event terms associated with discontinuation or serious consequences deserve the closest scrutiny, but other classifications should be at least spot-checked. The review should comment on how this issue was addressed.

7.1.5.3 Incidence of Common Adverse Events – Assessment of Various Databases

Applicants typically prepare a wide variety of tables of adverse event rates for individual studies and pools of various studies. Those tables generally include investigator causality assessments and severity ratings. The tables the reviewer considers useful should be appended to the review. Incidence rates for common adverse events may be estimated from the relatively small portion of the overall database that is contained in the controlled (especially placebo-controlled) trials. For these more common events, the ability to compare rates on drug with a control outweighs the disadvantage of basing the rate estimates on fewer subjects. In determining incidence rates for common

---

[17] Food and Drug Administration, *Coding Symbols for Thesaurus of Adverse Reaction Terms*, 5th ed., FDA, Rockville, MD, 1995.
[18] MedDRA (Medical Dictionary for Regulatory Activities), http://www.meddramsso.com/NewWeb2003/index.htm.

adverse events, the reviewer should identify the subset of trials in the Phases 2 and 3 database that will provide the best estimate of rates and develop tables of event rates based on that judgment.

- If possible, the reviewer should rely on pooled data from studies using the same comparator group (e.g., only placebo-controlled trials) and of roughly similar duration. If some of the trials also had an active control, rates for that group (pooled) can also be included (see Table 7.1.5.3.1). If different doses were used, both a pooled all doses group and individual dose groups can be shown. The best comparison is of the groups included in all studies (drug at a particular dose and placebo), but the others (active controls, individual dose groups) may also be useful (also see Section 7.4 for broader discussion of pooling).

- If there are not adequate numbers of patients in such trials to give meaningful rate estimates, the reviewer should consider pooling placebo-controlled trials, active control trials, and three arm trials (i.e., trials that do not all have the same control group). Even when this approach is needed overall, smaller subsets of studies, or even individual studies, can be used to examine high frequency events.

- Most applicants will construct adverse event tables by compiling and presenting the numbers and/or percentages of patients experiencing an adverse event in a study (or the absolute number of adverse events experienced in a group), without regard to the duration of treatment received. This is often satisfactory for relatively short-term studies. If studies of significantly different durations are pooled, however, or if there is a different discontinuation rate in the treatment arms and the risk of the adverse reaction persists over time, one must consider these durations to understand the real occurrence rate that patients will experience. One way to deal with the problem of different durations is to use the total person-time exposure for each treatment group and calculate the rate of the adverse event per period of exposure (# of patients with adverse event total person-time exposure), rather than the risk (# of patients with adverse event total number of patients). This is particularly useful for the more important adverse reactions and reactions that occur at a fairly constant rate over time, but the person-time approach can also be used when the hazard rate changes over time. In this case, however, the observation period must be broken into component periods (e.g., evaluating person-time rates for each treatment for month 1, month 2,…).

- If concurrently controlled data are unavailable, overall rates from well-monitored, single-arm databases can be used to provide some indication of rates that were observed in treated patients, but there is little ability to establish causality except insofar as reactions are predicted by the known pharmacology of the drug.

For the most part, attributions of causality by the investigators should be discounted, and adverse events should be assessed without regard to attribution. Also, in general, tables should give rates for all severities of a given effect, although in some cases (notably cytotoxic drugs), it is important to distinguish more and less severe reactions, as the former may be therapy-limiting or may affect the overall benefit-risk conclusion for the drug. For events with high background rates (e.g., headache, fatigue, and other events that occur frequently independent of drug therapy), however, display of all reported events can result in a high event rate that obscures drug-relatedness. This can be a particular problem when time on drug is prolonged. For example, it is common for studies of 4–6 weeks duration to report headache at a high (20–25%) rate. In that case, considering the severity or causality assessment of such events may allow a better assessment (e.g., if severe headaches are found only in the drug-treated group). Events that are more severe and for which subjects have multiple occurrences while on drug therapy are more likely drug-related. In determining incidence, however, both single occurrence and multiple occurrence events should be counted as one event.

Some categories of adverse events (e.g., decreased cognitive or sexual function) are notoriously difficult to detect without special efforts, such as targeted questionnaires. If the database includes special studies intended to identify these events, they should generally be given more credence than nontargeted studies, which tend to substantially underestimate rates (see Section 7.1.9). Incidence rates should be based on findings from the targeted studies.

7.1.5.4 *Common Adverse Event Tables*

The review should contain a table (or tables) that presents the best overall display of commonly occurring adverse events, generally those occurring at a rate of 1% or more (but lower rates can be presented for very large databases). The table, or tables, will form the basis for the adverse reaction table in labeling. The table may use a higher cutoff than 1% if doing this does not lose important information. Adverse events that are equally common on drug and placebo, or more common on placebo, are usually omitted. The frequency cutoff for inclusion of adverse events in the table (e.g., >1%) is inherently arbitrary. If one is used, the review should explain how the threshold was determined. It may also be informative to include tables that distinguish between common adverse events on the basis of severity. It is most common to group adverse events within body systems, but a display by descending frequency may also be useful.

7.1.5.5 *Identifying Common and Drug-Related Adverse Events*

For common adverse events, the reviewer should attempt to identify those events that can reasonably be considered drug-related. Although it is tempting to use hypothesis-testing methods, any reasonable correction for multiplicity would make a *finding* almost impossible, and studies are almost invariably underpowered for statistically valid detection of small differences. The most persuasive evidence for causality is a consistent difference from control across studies, and evidence of dose response. The reviewer may also consider specifying criteria for the minimum rate and the difference between drug and placebo rate that would be considered sufficient to establish that an event is drug-related (e.g., for a given dataset, events occurring at an incidence of at least 5% and for which the incidence is at least twice, or some other percentage greater than, the placebo incidence would be considered common and drug-related). The reviewer should be mindful that such criteria are inevitably arbitrary and sensitive to sample size.

7.1.5.6 *Additional Analyses and Explorations*

For adverse events that seem drug-related (the analyses suggested can have no value for unrelated events), the reviewer should perform the following additional analyses (see Section 7.4, General Methodology, for discussion of methods for the explorations and analyses identified below), as appropriate:

- Explorations for dose dependency. These are important. The reviewer should ordinarily rely on fixed dose studies, as titration studies tend to show that those who tolerate higher doses have lower adverse reaction rates, but in some cases titration studies may show a clearly increased rate of adverse reactions with dose. It may also be useful to evaluate safety as a function of weight-adjusted dose, body surface-adjusted dose, or cumulative dose. Dose increases may be associated with adverse reactions or the severity of adverse reactions.
- For events that occur commonly, explorations of time to onset.
- For common, troublesome events (e.g., somnolence, nausea) explorations of adaptation to develop information on the time course of, and tolerance for, such events.
- Explorations for demographic interactions (rates and comparisons with control for demographic and other subsets) for at least the more common and important adverse events. The applicant will have provided such analyses under 21 CFR 314.50(d)(5)(vi). Note that this analysis may require use of less optimal tables of pooled results (see Section 7.1.5.3).
- Explorations for drug–disease and drug–drug interactions if there is a strong signal for an interaction or good rationale for expecting an interaction.
- Selective exploration of certain adverse events in an attempt to better characterize them. For example, if rash appears to be drug-related, the reviewer may want to look more closely at individual cases of rash. The

applicant's line listing of all adverse events across the entire Phases 2–3 databases would be a good source for identifying individual cases of rash. If a subject dropped out because of rash, the applicant should have provided a narrative discussion of the event, which would also be a good source for attempting to better characterize the event. Although the data collected on nonserious adverse events is usually sparse, the reviewer could still request additional information from the applicant on commonly occurring adverse events that require further characterization.

- When adverse events of a given type vary markedly in severity, separate analyses of each severity may be useful.

A description of the methods used in such additional explorations should be provided, with all results, interpretations, and pertinent discussion. Where an applicant's analysis is considered inadequate, this should be noted and an alternate developed by the reviewer or requested from the applicant.

7.1.6 Less Common Adverse Events

In general, a fairly large database is needed to evaluate less common adverse events. To identify relatively rare events of significant concern, the reviewer has to examine the occurrence of adverse events over the entire Phases 2–3 database, including data for which there is no useful concurrent control. The overall database is typically heterogeneous, including uncontrolled exposure for varying durations and at varying doses, and is unlikely to lend itself to meaningful estimates of rates or assessment of causality (except where there has been re-challenge). Thus, it may be sufficient for the reviewer to group these data in gross categories of incidence and by body system. For example, it may be useful to categorize less common events in order of decreasing frequency within the following incidence ranges:

- Adverse events occurring at rates less than or equal to 1/100.
- Adverse events estimated to occur at rates between 1/100 and 1/1000.
- Adverse events estimated to occur at rates less than 1/1000.

The reviewer should then develop a condensed list of reactions to be included in the Adverse Reactions section of labeling.[19] This list should eliminate events that are common in the general population and not likely to be drug-related and adverse events characterized by terms that

---

[19] A draft guidance for industry and reviewers, *Content and Format of the Adverse Reactions Section of Labeling for Human Prescription Drugs and Biologics*, was issued in June 2000. Once finalized, it will represent the Agency's thinking on this topic.

are too vague to be helpful, unless the reviewer is able to identify a more meaningful term that was subsumed into the vague term when the adverse event was coded by the applicant (see Section 7.1.5.2 above).

Some of the reactions in the condensed list may be of particular concern, but insufficiently clear as to whether they are caused by the drug to lead to a Warning/Precaution in the labeling. In that case, it is useful to notify the safety evaluator in the Office of Drug Safety who will be monitoring the drug after marketing.

7.1.7 Laboratory Findings

The approach to review of laboratory findings (chemistry, hematology, and urinalysis) is generally similar to that suggested for the other categories of safety data. As considered in greater detail below, the review should identify laboratory tests performed in the clinical studies, describe the dataset from which laboratory findings information is obtained, describe the methods used to assess findings, discuss pertinent findings, and review the more important findings in depth. Laboratory findings discussed in detail in other sections of the review (e.g., Section 7.1.2 Other Serious Adverse Events, Section 7.1.3 Dropouts and Other Significant Adverse Events) need not be discussed in detail in this section. This section should refer to the more detailed discussions of such findings elsewhere in the review.

7.1.7.1 Overview of Laboratory Testing in the Development Program

The review should provide an overview of what laboratory testing (chemistry, hematology, and urinalysis) was carried out. It is preferable to summarize the overall approach, rather than provide detailed comments about laboratory testing for each study. The review should contain the following to the extent relevant to the data:

- Discussion of any discrepancies between planned analyses and analyses that were done (e.g., tests omitted or added, changes in planned frequency of testing).
- Discussion of procedures used to evaluate abnormal values (e.g., whether patients were followed until their values normalized, whether any patients were re-challenged, the procedures used for sample analysis (i.e., central or local labs, *windows* of time in which lab values were considered[20]).
- A summary table identifying the numbers of patients exposed to test drug who had baseline laboratory values and follow-up assessments.

---

[20] Applicants may consider only lab values obtained within a certain window around the protocol-specified date for collection. In some cases, the laboratory data obtained outside the window may be available, but the applicant may choose not to include it.

- Whether results of unscheduled lab tests were included in the principal analyses and tables.

The reviewer should note that laboratory tests obtained at *unscheduled visits* (e.g., when a patient is hospitalized for an adverse event) are often not included in the NDA/BLA laboratory database. In those cases, the only place a reviewer would learn of an abnormal laboratory value might be a narrative summary (or occasionally a CRF). Too often, however, the narrative summary includes only a preferred or verbatim term (e.g., *acute renal failure*) and does not include the laboratory value of interest (e.g., BUN/creatinine). In such cases, the laboratory data of interest should be requested from the applicant.

7.1.7.2 *Selection of Studies/Analyses for Drug-Control Comparisons of Laboratory Values*

Controlled comparisons generally provide the best data for deciding whether there is a signal of an effect of a drug on a laboratory test. Placebo-controlled trials are generally short-term, however, and therefore unsuitable for assessing late-developing abnormalities, so that longer term data also need to be examined. If there is no concomitant control, comparison may need to be made with similar populations outside the NDA (e.g., in other applications). In identifying the sample population for comparison of laboratory values, the reviewer should pool relevant studies. The review should explain how the studies to be pooled were selected. In comparing laboratory values, there are additional considerations when using pooled data (in addition to those discussed in Section 7.4.1 Methodology, Pooling), including:

- The methods of sample collection and handling in different studies.
- The assay methods used in different studies.
- The reference ranges used in different studies.

Several analyses may be needed. Separate analyses should be performed for patients with normal values at baseline, for patients with abnormal values at baseline, and for patients without baseline values. In general, there will need to be at least one analysis that includes all data (data from planned or unplanned visits, values collected as follow-up to abnormal findings).

7.1.7.3 *Standard Analyses and Explorations of Laboratory Data*

This review should generally include three standard approaches to the analysis of laboratory data. The first two analyses are based on comparative trial data. The third analysis should focus on all patients in the Phases 2–3 experience. Analyses are intended to be descriptive and should not be thought of as hypothesis testing. *p*-values or confidence intervals can provide some evidence of the strength of the finding, but unless the trials are designed for hypothesis testing (rarely the case), these should be thought of as descriptive. Generally, the magnitude of change is more important than the p-value for the difference.

7.1.7.3.1 Analyses Focused on Measures of Central Tendency

The central tendency analysis generally compares mean or median changes from baseline across treatment groups, and the review should contain the results of these analyses for all laboratory measurements. Although marked outliers are typically of greatest interest from a safety standpoint (see below), at times a potentially important effect may be revealed only in analyses looking at differences in mean change from baseline. For example, several drugs that cause modest decreases in uric acid because of a uricosuric effect have caused acute renal failure (ticrynafen, suprofen) in inadequately hydrated patients. Suprofen was withdrawn from the market for this reason. Mean changes in electrolyte levels can also signal risks.

It is generally useful to include as appendices tables providing data on central tendency (see Table 7.1.7.3.1.1). The reviewer should note and discuss signals that emerge from these tables and indicate those for which further study is needed, if any.

7.1.7.3.2 Analyses Focused on Outliers or Shifts from Normal to Abnormal

The review should focus on patients whose laboratory values deviate substantially from the reference range. Applicants usually include displays and analyses designed to detect such outliers. The relevant data would come from shift tables, scatter plots, box plots, cumulative distribution displays, and tables providing incidence of patients across treatment groups who had a potentially clinically important deviation from normal on one or more laboratory parameters while on treatment (see Table 7.1.7.3.2.1). In analyzing outliers, the reviewer should be aware of the following:

- Regression to the mean (and an apparent upward shift) can be expected if patients are screened for normality, giving a shift even if there is no drug effect; comparison with control groups is critical.
- If there are more measurements performed during treatment than baseline and abnormal values are randomly occurring, there is more opportunity for outliers during treatment. Again, comparison with a control group is critical.
- For important laboratory parameters, the reviewer should carefully consider the cutpoints used by the applicant to define *normal* and *abnormal*.
- If values used to identify outliers are too extreme, important findings may not be identified.

- If values used to identify outliers are not large enough, important findings may be obscured by grouping important outliers and trivial findings (e.g., values greater than 2 times upper limit of normal for transaminase are common in many datasets and may not distinguish hepatotoxic from nonhepatotoxic agents; 3-fold and higher elevations appear to be more discriminating).

Decisions about what criteria to use to identify outliers should, if possible, be made at the pre-NDA meeting. Because it is not possible to know in advance what criteria will be optimal for detecting between-group differences, it may be useful to conduct analyses using cutpoints other than those chosen by the applicant. In addition, it may be useful to consider between-group comparisons of the following:

- Cumulative or other distributions of data, rather than solely proportions of patients meeting some arbitrary criterion.
- Patients with large shifts within the normal reference range.
- Patients who meet outlier criteria for more than one variable simultaneously (e.g., transaminase and bilirubin).
- Patients having persistent abnormalities (more likely to be real deviations).

Analyses of outliers should serve as a source of signals for events to explore in more depth. The reviewer should discuss signals that emerge and indicate those for which further exploration is needed. The details of the explorations carried out and the results should be provided in Subsection 7.1.6.4 as described below.

7.1.7.3.3 Marked Outliers and Dropouts for Laboratory Abnormalities

The reviewer should carefully analyze individual patients with large changes in laboratory values. These changes are much more likely to identify significant problems than mean or median changes from baseline. Applicants typically provide a list that identifies patients with extreme changes, usually specified in advance. Individual patient data displays should be available to the reviewer for all such patients. Even for relatively uncommon events, it is helpful to compare rates in treatment and control groups.

Discontinuation of treatment for a laboratory abnormality may be considered a marker of perceived clinical importance of the finding. It is again useful to compare treatment groups, taking into account duration of treatments, for rates of discontinuation for particular laboratory abnormalities. Because of the importance of looking at dropouts for laboratory changes (even a small number of marked abnormalities, such as liver function or WBC count, may signal major problems), all such dropouts in the Phases 2–3 population should be identified. The reviewer should generally analyze and comment on each individual patient identified as dropping out for any significant laboratory abnormalities. In some cases, it is critical to note whether appropriate testing has been carried out to rule out nondrug-related mechanisms (e.g., viral hepatitis serological testing in patients with transaminase elevation or more severe liver injury) and whether appropriate additional tests have been performed (e.g., bilirubin in patients with transaminase elevation).

7.1.7.4 *Additional Analyses and Explorations*

Additional analyses may be appropriate for certain laboratory findings, including analyses for dose dependency, time dependency, and also drug–demographic, drug–disease, and drug–drug interactions (see Section 7.4 Methodology). The review should discuss the rationale for additional explorations, the methods used, and the results and interpretations.

7.1.7.5 *Special Assessments: Hepatotoxicity, QTc, Others*

Certain laboratory assessments are so critical to the safety assessment that they deserve special attention in any review. For example, hepatotoxicity has been an important cause of drug marketing withdrawals from the 1950s (iproniazid) to the present (ticrynafen, benoxaprofen, troglitizone, bromfenac) and has led to important limitations on the use of many more drugs (isoniazid, labetalol, trovafloxacin, tolcapone, nefazodone, felbamate). At present, it appears that a potential for severe hepatotoxicity may be signaled by a set of findings sometimes called *Hy's Law*, based on the observation by Hy Zimmerman, a major scholar of drug-induced liver injury, that a pure hepatocellular injury leading to jaundice had serious implications, a 10–50% mortality. Over the years, this observation has led to the following proposition:

In a drug development database, a potential for severe hepatotoxicity is signaled by the following set of findings:

1. An increased rate of transaminase elevations (3× ULN, 5× ULN, 10× ULN, etc.) in treated patients compared to control.
2. No significant evidence of obstruction (elevated AP), although some elevation may follow severe hepatocellular injury.
3. A very small number of cases (two, perhaps even one) of transaminase elevation accompanied by a rise in bilirubin to 2× ULN.

The explanation for the usefulness of this signal is the high capacity of the liver for bilirubin excretion; it takes a good deal of damage to the liver to impair bilirubin excretion (in the absence of obstruction). This signal has been present for troglitizone, bromfenac, and dilevalol (never approved in the United States, but hepatotoxic in Portugal).

Table 7.1.7.5.1 is an outline of a comprehensive assessment of available data pertinent to potential hepatotoxicity. A similar outline will be developed for assessment of electrocardiographic QT abnormalities, a risk factor for potentially fatal arrhythmias (see Section 7.1.9).

7.1.8 Vital Signs

Vital signs can be analyzed and reported using an approach essentially identical to that taken for laboratory data. This section should be organized in a similar manner to the laboratory section.

7.1.8.1 *Extent of Vital Signs Testing in the Development Program*

7.1.8.2 *Selection of Studies and Analyses for Overall Drug-Control Comparisons*

7.1.8.3 *Standard Analyses and Explorations of Vital Signs Data*

7.1.8.3.1 Analyses Focused on Measures of Central Tendency

7.1.8.3.2 Analyses Focused on Outliers or Shifts from Normal to Abnormal

7.1.8.3.3 Marked Outliers and Dropouts for Vital Signs Abnormalities

7.1.8.4 *Additional Analyses and Explorations*

7.1.9 Electrocardiograms

ECG data can be analyzed and reported using an essentially identical approach to that taken for laboratory data. The adequacy of the assessment (see Section 7.2) may be especially important in this case, given recent experience with drugs that prolong the QT interval and cause the ventricular tachycardia known as TdP. A guidance document on the design, conduct and interpretation of clinical studies assessing the effects of drugs on the QT interval is under development as a part of the ICH effort. The current version, a step 2 guidance (E14: Clinical Evaluation of QT/QTc Interval Prolongation and Pro-arrhythmic Potential for Non-Antiarrhythmic Drugs) can be found at http://www.ich.org. The safety review should provide in this section an overview of effects on the QT interval, organized in a similar manner to the laboratory section. This section of the safety review should summarize the results of any studies designed specifically to assess the effects of the drug on the QT interval.

7.1.9.1 Extent of ECG Testing in the Development Program, Including Brief Review of Preclinical Results

This section should describe the number of baseline and on-study ECGs obtained, who read the ECGs, and what methodology was used (e.g., automatic, blinded cardiologists).

7.1.9.2 Selection of Studies and Analyses for Overall Drug-Control Comparisons

7.1.9.3 Standard Analyses and Explorations of ECG Data

7.1.9.3.1 Analyses Focused on Measures of Central Tendency

7.1.9.3.2 Analyses Focused on Outliers or Shifts from Normal to Abnormal

7.1.9.3.3 Marked Outliers and Dropouts for ECG Abnormalities

7.1.9.4 Additional Analyses and Explorations

7.1.10 Immunogenicity

Data on the impact of immunogenicity (if applicable) on safety, efficacy, and/or clinical pharmacology and pharmacokinetics may be summarized in this section and referenced throughout the review.

All therapeutic proteins have the potential to elicit antibody responses. An antibody response to a protein may have no consequences or, in some cases, can lead to potentially serious sequelae. Adverse immune responses to a protein drug could result in one or more of the following outcomes:

- For a product that is intended as replacement for a missing endogenous substance, antibodies could neutralize the replacement product and generate a clinical deficiency syndrome.
- Neutralization of a protein product by *blocking* antibodies could reduce the efficacy of a life-saving product.
- Antibody development could result in a life-threatening hypersensitivity response.

Factors that tend to increase the likelihood of an immune response include whether the protein is highly conserved in nature (less likely if it is), whether the protein product is administered via the subcutaneous route (more likely if it is), and whether the protein intended for chronic use. This section of the review should assess the adequacy of the immunogenicity data provided to address these issues.

7.1.11 Human Carcinogenicity

Although formal studies in humans of the carcinogenic effects of drugs and biologics are uncommon, reflecting the expectation that induction of cancer would occur over a very long period of exposure, a systematic assessment of human tumors reported during drug development can provide useful safety information in some cases. Such an assessment would be appropriate where controlled studies are of long duration (e.g., more than a year), especially for drugs or biologics that have positive genotoxicity or animal carcinogenicity findings or are known immune modulators.

7.1.12 Special Safety Studies

The review should describe and discuss results of any studies designed to evaluate a specific safety concern or concerns. These studies may include the following:

- Studies to assess whether a drug has safety concerns common to its pharmacologic class (e.g., a study to assess effects of a benzodiazepine hypnotic on driving, respiration, memory, or next day psychomotor functioning).
- Studies in topical products (including systemic products delivered by a patch) to assess cumulative irritancy, contact sensitizing potential, photosensitivity, and photoallergenicity.
- Studies to characterize a drug's effect on QT interval, part of most modern development efforts
- Studies intended to demonstrate a safety advantage over therapeutic alternatives (less extrapyramidal effect for an anti-psychotic, less sedation for an anti-histamine, less cough from an angiotensin II blocker than an ACE inhibitor). Such studies must include the comparator agent (a failure to see the side effect in a placebo-controlled study is usually not informative without the active control to demonstrate assay sensitivity).
- Studies in special populations thought to be at increased risk and likely to use the drug.

In labeling, the results of these studies should, as appropriate, supersede data from less targeted studies (e.g., observational safety data collected from efficacy trials).

7.1.13 Withdrawal Phenomena/Abuse Potential

The review should contain a discussion of abuse potential and any apparent withdrawal symptoms. For therapeutic classes with a history of abuse potential and withdrawal phenomena (e.g., sedative/hypnotics and anxiolytics), studies are usually performed to assess these issues. The review should comment on the adequacy and findings of these studies. For other drugs, adverse events that emerge after discontinuation of the drug should be assessed to determine whether they may indicate a withdrawal phenomenon. If the applicant evaluated the potential for withdrawal phenomena, the review should indicate whether there was a prospective or post hoc assessment of withdrawal emergent signs and symptoms (during drug taper or following discontinuation) and discuss the implications of the approach used on the reliability of the findings.

7.1.14 Human Reproduction and Pregnancy Data

Although formal studies in humans of the effects of drugs on reproduction, pregnancy, or lactation are uncommon, the review should summarize any drug exposure in pregnant or nursing women, including any inadvertent exposure during the drug's development and exposure identified from secondary sources (e.g., post-marketing surveillance). If there is no information on drug exposure in pregnant or lactating women, the review should acknowledge that fact. The review should discuss positive and negative findings.

7.1.15 Assessment of Effect on Growth

Increasingly, clinical reviewers are presented with analyses of height and weight data collected during studies of pediatric subjects. These data are generally inadequate to allow for definitive conclusions about an effect of drug on growth for several reasons. Assessment of the effect of drug on growth requires accurate measurements, particularly for height, and in most studies, height is not measured accurately. Growth is a process that occurs over long periods of time, and controlled trials of several weeks duration may not provide a sufficient period of observation to assess the effect of drug on growth. Open label studies can offer longer periods of time to observe effects on growth, but the lack of a control group limits the ability to separate the effect of drug and underlying disease on growth. Review of height and weight data for possible effects on growth makes use, in part, on approaches described above in the laboratory data section. Analysis of changes in central tendency and outlier analysis, for example, apply to the evaluation of the effect of a drug on growth. There are, however, some distinctive issues that must be considered.

First, the sponsor should describe how weight and height were measured. The manner in which these measurements were made will bear on how much confidence the reviewer can have in the data provided. For example, a development program in which the measurement schedule and methodology were standardized and in which the study staff were trained in measurement, will result in more reliable data than a development program that did not standardize procedures. The review should therefore include a description of the measurement methodology.

Second, growth is not constant throughout childhood and varies by age and sex. Without consideration of these factors at baseline, absolute mean changes in weight and height can give misleading results. Adjustment of growth for age and sex can be done by conversion of a child's height and weight to a z-score, which is the number of standard deviations that an individual's measurement is from the mean for age and sex matched children in the general population. A decrease in mean z-score for a group is interpreted as evidence of a lag in growth compared to what would be predicted using general population data. In a controlled trial, differences in mean z-score changes from baseline between treatment groups may provide evidence of an effect of drug on growth. Declines in mean z-scores in open label studies are less easily interpreted because these could result from the effect of drug or could be caused by the disease for which the treatment is being studied.

Sponsors should provide analyses of height and weight data that assess measures of central tendency and outlier analyses using height and weight z-scores. Although results from these analyses will not provide definitive proof of drug-related effects on growth in most cases, they may help identify candidates for prospective studies of the effect of drug on growth in children. The review team should request such analyses at the pre-NDA meeting.

7.1.16 Overdose Experience

The review should summarize all overdose experience with a drug in humans (including both information provided by the applicant and information obtained from secondary sources) and describe the constellation of signs, symptoms, and other abnormalities one might expect to see in association with overdose. Phase 1 data should be reviewed to identify subjects who may have received higher doses than those used in later phases of study. In addition, patients with certain physiological differences that would compromise their ability to clear a drug (e.g., renal impairment, hepatic impairment, limited CYP4502D6 activity for a drug cleared by this isozyme) may provide data relevant to the clinical implications of overdose.

7.1.17 Post-marketing Experience

Relevant findings from post-marketing experience, if any, should be described briefly here and referenced in the summary section (Section 7.3).

7.2 ADEQUACY OF PATIENT EXPOSURE AND SAFETY ASSESSMENTS

Section 7.1 is an assessment of the adverse events seen during the development program. Section 7.2 should provide the reviewer's comments on the adequacy of drug exposure and the safety evaluations performed as part of the development program. This section addresses the regulatory question of whether or not *all tests reasonably applicable* were conducted to assess the safety of the new drug. Was there adequate experience with the drug in terms of overall numbers of patients and in appropriate demographic subsets of patients? Were doses and durations of exposure appropriate? Were all (or not all) appropriate tests performed in the exposed patients? Were all necessary and appropriate animal tests performed? Were all the appropriate clinical tests carried out (e.g., electrocardiographic assessment of effects on QT interval)? Was the drug adequately worked up metabolically? Were appropriate *in vitro* studies of drug–drug interaction carried out according to current guidelines? Were all potentially important findings adequately explored: for example, to what extent was psychomotor impairment specifically assessed in a drug that is sedating?

If important data are missing, this could influence the regulatory action on the drug. A critical task of the reviewer in this section is identification of specific concerns that need to be addressed by the applicant, either before approval or post-approval. Even more than for most other parts of the review, the reviewer needs to be conscious of recent developments and discuss issues broadly. Finally, this section is the place for detailed comments on the quality and completeness of the data provided.

The review should clearly describe the studies and overall extent of the data supporting the evaluation of safety. The reviewer should then make a judgment about the adequacy of the clinical experience with the new drug for assessing safety.

7.2.1 Description of Primary Clinical Data Sources (Populations Exposed and Extent of Exposure) Used to Evaluate Safety

In this section the reviewer should identify and characterize the primary safety data sources used in conducting the review. If these are described elsewhere in the review, this section can reference those sections. The primary source is generally the database derived from the applicant's development program. Studies in this program will generally have full study reports related to safety, or studies that are grouped for analysis of safety in an Integrated Summary of Safety; CRFs will be available. These studies usually will have been closely monitored. Secondary sources may also be available and may be of critical importance (e.g., for a drug already available in other countries), and there may be some parts of the database that have had limited analyses (i.e., only for deaths and adverse dropouts); these are described in Section 7.2.2.

Tables and graphs are useful in describing the data sources for the safety review. Generally, the reviewer should use the tables and graphs in this section to characterize the overall database. The detailed tables and other displays for this subsection may be included in an appendix to the review, but summary tables and narrative statements should be included here. The reviewer should also characterize the per patient data (narratives, CRFs, CRTs and electronically accessible databases for baseline information. See Section 7.4 for discussion of ability to link databases.

7.2.1.1 *Study Type and Design/Patient Enumeration*

The reviewer should include in an appendix a table, such as that illustrated in Table 7.2.1.1.1, enumerating all subjects and patients across the entire development program, Phases 1–3. This is a critical table that identifies the important patient pools and denominators for subsequent analyses and incidence estimates.

The reviewer should also include an appendix table that provides brief descriptive information for all individual studies, including study design (fixed dose vs. flexible dose, parallel vs. crossover), dosing schedule, study location (foreign vs. domestic), treatment groups and doses, sample sizes, patient population (elderly). Studies that were designed to assess a particular aspect of safety (e.g., ECG, ophthalmic) should be noted. Most NDAs/BLAs will include a table of all studies, as such a table is called for in the Clinical/Statistical guideline *and in the Common Technical Document.*

Applicants sometimes segregate certain clinical trials from their primary source data (see Section 7.2.2, secondary source data), especially foreign data. This may be appropriate, especially if there is a basis for believing that these data differ substantially in quality and/or completeness or in critical aspects of investigator practice from the data included in the primary source database. This is a matter of judgment, however, and cannot be assumed to be valid. An explanation should be provided in the review describing the basis for decisions about what data were included and what excluded from the primary source data.

An NDA/BLA generally includes data from patient samples that are at different levels of completeness in terms of data entry, information collected, and validation. Table 7.2.1.1.1 should include patient counts (or estimates) from all studies contributing data, regardless of these factors. Data cutoff dates or database *lock dates* for the various databases comprising the NDA/BLA should be identified at this point in the review. For example, the cutoff date for the overall safety database derived from completed studies might be more distant, while the cutoff date for submitting serious adverse events from all studies may generally be more recent.

These dates may likely need updating during the course of NDA/BLA review as more data become available.

7.2.1.2 Demographics

The reviewer should include appendix tables in a format similar to that illustrated in Table 7.2.1.2.1 (showing percent distribution within treatments of patients by age, gender, and race as well as weight in various groups), providing overall demographic information for Phase 1 and Phases 2–3 study pools separately. It may be appropriate to provide demographic displays for subsets within these larger pools at other points in the review.

7.2.1.3 Extent of Exposure (Dose/Duration)

There are many ways to summarize the dose and duration experience with a new drug. Either can be expressed as mean, median, maximum, with histograms or other displays that give the numbers exposed at various doses or for various durations. A particularly useful approach is to provide combined dose and duration information. It is suggested that the review contain tables in the format illustrated in Table 7.2.1.3, enumerating patients on the basis of mean daily dose of the NDA/BLA drug and duration of administration for Phase 1 and Phases 2–3 study pools separately. If the study used a titration design, the modal dose (if two different doses were used for the same duration, the larger, or maximal modal dose) may be the more useful summary statistic. It is particularly important to examine the subgroup of patients who received a dose at least as large as the dose intended for marketing.

It may also be useful to provide similar tables based on maximum dose, modal dose, dose expressed as mg/kg or mg/m^2, or even plasma concentrations, if such data are available.

It may also be useful to provide similar tables for various subgroups (e.g., males and females separately, various age groups separately, and patients with various co-morbid illnesses of interest separately). There should be similar displays for active control drugs if any were included in trials for the new drug.

Finally, it may be useful for the review to include an appendix table providing total person-time exposure data for the NDA/BLA drug, active control, and placebo, for the Phases 2–3 database.

7.2.2 Description of Secondary Clinical Data Sources Used to Evaluate Safety

Secondary source data are (1) data derived from studies not conducted under the applicant's investigational new drug (IND) and for which CRFs and full study reports are not available,[21] or studies so poorly conducted (e.g., poor ascertainment for adverse events), that they cannot be reasonably included in the primary source database, (2) post-marketing data, and (3) literature reports on studies not conducted under the IND. Often the applicant may have made the distinction between the data considered primary source data and other data, and the reviewer needs to examine the rationale for this distinction.

The secondary sources should be briefly described. It is worth emphasizing that secondary source data may be a critical source of information for review, despite the generally lower quality of these data, because they often provide the larger database needed to look for less common serious adverse events and may be reliable with respect to deaths and serious adverse events.

7.2.2.1 Other Studies

The NDA/BLA should be clear in describing exactly what other studies provided data and what the basis was for not integrating such data with the primary source data (e.g., no CRFs, no study reports, not adequately monitored). Lack of clarity in this should be noted by the reviewer.

7.2.2.2 Post-Marketing Experience

If post-marketing data are available, this section should describe briefly the type of information available for review. An example of such a description would be a comment that a line listing for (a specified number of) spontaneous reports from marketing in (country) was provided, along with narrative summaries for the serious adverse events among the reports and an estimate of product use in (country) during that time period. As is the case for most spontaneous reports, these reports are likely to be difficult to interpret. Important events will be described in appropriate sections (e.g., 7.1.1 and 7.1.2, Deaths and Other Serious Events).

7.2.2.3 Literature

Relevant literature may be incorporated in various sections of the NDA, but is ordinarily included in Section 5.4 of the Common Technical Document (*M4: The CTD – Efficacy*). The NDA/BLA may include a separate literature section or the literature may be provided or referenced as called for in various places in the Clinical/Statistical guideline in section II F, Other Studies and Information. The applicant should have provided a description of the search strategy to assess the world literature (e.g., databases used, key search words), the personnel who carried it out (their credentials)

---

[21] If CRFs are available from any such studies and the data quality is comparable to that of data from studies conducted under the applicant's IND, these data would ordinarily be included in the primary source database.

and whether the search relied on abstracts or full texts (including translations) of articles. A cutoff date for the literature search should also have been provided. A copy (translated as required) should have been submitted for any report or finding judged by the applicant to be potentially important.

This section of the review should describe what information from the literature search was provided for review, the extent to which the above description of an ideal presentation was met, and whether any missing information is important (and/or was obtained by the reviewer). Independent literature reviews conducted by the reviewer should be described here as well.

Actual safety findings should be described in appropriate sections of the safety review to present from the literature reports in this section of the review.

7.2.3 Adequacy of Overall Clinical Experience

In evaluating the adequacy of clinical experience with the drug, the reviewer should refer to current ICH guidance on extent and duration of exposure needed to assess safety[22] as well as the draft guidance on *Pre-Marketing Risk Assessment*.[23] The review should specifically address the following:

- Whether an adequate number of subjects were exposed to the drug, including adequate numbers of various demographic subsets and people with pertinent risk factors.
- Whether doses and durations of exposure were adequate to assess safety for the intended use.
- Whether the design of studies (open, active control, placebo control) was adequate to answer critical questions.
- Whether potential class effects were evaluated (e.g., for anti-arrhythmic effects, evaluation of the potential for pro-arrhythmic effects) and whether problems suggested by pre-clinical data were assessed.
- Whether patients excluded from the study limit the relevance of safety assessments (e.g., diabetics, people over 75, people with recent myocardial infarction, people with renal or hepatic functional impairment, or people on

other therapy). This may depend on the signals of toxicity that were observed in the patients who were studied.

7.2.4 Adequacy of Special Animal and/or *In Vitro* Testing

The clinical reviewer should not attempt a general assessment of the preclinical program, but rather, comment on whether preclinical testing was adequate to explore certain potential adverse reactions, using preclinical models based either on a drug's pharmacology or on clinical findings that emerged early in clinical development. For example, for a drug anticipated to cause QT prolongation because of its drug class or because QT prolongation was seen in Phase 1 studies, there are *in vitro* models to evaluate this potential. The reviewer should note whether such studies were done. If such studies were performed, the results would be summarized in the Pharmacology Review.

7.2.5 Adequacy of Routine Clinical Testing

The reviewer should comment on the adequacy of routine clinical testing of study subjects, including efforts to elicit adverse event data and monitor laboratory parameters, vital signs, and ECGs. In assessing the adequacy of clinical testing, the reviewer should consider the adequacy of the methods and tests used and the frequency of testing. The adequacy of specific testing intended to assess certain expected or observed reactions should be discussed under Section 7.2.7.

The reviewer should be alert to the absence of data in an NDA laboratory database for analytes that are typically included in routine laboratory monitoring. For example, it was discovered after approval that the NDA laboratory database for the anti-epileptic drug zonisamide did not have data on serum bicarbonate. It was later determined that this drug is associated with a nonanion gap metabolic acidosis. The serum bicarbonate data would have been helpful in identifying this adverse reaction earlier.

7.2.6 Adequacy of Metabolic, Clearance, and Interaction Workup

Knowledge of how a drug is metabolized and excreted is critical to anticipating safety problems in patients with impaired excretory or metabolic function and problems resulting from drug–drug interactions.

Drug–drug interaction assessment is a critical part of a modern drug development program and should evaluate the drug both as a substrate for interactions (interference with its clearance) and as an inducer or inhibitor of the clearance of other drugs. The reviewer should comment on the

[22] ICH *E1A The Extent of Population Exposure to Assess Clinical Safety: For Drugs Intended for Long-Term Treatment of Non-Life-Threatening Conditions* (http://www.fda.gov/cder/guidance/iche1a.pdf) recognizes possible differences in expected exposure (e.g., more patient exposure would be expected for drugs with small effects, or drugs that are used prophylactically in well populations, where only a small fraction of patients will benefit).

[23] A draft guidance *Premarketing Risk Assessment* was issued in May 2004. Once finalized, it will represent the Agency's thinking on this topic.

adequacy of *in vitro* and *in vivo* testing carried out by the applicant to identify the following:

- The enzymatic pathways responsible for clearance of the drug and the effects of inhibition of those pathways, notably CYP450 enzymes and P-glycoproteins.
- The effect of the drug on CYP450 enzymes (inhibition, induction) and the effects of the drug on the PK of model compounds.
- The major potential safety consequences of drug–drug interactions.

Details of these assessments will be found in the Clinical Pharmacology Review and in the summary of that evaluation in the Medical Officer's Review.

7.2.7 Adequacy of Evaluation for Potential Adverse Reactions for Any New Drug and Particularly for Drugs in the Class Represented by New Drug; Recommendations for Further Study

The reviewer should discuss the adequacy of the applicant's efforts to detect specific adverse reactions that are potentially problematic and might be expected with a drug of any class (e.g., QT prolongation or hepatotoxicity) or that are predicted on the basis of the drug class (e.g., sexual dysfunction with SSRI anti-depressants). The reviewer should also discuss whether the applicant should have made efforts to assess certain events that it did not assess. The reviewer should also discuss pertinent negative findings (absence of findings) for a drug in this section of the review (see examples below).

The adverse events that warrant specific attention will vary depending on the characteristics of the drug and the drug class. The known pharmacology of the drug would suggest some evaluations (e.g., first dose effects for peripheral alpha blockers, tolerance and withdrawal effects for central alpha agonists, urinary retention with anti-cholinergics, QT prolongation with type III anti-arrhythmics, extrapyramidal effects with anti-psychotics, muscle pain with statins), while experience with other members of the class would suggest others (e.g., hepatotoxicity with thiazolidinedione peroxisome proliferator-activated receptor (PPAR) gamma agonists (glitizones), tendon problems with fluoroquinolones). There should be a subheading for each adverse reaction that warrants special consideration (even if not observed) and, under each subheading, a discussion of what was done to detect the reaction and the adequacy of the approach. The following list of potential adverse reactions, and some of the drug and therapeutic classes that might trigger higher interest in them, may be a useful starting point in assembling a list (it is also important to examine labeling for other members of the drug's pharmacologic class):

- Hepatotoxicity (NSAIDs, thiazolidinedione PPAR gamma agonists)

- Pancreatic toxicity
- QT prolongation (any anti-arrhythmic, anti-psychotic, anti-histamine, fluoroquinolone)
- Vasodilator effects, such as hypotension (alpha blockers) or edema (dihydropyridine calcium channel blockers)
- Withdrawal effects (beta blockers, central alpha agonists, SSRIs, narcotics)
- Orthostatic hypotension (any anti-hypertensive, anti-psychotics)
- Hypertension (any sympathomimetic or phosphodiesterase inhibitor)
- Tachycardia
- Neutropenia (drugs related to ticlopidine, procainamide, clozapine)
- Bleeding (drugs inhibiting any aspect of clotting or platelet function, NSAIDs)
- Aplastic anemia
- Increased coagulation times
- Muscle injury (any HMG CoA reductase inhibitor (statin) or other lipid-lowering drug)
- Sedation (any psychotropic drug)
- CNS stimulation
- Anti-cholinergic activity
- Allergic reactions
- Sexual dysfunction (any anti-depressant, sedating drug)
- Elevated intra-ocular pressure
- Cataracts
- Retinopathy
- Worsening glucose tolerance/diabetes (diuretics, atypical anti-psychotics)
- Pro-arrhythmic effects and increased mortality (most nonbeta blocker anti-arrhythmics)
- Increased congestive heart failure (CHF) and SD mortality (any inotrope, some negative inotropes such as calcium channel blockers)
- Nephropathy (NSAIDs)

Example 1: If orthostatic hypotension was an expected adverse reaction, but was not observed, the reviewer should determine whether the applicant made efforts to detect it and, if so, whether the applicant's approach (e.g., timing and frequency of vital signs testing) was adequate to detect it.

Example 2: If QT prolongation was observed in Phase 1 studies, the reviewer should ascertain whether the applicant made efforts, beyond routine ECG testing, in Phases 2 and 3 to explore the consequences in patients of the observed QT prolongation and, if so, whether those efforts were adequate, including adequate exposure to higher doses. For example, how did the applicant follow-up patients who experienced clinical events that may be manifestations of TdP (e.g., syncope, dizziness, or palpitations)? Holter monitoring, for example, might have been appropriate in such patients.

7.2.8 Assessment of Quality and Completeness of Data

The reviewer should provide general overall assessments of the quality and completeness of the data available for conducting the safety review and describe the bases for these assessments. More than that, attention to completeness and quality of assessment is important throughout the review. The reviewer should recognize that quality may *differ from* the primary source data and for data over which the applicant had less control. The following examples illustrate some of the ways in which applicants can differ in the quality and completeness of data they provide:

- Applicants may differ in what they include in a CRF. For example, if additional laboratory data are collected at unscheduled visits or after the normal end of a trial, some do not include these data. Such data may be stored in some other place (a *correspondence file*). Sometimes additional information is attached to the front of the CRF as *queries*. If CRFs do not indicate any additional testing beyond the routine assessments, the reviewer should ascertain whether additional testing was done to reassess abnormal values before the next routine visit (e.g., at an unscheduled visit). If the CRFs do not indicate that additional testing was performed, the reviewer should ask the applicant if additional laboratory data are available.
- If it is apparent that the CRF contains insufficient information about an adverse event (e.g., if a patient was hospitalized for an adverse event), the reviewer needs to determine whether there is additional information available. Such an observation also raises the general question of whether all pertinent data have been included in CRFs.
- The reviewer should be concerned about patients with abnormal clinical or laboratory findings who are lost to follow-up, particularly if there are significant numbers of such patients. In these situations, the reviewer may consider asking the applicant to attempt to obtain the needed follow-up information. If the information cannot be obtained, it may be appropriate to perform sensitivity analyses to assess the possible impact of missing data, assuming a worst-case outcome.
- The reviewer should be particularly alert to situations in which applicants make changes in CRFs to reclassify adverse events or reasons for subjects dropping out without the investigator's agreement. There is greater concern where serious adverse events are reclassified and reclassifications are done without blinding. The reviewer should ask the applicants about procedures used (if unclear) and attempt to assess the impact of multiple changes on the safety evaluation.
- For electronic data, the reviewer should clarify what information is, and is not, included in the electronic files. For example, if a reviewer is relying on electronic files from the CRFs, it is important to know what, if any, information from the CRFs was not included. A separate file may be needed for any missing data.

7.2.9 Additional Submissions, Including Safety Update

The initial NDA/BLA submission may not contain all information pertinent to the safety evaluation. Further data submissions may be planned at the time of initial submission and filing (e.g., results of additional long-term follow-up), may represent responses to specific questions or discipline review letters, or may be part of the safety update required under regulations (21 CFR 314.50(d)(5)(vi)(b)). It is critical to review these data to determine whether safety conclusions are affected, particularly with respect to serious or fatal events.

This section should:

- Describe safety submissions, noting whether the results have been incorporated into the rest of the review or are considered in this section.
- For those safety matters not incorporated into the rest of the review, discuss any data with important implications for safety. In general, this will involve deaths, adverse dropouts and other serious events, and these should be considered as in Sections 7.1.1, 7.1.2, 7.1.3, as appropriate to the (usually) small numbers. Only if these events alter the overall safety picture will a more detailed discussion of the entire area (e.g., deaths, liver injury) be needed.

Any reports of important changes in foreign labeling or new studies that give insight into more common events should also be noted.

7.3 SUMMARY OF SELECTED ADVERSE REACTIONS, IMPORTANT LIMITATIONS OF DATA, AND CONCLUSIONS

This section of the review should briefly summarize each of the adverse reactions that the reviewer considers important and drug-related (i.e., this should constitute a *problem list* for the drug). For each adverse reaction, there should be a separate subheading followed by a brief summary of the reaction and references to sections of the review (e.g., other parts of the safety section, Clinical Pharmacology, studies described in the Efficacy section) containing more detailed information about the adverse reaction generally, or specific aspects of the reaction. The review should integrate by reference all relevant details about the reaction, including patient identifying numbers for certain patients (e.g., for deaths). Below is a sample summary section entry for QT prolongation:

QT Prolongation

Dose-related QT prolongation compared to control was seen in all controlled trials, with a mean change of 20 msec at 100 mg/day (peak), the recommended maximum dose, and smaller changes at lower doses; 5% of patients had QTc values over 500 msec at some point, compared with ___ percent on placebo. The drug's metabolism is predominately via CYP4503A4, so that moderate inhibitors of this enzyme could lead to greater QTc prolongation. The QTc effects of doses greater than 100 mg have not been studied.

- See Section 7.1.1 (Deaths) at page __ for discussion of deaths that may be related to QT prolongation and detailed discussion of the finding.
- See Section 7.1.9 (ECGs) at page __ for discussion of ECG changes.
- See Section 7.1.10 (Special Studies) at page __ for dose response study of QT prolongation (doses of 10, 40, and 100 mg).
- See Section 7.2.4 (Metabolic and Interaction Workup) at page __ for discussion of the adequacy of the applicant's *in vivo* and *in vitro* assessments of the metabolism of (drug) and potential relation of drug–drug interactions to QT prolongation.
- See Section 3.2 (Animal Pharmacology/Toxicology) at page __ for discussion of the animal models used to evaluate effects on K channels, and QT prolongation.
- See Section 7.2.1.1.2.3 (Literature) at page __ for published articles about similar products and methodological suggestions.
- See Section 7.1.13 (Overdose) at page __.
- Patient ID numbers for possibly relevant deaths: _____, _____, _____.

As the QT prolongation example shows, it is useful to identify the various sections of the clinical review that can be referenced for additional details about an identified adverse event. If the review is converted into a PDF file, bookmarking can be used to electronically link the text in the problem list to earlier sections of the review.

In addition, in this section the reviewer should provide summary recommendations for further studies, with a reference to Section 7.2 for more details.

The review should also provide overall conclusions about the safety of the drug, including:

- Overall assessment of the available safety information, referring both to what it has shown and its adequacy.
- The limitations of the available data.
- Additional information needed, including both further analyses and additional studies.

- Comparison, to the extent possible, of the safety of the drug under review to the safety of other available products, and the basis for that comparison (direct comparative data vs. clinical opinion).
- Whether a risk management program (beyond labeling) is needed and why.
- Analysis of likely uses beyond labeling, (e.g., in more severe patients, in other diseases, in children).
- Whether there is a need for post-marketing safety studies.

7.4 GENERAL METHODOLOGY

This section of the guidance describes analytical methods that have general application to the safety review and provides a location in the review for any general discussion of methodological issues not discussed elsewhere, organized by the subsections listed here, with additional sections as needed. It is important to consider early in the review whether the available patient level data will allow the analyses the reviewer intends. For example, in examining whether particular baseline risk factors are related to an adverse event, the reviewer will either need to extract the baseline characteristics from case report tabulations or be sure the information is available in a retrievable form. Similarly, it may be important to link individual safety observations with other on therapy data, such as dose, duration of treatment, concomitant therapy, other adverse events, lab data or effectiveness results (it is obviously best if such issues are considered at pre-NDA/BLA meetings).

7.4.1 Pooling Data Across Studies to Estimate and Compare Incidence

7.4.1.1 *Pooled Data vs. Individual Study Data*

Before estimating the incidence of adverse events, the reviewer must select the patient sample of interest. Pooling data from different studies can improve the precision of an incidence estimate (i.e., narrow the confidence intervals by enlarging the sample size). Better precision is particularly important for lower frequency events, which can be difficult to detect and may not occur in some studies. Pooling can also provide the larger database that will permit explorations of possible drug–demographic or drug–disease interactions in subgroups of the population. Pooling can also, however, obscure real potentially meaningful differences between studies. The review should explain why any pooling used in the review was chosen. When making decisions about pooling, the reviewer should consider the following:

- It is most appropriate to combine data from studies that are of similar design, that is, similar in dose, duration, choice of control, methods of ascertainment, and population (checklist vs. general inquiries vs. no prompt at all; in psychiatric drug trials it is typical for obsessive compulsive patients to spontaneously report adverse events more frequently than schizophrenic patients. It is also possible that different populations may have different vulnerabilities to a drug, and therefore, different risk profiles.) When the studies are similar in design but differ in duration, it may be critical to account for exposure duration and to look for time-dependent events.

- Even when the pooled analysis is the primary one, it is important to explore the range of incidences across the studies being pooled. For a specific adverse event, if the incidence differs substantially across the individual studies in a pool, the pooled value should not be used, as it is probably not meaningful and, in some cases, could obscure important information about predictors for that event. (In one case, for example, several studies were combined and a reassuringly low estimate of phototoxicity was obtained. Subsequent examination of individual study results found one study with a substantial rate of phototoxicity. The study was the only outpatient study done (i.e., the only one in which patients had an opportunity to be exposed to sunlight). In some situations, the incidence may be best described by the range in the various studies. For the phototoxicity example above, however, the most relevant data are those from the outpatient study, the only study that was conducted under conditions pertinent to intended use.

- In some cases, observed differences in rates in various studies can be explained (e.g., better ascertainment, different populations), so that a consistent rate can be determined from a subset of studies.

- Formal tests for extreme values may be useful to assess appropriateness of assay pooled data (e.g., test of heterogeneity such as the Breslow–Day Chi-square test could be used). Alternatively, the reviewer might use a more subjective approach, such as determining if the direction of the difference is always the same across studies, or use a graphic display of incidence by study to informally consider the extent of variability and to identify outliers; outliers may be important in identifying subgroups of patients who are at particular risk for certain adverse reactions.

7.4.1.2 *Combining Data*

In pooling data, usually the numerator events and denominators for the selected studies are simply combined. Other more formal weighting methods can be used (e.g., weighting studies on the basis of study size or inversely to their variance). The review should describe how the pooling was performed, as well as the rationale for selection of the method used.

7.4.2 Explorations for Predictive Factors

Adverse reaction rates may differ considerably from one patient population to another and may change over time. Factors that may affect the safety profile of a drug should be explored during the review. Explorations for common predictive factors, such as dose, plasma level, duration of treatment and concomitant medications, and patient-predictive factors such as age, sex, race, concomitant illnesses, are considered below. In general, these explorations are meaningful only for adverse events that appear to be drug-related (see Section 7.4.3).

7.4.2.1 *Explorations for Dose Dependency for Adverse Findings*

If data from randomized, parallel, fixed-dose studies (or data from studies in which patients were randomized to fixed dose ranges), are available, they should be analyzed for evidence of dose dependency for any adverse reactions. If plasma concentration data are available, it may be useful to explore plasma concentration effect relationships as well. It may also be useful to reconfigure dose as mg/kg or mg/m^2, to decrease the effect of size or weight differences on drug exposure. Dose–response relationships should also be examined in demographic subgroups (e.g., females, blacks, elderly patients). Dose-dependency analyses are usually performed by simple inspection of incidence rates across different doses or different weight or body surface area-adjusted doses. Formal statistical testing can also be used. If formal statistical tests are performed for a study that includes placebo control as well as different doses, and a drug-placebo difference is apparent, it may be desirable to focus on between-dose group differences.

Flexible Dose Titration Studies

Although it is tempting to try to extract dose-response or plasma level-response data from flexible dose (titration) studies, and the ICH dose-response guideline[24] encourages this, there are many potential problems with such analyses. In particular, many adverse reactions show considerable time dependency, some occurring early, some late. It is easy to confound dose (or plasma concentration) with duration when dose is increased over time. In some cases, such as anti-cancer drugs or drugs that are known to produce anti-cholinergic or sedating reactions, the drug is dose-adjusted to toxicity, which will often obscure any dose–response relationship. In addition, if dose is increased only in patients without adverse effects (i.e., subjects who are resistant to them), the higher doses will be associated with lower adverse effect rates. On the other hand, if dose

---

[24] See ICH *E4Dose-Response Information to Support Drug Registration* (http://www.fda.gov/cder/guidance/iche4.pdf).

is titrated to clinical effect, and adverse reactions occur late (so that they do not affect the dose given), analysis of the rate with respect to dose may be useful. For example, erythropoietin, used to treat anemia in patients with chronic renal failure or cancer, is titrated to maintain hemoglobin within a specific range. Given the delayed therapeutic response (erythropoiesis), analysis of adverse events by dose or cumulative dose prior to a reaction can give insight into dose-related toxicity.

Cumulative Dose Dependency

For certain adverse reactions, it may be possible to demonstrate a relationship between cumulative dose and the occurrence of the reaction (e.g., liver fibrosis and cirrhosis with methotrexate, cardiotoxicity with doxorubicin, renal toxicity with Amphotericin B). For drugs that are used chronically, the reviewer should consider the possibility that cumulative dose may predict toxicity and discuss this in the review.

7.4.2.2 Explorations of Time Dependency for Adverse Findings

The reviewer should explore time dependency of adverse reactions in two ways – time to onset of the finding and duration of the finding:

Time of Onset

Although most adverse reactions occur early in treatment and may be best characterized by a crude incidence rate (number with the reaction divided by number exposed), others may occur only after some delay of weeks, months, or longer. A crude incidence rate, based on a patient population exposed predominantly for short periods, will understate the importance of such adverse reactions for chronically used drugs. For important adverse reactions that occur later in treatment, there should be explorations of the time dependency of the reaction. Possible methods include:

- A life table (Kaplan–Meier graph) describing risk as a function of duration of exposure (i.e., cumulative incidence).
- Plotting risk for discrete time intervals over the observation period (i.e., a hazard rate curve) reveals how risk changes over time.
- Adjusting for duration of exposure by expressing the adverse reaction rate in terms of person-time (person-time is duration of exposure summed across all patients, e.g., 2 patients each exposed for 6 months = 1 patient-exposure-year). This approach is useful only when one can safely assume that the hazard rate is constant over time.

Duration of Adverse Event

Certain adverse events that occur at initiation of treatment may *appear* to diminish in frequency with continued use.

Possible expanations for this phenomenon include adaptation or tolerance, decreased reporting of the event even by patients though it is still occurring at the same rate, and reduced dose or dropping out in patients with the event. For drugs used chronically and for which there was an adverse event that seemed to diminish in frequency over time, it may be useful to characterize and quantify the change. It would be important, for adverse events of interest, to determine whether the decreased rate simply reflected discontinuation by affected patients or real adaptation. One way to make this distinction is to identify a cohort that experienced an event of interest during a specified period of a trial, but nonetheless completed the trial, and observe the rate of the event in that cohort over time. This cohort of survivors could be compared to a similar cohort of placebo recipients who experienced the same event at baseline. The same approach could be used for adverse events occurring later in treatment. It is usually sufficient to do such analyses for those adverse reactions that are relatively common and likely to be drug-related (see Section 7.1.5.4 for methods to identify drug-related events).

7.4.2.3 Explorations for Drug–Demographic Interactions

Numerous methods can be used to analyze age, gender, and race implications for safety, and applicants must present analyses of safety information for these population subsets. In most cases, there will be pharmacokinetic information available for some or all of these subsets, which may help in interpreting adverse event rates. In some cases, it may be useful to construct subgroups based on more than one factor. For example, bleeding is the principal risk associated with use of thrombolytic agents in patients with AMI. Women tend to have more bleeding than men, and risk is inversely related to weight. Thus, an analysis by gender weight subgroups can identify the group at greatest risk of bleeding (thin women). It may also be useful to consider age–gender or race–gender subgroups. Formal analysis should be limited to events considered common (e.g., occurring at an incidence of at least 2%) and that occur at a clearly greater rate on drug than placebo. In small studies or for low frequency events, there will usually not be sufficient power to detect differences between groups, so that these analyses will usually be based on pooled data. In general, these analyses are descriptive, comparing risk of an event in one subset with the risk in another (men vs. women, old vs. young, black vs. white); as these comparisons obviously do not reflect randomization to the subset (baseline characteristic) of interest, formal statistical comparisons are usually not warranted. For these descriptive comparisons, two approaches deserve consideration; when the control rates of adverse events differ for population subsets these approaches can provide quite different results: (1) evaluation of relative risk (RR) (cumulative risk on drug/cumulative risk on comparison drug or placebo) and

(2) evaluation of attributable risk (AR) (cumulative risk on drug-cumulative risk on comparison drug or placebo).

When background event rates differ by demographic subgroup, relative risk analysis will provide a quantitative estimate of the difference in effect of the drug, but the AR may be a better estimate of the importance of the risk in the subsets. To illustrate, consider a comparison of drug-induced nausea for males vs. females. Suppose the rate of nausea on placebo is 1% for men and 3% for women and that on drug it is 3% for men and 9% for women. The risk ratios (RR) for both sexes are 3 and the relative risk for men and women (RRf/RRm) is one (no difference), yet the AR is much greater for women than men (6% vs. 2%), a finding of possible importance in treatment. Such a difference has been observed for several adverse reactions of amlodipine, a calcium channel blocker, and is described in labeling as a gender difference, even though the RR's are the same.

7.4.2.4 *Explorations for Drug–Disease Interactions*

The reviewer should be alert to the possibility that co-morbidity will affect the adverse reaction profile of the drug (i.e., a drug–disease interaction). Such interactions can arise from abnormalities of excretory function (renal or hepatic disease), and typically, the applicant will have carried out formal pharmacokinetic studies in patients with hepatic and renal disease to indicate the potential for such reactions. The reviewer needs to consider, in that case, whether PK differences are manifested as differences in adverse reaction rates. Apart from differences in adverse reaction rates related to PK differences, differences in rates can also reflect true differences in susceptibility to adverse reactions (i.e., real pharmacodynamic differences). In general, the same methods described for exploring drug–demographic interactions can be applied here.

7.4.2.5 *Explorations for Drug–Drug Interactions*

The clinical reviewer should be alert to the potential of drug–drug interactions to affect the safety profile of the drug. Again, these interactions could be either pharmacokinetic (affecting elimination of the drug) or pharmacodynamic, in either case leading to observed differences in adverse reaction rates for the subgroups receiving or not receiving co-administered drugs. Typically, there will be formal interaction studies to evaluate potential pharmacokinetic effects of concomitant therapy on drugs metabolized by CYP450 enzymes, but PK interactions can also occur through effects on renal excretion and transport (P-glycoprotein) proteins. True pharmacodynamic interactions are less frequently recognized but can be important (e.g., marked hypotension when sildenafil is given with organic nitrates). In general, the same methods described for exploring drug–demographic interactions can be applied here.

7.4.3 Causality Determination

In assessing the critical question of whether an adverse event is caused by a drug, whether the drug is capable of causing that adverse event in the population is usually of greater interest than whether the drug caused the event in each patient who reported the event, but the approach to causality is distinctly different for relatively common events and relatively rare, serious events.

Common Events
Where events are common and occur in multiple patients in controlled trials, it is usually not necessary or helpful to consider each case individually. Rather, all reported cases can be considered potentially drug-related, and causality is assessed by comparing the rates of reports in patients treated with test drug and in control groups. If an event is clearly more frequent with test drug than the control, it can be attributed to treatment with the test drug.

Uncommon, Serious Events
Causality judgments are much more difficult for uncommon (e.g., <1/1000) serious events where there are, in most cases, no useful comparisons to control groups. The reviewer therefore must form a judgment as to the plausibility of drug-relatedness for the individual cases.

- The following questions should be considered:
  1. Was the patient in fact exposed to drug and did the adverse event occur after drug exposure?
  2. Did the patient have a clinical experience that meets the criteria for the adverse event of interest? (Establishing a standard case definition may be helpful here.)
  3. Is there a reasonably compelling alternative explanation for the event? (For example, recent benzene exposure for a case of aplastic anemia; the event is a well-recognized consequence of the patient's underlying illness.)
  4. Is the adverse event of a type commonly associated with drug exposure, such as hematologic, hepatic, renal, dermatologic or pro-arrhythmic events? (But also see below caution about discarding events that do not seem plausibly drug-related.)
- After assessing individual cases to identify events that could be drug-related and for which there are no compelling alternative explanations, the reviewer should compare the observed rate of occurrence of the event in the database with a best estimate about the background rate for the event for the population being studied. For an event like aplastic anemia, with a background rate of perhaps 1 per million person years, finding even one case suggests a causal relationship. For events that occur more frequently in the absence of drug therapy

(e.g., MI, stroke, sudden death, seizure, which could occur at rates of 0.1–1%, depending on the population), the finding of one or two cases may be very difficult to interpret in the absence of a substantial controlled trial database.

- The reviewer should also evaluate any other information about the drug that bears on causality including:
  1. Whether the drug is a member of a class of drugs known to be causally associated with the event of interest.
  2. Presence of other adverse events in the database that may be associated with the event of interest (e.g., a general finding of drug associated transaminitis or animal findings suggestive of hepatotoxicity would substantially strengthen the signal generated by the finding of a single case of hepatic failure).
  3. Positive re-challenge with the drug (although it would be unusual to deliberately re-challenge for a serious event, there may occasionally be inadvertent re-exposures that are informative).

- Caution concerning relative plausibility of uncommon, serious events.

The reviewer should be cautious about dismissing uncommon, serious events *that don't seem plausibly drug-related* and should consider differences in common less serious adverse reactions that might predict the uncommon serious reactions with longer use. There are numerous examples of uncommon, serious adverse reactions that are uniquely associated with a drug or drug class:

- Tendon rupture associated with the quinolone antibiotics
- Heart valve lesions associated with fenfluramine
- Practolol syndrome
- Retroperitoneal fibrosis with Sansert
- Pulmonary hypertension with Aminorex (a European weight loss drug), and various other drugs
- Suicidal ideation with interferons, Accutane
- Intussusception with rotovirus vaccine
- Pulmonary fibrosis with amiodarone.

LIST OF TABLES

TABLE 7.0.1   Index for Linking Identified Patients with Supplementary Patient Information in the NDA (CRFs, Narrative Summaries, and Patient Data Listings)   445

TABLE 7.1.1.1   Deaths Listing Treatment = New Drug Cutoff Date   445

TABLE 7.1.1.2   Mortality by Treatment Group for Pool of Phases 2–3 Studies with New Drug Cutoff Date   446

TABLE 7.1.2.1   Serious Adverse Event Listing New Drug Clinical Trials Source: Phases 2–3 Trials Sorting A: Randomized Treatment, Trial #, Investigator/Center #, Patient # Treatment = New Drug Cutoff Date   447

TABLE 7.1.3.1.1   Dropout Profile: Incidence of Dropout by Treatment Group and Reason for Phases 2–3 Studies with New Drug Cutoff Date   448

TABLE 7.1.3.2.1   Adverse Event Dropout Listing New Drug Clinical Trials Source: Phases 2–3 Database Sorting A: Randomized Treatment, Trial #, Investigator/Center #, Patient # Treatment = New Drug Cutoff Date   449

TABLE 7.1.5.2.1   Treatment Emergent Adverse Event Listing New Drug Clinical Trials Source: Phases 2–3 Database Sorting A: Randomized Treatment, Trial #, Investigator/Center #, Patient # Treatment = New Drug Cutoff Date   451

TABLE 7.1.5.3.1   Treatment-Emergent Adverse Event Incidence for Pool of 6-Week Placebo-Controlled Trials Cutoff Date   452

TABLE 7.1.7.3.1.1 Mean Change from Baseline for Serum Chemistry Parameters in Pool of Placebo-Controlled Studies Cutoff Date   453

TABLE 7.1.7.3.2.1 Incidence of Potentially Clinically Significant Changes in Serum Chemistry Parameters for Pool of Placebo Controlled Studies for New Drug Cutoff Date   454

TABLE 7.1.7.5.1   Hepatotoxicity Evaluation   456

TABLE 7.2.1.1.1   Enumeration of Subjects/Patients for New Drug Development Program Cutoff Date   457

TABLE 7.2.1.2.1   Demographic Profile for Phases 2–3 Studies with New Drug Cutoff Date   458

TABLE 7.2.1.3.1   Number (Percent) of Patients Receiving New Drug According to Mean Daily Dose and Duration of Therapy in Phases 2–3 Studies (N = 2500) Cutoff Date   459

TABLE 7.0.1 Index for Linking Identified Patients with Supplementary Patient Information in the NDA (CRFs, Narrative Summaries, and Patient Data Listings)[1]

		Case report forms		Narrative summaries		Patient data listings	
Study number[2]	Patient number[3]	Volume[4]	Pages[5]	Volume	Pages	Volume	Pages

[1] Separate indices should be provided for patients exposed to new drug, active control drugs, and placebo.
[2] Study numbers should be numerically ordered and tabbed as separate sections within the index.
[3] Patient numbers should be numerically ordered within each study section.
[4] The volume number provided in this index should be the unique volume number assigned to the volume as part of the complete NDA, and not a separate volume number assigned to the volume as part of a section of the NDA.
[5] The page numbers provided in this index should be the unique page numbers assigned for the entire volume, and not separate page numbers assigned to the separate sections that might be included in any particular volume.

TABLE 7.1.1.1 Deaths Listing[1,2,3] Treatment = New Drug[4] Cutoff Date[5]

Trial	Center	Patient	Age (years)	Sex	Dose[6] (mg)	Time[7] (days)	Source[8]	Person-time[9]	Description[10]

[1] A footnote should describe the rule for including deaths in the table (e.g., all deaths that occurred during a period of drug exposure or within a period of up to 30 days following discontinuation from drug and also those occurring later but resulting from adverse events that had an onset during drug exposure or during the 30-day follow-up period). Other rules may be equally appropriate.
[2] Deaths occurring outside the time window for this table should be listed elsewhere.
[3] This table should be provided by the sponsor in electronic format. The exact design of the table and the preferred electronic format should be established in discussions between the sponsor and the reviewing division.
[4] Similar lists should be provided for patients exposed to placebo and active control drugs.
[5] This is the data lock date for entering data into this table (i.e., the date beyond which additional exposed patients were not available for entry). Generally this date should be no more than several months prior to the submission date for an NDA. This date as well as this table may likely need to be updated during the course of NDA review as more data become available.
[6] Dose at time of death, or if death occurred after discontinuation, note that, as well as last dose before discontinuation.
[7] Days on drug at time of death; or if death occurred after discontinuation, note how many days on drug before discontinuation and also how many days off drug at time of death.
[8] This listing should include all deaths meeting the inclusion rule, whether arising from a clinical trial or from any secondary source (e.g., post-marketing experience). The source should be identified in this column (i.e., 1^0 for deaths arising from primary source clinical trials and 2^0 for those arising from secondary sources).
[9] This column should identify patients (yes/no) for whom person-time data are available, so the reviewer can know which patients were included in the mortality rate calculations.
[10] Since narrative summaries should be available for all deaths, the description can be very brief (e.g., myocardial infarction, stroke, pancreatic cancer, suicide by drowning).

TABLE 7.1.1.2 Mortality by Treatment Group for Pool of Phases 2–3 Studies with New Drug[1,2,3] Cutoff Date[4]

Treatment group[5]	Total number of patients[6]	Total number of deaths[7]	Crude mortality[8]	Patient exposure years (PEY)[9]	Total deaths with person-time[10]	Mortality per 100 PEY[11]
New drug						
Active control						
Placebo						

[1] This table provides data comparing overall mortality across treatment groups for the pool of all Phases 2–3 studies in the development program. Similar tables may be appropriate for other subgroups within the Phases 2–3 program (e.g., a table may be provided for a pool of all similarly designed short-term placebo controlled trials). Similar tables may be appropriate for certain individual trials of interest. All deaths should be counted, regardless of the investigator's or the sponsor's judgment about causality, including (1) any deaths occurring during participation in any of the studies in the target pool, (2) any deaths occurring after a patient leaves any of the targeted studies, whether prematurely or after completion to the nominal endpoint, if the death is (a) any deaths initiated during the study, regardless of when it actually occurs, or (b) occurs within 4 weeks of a patient leaving a study, or longer for drugs with particularly long elimination half-lives or from drug classes with known late occurring effects. The actual rule used for including deaths should be provided in a footnote to the table. In case there are substantial deaths of specific causes, it may be appropriate to provide data for cause specific mortality as well.

[2] Patients participating in crossover trials should be enumerated for each of the pertinent columns of the table (e.g., a patient receiving treatment in each of the three arms of a 3-way crossover study comparing new drug, active control, and placebo would be included in all three columns.

[3] This table should be provided by the sponsor in electronic format. The exact design of the table and the preferred electronic format should be established in discussions between the sponsor and the reviewing division.

[4] This is the data lock date for entering data into this table (i.e., the date beyond which additional exposed patients were not available for entry. Generally, this date should, be no more than several months prior to the submission date for an NDA. This date as well as this table may likely need to be updated during the course of NDA review as more data become available.

[5] In the sample table, only 1 row is provided for an active control group. One such category may suffice for certain NDAs, but may not for others, and the decision regarding how to categorize active control patients should be made in consultation with the reviewing division. Similarly, for this table, only 1 row is provided for new drug, with the implication that all new drug patients, regardless of dose, should be included in the calculations for that column. Other approaches (e.g., distinguishing patients on the basis of dose) may be equally appropriate.

[6] The N's in these rows should match the N's in Table 5 1.1.1, and if not, an explanation should be provided in a footnote.

[7] This is the total number of deaths for each group.

[8] This is simply the total number of deaths divided by the total number of patients exposed in each group.

[9] This column should provide person-time in patient exposure years (PEY). This table assumes a constant hazard rate; however, in certain situations, it may be appropriate to stratify by increments of exposure.

[10] This is the subset of total deaths for which person-time is available.

[11] This is the number of deaths for whom person-time is available divided by PEY for each group, and multiplied by 100.

TABLE 7.1.2.1 Serious Adverse Event Listing[1,2,3] New Drug Clinical Trials Source: Phases 2–3 Trials[4] Sorting A: Randomized Treatment, Trial #, Investigator/Center #, Patient #, Patient #[5] Treatment = New Drug[6] Cutoff Date[7]

Trial	Center	Patient	Age (years)	Sex	Dose[8] (mg)	Time[9] (days)	Body system	Preferred term	Adverse event[10]	W/D[11]

[1] This is a line listing of all reported adverse events that met the sponsor's definition of being a serious adverse event, regardless of whether or not considered drug related, for all patients participating in the Phases 2–3 trials in the development program. This listing is a critical component of the integrated safety summary.

[2] The variables included in this listing include:
- Trial #
- Center #
- Patient # (a unique number that identifies this patient in the NDA database)
- Age
- Sex
- Dose (in mg) at time of event onset
- Time, that is, duration, of exposure (in days) at time of event onset
- Body system category for event (using COSTART or other thesaurus)
- Preferred term for event
- Adverse event as reported by investigator and/or patient
- An indication of whether or not the event led to withdrawal
- Serious adverse event type (e.g., fatal, life-threatening).

The following additional variables may be considered for inclusion as well:
- Race
- Weight
- Height
- Dose expressed as mg/kg, mg/mm^2, or even plasma concentration, if available
- Other drug treatment
- Severity of adverse event (mild, moderate, severe)
- Action taken (e.g., none, decrease dose, discontinue treatment)
- Outcome
- Causality assessment by investigator (definitely, probably, possibly, unlikely related)
- Location in NDA of CRF (e.g., patient narrative summary)

[3] The exact design of the table and whether or not it needs to be provided in electronic format should be established in discussions between the sponsor and the reviewing division.

[4] Similar listings may be provided for individual studies as part of full reports for such studies, and possibly for other pools that are subsets of this larger pool.

[5] It is essential to provide this listing in two different forms (i.e., sorting A (by patient) and sorting B (by adverse event)). This listing is for sorting A, by patient, and permits the reviewer to explore all the serious adverse events reported for each individual patient. Sorting B (by adverse event) should be as follows: Randomized treatment, body system, preferred term, adverse event, trial, center, patient #, age, sex, dose, time, W/D. Sorting B permits the reviewer to explore all the reported serious adverse events of a similar type.

[6] This sample listing is for all new drug patients across all studies in the Phases 2–3 development program. Similar listings should be provided for active control and placebo patients.

[7] This is the data lock date for entering data into this table (i.e., the date beyond which additional exposed patients were not available for entry). Generally, this date should be no more than several months prior to the submission date for an NDA. This date as well as this table may likely need to be updated during the course of NDA review as more data become available.

[8] This column should include the dose being administered (in mg/day) at the time the event occurred.

[9] This column should include the time (i.e., duration of exposure (in days)) at the time the event occurred. If the event occurred after discontinuation of drug, a footnote should note how long after discontinuation.

[10] This column should include the adverse event in the language reported by the investigator and/or patient (i.e., before coding).

[11] This column should include an indication of whether or not the adverse event led to discontinuation of the assigned treatment.

TABLE 7.1.3.1.1   Dropout Profile: Incidence of Dropout by Treatment Group and Reason for Phases 2–3 Studies with New Drug[1,2,3] Cutoff Date[4]

Reasons for dropout[5]	Treatment groups[6]		
	New drug N =	Placebo N =	Active control N =
Lack of efficacy	%[7]	%	%
Adverse event	%	%	%
Lost to follow-up	%	%	%
Other	%	%	%
Total dropouts	%	%	%

[1] This sample table should be based on a pool of all trials in the Phases 2–3 development program. Similar tables may be appropriate for other subgroups within the Phases 2–3 program (e.g., a table should be provided for a pool of all similarly designed short-term placebo controlled trials). Similar tables may be appropriate for certain individual trials of interest.

[2] Patients participating in crossover trials should be enumerated for each of the pertinent columns of the table (e.g., a patient receiving treatment in each of the three arms of a 3-way crossover study comparing new drug, active control, and placebo would be included in all three columns).

[3] This table should be provided by the sponsor in electronic format. The exact design of the table and the preferred electronic format should be established in discussions between the sponsor and the reviewing division.

[4] This is the data lock date for entering data into this table (i.e., the date beyond which additional exposed patients were not available for entry). Generally this date should be no more than several months prior to the submission date for an NDA. This date as well as this table may likely need to be updated during the course of NDA review as more data become available.

[5] This sample table includes four categories for dropout, but a more detailed breakdown may be of interest as well.

- The adverse event category here would include all patients identified as dropping out for adverse events, regardless of whether or not the events were judged by the investigator or sponsor to be drug related and regardless of what other reasons may have been identified in association with dropout. Patients identified as dropping out for inter-current illness would ordinarily be included under this adverse event category. Similarly, a patient identified as dropping out for an adverse event and lack of efficacy would also ordinarily be included under this adverse event category.
- Lost-to-follow up is an important outcome to track, since it reflects on the overall conduct of the studies.
- The other category is intended to include all other reasons that may generally be considered nontreatment related. This category is often identified as administrative, and includes such reasons as patient refused further participation, patient moved away, patient improved, patient not eligible, protocol violation, unknown.
- Decisions about what categories to include should be made in consultation with the reviewing division.

[6] In the sample table, only 1 column is provided for an active control group. One such category may suffice for certain NDAs, but may not for others, and the decision regarding how to categorize active control patients should be made in consultation with the reviewing division. Similarly, for this table, only 1 column is provided for new drug, with the implication that all new drug patients, regardless of dose, should be included in the calculations for that column. Other approaches (e.g., distinguishing patients on the basis of dose) may be equally appropriate. The N's in these column headings should match the N's in Table 5.1.1.1., and if not, an explanation should be provided in a footnote.

[7] Numbers for this table should be rounded to the nearest integer.

TABLE 7.1.3.2.1 Adverse Event Dropout Listing[1,2,3] New Drug Clinical Trials Source: Phases 2–3 Database[4] Sorting A: Randomized Treatment, Trial #, Investigator/Center #, Patient #[5] Treatment = New Drug[6] Cutoff Date[7]

Trial	Center	Patient	Age (years)	Sex	Dose[8] (mg)	Time[9] (days)	Body system	Preferred term	Adverse event[10]	Serious[11]	Outcome[12]

(Continued)

TABLE 7.1.3.2.1 (Continued)

[1] This is a line listing of all reported adverse events identified as leading to discontinuation, regardless of whether or not they were considered drug related, for all patients participating in trials identified as sources for this listing. Thus, all events categorized as inter-current illness leading to discontinuation would, nevertheless, be included in this listing, and any judgments about attribution can be included in the narrative summary. This listing is a critical component of the integrated safety summary.

[2] The variables included in this listing include:

– Trial #
– Center #
– Patient # (a unique number that identifies this patient in the NDA database)
– Age
– Sex
– Dose (in mg) at time of event onset
– Time (i.e., duration, of exposure (in days) at time of event onset)
– Body system category for event (using COSTART or other thesaurus)
– Preferred term for event
– Adverse event as reported by investigator and/or patient
– An indication of whether or not the event met definition for serious
– Outcome

The following additional variables may be considered for inclusion as well:

– Race
– Weight
– Height
– Dose expressed as mg/kg, mg/mm^2, or even plasma concentration, if available
– Other drug treatment
– Severity of adverse event (mild, moderate, severe)
– Action taken (e.g., none; decrease dose, discontinue treatment)
– Causality assessment by investigator (related, not related)
– Location in NDA of CRF (patient narrative summary)

[3] The exact design of the table and whether or not it needs to be provided in electronic format should be established in discussions between the sponsor and the reviewing division.

[4] Similar listings may be provided for individual studies as part of full reports for such studies and, possibly, for other pools that are subsets of this larger pool.

[5] It is essential to provide this listing in two different forms (i.e., sorting A (by patient) and sorting B (by adverse event)). This listing is for sorting A, by patient, and permits the reviewer to explore all the adverse events reported as leading to discontinuation for each individual patient. Sorting B (by adverse event) should be as follows: Randomized treatment, body system, preferred term, adverse event, trial, center, patient #, age, sex, dose, time, serious. sorting B permits the reviewer to explore all the adverse events of a similar type reported as leading to discontinuation.

[6] This sample listing is for all new drug patients across all studies in the Phases 2–3 development program. Similar listings should be provided for active control and placebo patients.

[7] This is the data lock date for entering data into this table (i.e., the date beyond which additional exposed patients were not available for entry). Generally this date should be no more than several months prior to the submission date for an NDA. This date as well as this table may likely need to be updated during the course of NDA review as more data become available.

[8] This column should include the dose being administered (in mg/day) at the time the event occurred.

[9] This column should include the time (i.e., duration of exposure (in days)), at the time the event occurred.

[10] This column should include the adverse event in the language reported by the investigator and/or patient, that is, before coding.

[11] This column should include an indication of whether or not the adverse event met the criteria for serious as defined for the development program overall.

[12] This column should categorize the outcome upon follow-up evaluation for the adverse event leading to discontinuation, as follows:

(R) Resolved
(P) Persisting
(U) Unknown

TABLE 7.1.5.2.1 Treatment Emergent Adverse Event Listing[1,2,3] New Drug Clinical Trials Source: Phases 2–3 Database[4] Sorting A: Randomized Treatment, Trial #, Investigator/Center #, Patient #[5] Treatment = New Drug[6] Cutoff Date[7]

Trial	Center	Patient	Age (years)	Sex	Dose[8] (mg)	Time[9] (days)	Body system	Preferred term	Adverse event[10]	Serious[11]	W/D[12]

[1] This is a line listing of all reported treatment emergent adverse events, regardless of whether or not they were considered drug related, for all patients participating in trials identified as sources for this listing. A footnote should identify all studies contributing to this pool.

[2] The variables included in this listing:

  – Trial #
  – Center #
  – Patient # (a unique number that identifies this patient in the NDA database)
  – Age
  – Sex
  – Dose (in mg) at time of event onset
  – Time (i.e., duration of exposure (in days) at time of event onset)
  – Body system category for event (using COSTART or other thesaurus)
  – Preferred term for event
  – Adverse event as reported by investigator and/or patient
  – An indication of whether or not the event met definition for serious
  – An indication of whether or not the event led to withdrawal

The following additional variables may be considered for inclusion as well:

  – Race
  – Weight
  – Height
  – Dose expressed as mg/kg, mg/mm², or even plasma concentration, if available
  – Other drug treatment
  – Duration of adverse event
  – Timing of adverse event relative to last dose
  – Severity of adverse event (mild, moderate, severe)
  – Action taken (none, decrease dose, discontinue treatment)
  – Outcome
  – Causality assessment by investigator (definitely, probably, possibly, or unlikely related)
  – Location in NDA of CRF, patient narrative summary

[3] The exact design of the table and whether or not it needs to be provided in electronic format should be established in discussions between the sponsor and the reviewing division.

[4] Similar listings may be provided for individual studies as part of full reports for such studies, and possibly for other pools that are subsets of this larger pool.

[5] It is essential to provide this listing in two different forms (i.e., sorting A (by patient) and sorting B (by adverse event)). This listing is for sorting A, by patient, and permits the reviewer to explore all the adverse events reported for each individual patient. Sorting B (by adverse event (i.e., 1 row for each occurrence of each adverse event)) should be as follows: Randomized treatment, body system, preferred term, adverse event, trial, center, patient #, age, sex, dose, time, serious, W/D. Sorting B permits the reviewer to explore all the reported adverse events of a similar type.

[6] This sample listing is for new drug patients (i.e., for all patients exposed to new drug in the Phases 2–3 studies that are part of the Integrated Primary Database). Similar listings should be provided for active control and placebo patients.

[7] This is the data lock date for entering data into this table (i.e., the date beyond which additional exposed patients were not available for entry). Generally this date should be no more than several months prior to the submission date for an NDA. This date as well as this table may likely need to be updated during the course of NDA review as more data become available.

[8] This column should include the dose being administered (in mg/day) at the time the event occurred.

[9] This column should include the time (i.e., duration of exposure (in days)), at the time the event occurred.

[10] This column should include the adverse event in the language reported by the investigator and/or patient (i.e., before coding).

[11] This column should include an indication of whether or not the adverse event met the criteria for serious as defined for the development program overall.

[12] This column should include an indication of whether or not the adverse event led to discontinuation of the assigned treatment.

TABLE 7.1.5.3.1 Treatment-Emergent Adverse Event Incidence for Pool of 6-Week Placebo-Controlled Trials[1–10] Cutoff Date[11]

Body system/Adverse event[12–14]	Percentage of patients reporting event[15]		
	New drug N[16] =	Active control N =	Placebo N =
Body as a whole			
Headache			
Etc.			
Cardiovascular system			
Postural hypotension			
Etc.			
Gastrointestinal system			
Constipation			
Etc.			
●			
●			
Urogenital system			
Impotence[17]			
Etc.			
●			
●			

[1] This table compares the incidence of treatment emergent adverse events across treatment groups for a pool of similarly designed placebo-controlled trials of new drug. Generally, an arbitrary threshold incidence for new drug patients is used as a criterion for selecting adverse events to include; ≥1% for new drug is a commonly used rule, but others may be equally appropriate. The criterion used should be noted in the table title or in a footnote.

[2] Study pools other than those described for this sample table may be equally appropriate, and similar tables useful for individual trials may also be of interest.

[3] In the sample table, only 1 column is provided for an active control group. One such category may suffice for certain NDAs, but may not for others, and the decision regarding how to categorize active control patients should be made in consultation with the reviewing division.

[4] Similarly, for this table, only 1 column is provided for new drug, with the implication that all new drug patients, regardless of dose, should be included in the calculations for that column. Other approaches (e.g., dividing patients on the basis of dose), may be equally appropriate. If the studies used were fixed-dose studies, it is generally most informative to preserve the dose categories in constructing this table. However, dose categories that are not relevant to the doses that are being recommended for use may reasonably be omitted from this table. It is generally not useful to try to artificially construct dose categories from dose titration studies, since there is often confounding of dose and time.

[5] Data are often available on the investigator's opinion regarding whether or not any particular adverse event was in fact related to the drug being taken. Some reviewers consider this useful information and may construct tables that include only those events considered possibly, probably, or definitely drug-related by the investigator. Others ignore such judgments and include all reported adverse events, with the view that the control groups, especially placebo if present, should permit one to make causality decisions, regardless of the investigators' judgments about drug-relatedness. Either approach can be acceptable, but it is critical that a footnote indicate clearly when adverse events are not included due to investigators' judgments that they were not drug-related, since this approach may reduce the adverse event rates that appear in the table.

[6] Data are also often available on the intensity of the reported adverse events, generally including categories of mild, moderate, or severe. Adverse event tables may ignore such classifications and pool all events together, or some attempt may be made to focus only on a subset of reported events (e.g., only those classified as severe). Again, either approach is acceptable, but it is important to describe in a footnote what approach was taken.

[7] Not uncommonly, a new drug is developed for more than one indication. If adverse event rates appear to be to occur at similar rates across the indications, it may be reasonable to pool the data in creating an adverse events table, possibly one providing greater precision. However, it is not inconceivable that adverse event rates may vary depending on the population studied, and if this appears to be the case, pooling may not be appropriate.

[8] Adverse events that occur at a rate for placebo that is ≥ the rate for new drug should be removed from the table and noted only as a footnote.

[9] Patients participating in crossover trials should be included in the calculations for each of the pertinent columns of the table (e.g., a patient receiving treatment in each of the three arms of a 3-way crossover study comparing new drug, active control, and placebo would be included in the calculations for all three columns).

[10] This table should be provided by the sponsor in electronic format. The exact design of the table and the preferred electronic format should be established in discussions between the sponsor and the reviewing division.

[11] This is the data lock date for entering data into this table (i.e., the date beyond which additional exposed patients were not available for entry). Generally this date should be no more than several months prior to the submission date for an NDA. This date as well as this table may likely need to be updated during the course of NDA review as more data become available.

[12] Adverse events should be organized under body system categories.

[13] Within each body system category, adverse events should be ordered according to decreasing frequency.

[14] Adverse events during exposure are generally obtained by spontaneous report and recorded by clinical investigators using terminology of their own choosing. Consequently, it is not possible to provide a meaningful estimate of the proportion of individuals experiencing adverse events without first grouping similar types of events into a smaller number of standardized event categories. Generally a table of this type should use these preferred adverse event terms, and a footnote should identify the system used for coding investigator terms. Adverse event terms that convey no useful information (e.g., joint disorder), should be replaced by more clinically useful terms or deleted.

[15] Percentages should be rounded to the nearest integer. Although not strictly hypothesis testing, p-values give some feeling for the strength of the finding and should be produced for all new drug/placebo pairwise comparisons and any p-values meeting a $p < 0.05$ level of significance should be noted by an asterisk (*) as a superscript to the %.

[16] The N for each column should be provided at the column heading, so that only the percentage of patients having that adverse event need be included in the table, and not the actual number.

[17] The rates for gender specific adverse events (e.g., impotence) should be determined using the appropriate gender specific denominator, and this fact should be indicated with a footnote.

TABLE 7.1.7.3.1.1 Mean Change from Baseline for Serum Chemistry Parameters[1] in Pool of Placebo-Controlled Studies[2,3,4] Cutoff Date[5]

Serum chemistry parameters and units of measure[6]	Treatment groups[7,8]								
	New drug			Placebo			Active control		
	N[9]	BL[10]	Change from BL[11]	N	BL	Change from BL	N	BL	Change from BL
Albumin (g/dL)									
Alkaline phosphatase (U/L)									
Bilirubin, total (mg/dL)									
BUN (mg/dL)									
CK (U/L)									
Calcium (mg/dL)									
Cholesterol (mg/dL)									
Creatinine (mg/dL)									
GGT (U/L)									
Glucose (mg/dL)									
LDH (U/L)									
Phosphorus (mg/dL)									
Potassium (mmol/L)									
Sodium (mmol/L)									
Triglycerides (mg/dL)									
Uric Acid (mg/dL)									

[1] This table provides data comparing the mean change from baseline across treatment groups for serum chemistry parameters. An acceptable alternative would be to provide median change from baseline. The post-measurement is generally the worst value during treatment.

[2] This sample table is based on a pool of similarly designed placebo controlled trials. Other pools, as well as individual trials may also be of interest.

[3] Patients participating in crossover trials should be enumerated for each of the pertinent columns of the table (e.g., a patient receiving treatment in each of the three arms of a 3-way crossover study comparing new drug, active control, and placebo would be included in all three columns).

[4] This table should be provided by the sponsor in electronic format. The exact design of the table and the preferred electronic format should be established in discussions between the sponsor and the reviewing division.

[5] This is the data lock date for entering data into this table (i.e., the date beyond which additional exposed patients were not available for entry). Generally this date should be no more than several months prior to the submission date for an NDA. This date as well as this table may likely need to be updated during the course of NDA review as more data become available.

[6] The parameters included in this list are for illustration. In general, the list should include all those serum chemistry parameters measured in whatever pool of studies is the focus of the table. Similarly, the units of measure are for illustration, and these details should be worked out in consultation with the reviewing division.

[7] In the sample table, only 1 column is provided for an active control group. One such category may suffice for certain NDAs, but may not for others, and the decision regarding how to categorize active control patients should be made in consultation with the reviewing division.

[8] Similarly, for this table, only 1 column is provided for new drug, with the implication that all new drug patients, regardless of dose, should be included in the calculations for that column. Other approaches (e.g., dividing patients on the basis of dose), may be equally appropriate. If the studies used were fixed-dose studies, it is generally most informative to preserve the dose categories in constructing this table. However, dose categories that are not relevant to the doses that are being recommended for use may reasonably be omitted from this table. It is generally not useful to try to artificially construct dose categories from dose titration studies, since there is often confounding of dose and time.

[9] N represents the number of patients who had the serum chemistry parameter of interest assessed at baseline and at least one follow-up time.

[10] This column should provide the baseline means for all the serum chemistry parameters of interest.

[11] This column should provide the mean change from baseline to patient's worst on drug value for each of the serum chemistry parameters of interest. While not hypothesis testing, p-values provide some measures of the strength of the finding and should be produced for all new drug/placebo pairwise comparisons and any p-values meeting a $p < 0.05$ level of significance criterion should be noted by an asterisk (*) as a superscript to the mean change from baseline.

TABLE 7.1.7.3.2.1 Incidence of Potentially Clinically Significant Changes in Serum Chemistry Parameters[1] for Pool of Placebo Controlled Studies for New Drug[2,3,4] Cutoff Date[5]

Serum chemistry parameters and PCS criteria[7] L = Low; H = High; ULN = Upper limits of normal	Treatment groups[6]											
	New drug			Placebo			Active control					
	Total Pts[8]	Abnormal		Total Pts	Abnormal		Total Pts	Abnormal				
		Nbr[9]	%[10]		Nbr	%		Nbr	%				
Albumin-L (<2.5 g/dL)												
Alkaline Phosphatase-H (>400 U/L)												
Bilirubin, total-H (>2 mg/dL)												
BUN-H (>30 mg/dL)												
CK-H (>3 × ULN)												
Calcium-L (<7 mg/dL)												
Calcium-H (>12 mg/dL)												
Cholesterol-H (>300 mg/dL)												
Creatinine-H (>2 mg/dL)												
GGT-H (>3 × ULN)												
Glucose-L (<50 mg/dL)												
Glucose-H (>250 mg/dL)												
LDH-H (>3 × ULN)												
Phosphorus-L (<2.0 mg/dL)												
Phosphorus-H (>5.0 mg/dL)												
Potassium-L (<3.0 mmol/L)												
Potassium-H (>5.5 mmol/L)												

SGOT/AST-H (>3 × ULN)

SGPT/ALT-H (>3 × ULN)

Sodium-L (<130 mmol/L)

Sodium-H (>150 mmol/L)

Triglycerides-H (>300 mg/dL)

Uric acid (F)-H (>8.0 mg/dL)

Uric acid (M)-H (>10.0 mg/dL)

[1] This table provides data comparing the incidence across treatment groups of patients who were normal at baseline meeting criteria of having had a change on any of the listed serum chemistry parameters of potential clinical significance (PCS). Separate listings should be provided for patients who were abnormal at baseline and met these PCS criteria.

[2] This sample table is based on a pool of similarly designed placebo controlled trials. Other pools, as well as individual trials may also be of interest.

[3] Patients participating in crossover trials should be enumerated for each of the pertinent columns of the table (e.g., a patient receiving treatment in each of the three arms of a 3-way crossover study comparing new drug, active control, and placebo would be included in all three columns).

[4] This table should be provided by the sponsor in electronic format. The exact design of the table and the preferred electronic format should be established in discussions between the sponsor and the reviewing division.

[5] This is the data lock date for entering data into this table (i.e., the date beyond which additional exposed patients were not available for entry. Generally this date should be no more than several months prior to the submission date for an NDA. This date as well as this table may likely need to be updated during the course of NDA review as more data become available.

[6] In the sample table, only 1 column is provided for an active control group. One such category may suffice for certain NDAs, but may not for others, and the decision regarding how to categorize active control patients should be made in consultation with the reviewing division. Similarly, for this table, only 1 column is provided for new drug, with the implication that all new drug patients, regardless of dose, should be included in the calculations for that column. Other approaches (e.g., distinguishing patients on the basis of dose), may be equally appropriate.

[7] The parameters included in this list are for illustration. In general, the list should include all those serum chemistry parameters measured in whatever pool of studies is the focus of the table. Similarly, the proposed criteria for potentially clinically significant are for illustration, and these details should be worked out in consultation with the reviewing division.

[8] The total number of patients for each parameter should represent the number of patients for the treatment group who (1) had that parameter assessed at baseline and at least one follow-up time and (2) for whom the baseline assessment was normal.

[9] The number abnormal represents the subset of the total number who met the criterion in question at least once during treatment. A separate listing should provide patient identification for those patients meeting the criterion.

[10] Percentage of the total number meeting the criterion should be rounded to the nearest integer. While not strictly hypothesis testing, p-values should be produced for all new drug/placebo pairwise comparisons and any p-values meeting a $p < 0.05$ level of significance should be noted by an asterisk (*) as a superscript to the %.

TABLE 7.1.7.5.1   Hepatotoxicity Evaluation

I.   Data Collection
   A.   Overview of liver chemistry data (tests performed, frequency, specific follow-up plans for abnormal values)
   B.   Specific follow-up plan if chemistry is elevated at end of treatment
   C.   Re-challenge plan, if any
   D.   Exclusions from studies because of liver chemistry abnormalities, if any

II.   Observations
   A.   Abnormal liver chemistries seen in controlled trials (separate for pooled placebo controlled, active controlled) with greater than 2-week exposure. Rates can be given as events/exposed; positive findings can be also analyzed as events per patient year and examined for rates over time
      1.   Rates of 3×, 5×, 10×, 20× ULN elevations of AST (SGOT), ALT (SGPT), and either ALT or AST
      2.   Rates of any elevations of bilirubin; rate of elevated bilirubin to >1.5× ULN
      3.   Rates of alkaline phosphatase (AP)≥1.5 × ULN
      4.   Rates of elevated transaminase accompanied by elevated bilirubin

All rates should be given for both drug and control group

   B.   For total database with exposure ≥2 weeks (i.e., including uncontrolled). Same as for controlled database (1–4)
   C.   Individual events
      1.   Listing of patients with any elevated transaminase (>3 × ULN), without more than slight AP elevation, associated with increase in bilirubin to >ULN
      2.   Show time course of enzyme and bilirubin elevations
      3.   For such patients, review clinical situation
         a.   Ethanol history
         b.   Evidence viral hepatitis
         c.   Symptoms and course – follow-up is particularly important to detect underlying liver disease
         d.   Special studies, notably Bx
         e.   Possible confounding, including concomitant illness, concomitant medications (known hepatotoxins, including acetaminophen)

III.   Possible problems/signals
   A.   Any patient with elevated transaminase (to at least 3× ULN, generally higher), no evidence of obstruction (elevated AP) and even modestly (2× ULN) elevated bilirubin. Greater elevation of bilirubin is stronger signal
   B.   Greater rate than control of 3×, 5×, 10×, etc. elevations of transaminase

TABLE 7.2.1.1.1 Enumeration of Subjects/Patients for New Drug Development Program[1,2,3,4] Cutoff Date[5]

Study groups	Treatment groups		
	New drug	Active control[6]	Placebo
Completed Phase 1 (Clinical Pharmacology)			
Single dose	120	30	30
Multiple dose	60	30	30
Phase 1 subtotal	180	60	60
Completed Phases 2–3 (Studies of Proposed Indication)			
Placebo control[7]			
Fixed dose	500	150	150
Flexible dose	100	100	100
Active control			
Fixed dose	200	100	0
Flexible dose	100	100	0
Uncontrolled			
Short term	100	0	0
Long term	700	0	0
Phases 2–3 subtotal	1200[8]	450	250
Ongoing Phases 2–3 Studies (Studies of Proposed Indication)			
Placebo control			
Flexible dose	150[9]	0	150[9]
SD subtotal	120	30	30
MD subtotal	1410	480	430
Grand total	1530	510	460

[1] *This table provides a count by study type of the subjects/patients exposed to new drug, active control, and placebo across the entire set of studies in the development program that contributed safety and efficacy data for new drug. It should include all subjects/patients known or assumed to have received even a single dose of assigned treatment. It should exclude subjects/patients who are known not to have received any of the assigned treatments or for whom no follow-up information is available subsequent to the assumed receipt of assigned treatment. A separate listing of all such patients should be provided. (Note: If this list includes more than a few patients, this may indicate a potentially important problem in the conduct of studies.)*

In creating this table, it is necessary to classify and group studies on the basis of several characteristics. For the purposes of this table, the following characteristics and distinctions were deemed important:

   – Phase 1 vs. Phases 2–3
   – Completed vs. ongoing and blinded
   – Single dose vs. multiple dose
   – Controlled vs. uncontrolled
   – Short-term vs. long-term
   – Placebo-controlled vs. active-controlled
   – Fixed dose vs. flexible dose

Obviously, there are other features that may be important as well, and that could lead to additional breakdowns within the table or to separate tables (e.g., different indications, inpatient vs. outpatient status, differences in the quality and completeness of data collected across different studies, foreign vs. domestic). The characteristics to be used in classifying studies for the purpose of this table should be decided in consultation with the designated reviewing division at FDA.

In addition to this table that enumerates patients by category of study, it would be useful to have a table that enumerates patients by each individual study in the development program. This would be an expanded version of the above table that enumerates patients for each study (i.e., each of the categories in the above table would identify and provide data for the individual studies comprising that category). Sponsors ordinarily provide such a table.

[2] *Patients participating in crossover trials should be counted in each of the pertinent columns of the table (e.g., a patient receiving treatment in each of the three arms of a 3-way crossover study comparing new drug, active control, and placebo would be counted in all three columns).*

[3] *Footnotes to this table should identify by study number all those studies comprising the various study groupings for this table. For example, in the sample table, the fixed dose placebo controlled trials contributing to the counts for that category should be listed in a footnote, and similarly for all other categories.*

[4] *This table should be provided by the sponsor in electronic format. The exact design of the table and the preferred electronic format should be established in discussions between the sponsor and the reviewing division.*

[5] *This is the data lock date for entering data into this table (i.e., the date beyond which additional exposed patients were not available for entry). Generally this date should be no more than several months prior to the submission date for an NDA. This date as well as this table likely need to be updated during the course of NDA review as more data become available.*

(Continued)

TABLE 7.2.1.1.1   (*Continued*)

[6] *In the sample table, only 1 column is provided for an active control group. One such category may suffice for certain NDAs, but may not for others, and the decision regarding how to categorize active control patients should be made in consultation with the reviewing division.*

[7] *In this table, a decision was made to pool all studies having a placebo arm, whether or not an active control arm was also included. Thus, the active control category includes only those active control studies that did not have a placebo control arm. Other approaches to grouping studies may be equally appropriate.*

[8] *The intent of this table is to provide a count of unique subjects/patients exposed to new drug, etc. in the development program. Since patients often participate in more than 1 study in a development program, it is necessary to have an approach to avoid counting patients more than once for the subtotals and grand totals. The approach used in this table is to include in parentheses in the pertinent cells of the table a count of the patients in that cell total who have already been counted by virtue of having participated in a previous study (e.g., a patient in an open extension trial should have been previously counted in an acute, controlled phase). The subtotals of unique individuals exposed to the assigned treatment can then be calculated by subtracting the sum of all numbers in parentheses from the sum of all the cell totals for each column (e.g., in this table, the completed Phases 2–3 subtotal for new drug is 1700 less the 500 patients already counted in short-term controlled trials, or 1200).*

[9] *Frequently, some studies may be ongoing and blinded at the time of NDA submission, even though some individual patients having experienced serious adverse events may have been unblinded. In these instances, the table should include estimates of the numbers of patients exposed to new drug, etc. from these studies, since exact counts may not be available. Footnotes should indicate when the table entries are based on estimates rather than exact counts.*

TABLE 7.2.1.2.1   Demographic Profile for Phases 2–3 Studies with New Drug[1,2,3,4,5] Cutoff Date[6]

Demographic parameters	Treatment groups[7,8]		
	New drug N =	Placebo N =	Active control N =
Age (years)			
Mean			
Range			
Groups[9]			
<40	%	%	%
40–64	%	%	%
>65	%	%	%
Sex			
Female	%	%	%
Male	%	%	%
Race[10]			
Caucasian	%	%	%
Non-Caucasian	%	%	%
Weight (kg)			
Mean			
Range			

[1] *This table should be based on a pool of all trials in the Phases 2–3 development program. Similar tables may be appropriate for other subgroups within the Phases 2–3 program and also for certain individual trials of interest. The specific trials included should be listed.*

[2] *Patients participating in crossover trials should be included in the calculations for each of the pertinent columns of the table (e.g., a patient receiving treatment in each of the three arms of a 3-way crossover study comparing new drug, active control, and placebo would be included in the calculations for all three columns).*

[3] *Numbers for this table should be rounded to the nearest integer.*

[4] *This sample table includes four demographic categories of obvious interest, however, others may be of interest as well (e.g., height, severity on baseline measures of disease severity). It may also be of interest to look at combinations of characteristics, such as gender and age (e.g., women under 50).*

[5] *This table should be provided by the sponsor in electronic format. The exact design of the table and the preferred electronic format should be established in discussions between the sponsor and the reviewing division.*

[6] *This is the data lock date for entering data into this table (i.e., the date beyond which additional exposed patients were not available for entry). Generally this date should be no more than several months prior to the submission date for an NDA. This date as well as this table may likely need to be updated during the course of NDA review as more data become available.*

[7] *In the sample table, only 1 column is provided for an active control group. One such category may suffice for certain NDAs, but may not for others, and the decision regarding how to categorize active control patients should be made in consultation with the reviewing division. Similarly, for this table, only 1 column is provided for new drug, with the implication that all new drug patients, regardless of dose, should be included in the calculations for that column. Other approaches (e.g., distinguishing patients on the basis of dose), may be equally appropriate.*

[8] *If, as is often the case, the Ns available for calculating any particular demographic parameter are less than the Ns in the column headings, these Ns should be provided, along with an explanation, in footnotes.*

[9] *If there are pediatric exposures, these should be broken out as well.*

[10] *Other approaches to racial categorization may be substituted for that proposed in this sample table.*

TABLE 7.2.1.3.1 Number (Percent) of Patients Receiving New Drug According to Mean[1,2,3,4,5,6,7] Daily Dose and Duration of Therapy in Phases 2–3 Studies (N = 2500) Cutoff Date[8]

Duration (Weeks)	Dose[9] (mg)						Total (AnyDos)	(%)
	0<Dos≤5	5<Dos≤10	10<Dos≤20	20<Dos≤30	30<Dos≤50	50<Dos		
0<Dur≤1	6	19	31	31	25	13	125	(5%)
1≤Dur<2	6	19	31	31	25	13	125	(5%)
2≤Dur<4	13	37	62	63	50	25	250	(10%)
4≤Dur<12	31	94	156	156	125	63	625	(25%)
12≤Dur<24	25	75	125	125	100	50	500	(20%)
24<Dur≤48	25	75	125	125	100	50	500	(20%)
48≤Dur<96	13	37	62	63	50	25	250	(10%)
96≤Dur	6	19	31	31	25	13	125	(5%)
Total (AnyDur)	125	375	623	625	500	252	2500	(100%)
(%)	(5%)	(15%)	(25%)	(25%)	(20%)	(10%)	(100%)	

[1] This table is calculated by first categorizing patients on the basis of the interval of exposure for each (e.g., a patient exposed for 6 weeks would be counted in the 4<Dur<12 row). The mean daily dose is then calculated for each patient for dose categorization (e.g., a 6-week patient with a mean daily dose of 15 mg would be counted in the 10<Dos≤20 column). Patients are enumerated in only 1 cell of the matrix (i.e., this is a mutually exclusive display). The dose and duration intervals need to be designed specifically for the drug of interest. The specific trials included should be listed. As with any table summarizing data from disparate sources, it does not address all information needs, and it should be interpreted with caution (e.g., mean doses in the 4–12 row refer to mean doses over 0–12 weeks, not 4–12 as one might think). Nevertheless, the information provided provides useful information.

[2] Similar tables can be prepared for median, for modal, and for maximum dose.

[3] The same table can be generated for any individual study or for any pool of studies.

[4] The same table can be generated for any subgroup of interest (e.g., on the basis of age, sex, race, co-morbid condition, concomitant medications, or any combination of these factors).

[5] Similar tables should be provided for active control drugs and placebo.

[6] If the total N for this table does not match the total N from Table 5.1.1.1, as may be the case (e.g., if dose or duration data are not available for all exposed patients counted in Table 5.1.1.1, a footnote should provide an explanation for the discrepancy).

[7] This table should be provided by the sponsor in electronic format. The exact design of the table and the preferred electronic format should be established in discussions between the sponsor and the reviewing division.

[8] This is the data lock date for entering data into this table (i.e., the date beyond which additional exposed patients were not available for entry). Generally this date should be no more than several months prior to the submission date for an NDA. This date as well as this table may likely need to be updated during the course of NDA review as more data become available.

[9] Dose may also be expressed as mg/kg, mg/m², or in terms of plasma concentration if such data are available.

Common Terminology Criteria for Adverse Events v3.0 (CTCAE)

Published Date: August 9, 2006

Quick Reference

The NCI Common Terminology Criteria for Adverse Events v3.0 is a descriptive terminology which can be utilized for Adverse Event (AE) reporting. A grading (severity) scale is provided for each AE term.

Components and Organization

CATEGORY

A CATEGORY is a broad classification of AEs based on anatomy and/or pathophysiology. Within each CATEGORY, AEs are listed accompanied by their descriptions of severity (grade).

Adverse Event Terms

An AE is any unfavorable and unintended sign (including an abnormal laboratory finding), symptom, or disease temporally associated with the use of a medical treatment or procedure that may or may *not* be considered related to the medical treatment or procedure. An AE is a term that is a unique representation of a specific event used for medical documentation and scientific analyses. Each AE term is mapped to a MedDRA term and code. AEs are listed alphabetically within CATEGORIES.

Short AE Name

The "Short Name" column is new and it is used to simplify documentation of AE names on Case Report Forms.

Supra-ordinate Terms

A supra-ordinate term is located within a CATEGORY and is a grouping term based on disease process, signs, symptoms, or diagnosis. A supra-ordinate term is followed by the word "*Select*" and is accompanied by specific AEs that are all related to the supra-ordinate term. Supra-ordinate terms provide clustering and consistent representation of grade for related AEs. Supra-ordinate terms are not AEs, are not mapped to a MedDRA term and code, cannot be graded and cannot be used for reporting.

Remark

A "Remark" is a clarification of an AE.

Also Consider

An "Also Consider" indicates additional AEs that are to be graded if they are clinically significant.

Navigation Note

A "Navigation Note" indicates the location of an AE term within the CTCAE document. It lists signs/symptoms alphabetically and the CTCAE term will appear in the same CATEGORY unless the "Navigation Note" states differently.

Grades

Grade refers to the severity of the AE. The CTCAE v3.0 displays Grades 1 through 5 with unique clinical descriptions of severity for each AE based on this general guideline:

Grade 1	Mild AE
Grade 2	Moderate AE
Grade 3	Severe AE
Grade 4	Life-threatening or disabling AE
Grade 5	Death related to AE

A Semi-colon indicates "or" within the description of the grade. An "Em dash" (—) indicates a grade not available.

Not all grades are appropriate for all AEs. Therefore, some AEs are listed with fewer than five options for grade selection.

Grade 5

Grade 5 (Death) is not appropriate for some AEs and therefore is not an option.

The DEATH CATEGORY is new. Only one Supra-ordinate term is listed in this CATEGORY: "Death not associated with CTCAE term – *Select*" with four AE options: Death NOS; Disease progression NOS; Multi-organ failure; Sudden death.

Important:

- Grade 5 is the only appropriate grade
- This AE is to be used in the situation where a death
  1. cannot be reported using a CTCAE v3.0 term associated with Grade 5, or
  2. cannot be reported within a CTCAE CATEGORY as "Other (Specify)"

Contents

ALLERGY/IMMUNOLOGY...463

AUDITORY/EAR 464

BLOOD/BONE MARROW...466

CARDIAC ARRHYTHMIA...467

CARDIAC GENERAL 469

COAGULATION 472

CONSTITUTIONAL SYMPTOMS 473

DEATH 475

DERMATOLOGY/SKIN...476

ENDOCRINE 479

GASTROINTESTINAL...481

GROWTH AND DEVELOPMENT 491

HEMORRHAGE/BLEEDING 492

HEPATOBILIARY/PANCREAS 496

INFECTION 497

LYMPHATICS 500

METABOLIC/LABORATORY 502

MUSCULOSKELETAL/SOFT TISSUE..505

NEUROLOGY...509

OCULAR/VISUAL 514

PAIN..517

PULMONARY/UPPER RESPIRATORY 518

RENAL/GENITOURINARY..522

SECONDARY MALIGNANCY 525

SEXUAL/REPRODUCTIVE FUNCTION 526

SURGERY/INTRA-OPERATIVE INJURY 528

SYNDROMES 530

VASCULAR..532

Adverse Event	Short Name	Grade 1	Grade 2	Grade 3	Grade 4	Grade 5
Allergic reaction/ hypersensitivity (including drug fever)	Allergic reaction	Transient flushing or rash; drug fever <38°C (<100.4°F)	Rash; flushing; urticaria; dyspnea; drug fever ≥38°C (≥100.4°F)	Symptomatic bronchospasm, with or without urticaria; parenteral medication(s) indicated; allergy-related edema/angioedema; hypotension	Anaphylaxis	Death

REMARK: Urticaria with manifestations of allergic or hypersensitivity reaction is graded as Allergic reaction/hypersensitivity (including drug fever).

ALSO CONSIDER: Cytokine release syndrome/acute infusion reaction.

Adverse Event	Short Name	Grade 1	Grade 2	Grade 3	Grade 4	Grade 5
Allergic rhinitis (including sneezing, nasal stuffiness, postnasal drip)	Rhinitis	Mild, intervention not indicated	Moderate, intervention indicated	—	—	—

REMARK: Rhinitis associated with obstruction or stenosis is graded as Obstruction/stenosis of airway – Select in the PULMONARY/UPPER RESPIRATORY CATEGORY.

Adverse Event	Short Name	Grade 1	Grade 2	Grade 3	Grade 4	Grade 5
Autoimmune reaction	Autoimmune reaction	Asymptomatic and serologic or other evidence of autoimmune reaction, with normal organ function and intervention not indicated	Evidence of autoimmune reaction involving a non-essential organ or function (e.g., hypothyroidism)	Reversible autoimmune reaction involving function of a major organ or other adverse event (e.g., transient colitis or anemia)	Autoimmune reaction with life-threatening consequences	Death

ALSO CONSIDER: Colitis; Hemoglobin; Hemolysis (e.g., immune hemolytic anemia, drug-related hemolysis); Thyroid function, low (hypothyroidism).

Adverse Event	Short Name	Grade 1	Grade 2	Grade 3	Grade 4	Grade 5
Serum sickness	Serum sickness	—	—	Present	—	Death

NAVIGATION NOTE: Splenic function is graded in the BLOOD/BONE MARROW CATEGORY.

NAVIGATION NOTE: Urticaria as an isolated symptom is graded as Urticaria (hives, welts, wheals) in the DERMATOLOGY/SKIN CATEGORY.

Adverse Event	Short Name	Grade 1	Grade 2	Grade 3	Grade 4	Grade 5
Vasculitis	Vasculitis	Mild, intervention not indicated	Symptomatic, non-steroidal medical intervention indicated	Steroids indicated	Ischemic changes; amputation indicated	Death
Allergy/Immunology – Other (Specify, __)	Allergy – Other (Specify)	Mild	Moderate	Severe	Life-threatening; disabling	Death

AUDITORY/EAR

Adverse Event	Short Name	Grade				
		1	2	3	4	5
NAVIGATION NOTE: Earache (otalgia) is graded as Pain – *Select in the PAIN CATEGORY.*						
Hearing: patients with/without baseline audiogram and enrolled in a monitoring program[1]	Hearing (monitoring program)	Threshold shift or loss of 15 – 25 dB relative to baseline, averaged at 2 or more contiguous test frequencies in at least one ear; or subjective change in the absence of a Grade 1 threshold shift	Threshold shift or loss of >25 – 90 dB, averaged at 2 contiguous test frequencies in at least one ear	Adult only: Threshold shift of >25 – 90 dB, averaged at 3 contiguous test frequencies in at least one ear Pediatric: Hearing loss sufficient to indicate therapeutic intervention, including hearing aids (e.g., ≥20 dB bilateral HL in the speech frequencies; ≥30 dB unilateral HL; and requiring additional speech-language related services)	Adult only: Profound bilateral hearing loss (>90 dB) Pediatric: Audiologic indication for cochlear implant and requiring additional speech-language related services	—
REMARK: Pediatric recommendations are identical to those for adults, unless specified. For children and adolescents (≤18 years of age) without a baseline test, pre-exposure/pre-treatment hearing should be considered to be <5 dB loss.						
Hearing: patients without baseline audiogram and not enrolled in a monitoring program[1]	Hearing (without monitoring program)	—	Hearing loss not requiring hearing aid or intervention (i.e., not interfering with ADL)	Hearing loss requiring hearing aid or intervention (i.e., interfering with ADL)	Profound bilateral hearing loss (>90 dB)	—
REMARK: Pediatric recommendations are identical to those for adults, unless specified. For children and adolescents (≤18 years of age) without a baseline test, pre-exposure/pre-treatment hearing should be considered to be <5 dB loss.						
Otitis, external ear (non-infectious)	Otitis, external	External otitis with erythema or dry desquamation	External otitis with moist desquamation, edema, enhanced cerumen or discharge; tympanic membrane perforation; tympanostomy	External otitis with mastoiditis; stenosis or osteomyelitis	Necrosis of soft tissue or bone	Death
ALSO CONSIDER: Hearing: patients with/without baseline audiogram and enrolled in a monitoring program[1]; Hearing: patients without baseline audiogram and not enrolled in a monitoring program[1].						
Otitis, middle ear (non-infectious)	Otitis, middle	Serous otitis	Serous otitis, medical intervention indicated	Otitis with discharge; mastoiditis	Necrosis of the canal soft tissue or bone	Death

AUDITORY/EAR

Adverse Event	Short Name	Grade				
		1	2	3	4	5
Tinnitus	Tinnitus	—	Tinnitus not interfering with ADL	Tinnitus interfering with ADL	Disabling	—
ALSO CONSIDER: Hearing: patients with/without baseline audiogram and enrolled in a monitoring program[1]; Hearing: patients without baseline audiogram and not enrolled in a monitoring program[1].						
Auditory/Ear – Other (Specify, ___)	Auditory/Ear – Other (Specify)	Mild	Moderate	Severe	Life-threatening; disabling	Death

[1] Drug-induced ototoxicity should be distinguished from age-related threshold decrements or unrelated cochlear insult. When considering whether an adverse event has occurred, it is first necessary to classify the patient into one of two groups. (1) The patient is under standard treatment/enrolled in a clinical trial <2.5 years, and has a 15 dB or greater threshold shift averaged across two contiguous frequencies; or (2) The patient is under standard treatment/enrolled in a clinical trial >2.5 years, and the difference between the expected age-related and the observed threshold shifts is 15 dB or greater averaged across two contiguous frequencies. Consult standard references for appropriate age- and gender-specific hearing norms, for example Morrell, C.H. *et al.* (1996). Age- and gender-specific reference ranges for hearing level and longitudinal changes in hearing level. *Journal of the Acoustical Society of America*, **100**,1949–1967 ; or Shotland, L.I. *et al.* (2001). Recommendations for cancer prevention trials using potentially ototoxic test agents. *Journal of Clinical Oncology*, **19**, 1658–1663.

In the absence of a baseline prior to initial treatment, subsequent audiograms should be referenced to an appropriate database of normals.

ANSI (1996) American National Standard: Determination of occupational noise exposure and estimation of noise-induced hearing impairment, ANSI S 3.44–1996. (Standard S 3.44). New York: American National Standards Institute. The recommended ANSI S3.44 database is Annex B.

BLOOD/BONE MARROW

Adverse Event	Short Name	1	2	Grade 3	4	5
Bone marrow cellularity	Bone marrow cellularity	Mildly hypocellular or ≤25% reduction from normal cellularity for age	Moderately hypocellular or >25 – ≤50% reduction from normal cellularity for age	Severely hypocellular or >50 – ≤75% reduction cellularity from normal for age	—	Death
CD4 count	CD4 count	<LLN – 500/mm³ <LLN – 0.5 x 10⁹/L	<500 – 200/mm³ <0.5 – 0.2 x 10⁹/L	<200 – 50/mm³ <0.2 x 0.05 – 10⁹/L	<50/mm³ <0.05 x 10⁹/L	Death
Haptoglobin	Haptoglobin	<LLN	—	Absent	—	Death
Hemoglobin	Hemoglobin	<LLN – 10.0 g/dL <LLN – 6.2 mmol/L <LLN – 100 g/L	<10.0 – 8.0 g/dL <6.2 – 4.9 mmol/L <100 – 80g/L	<8.0 – 6.5 g/dL <4.9 – 4.0 mmol/L <80 – 65 g/L	<6.5 g/dL <4.0 mmol/L <65 g/L	Death
Hemolysis (e.g., immune hemolytic anemia, drug-related hemolysis)	Hemolysis	Laboratory evidence of hemolysis only (e.g., direct antiglobulin test [DAT, Coombs'] schistocytes)	Evidence of red cell destruction and ≥2 gm decrease in hemoglobin, no transfusion	Transfusion or medical intervention (e.g., steroids) indicated	Catastrophic consequences of hemolysis (e.g., renal failure, hypotension, bronchospasm, emergency splenectomy)	Death

ALSO CONSIDER: Haptoglobin; Hemoglobin.

Adverse Event	Short Name	1	2	Grade 3	4	5
Iron overload	Iron overload	—	Asymptomatic iron overload, intervention not indicated	Iron overload, intervention indicated	Organ impairment (e.g., endocrinopathy, cardiopathy)	Death
Leukocytes (total WBC)	Leukocytes	<LLN – 3000/mm³ <LLN – 3.0 x 10⁹/L	<3000–2000/mm³ <3.0 – 2.0 x 10⁹/L	<2000 – 1000/mm³ <2.0 – 1.0 x 10⁹/L	<1000/mm³ <1.0 x 10⁹/L	Death
Lymphopenia	Lymphopenia	<LLN – 800/mm³ <LLN x 0.8 – 10⁹/L	<800 – 500/mm³ <0.8 – 0.5 x 10⁹/L	<500 – 200 mm³ <0.5 – 0.2 x 10⁹/L	<200/mm³ <0.2 x 10⁹/L	Death
Myelodysplasia	Myelodysplasia	—	—	Abnormal marrow cytogenetics (marrow blasts ≤5%)	RAEB or RAEB-T (marrow blasts >5%)	Death
Neutrophils/granulocytes (ANC/AGC)	Neutrophils	<LLN – 1500/mm³ <LLN – 1.5 x 10⁹/L	<1500 – 1000/mm³ <1.5 – 1.0 x 10⁹/L	<1000 – 500/mm³ <1.0 – 0.5 x 10⁹/L	<500/mm³ <0.5 x 10⁹/L	Death
Platelets	Platelets	<LLN – 75,000/mm³ <LLN – 75.0 x 10⁹/L	<75,000 – 50,000/mm³ <75.0 – 50.0 x 10⁹/L	<50,000 – 25,000/mm³ <50.0 – 25.0 x 10⁹/L	<25,000/mm³ <25.0 x 10⁹/L	Death
Splenic function	Splenic function	Incidental findings (e.g., Howell-Jolly bodies)	Prophylactic antibiotics indicated	—	Life-threatening consequences	Death
Blood/Bone Marrow – Other (Specify, __)	Blood – Other (Specify)	Mild	Moderate	Severe	Life-threatening; disabling	Death

CARDIAC ARRHYTHMIA

Adverse Event	Short Name	Grade				
		1	2	3	4	5
Conduction abnormality/ atrioventricular heart block – Select: – Asystole – AV Block-First degree – AV Block-Second degree Mobitz Type I (Wenckebach) – AV Block-Second degree Mobitz Type II – AV Block-Third degree (Complete AV block) – Conduction abnormality NOS – Sick Sinus Syndrome – Stokes-Adams Syndrome – Wolff-Parkinson-White Syndrome	Conduction abnormality – Select	Asymptomatic, intervention not indicated	Non-urgent medical intervention indicated	Incompletely controlled medically or controlled with device (e.g., pacemaker)	Life-threatening (e.g., arrhythmia associated with CHF, hypotension, syncope, shock)	Death
Palpitations	Palpitations	Present	Present with associated symptoms (e.g., lightheadedness, shortness of breath)	—	—	—
REMARK: Grade palpitations only in the absence of a documented arrhythmia.						
Prolonged QTc interval	Prolonged QTc	QTc >0.45 – 0.47 second	QTc >0.47 – 0.50 second; ≥0.06 second above baseline	QTc >0.50 second	QTc >0.50 second; life-threatening signs or symptoms (e.g., arrhythmia, CHF, hypotension, shock syncope); Torsade de pointes	Death
Supraventricular and nodal arrhythmia – Select: – Atrial fibrillation – Atrial flutter – Atrial tachycardia/Paroxysmal Atrial Tachycardia – Nodal/Junctional – Sinus arrhythmia – Sinus bradycardia – Sinus tachycardia – Supraventricular arrhythmia NOS – Supraventricular extrasystoles (Premature Atrial Contractions; Premature Nodal/Junctional Contractions) – Supraventricular tachycardia	Supraventricular arrhythmia – Select	Asymptomatic, intervention not indicated	Non-urgent medical intervention indicated	Symptomatic and incompletely controlled medically, or controlled with device (e.g., pacemaker)	Life-threatening (e.g., arrhythmia associated with CHF, hypotension, syncope, shock)	Death

NAVIGATION NOTE: Syncope is graded as Syncope (fainting) in the NEUROLOGY CATEGORY.

CARDIAC ARRHYTHMIA

Adverse Event	Short Name	Grade				
		1	2	3	4	5
Vasovagal episode	Vasovagal episode	—	Present without loss of consciousness	Present with loss of consciousness	Life-threatening consequences	Death
Ventricular arrhythmia – Select: – Bigeminy – Idioventricular rhythm – PVCs – Torsade de pointes – Trigeminy – Ventricular arrhythmia NOS – Ventricular fibrillation – Ventricular flutter – Ventricular tachycardia	Ventricular arrhythmia – Select	Asymptomatic, no intervention indicated	Non-urgent medical intervention indicated	Symptomatic and incompletely controlled medically or controlled with device (e.g., defibrillator)	Life-threatening (e.g., arrhythmia associated with CHF, hypotension, syncope, shock)	Death
Cardiac Arrhythmia – Other (Specify, __)	Cardiac Arrhythmia – Other (Specify)	Mild	Moderate	Severe	Life-threatening; disabling	Death

CARDIAC GENERAL

Adverse Event	Short Name	1	2	3	4	5
				Grade		

NAVIGATION NOTE: Angina is graded as Cardiac ischemia/infarction in the CARDIAC GENERAL CATEGORY.

Adverse Event	Short Name	1	2	3	4	5
Cardiac ischemia/infarction	Cardiac ischemia/infarction	Asymptomatic arterial narrowing without ischemia	Asymptomatic and testing suggesting ischemia; stable angina	Symptomatic and testing consistent with ischemia; unstable angina; intervention indicated	Acute myocardial infarction	Death
Cardiac troponin I (cTnI)	cTnI	—	—	Levels consistent with unstable angina as defined by the manufacturer	Levels consistent with myocardial infarction as defined by the manufacturer	Death
Cardiac troponin T (cTnT)	cTnT	0.03 – <0.05 ng/mL	0.05 – <0.1 ng/mL	0.1 – <0.2 ng/mL	0.2 ng/mL	Death
Cardiopulmonary arrest, cause unknown (non-fatal)	Cardiopulmonary arrest	—	—	—	Life-threatening	—

REMARK: Grade 4 (non-fatal) is the only appropriate grade. CTCAE provides three alternatives for reporting Death:

1. A CTCAE term associated with Grade 5.
2. A CTCAE 'Other (Specify, ___)' within any CATEGORY.
3. Death not associated with CTCAE term – *Select* in the DEATH CATEGORY.

NAVIGATION NOTE: Chest pain (non-cardiac and non-pleuritic) is graded as Pain – *Select* in the PAIN CATEGORY.

NAVIGATION NOTE: CNS ischemia is graded as CNS cerebrovascular ischemia in the NEUROLOGY CATEGORY.

Adverse Event	Short Name	1	2	3	4	5
Hypertension	Hypertension	Asymptomatic, transient (<24 hrs) increase by >20 mmHg (diastolic) or to >150/100 if previously WNL; intervention not indicated Pediatric: Asymptomatic, transient (<24 hrs) BP increase >ULN; intervention not indicated	Recurrent or persistent (≥24 hrs) or symptomatic increase by >20 mmHg (diastolic) or to >150/100 if previously WNL; monotherapy may be indicated Pediatric: Recurrent or persistent (≥24 hrs) BP >ULN; monotherapy may be indicated	Requiring more than one drug or more intensive therapy than previously Pediatric: Same as adult	Life-threatening consequences (e.g., hypertensive crisis) Pediatric: Same as adult	Death

REMARK: Use age and gender-appropriate normal values >95th percentile ULN for pediatric patients.

CARDIAC GENERAL

Adverse Event	Short Name	Grade				
		1	2	3	4	5
Hypotension	Hypotension	Changes, intervention not indicated	Brief (<24 hrs) fluid replacement or other therapy; no physiologic consequences	Sustained (≥24 hrs) therapy, resolves without persisting physiologic consequences	Shock (e.g., acidemia; impairment of vital organ function)	Death
ALSO CONSIDER: Syncope (fainting).						
Left ventricular diastolic dysfunction	Left ventricular diastolic dysfunction	Asymptomatic diagnostic finding; intervention not indicated	Asymptomatic, intervention indicated	Symptomatic CHF responsive to intervention	Refractory CHF, poorly controlled; intervention such as ventricular assist device or heart transplant indicated	Death
Left ventricular systolic dysfunction	Left ventricular systolic dysfunction	Asymptomatic, resting ejection fraction (EF) <60 – 50%; shortening fraction (SF) <30 – 24%	Asymptomatic, resting EF <50 – 40%; SF <24 – 15%	Symptomatic CHF responsive to intervention; EF <40 – 20% SF <15%	Refractory CHF or poorly controlled; EF <20%; intervention such as ventricular assist device, ventricular reduction surgery, or heart transplant indicated	Death

NAVIGATION NOTE: Myocardial infarction is graded as Cardiac ischemia/infarction in the CARDIAC GENERAL CATEGORY.

Adverse Event	Short Name	1	2	3	4	5
Myocarditis	Myocarditis	—	—	CHF responsive to intervention	Severe or refractory CHF	Death
Pericardial effusion (non–malignant)	Pericardial effusion	Asymptomatic effusion	—	Effusion with physiologic consequences	Life-threatening consequences (e.g., tamponade); emergency intervention indicated	Death
Pericarditis	Pericarditis	Asymptomatic, ECG or physical exam (rub) changes consistent with pericarditis	Symptomatic pericarditis (e.g., chest pain)	Pericarditis with physiologic consequences (e.g., pericardial constriction)	Life-threatening consequences; emergency intervention indicated	Death

NAVIGATION NOTE: Pleuritic pain is graded as Pain – Select in the PAIN CATEGORY.

Adverse Event	Short Name	1	2	3	4	5
Pulmonary hypertension	Pulmonary hypertension	Asymptomatic without therapy	Asymptomatic, therapy indicated	Symptomatic hypertension, responsive to therapy	Symptomatic hypertension, poorly controlled	Death
Restrictive cardiomyopathy	Restrictive cardiomyopathy	Asymptomatic, therapy not indicated	Asymptomatic, therapy indicated	Symptomatic CHF responsive to intervention	Refractory CHF, poorly controlled; intervention such as ventricular assist device, or heart transplant indicated	Death

Adverse Event	Short Name	Grade				
		1	2	3	4	5
Right ventricular dysfunction (cor pulmonale)	Right ventricular dysfunction	Asymptomatic without therapy	Asymptomatic; therapy indicated	Symptomatic cor pulmonale, responsive to intervention	Symptomatic cor pulmonale poorly controlled; intervention such as ventricular assist device, or heart transplant indicated	Death
Valvular heart disease	Valvular heart disease	Asymptomatic valvular thickening with or without mild valvular regurgitation or stenosis; treatment other than endocarditis prophylaxis not indicated	Asymptomatic; moderate regurgitation or stenosis by imaging	Symptomatic; severe regurgitation or stenosis; symptoms controlled with medical therapy	Life-threatening; disabling; intervention (e.g., valve replacement, valvuloplasty) indicated	Death
Cardiac General – Other (Specify, ___)	Cardiac General – Other (Specify)	Mild	Moderate	Severe	Life-threatening; disabling	Death

COAGULATION

Adverse Event	Short Name	Grade				
		1	2	3	4	5
DIC (disseminated intravascular coagulation)	DIC	—	Laboratory findings with no bleeding	Laboratory findings and bleeding	Laboratory findings, life-threatening or disabling consequences (e.g., CNS hemorrhage, organ damage, or hemodynamically significant blood loss)	Death

REMARK: DIC (disseminated intravascular coagulation) must have increased fibrin split products or D-dimer.

ALSO CONSIDER: Platelets.

Fibrinogen	Fibrinogen	<1.0 – 0.75 x LLN or <25% decrease from baseline	<0.75 – 0.5 x LLN or 25 – <50% decrease from baseline	<0.5 – 0.25 x LLN or 50 – <75% decrease from baseline	<0.25 x LLN or 75% decrease from baseline or absolute value <50 mg/dL	Death

REMARK: Use % decrease only when baseline is <LLN (local laboratory value).

INR (International Normalized Ratio of prothrombin time)	INR	>1 – 1.5 x ULN	>1.5 – 2 x ULN	>2 x ULN	—	—

ALSO CONSIDER: Hemorrhage, CNS; Hemorrhage, GI – *Select*; Hemorrhage, GU – *Select*; Hemorrhage, pulmonary/upper respiratory – *Select*.

PTT (Partial Thromboplastin Time)	PTT	>1 – 1.5 x ULN	>1.5 – 2 x ULN	>2 x ULN	—	—

ALSO CONSIDER: Hemorrhage, CNS; Hemorrhage, GI – *Select*; Hemorrhage, GU – *Select*; Hemorrhage, pulmonary/upper respiratory – *Select*.

Thrombotic microangiopathy (e.g., thrombotic thrombocytopenic purpura [TTP] or hemolytic uremic syndrome [HUS])	Thrombotic microangiopathy	Evidence of RBC destruction (schistocytosis) without clinical consequences	—	Laboratory findings present with clinical consequences (e.g., renal insufficiency, petechiae)	Laboratory findings and life-threatening or disabling consequences, (e.g., CNS hemorrhage/ bleeding or thrombosis/ embolism or renal failure)	Death

REMARK: **Must** have microangiopathic changes on blood smear (e.g., schistocytes, helmet cells, red cell fragments).

ALSO CONSIDER: Creatinine; Hemoglobin; Platelets.

Coagulation – Other (Specify, ___)	Coagulation – Other (Specify)	Mild	Moderate	Severe	Life-threatening; disabling	Death

CONSTITUTIONAL SYMPTOMS

Adverse Event	Short Name	Grade				
		1	2	3	4	5
Fatigue (asthenia, lethargy, malaise)	Fatigue	Mild fatigue over baseline	Moderate or causing difficulty performing some ADL	Severe fatigue interfering with ADL	Disabling	—
Fever (in the absence of neutropenia, where neutropenia is defined as ANC <1.0 x 10⁹/L)	Fever	38.0 – 39.0°C (100.4 – 102.2°F)	>39.0 – 40.0°C (102.3 – 104.0°F)	>40.0°C (>104.0°F) for ≤24 hrs	>40.0°C (>104.0°F) for >24 hrs	Death

REMARK: The temperature measurements listed are oral or tympanic.

ALSO CONSIDER: Allergic reaction/hypersensitivity (including drug fever).

NAVIGATION NOTE: Hot flashes are graded as Hot flashes/flushes in the ENDOCRINE CATEGORY.

Adverse Event	Short Name	1	2	3	4	5
Hypothermia	Hypothermia	—	35 – >32°C 95 – >89.6°F	32 – >28°C 89.6 – >82.4° F	≤28 °C 82.4°F or life-threatening consequences (e.g., coma, hypotension, pulmonary edema, acidemia, ventricular fibrillation)	Death
Insomnia	Insomnia	Occasional difficulty sleeping, not interfering with function	Difficulty sleeping, interfering with function but not interfering with ADL	Frequent difficulty sleeping, interfering with ADL	Disabling	—

REMARK: If pain or other symptoms interfere with sleep, do NOT grade as insomnia. Grade primary event(s) causing insomnia.

Adverse Event	Short Name	1	2	3	4	5
Obesity²	Obesity	—	BMI 25 – 29.9 kg/m²	BMI 30 – 39.99 kg/m²	BMI ≥40 kg/m²	—

REMARK: BMI = (weight [kg]) / (height [m])²

Adverse Event	Short Name	1	2	3	4	5
Odor (patient odor)	Patient odor	Mild odor	Pronounced odor	—	—	—
Rigors/chills	Rigors/chills	Mild	Moderate, narcotics indicated	Severe or prolonged, not responsive to narcotics	—	—

²sNHLBI Obesity Task Force (1998). "Clinical Guidelines on the Identification, Evaluation, and Treatment of Overweight and Obesity in Adults," The Evidence Report. *Obesity Research*, **6**, 51S–209S.

CONSTITUTIONAL SYMPTOMS

Adverse Event	Short Name	Grade				
		1	2	3	4	5
Sweating (diaphoresis)	Sweating	Mild and occasional	Frequent or drenching	—	—	—
ALSO CONSIDER: Hot flashes/flushes.						
Weight gain	Weight gain	5 – <10% of baseline	10 – <20% of baseline	≥20% of baseline	—	
REMARK: Edema, depending on etiology, is graded in the CARDIAC GENERAL or LYMPHATICS CATEGORIES.						
ALSO CONSIDER: Ascites (non-malignant); Pleural effusion (non-malignant).						
Weight loss	Weight loss	5 to <10% from baseline; intervention not indicated	10 – <20% from baseline; nutritional support indicated	≥20% from baseline; tube feeding or TPN indicated	—	
Constitutional Symptoms – Other (Specify, __)	Constitutional Symptoms – Other (Specify)	Mild	Moderate	Severe	Life-threatening; disabling	Death

Adverse Event	Short Name	Grade				
		1	2	3	4	5
Death not associated with CTCAE term – *Select*: – Death NOS – Disease progression NOS – Multi-organ failure – Sudden death	Death not associated with CTCAE term – *Select*	—	—	—	—	Death

REMARK: Grade 5 is the only appropriate grade. 'Death not associated with CTCAE term – *Select*' is to be used where a death:

1. Cannot be attributed to a CTCAE term associated with Grade 5.
2. Cannot be reported within any CATEGORY using a CTCAE 'Other (Specify, __)'.

DERMATOLOGY/SKIN

Adverse Event	Short Name	Grade				
		1	2	3	4	5
Atrophy, skin	Atrophy, skin	Detectable	Marked	—	—	—
Atrophy, subcutaneous fat	Atrophy, subcutaneous fat	Detectable	Marked	—	—	—
ALSO CONSIDER: Induration/fibrosis (skin and subcutaneous tissue).						
Bruising (in absence of Grade 3 or 4 thrombocytopenia)	Bruising	Localized or in a dependent area	Generalized	—	—	—
Burn	Burn	Minimal symptoms; intervention not indicated	Medical intervention; minimal debridement indicated	Moderate to major debridement or reconstruction indicated	Life-threatening consequences	Death
REMARK: Burn refers to all burns including radiation, chemical, etc.						
Cheilitis	Cheilitis	Asymptomatic	Symptomatic, not interfering with ADL	Symptomatic, interfering with ADL	—	—
Dry skin	Dry skin	Asymptomatic	Symptomatic, not interfering with ADL	Interfering with ADL	—	—
Flushing	Flushing	Asymptomatic	Symptomatic	—	—	—
Hair loss/alopecia (scalp or body)	Alopecia	Thinning or patchy	Complete	—	—	—
Hyperpigmentation	Hyperpigmentation	Slight or localized	Marked or generalized	—	—	—
Hypopigmentation	Hypopigmentation	Slight or localized	Marked or generalized	—	—	—
Induration/fibrosis (skin and subcutaneous tissue)	Induration	Increased density on palpation	Moderate impairment of function not interfering with ADL; marked increase in density and firmness on palpation with or without minimal retraction	Dysfunction interfering with ADL; very marked density, retraction or fixation	—	
ALSO CONSIDER: Fibrosis-cosmesis; Fibrosis-deep connective tissue.						
Injection site reaction/ extravasation changes	Injection site reaction	Pain; itching; erythema	Pain or swelling, with inflammation or phlebitis	Ulceration or necrosis that is severe; operative intervention indicated	—	
ALSO CONSIDER: Allergic reaction/hypersensitivity (including drug fever); Ulceration.						

DERMATOLOGY/SKIN

Adverse Event	Short Name	Grade				
		1	2	3	4	5
Nail changes	Nail changes	Discoloration; ridging (koilonychias); pitting	Partial or complete loss of nail(s); pain in nailbed(s)	Interfering with ADL	—	—

NAVIGATION NOTE: Petechiae is graded as Petechiae/purpura (hemorrhage/bleeding into skin or mucosa) in the HEMORRHAGE/BLEEDING CATEGORY.

Adverse Event	Short Name	1	2	3	4	5
Photosensitivity	Photosensitivity	Painless erythema	Painful erythema	Erythema with desquamation	Life-threatening; disabling	Death
Pruritus/itching	Pruritus	Mild or localized	Intense or widespread	Intense or widespread and interfering with ADL	—	—

ALSO CONSIDER: Rash/desquamation.

Adverse Event	Short Name	1	2	3	4	5
Rash/desquamation	Rash	Macular or papular eruption or erythema without associated symptoms	Macular or papular eruption or erythema with pruritus or other associated symptoms; localized desquamation or other lesions covering <50% of body surface area (BSA)	Severe, generalized erythroderma or macular, papular or vesicular eruption; desquamation ≥50% BSA	Generalized exfoliative, ulcerative, or bullous dermatitis	Death

REMARK: Rash/desquamation may be used for GVHD.

Adverse Event	Short Name	1	2	3	4	5
Rash: acne/acneiform	Acne	Intervention not indicated	Intervention indicated	Associated with pain, disfigurement, ulceration, or desquamation	—	Death
Rash: dermatitis associated with radiation – Select: – Chemoradiation – Radiation	Dermatitis – Select	Faint erythema or dry desquamation	Moderate to brisk erythema; patchy moist desquamation, mostly confined to skin folds and creases; moderate edema	Moist desquamation other than skin folds and creases; bleeding induced by minor trauma or abrasion	Skin necrosis or ulceration of full thickness dermis; spontaneous bleeding from involved site	Death
Rash: erythema multiforme (e.g., Stevens-Johnson syndrome, toxic epidermal necrolysis)	Erythema multiforme	—	Scattered, but not generalized eruption	Severe (e.g., generalized rash or painful stomatitis); IV fluids, tube feedings, or TPN indicated	Life-threatening; disabling	Death
Rash: hand-foot skin reaction	Hand-foot	Minimal skin changes or dermatitis (e.g., erythema) without pain	Skin changes (e.g., peeling, blisters, bleeding, edema) or pain, not interfering with function	Ulcerative dermatitis or skin changes with pain interfering with function	—	—

DERMATOLOGY/SKIN

Adverse Event	Short Name	Grade				
		1	2	3	4	5
Skin breakdown/decubitus ulcer	Decubitus	—	Local wound care; medical intervention indicated	Operative debridement or other invasive intervention indicated (e.g., hyperbaric oxygen)	Life-threatening consequences; major invasive intervention indicated (e.g., tissue reconstruction, flap, or grafting)	Death

REMARK: Skin breakdown/decubitus ulcer is to be used for loss of skin integrity or decubitus ulcer from pressure or as the result of operative or medical intervention.

Striae	Striae	Mild	Cosmetically significant	—	—	—
Telangiectasia	Telangiectasia	Few	Moderate number	Many and confluent	—	—
Ulceration	Ulceration	—	Superficial ulceration <2 cm size; local wound care; medical intervention indicated	Ulceration ≥2 cm size; operative debridement, primary closure or other invasive intervention indicated (e.g., hyperbaric oxygen)	Life-threatening consequences; major invasive intervention indicated (e.g., complete resection, tissue reconstruction, flap, or grafting)	Death
Urticaria (hives, welts, wheals)	Urticaria	Intervention not indicated	Intervention indicated for <24 hrs	Intervention indicated for ≥24 hrs	—	—

ALSO CONSIDER: Allergic reaction/hypersensitivity (including drug fever).

Wound complication, non-infectious	Wound complication, non-infectious	Incisional separation of ≤25% of wound, no deeper than superficial fascia	Incisional separation >25% of wound with local care; asymptomatic hernia	Symptomatic hernia without evidence of strangulation; fascial disruption/dehiscence without evisceration; primary wound closure or revision by operative intervention indicated; hospitalization or hyperbaric oxygen indicated	Symptomatic hernia with evidence of strangulation; fascial disruption with evisceration; major reconstruction flap, grafting, resection, or amputation indicated	Death

REMARK: Wound complication, non-infectious is to be used for separation of incision, hernia, dehiscence, evisceration, or second surgery for wound revision.

Dermatology/Skin – Other (Specify, ___)	Dermatology – Other (Specify)	Mild	Moderate	Severe	Life-threatening; disabling	Death

ENDOCRINE

Adverse Event	Short Name	Grade				
		1	2	3	4	5
Adrenal insufficiency	Adrenal insufficiency	Asymptomatic, intervention not indicated	Symptomatic, intervention indicated	Hospitalization	Life-threatening; disabling	Death

REMARK: Adrenal insufficiency includes any of the following signs and symptoms: abdominal pain, anorexia, constipation, diarrhea, hypotension, pigmentation of mucous membranes, pigmentation of skin, salt craving, syncope (fainting), vitiligo, vomiting, weakness, weight loss. Adrenal insufficiency must be confirmed by laboratory studies (low cortisol frequently accompanied by low aldosterone).

ALSO CONSIDER: Potassium, serum-high (hyperkalemia); Thyroid function, low (hypothyroidism).

Adverse Event	Short Name	1	2	3	4	5
Cushingoid appearance (e.g., moon face, buffalo hump, centripetal obesity, cutaneous striae)	Cushingoid	—	Present	—	—	—

ALSO CONSIDER: Glucose, serum-high (hyperglycemia); Potassium, serum-low (hypokalemia).

Adverse Event	Short Name	1	2	3	4	5
Feminization of male	Feminization of male	—	—	Present	—	—

NAVIGATION NOTE: Gynecomastia is graded in the SEXUAL/REPRODUCTIVE FUNCTION CATEGORY.

Adverse Event	Short Name	1	2	3	4	5
Hot flashes/flushes[3]	Hot flashes	Mild	Moderate	Interfering with ADL	—	—
Masculinization of female	Masculinization of female	—	—	Present	—	—
Neuroendocrine: ACTH deficiency	ACTH	Asymptomatic	Symptomatic, not interfering with ADL; intervention indicated	Symptoms interfering with ADL; hospitalization indicated	Life-threatening consequences (e.g., severe hypotension)	Death
Neuroendocrine: ADH secretion abnormality (e.g., SIADH or low ADH)	ADH	Asymptomatic	Symptomatic, not interfering with ADL; intervention indicated	Symptoms interfering with ADL	Life-threatening consequences	Death
Neuroendocrine: gonadotropin secretion abnormality	Gonadotropin	Asymptomatic	Symptomatic, not interfering with ADL; intervention indicated	Symptoms interfering with ADL; osteopenia; fracture; infertility	—	—
Neuroendocrine: growth hormone secretion abnormality	Growth hormone	Asymptomatic	Symptomatic, not interfering with ADL; intervention indicated	—	—	—
Neuroendocrine: prolactin hormone secretion abnormality	Prolactin	Asymptomatic	Symptomatic, not interfering with ADL; intervention indicated	Symptoms interfering with ADL; amenorrhea; galactorrhea	—	Death

[3] Sloan, J.A., Loprinzi, C.L., Novotny, P.J., Barton, D.L., Lavasseur, B.I., Windschitl, H.J. (2001). Methodologic lessons learned from Hot Flash Studies. *Journal of Clinical Oncology*, 19 (23), 4280–4290.

Adverse Event	Short Name	Grade				
		1	2	3	4	5
Pancreatic endocrine: glucose intolerance	Diabetes	Asymptomatic, intervention not indicated	Symptomatic; dietary modification or oral agent indicated	Symptoms interfering with ADL; insulin indicated	Life-threatening consequences (e.g., ketoacidosis, hyperosmolar non-ketotic coma)	Death
Parathyroid function, low (hypoparathyroidism)	Hypoparathyroidism	Asymptomatic, intervention not indicated	Symptomatic; intervention indicated	—	—	—
Thyroid function, high (hyperthyroidism, thyrotoxicosis)	Hyperthyroidism	Asymptomatic, intervention not indicated	Symptomatic, not interfering with ADL; thyroid suppression therapy indicated	Symptoms interfering with ADL; hospitalization indicated	Life-threatening consequences (e.g., thyroid storm)	Death
Thyroid function, low (hypothyroidism)	Hypothyroidism	Asymptomatic, intervention not indicated	Symptomatic, not interfering with ADL; thyroid replacement indicated	Symptoms interfering with ADL; hospitalization indicated	Life-threatening myxedema coma	Death
Endocrine – Other (Specify, ___)	Endocrine – Other (Specify)	Mild	Moderate	Severe	Life-threatening; disabling	Death

GASTROINTESTINAL

Adverse Event	Short Name	Grade				
		1	2	3	4	5

NAVIGATION NOTE: Abdominal pain or cramping is graded as Pain – *Select* in the PAIN CATEGORY.

Adverse Event	Short Name	1	2	3	4	5
Anorexia	Anorexia	Loss of appetite without alteration in eating habits	Oral intake altered without significant weight loss or malnutrition; oral nutritional supplements indicated	Associated with significant weight loss or malnutrition (e.g., inadequate oral caloric and/or fluid intake); IV fluids, tube feedings or TPN indicated	Life-threatening consequences	Death

ALSO CONSIDER: Weight loss.

Adverse Event	Short Name	1	2	3	4	5
Ascites (non-malignant)	Ascites	Asymptomatic	Symptomatic, medical intervention indicated	Symptomatic, invasive procedure indicated	Life-threatening consequences	Death

REMARK: Ascites (non-malignant) refers to documented non-malignant ascites or unknown etiology, but unlikely malignant, and includes chylous ascites.

Adverse Event	Short Name	1	2	3	4	5
Colitis	Colitis	Asymptomatic, pathologic or radiographic findings only	Abdominal pain; mucus or blood in stool	Abdominal pain, fever, change in bowel habits with ileus; peritoneal signs	Life-threatening consequences (e.g., perforation, bleeding, ischemia, necrosis, toxic megacolon)	Death

ALSO CONSIDER: Hemorrhage, GI – *Select*.

Adverse Event	Short Name	1	2	3	4	5
Constipation	Constipation	Occasional or intermittent symptoms; occasional use of stool softeners, laxatives, dietary modification, or enema	Persistent symptoms with regular use of laxatives or enemas indicated	Symptoms interfering with ADL; obstipation with manual evacuation indicated	Life-threatening consequences (e.g., obstruction, toxic megacolon)	Death

ALSO CONSIDER: Ileus, GI (functional obstruction of bowel, i.e., neuroconstipation); Obstruction, GI – *Select*.

Adverse Event	Short Name	1	2	3	4	5
Dehydration	Dehydration	Increased oral fluids indicated; dry mucous membranes; diminished skin turgor	IV fluids indicated <24 hrs	IV fluids indicated ≥24 hrs	Life-threatening consequences (e.g., hemodynamic collapse)	Death

ALSO CONSIDER: Diarrhea; Hypotension; Vomiting.

Adverse Event	Short Name	1	2	3	4	5
Dental: dentures or prosthesis	Dentures	Minimal discomfort, no restriction in activities	Discomfort preventing use in some activities (e.g., eating), but not others (e.g., speaking)	Unable to use dentures or prosthesis at any time	—	—

GASTROINTESTINAL

Adverse Event	Short Name	Grade				
		1	2	3	4	5
Dental: periodontal disease	Periodontal	Gingival recession or gingivitis; limited bleeding on probing; mild local bone loss	Moderate gingival recession or gingivitis; multiple sites of bleeding on probing; moderate bone loss	Spontaneous bleeding; severe bone loss with or without tooth loss; osteonecrosis of maxilla or mandible	—	—

REMARK: Severe periodontal disease leading to osteonecrosis is graded as Osteonecrosis (avascular necrosis) in the MUSCULOSKELETAL CATEGORY.

Adverse Event	Short Name	1	2	3	4	5
Dental: teeth	Teeth	Surface stains; dental caries; restorable, without extractions	Less than full mouth extractions; tooth fracture or crown amputation or repair indicated	Full mouth extractions indicated	—	—
Dental: teeth development	Teeth development	Hypoplasia of tooth or enamel not interfering with function	Functional impairment correctable with oral surgery	Maldevelopment with functional impairment not surgically correctable	—	—
Diarrhea	Diarrhea	Increase of <4 stools per day over baseline; mild increase in ostomy output compared to baseline	Increase of 4 – 6 stools per day over baseline; IV fluids indicated <24hrs; moderate increase in ostomy output compared to baseline; not interfering with ADL	Increase of ≥7 stools per day over baseline; incontinence; IV fluids ≥24 hrs; hospitalization; severe increase in ostomy output compared to baseline; interfering with ADL	Life-threatening consequences (e.g., hemodynamic collapse)	Death

REMARK: Diarrhea includes diarrhea of small bowel or colonic origin, and/or ostomy diarrhea.

ALSO CONSIDER: Dehydration; Hypotension.

Adverse Event	Short Name	1	2	3	4	5
Distension/bloating, abdominal	Distension	Asymptomatic	Symptomatic, but not interfering with GI function	Symptomatic, interfering with GI function	—	—

ALSO CONSIDER: Ascites (non-malignant); Ileus, GI (functional obstruction of bowel, i.e., neuroconstipation); Obstruction, GI – Select.

Adverse Event	Short Name	Grade				
		1	2	3	4	5
Dry mouth/salivary gland (xerostomia)	Dry mouth	Symptomatic (dry or thick saliva) without significant dietary alteration; unstimulated saliva flow >0.2 ml/min	Symptomatic and significant oral intake alteration (e.g., copious water, other lubricants, diet limited to purees and/or soft, moist foods); unstimulated saliva 0.1 to 0.2 ml/min	Symptoms leading to inability to adequately aliment orally; IV fluids, tube feedings, or TPN indicated; unstimulated saliva <0.1 ml/min	—	—

REMARK: Dry mouth/salivary gland (xerostomia) includes descriptions of grade using both subjective and objective assessment parameters. Record this event consistently throughout a patient's participation on study. If salivary flow measurements are used for initial assessment, subsequent assessments must use salivary flow.

ALSO CONSIDER: Salivary gland changes/saliva.

Adverse Event	Short Name	1	2	3	4	5
Dysphagia (difficulty swallowing)	Dysphagia	Symptomatic, able to eat regular diet	Symptomatic and altered eating/swallowing (e.g., altered dietary habits, oral supplements); IV fluids indicated <24 hrs	Symptomatic and severely altered eating/swallowing (e.g., inadequate oral caloric or fluid intake); IV fluids, tube feedings, or TPN indicated ≥24 hrs	Life-threatening consequences (e.g., obstruction, perforation)	Death

REMARK: Dysphagia (difficulty swallowing) is to be used for swallowing difficulty from oral, pharyngeal, esophageal, or neurologic origin. Dysphagia requiring dilation is graded as Stricture/stenosis (including anastomotic), GI – Select.

ALSO CONSIDER: Dehydration; Esophagitis.

Adverse Event	Short Name	1	2	3	4	5
Enteritis (inflammation of the small bowel)	Enteritis	Asymptomatic, pathologic or radiographic findings only	Abdominal pain; mucus or blood in stool	Abdominal pain, fever, change in bowel habits with ileus; peritoneal signs	Life-threatening consequences (e.g., perforation, bleeding, ischemia, necrosis)	Death

ALSO CONSIDER: Hemorrhage, GI – Select; Typhlitis (cecal inflammation).

Adverse Event	Short Name	1	2	3	4	5
Esophagitis	Esophagitis	Asymptomatic pathologic, radiographic, or endoscopic findings only	Symptomatic; altered eating/swallowing (e.g., altered dietary habits, oral supplements); IV fluids indicated <24 hrs	Symptomatic and severely altered eating/swallowing (e.g., inadequate oral caloric or fluid intake); IV fluids, tube feedings, or TPN indicated ≥24 hrs	Life-threatening consequences	Death

REMARK: Esophagitis includes reflux esophagitis.

ALSO CONSIDER: Dysphagia (difficulty swallowing).

GASTROINTESTINAL

Adverse Event	Short Name	Grade 1	2	3	4	5
Fistula, GI – Select: – Abdomen NOS – Anus – Biliary tree – Colon/cecum/appendix – Duodenum – Esophagus – Gallbladder – Ileum – Jejunum – Oral cavity – Pancreas – Pharynx – Rectum – Salivary gland – Small bowel NOS – Stomach	Fistula, GI – Select	Asymptomatic, radiographic findings only	Symptomatic; altered GI function (e.g., altered dietary habits, diarrhea, or GI fluid loss); IV fluids indicated <24 hrs	Symptomatic and severely altered GI function (e.g., altered dietary habits, diarrhea, or GI fluid loss); tube feedings, or TPN indicated ≥24 hrs	Life-threatening consequences	Death

REMARK: A fistula is defined as an abnormal communication between two body cavities, potential spaces, and/or the skin. The site indicated for a fistula should be the site from which the abnormal process is believed to have originated. For example, a tracheo-esophageal fistula arising in the context of a resected or irradiated esophageal cancer is graded as Fistula, GI – esophagus.

Adverse Event	Short Name	Mild	Moderate	3	4	5
Flatulence	Flatulence	Mild	Moderate	—	—	—
Gastritis (including bile reflux gastritis)	Gastritis	Asymptomatic radiographic or endoscopic findings only	Symptomatic; altered gastric function (e.g., inadequate oral caloric or fluid intake); IV fluids indicated <24 hrs	Symptomatic and severely altered gastric function (e.g., inadequate oral caloric or fluid intake); IV fluids, tube feedings, or TPN indicated ≥24 hrs	Life-threatening consequences; operative intervention requiring complete organ resection (e.g., gastrectomy)	Death

ALSO CONSIDER: Hemorrhage, GI – Select; Ulcer, GI – Select.

NAVIGATION NOTE: Head and neck soft tissue necrosis is graded as Soft tissue necrosis – Select in the MUSCULOSKELETAL/SOFT TISSUE CATEGORY.

Adverse Event	Short Name	Mild	Moderate	Severe	4	5
Heartburn/dyspepsia	Heartburn	Mild	Moderate	Severe	—	—
Hemorrhoids	Hemorrhoids	Asymptomatic	Symptomatic; banding or medical intervention indicated	Interfering with ADL; interventional radiology, endoscopic, or operative intervention indicated	Life-threatening consequences	Death

GASTROINTESTINAL

Adverse Event	Short Name	Grade				
		1	2	3	4	5
Ileus, GI (functional obstruction of bowel, i.e., neuroconstipation)	Ileus	Asymptomatic, radiographic findings only	Symptomatic; altered GI function (e.g., altered dietary habits); IV fluids indicated <24 hrs	Symptomatic and severely altered GI function; IV fluids, tube feeding, or TPN indicated ≥24 hrs	Life-threatening consequences	Death

REMARK: Ileus, GI is to be used for altered upper or lower GI function (e.g., delayed gastric or colonic emptying).

ALSO CONSIDER: Constipation; Nausea; Obstruction, GI – *Select*; Vomiting.

| Incontinence, anal | Incontinence, anal | Occasional use of pads required | Daily use of pads required | Interfering with ADL; operative intervention indicated | Permanent bowel diversion indicated | Death |

REMARK: Incontinence, anal is to be used for loss of sphincter control as sequelae of operative or therapeutic intervention.

| Leak (including anastomotic), GI – *Select*:
 – Biliary tree
 – Esophagus
 – Large bowel
 – Leak NOS
 – Pancreas
 – Pharynx
 – Rectum
 – Small bowel
 – Stoma
 – Stomach | Leak, GI – *Select* | Asymptomatic radiographic findings only | Symptomatic; medical intervention indicated | Symptomatic and interfering with GI function; invasive or endoscopic intervention indicated | Life-threatening consequences | Death |

REMARK: Leak (including anastomotic), GI – *Select* is to be used for clinical signs/symptoms or radiographic confirmation of anastomotic or conduit leak (e.g., biliary, esophageal, intestinal, pancreatic, pharyngeal, rectal), but without development of fistula.

| Malabsorption | Malabsorption | — | Altered diet; oral therapies indicated (e.g., enzymes, medications, dietary supplements) | Inability to aliment adequately via GI tract (i.e., TPN indicated) | Life-threatening consequences | Death |

GASTROINTESTINAL

Adverse Event	Short Name	Grade				
		1	2	3	4	5
Mucositis/stomatitis (clinical exam) – *Select*: – Anus – Esophagus – Large bowel – Larynx – Oral cavity – Pharynx – Rectum – Small bowel – Stomach – Trachea	Mucositis/stomatitis (clinical exam) – *Select*	Erythema of the mucosa	Patchy ulcerations or pseudomembranes	Confluent ulcerations or pseudomembranes; bleeding with minor trauma	Tissue necrosis; significant spontaneous bleeding; life-threatening consequences	Death

REMARK: Mucositis/stomatitis (functional/symptomatic) may be used for mucositis of the upper aero-digestive tract caused by radiation, agents, or GVHD.

Adverse Event	Short Name	1	2	3	4	5
Mucositis/stomatitis (functional/symptomatic) – *Select*: – Anus – Esophagus – Large bowel – Larynx – Oral cavity – Pharynx – Rectum – Small bowel – Stomach – Trachea	Mucositis/stomatitis (functional/symptomatic) – *Select*	<u>Upper aerodigestive tract sites:</u> Minimal symptoms, normal diet; minimal respiratory symptoms but not interfering with function <u>Lower GI sites:</u> Minimal discomfort, intervention not indicated	<u>Upper aerodigestive tract sites:</u> Symptomatic but can eat and swallow modified diet; respiratory symptoms interfering with function but not interfering with ADL <u>Lower GI sites:</u> Symptomatic, medical intervention indicated but not interfering with ADL	<u>Upper aerodigestive tract sites:</u> Symptomatic and unable to adequately aliment or hydrate orally; respiratory symptoms interfering with ADL <u>Lower GI sites:</u> Stool incontinence or other symptoms interfering with ADL	Symptoms associated with life-threatening consequences	Death
Nausea	Nausea	Loss of appetite without alteration in eating habits	Oral intake decreased without significant weight loss, dehydration or malnutrition; IV fluids indicated <24 hrs	Inadequate oral caloric or fluid intake; IV fluids, tube feedings, or TPN indicated ≥24 hrs	Life-threatening consequences	Death

ALSO CONSIDER: Anorexia; Vomiting.

GASTROINTESTINAL

Adverse Event	Short Name	Grade				
		1	2	3	4	5
Necrosis, GI – Select: – Anus – Colon/cecum/appendix – Duodenum – Esophagus – Gallbladder – Hepatic – Ileum – Jejunum – Oral – Pancreas – Peritoneal cavity – Pharynx – Rectum – Small bowel NOS – Stoma – Stomach	Necrosis, GI – Select	—	—	Inability to aliment adequately by GI tract (e.g., requiring enteral or parenteral nutrition); interventional radiology, endoscopic, or operative intervention indicated	Life-threatening consequences; operative intervention requiring complete organ resection (e.g., total colectomy)	Death

ALSO CONSIDER: Visceral arterial ischemia (non-myocardial).

Adverse Event	Short Name	1	2	3	4	5
Obstruction, GI – Select: – Cecum – Colon – Duodenum – Esophagus – Gallbladder – Ileum – Jejunum – Rectum – Small bowel NOS – Stoma – Stomach	Obstruction, GI – Select	Asymptomatic radiographic findings only	Symptomatic; altered GI function (e.g., altered dietary habits, vomiting, diarrhea, or GI fluid loss); IV fluids indicated <24 hrs	Symptomatic and severely altered GI function (e.g., altered dietary habits, vomiting, diarrhea, or GI fluid loss); IV fluids, tube feedings, or TPN indicated ≥24 hrs; operative intervention indicated	Life-threatening consequences; operative intervention requiring complete organ resection (e.g., total colectomy)	Death

NAVIGATION NOTE: Operative injury is graded as Intra-operative injury – *Select Organ or Structure* in the SURGERY/INTRA-OPERATIVE INJURY CATEGORY.

NAVIGATION NOTE: Pelvic pain is graded as Pain – *Select* in the PAIN CATEGORY.

GASTROINTESTINAL

Adverse Event	Short Name	Grade				
		1	2	3	4	5
Perforation, GI – Select: – Appendix – Biliary tree – Cecum – Colon – Duodenum – Esophagus – Gallbladder – Ileum – Jejunum – Rectum – Small bowel NOS – Stomach	Perforation, GI – Select	Asymptomatic radiographic findings only	Medical intervention indicated; IV fluids indicated <24 hrs	IV fluids, tube feedings, or TPN indicated ≥24 hrs; operative intervention indicated	Life-threatening consequences	Death
Proctitis	Proctitis	Rectal discomfort, intervention not indicated	Symptoms not interfering with ADL; medical intervention indicated	Stool incontinence or other symptoms interfering with ADL; operative intervention indicated	Life-threatening consequences (e.g., perforation)	Death
Prolapse of stoma, GI	Prolapse of stoma, GI	Asymptomatic	Extraordinary local care or maintenance; minor revision indicated	Dysfunctional stoma; major revision indicated	Life-threatening consequences	Death

REMARK: Other stoma complications may be graded as Fistula, GI – *Select*; Leak (including anastomotic), GI – *Select*; Obstruction, GI – *Select*; Perforation, GI – *Select*; Stricture/stenosis (including anastomotic), GI – *Select*.

NAVIGATION NOTE: Rectal or perirectal pain (proctalgia) is graded as Pain – *Select* in the PAIN CATEGORY.

Adverse Event	Short Name	Grade				
		1	2	3	4	5
Salivary gland changes/saliva	Salivary gland changes	Slightly thickened saliva; slightly altered taste (e.g., metallic)	Thick, ropy, sticky saliva; markedly altered taste; alteration in diet indicated; secretion-induced symptoms not interfering with ADL	Acute salivary gland necrosis; severe secretion-induced symptoms interfering with ADL	Disabling	—

ALSO CONSIDER: Dry mouth/salivary gland (xerostomia); Mucositis/stomatitis (clinical exam) – *Select*; Mucositis/stomatitis (functional/symptomatic) – *Select*; Taste alteration (dysgeusia).

NAVIGATION NOTE: Splenic function is graded in the BLOOD/BONE MARROW CATEGORY.

GASTROINTESTINAL

Adverse Event	Short Name	Grade				
		1	2	3	4	5
Stricture/stenosis (including anastomotic), GI – Select: – Anus – Biliary tree – Cecum – Colon – Duodenum – Esophagus – Ileum – Jejunum – Pancreas/pancreatic duct – Pharynx – Rectum – Small bowel NOS – Stoma – Stomach	Stricture, GI – Select	Asymptomatic radiographic findings only	Symptomatic; altered GI function (e.g., altered dietary habits, vomiting, bleeding, diarrhea); IV fluids indicated <24 hrs	Symptomatic and severely altered GI function (e.g., altered dietary habits, diarrhea, or GI fluid loss); IV fluids, tube feedings, or TPN indicated ≥24 hrs; operative intervention indicated	Life-threatening consequences; operative intervention requiring complete organ resection (e.g., total colectomy)	Death
Taste alteration (dysgeusia)	Taste alteration	Altered taste but no change in diet	Altered taste with change in diet (e.g., oral supplements); noxious or unpleasant taste; loss of taste	—	—	—
Typhlitis (cecal inflammation)	Typhlitis	Asymptomatic, pathologic or radiographic findings only	Abdominal pain; mucus or blood in stool	Abdominal pain, fever, change in bowel habits with ileus; peritoneal signs	Life-threatening consequences (e.g., perforation, bleeding, ischemia, necrosis); operative intervention indicated	Death

ALSO CONSIDER: Colitis; Hemorrhage, GI – Select; Ileus, GI (functional obstruction of bowel, i.e., neuroconstipation).

GASTROINTESTINAL

Adverse Event	Short Name	Grade				
		1	2	3	4	5
Ulcer, GI – Select: – Anus – Cecum – Colon – Duodenum – Esophagus – Ileum – Jejunum – Rectum – Small bowel NOS – Stoma – Stomach	Ulcer, GI – Select	Asymptomatic, radiographic or endoscopic findings only	Symptomatic; altered GI function (e.g., altered dietary habits, oral supplements); IV fluids indicated <24 hrs	Symptomatic and severely altered GI function (e.g., inadequate oral caloric or fluid intake); IV fluids, tube feedings, or TPN indicated ≥24 hrs	Life-threatening consequences	Death
ALSO CONSIDER: Hemorrhage, GI – Select.						
Vomiting	Vomiting	1 episode in 24 hrs	2 – 5 episodes in 24 hrs; IV fluids indicated <24 hrs	≥6 episodes in 24 hrs; IV fluids, or TPN indicated ≥24 hrs	Life-threatening consequences	Death
ALSO CONSIDER: Dehydration.						
Gastrointestinal – Other (Specify, __)	GI – Other (Specify)	Mild	Moderate	Severe	Life-threatening; disabling	Death

GROWTH AND DEVELOPMENT

Adverse Event	Short Name	Grade				
		1	2	3	4	5
Bone age (alteration in bone age)	Bone age	—	±2 SD (standard deviation) from normal	—	—	—
Bone growth: femoral head; slipped capital femoral epiphysis	Femoral head growth	Mild valgus/varus deformity	Moderate valgus/varus deformity, symptomatic, interfering with function but not interfering with ADL	Mild slipped capital femoral epiphysis; operative intervention (e.g., fixation) indicated; interfering with ADL	Disabling; severe slipped capital femoral epiphysis >60%; avascular necrosis	—
Bone growth: limb length discrepancy	Limb length	Mild length discrepancy <2 cm	Moderate length discrepancy 2 – 5 cm; shoe lift indicated	Severe length discrepancy >5 cm; operative intervention indicated; interfering with ADL	Disabling; epiphysiodesis	—
Bone growth: spine kyphosis/lordosis	Kyphosis/lordosis	Mild radiographic changes	Moderate accentuation; interfering with function but not interfering with ADL	Severe accentuation; operative intervention indicated; interfering with ADL	Disabling (e.g., cannot lift head)	—
Growth velocity (reduction in growth velocity)	Reduction in growth velocity	10 – 29% reduction in growth from the baseline growth curve	30 – 49% reduction in growth from the baseline growth curve	≥50% reduction in growth from the baseline growth curve	—	—
Puberty (delayed)	Delayed puberty	—	No breast development by age 13 yrs for females; no Tanner Stage 2 development by age 14.5 yrs for males	No sexual development by age 14 yrs for girls, age 16 yrs for boys; hormone replacement indicated	—	—

REMARK: Do not use testicular size for Tanner Stage in male cancer survivors.

Adverse Event	Short Name	Grade				
Puberty (precocious)	Precocious puberty	—	Physical signs of puberty <7 years for females, <9 years for males	—	—	—
Short stature	Short stature	Beyond two standard deviations of age and gender mean height	Altered ADL	—	—	—

REMARK: Short stature is secondary to growth hormone deficiency.

ALSO CONSIDER: Neuroendocrine: growth hormone secretion abnormality.

Adverse Event	Short Name	Grade				
Growth and Development – Other (Specify, __)	Growth and Development – Other (Specify)	Mild	Moderate	Severe	Life-threatening; disabling	Death

HEMORRHAGE/BLEEDING

Adverse Event	Short Name	Grade				
		1	2	3	4	5
Hematoma	Hematoma	Minimal symptoms, invasive intervention not indicated	Minimally invasive evacuation or aspiration indicated	Transfusion, interventional radiology, or operative intervention indicated	Life-threatening consequences; major urgent intervention indicated	Death

Remark: Hematoma refers to extravasation at wound or operative site or secondary to other intervention. Transfusion implies pRBC.

Also Consider: Fibrinogen; INR (International Normalized Ratio of prothrombin time); Platelets; PTT (Partial Thromboplastin Time).

Adverse Event	Short Name	1	2	3	4	5
Hemorrhage/bleeding associated with surgery, intra-operative or postoperative	Hemorrhage with surgery	—	—	Requiring transfusion of 2 units non-autologous (10 cc/kg for pediatrics) pRBCs beyond protocol specification; postoperative interventional radiology, endoscopic, or operative intervention indicated	Life-threatening consequences	Death

Remark: Postoperative period is defined as ≤72 hours after surgery. Verify protocol-specific acceptable guidelines regarding pRBC transfusion.

Also Consider: Fibrinogen; INR (International Normalized Ratio of prothrombin time); Platelets; PTT (Partial Thromboplastin Time).

Adverse Event	Short Name	1	2	3	4	5
Hemorrhage, CNS	CNS hemorrhage	Asymptomatic, radiographic findings only	Medical intervention indicated	Ventriculostomy, ICP monitoring, intraventricular thrombolysis, or operative intervention indicated	Life-threatening consequences; neurologic deficit or disability	Death

Also Consider: Fibrinogen; INR (International Normalized Ratio of prothrombin time); Platelets; PTT (Partial Thromboplastin Time).

HEMORRHAGE/BLEEDING

Adverse Event	Short Name	Grade				
		1	2	3	4	5
Hemorrhage, GI – Select: – Abdomen NOS – Anus – Biliary tree – Cecum/appendix – Colon – Duodenum – Esophagus – Ileum – Jejunum – Liver – Lower GI NOS – Oral cavity – Pancreas – Peritoneal cavity – Rectum – Stoma – Stomach – Upper GI NOS – Varices (esophageal) – Varices (rectal)		Mild, intervention (other than iron supplements) not indicated	Symptomatic and medical intervention or minor cauterization indicated	Transfusion, interventional radiology, endoscopic, or operative intervention indicated; radiation therapy (i.e., hemostasis of bleeding site)	Life-threatening consequences; major urgent intervention indicated	Death

REMARK: Transfusion implies pRBC.

ALSO CONSIDER: Fibrinogen; INR (International Normalized Ratio of prothrombin time); Platelets; PTT (Partial Thromboplastin Time).

Adverse Event	Short Name	Grade				
		1	2	3	4	5
Hemorrhage, GU – *Select*: – Bladder – Fallopian tube – Kidney – Ovary – Prostate – Retroperitoneum – Spermatic cord – Stoma – Testes – Ureter – Urethra – Urinary NOS – Uterus – Vagina – Vas deferens	Hemorrhage, GU	Minimal or microscopic bleeding; intervention not indicated	Gross bleeding, medical intervention, or urinary tract irrigation indicated	Transfusion, interventional radiology, endoscopic, or operative intervention indicated; radiation therapy (i.e., hemostasis of bleeding site)	Life-threatening consequences; major urgent intervention indicated	Death

REMARK: Transfusion implies pRBC.

ALSO CONSIDER: Fibrinogen; INR (International Normalized Ratio of prothrombin time); Platelets; PTT (Partial Thromboplastin Time).

| Hemorrhage, pulmonary/ upper respiratory – *Select*:
– Bronchopulmonary NOS
– Bronchus
– Larynx
– Lung
– Mediastinum
– Nose
– Pharynx
– Pleura
– Respiratory tract NOS
– Stoma
– Trachea | Hemorrhage pulmonary – *Select* | Mild, intervention not indicated | Symptomatic and medical intervention indicated | Transfusion, interventional radiology, endoscopic, or operative intervention indicated; radiation therapy (i.e., hemostasis of bleeding site) | Life-threatening consequences; major urgent intervention indicated | Death |

REMARK: Transfusion implies pRBC.

ALSO CONSIDER: Fibrinogen; INR (International Normalized Ratio of prothrombin time); Platelets; PTT (Partial Thromboplastin Time).

| Petechiae/purpura (hemorrhage/bleeding into skin or mucosa) | Petechiae | Few petechiae | Moderate petechiae; purpura | Generalized petechiae or purpura | — | — |

ALSO CONSIDER: Fibrinogen; INR (International Normalized Ratio of prothrombin time); Platelets; PTT (Partial Thromboplastin Time).

HEMORRHAGE/BLEEDING

Adverse Event	Short Name	Grade				
		1	2	3	4	5
NAVIGATION NOTE: Vitreous hemorrhage is graded in the OCULAR/VISUAL CATEGORY.						
Hemorrhage/Bleeding – Other (Specify, __)	Hemorrhage – Other (Specify)	Mild without transfusion	—	Transfusion indicated	Catastrophic bleeding, requiring major non-elective intervention	Death

HEPATOBILIARY/PANCREAS

Adverse Event	Short Name	Grade				
		1	2	3	4	5
NAVIGATION NOTE: Biliary tree damage is graded as Fistula, GI – Select; Leak (including anastomotic), GI – Select; Necrosis, GI – Select; Obstruction, GI – Select; Perforation, GI – Select; Stricture/stenosis (including anastomotic), GI – Select in the GASTROINTESTINAL CATEGORY.						
Cholecystitis	Cholecystitis	Asymptomatic, radiographic findings only	Symptomatic, medical intervention indicated	Interventional radiology, endoscopic, or operative intervention indicated	Life-threatening consequences (e.g., sepsis or perforation)	Death
ALSO CONSIDER: Infection (documented clinically or microbiologically) with Grade 3 or 4 neutrophils – Select; Infection with normal ANC or Grade 1 or 2 neutrophils – Select; Infection with unknown ANC – Select.						
Liver dysfunction/failure (clinical)	Liver dysfunction	—	Jaundice	Asterixis	Encephalopathy or coma	Death
REMARK: Jaundice is not an AE, but occurs when the liver is not working properly or when a bile duct is blocked. It is graded as a result of liver dysfunction/failure or elevated bilirubin.						
ALSO CONSIDER: Bilirubin (hyperbilirubinemia).						
Pancreas, exocrine enzyme deficiency	Pancreas, exocrine enzyme deficiency	—	Increase in stool frequency, bulk, or odor; steatorrhea	Sequelae of absorption deficiency (e.g., weight loss)	Life-threatening consequences	Death
ALSO CONSIDER: Diarrhea.						
Pancreatitis	Pancreatitis	Asymptomatic, enzyme elevation and/or radiographic findings	Symptomatic, medical intervention indicated	Interventional radiology or operative intervention indicated	Life-threatening consequences (e.g., circulatory failure, hemorrhage, sepsis)	Death
ALSO CONSIDER: Amylase.						
NAVIGATION NOTE: Stricture (biliary tree, hepatic or pancreatic) is graded as Stricture/stenosis (including anastomotic), GI – Select in the GASTROINTESTINAL CATEGORY.						
Hepatobiliary/Pancreas – Other (Specify, ___)	Hepatobiliary – Other (Specify)	Mild	Moderate	Severe	Life-threatening; disabling	Death

Adverse Event	Short Name	Grade				
		1	2	3	4	5
Colitis, infectious (e.g., Clostridium difficile)	Colitis, infectious	Asymptomatic, pathologic or radiographic findings only	Abdominal pain with mucus and/or blood in stool	IV antibiotics or TPN indicated	Life-threatening consequences (e.g., perforation, bleeding, ischemia, necrosis or toxic megacolon); operative resection or diversion indicated	Death
ALSO CONSIDER: Hemorrhage, GI – *Select*; Typhlitis (cecal inflammation).						
Febrile neutropenia (fever of unknown origin without clinically or microbiologically documented infection) (ANC <1.0 x 10⁹/L, fever ≥38.5°C)	Febrile neutropenia	—	—	Present	Life-threatening consequences (e.g., septic shock, hypotension, acidosis, necrosis)	Death
ALSO CONSIDER: Neutrophils/granulocytes (ANC/AGC).						
Infection (documented clinically or microbiologically) with Grade 3 or 4 neutrophils (ANC <1.0 x 10⁹/L) – *Select* 'Select' AEs appear at the end of the CATEGORY.	Infection (documented clinically or microbiologically) with Grade 3 or 4 ANC – *Select*	—	Localized, local intervention indicated	IV antibiotic, antifungal, or antiviral intervention indicated; interventional radiology or operative intervention indicated	Life-threatening consequences (e.g., septic shock, hypotension, acidosis, necrosis)	Death
REMARK: Fever with Grade 3 or 4 neutrophils in the absence of documented infection is graded as Febrile neutropenia (fever of unknown origin without clinically or microbiologically documented infection).						
ALSO CONSIDER: Neutrophils/granulocytes (ANC/AGC).						
Infection with normal ANC or Grade 1 or 2 neutrophils – *Select* 'Select' AEs appear at the end of the CATEGORY.	Infection with normal ANC – *Select*	—	Localized, local intervention indicated	IV antibiotic, antifungal, or antiviral intervention indicated; interventional radiology or operative intervention indicated	Life-threatening consequences (e.g., septic shock, hypotension, acidosis, necrosis)	Death

Adverse Event	Short Name	Grade				
		1	2	3	4	5
Infection with unknown ANC – Select 'Select' AEs appear at the end of the CATEGORY.	Infection with unknown ANC – Select	—	Localized, local intervention indicated	IV antibiotic, antifungal, or antiviral intervention indicated; interventional radiology or operative intervention indicated	Life-threatening consequences (e.g., septic shock, hypotension, acidosis, necrosis)	Death
REMARK: Infection with unknown ANC – Select is to be used in the rare case when ANC is unknown.						
Opportunistic infection associated with ≥Grade 2 Lymphopenia ALSO CONSIDER: Lymphopenia.	Opportunistic infection	—	Localized, local intervention indicated	IV antibiotic, antifungal, or antiviral intervention indicated; interventional radiology or operative intervention indicated	Life-threatening consequences (e.g., septic shock, hypotension, acidosis, necrosis)	Death
Viral hepatitis	Viral hepatitis	Present; transaminases and liver function normal	Transaminases abnormal, liver function normal	Symptomatic liver dysfunction; fibrosis by biopsy; compensated cirrhosis	Decompensated liver function (e.g., ascites, coagulopathy, encephalopathy, coma)	Death
REMARK: Non-viral hepatitis is graded as Infection – Select. ALSO CONSIDER: Albumin, serum-low (hypoalbuminemia); ALT, SGPT (serum glutamic pyruvic transaminase); AST, SGOT (serum glutamic oxaloacetic transaminase); Bilirubin (hyperbilirubinemia); Encephalopathy.						
Infection – Other (Specify, __)	Infection – Other (Specify)	Mild	Moderate	Severe	Life-threatening; disabling	Death

INFECTION – SELECT

AUDITORY/EAR
– External ear (otitis externa)
– Middle ear (otitis media)

CARDIOVASCULAR
– Artery
– Heart (endocarditis)
– Spleen
– Vein

DERMATOLOGY/SKIN
– Lip/perioral
– Peristomal
– Skin (cellulitis)
– Ungual (nails)

GASTROINTESTINAL
– Abdomen NOS
– Anal/perianal
– Appendix
– Cecum
– Colon
– Dental-tooth
– Duodenum
– Esophagus
– Ileum
– Jejunum
– Oral cavity-gums (gingivitis)
– Peritoneal cavity
– Rectum
– Salivary gland
– Small bowel NOS
– Stomach

GENERAL
– Blood
– Catheter-related
– Foreign body (e.g., graft, implant, prosthesis, stent)
– Wound

HEPATOBILIARY/PANCREAS
– Biliary tree
– Gallbladder (cholecystitis)
– Liver
– Pancreas

LYMPHATIC
– Lymphatic

MUSCULOSKELETAL
– Bone (osteomyelitis)
– Joint
– Muscle (infection myositis)
– Soft tissue NOS

NEUROLOGY
– Brain (encephalitis, infectious)
– Brain + Spinal cord (encephalomyelitis)
– Meninges (meningitis)
– Nerve-cranial
– Nerve-peripheral
– Spinal cord (myelitis)

OCULAR
– Conjunctiva
– Cornea
– Eye NOS
– Lens

PULMONARY/UPPER RESPIRATORY
– Bronchus
– Larynx
– Lung (pneumonia)
– Mediastinum NOS
– Mucosa
– Neck NOS
– Nose
– Paranasal
– Pharynx
– Pleura (empyema)
– Sinus
– Trachea
– Upper aerodigestive NOS
– Upper airway NOS

RENAL/GENITOURINARY
– Bladder (urinary)
– Kidney
– Prostate
– Ureter
– Urethra
– Urinary tract NOS

SEXUAL/REPRODUCTIVE FUNCTION
– Cervix
– Fallopian tube
– Pelvis NOS
– Penis
– Scrotum
– Uterus
– Vagina
– Vulva

Adverse Event	Short Name	Grade				
		1	2	3	4	5
Chyle or lymph leakage	Chyle or lymph leakage	Asymptomatic, clinical or radiographic findings	Symptomatic, medical intervention indicated	Interventional radiology or operative intervention indicated	Life-threatening complications	Death
ALSO CONSIDER: Chylothorax.						
Dermal change lymphedema, phlebolymphedema	Dermal change	Trace thickening or faint discoloration	Marked discoloration; leathery skin texture; papillary formation	—	—	—
REMARK: Dermal change lymphedema, phlebolymphedema refers to changes due to venous stasis.						
ALSO CONSIDER: Ulceration.						
Edema: head and neck	Edema: head and neck	Localized to dependent areas, no disability or functional impairment	Localized facial or neck edema with functional impairment	Generalized facial or neck edema with functional impairment (e.g., difficulty in turning neck or opening mouth compared to baseline)	Severe with ulceration or cerebral edema; tracheotomy or feeding tube indicated	Death
Edema: limb	Edema: limb	5 – 10% inter-limb discrepancy in volume or circumference at point of greatest visible difference; swelling or obscuration of anatomic architecture on close inspection; pitting edema	>10 – 30% inter-limb discrepancy in volume or circumference at point of greatest visible difference; readily apparent obscuration of anatomic architecture; obliteration of skin folds; readily apparent deviation from normal anatomic contour	>30% inter-limb discrepancy in volume; lymphorrhea; gross deviation from normal anatomic contour; interfering with ADL	Progression to malignancy (i.e., lymphangiosarcoma); amputation indicated; disabling	Death
Edema: trunk/genital	Edema: trunk/genital	Swelling or obscuration of anatomic architecture on close inspection; pitting edema	Readily apparent obscuration of anatomic architecture; obliteration of skin folds; readily apparent deviation from normal anatomic contour	Lymphorrhea; interfering with ADL; gross deviation from normal anatomic contour	Progression to malignancy (i.e., lymphangiosarcoma); disabling	Death
Edema: viscera	Edema: viscera	Asymptomatic; clinical or radiographic findings only	Symptomatic; medical intervention indicated	Symptomatic and unable to aliment adequately orally; interventional radiology or operative intervention indicated	Life-threatening consequences	Death

LYMPHATICS

Adverse Event	Short Name	Grade				
		1	2	3	4	5
Lymphedema-related fibrosis	Lymphedema-related fibrosis	Minimal to moderate redundant soft tissue, unresponsive to elevation or compression, with moderately firm texture or spongy feel	Marked increase in density and firmness, with or without tethering	Very marked density and firmness with tethering affecting ≥40% of the edematous area	—	—
Lymphocele	Lymphocele	Asymptomatic, clinical or radiographic findings only	Symptomatic; medical intervention indicated	Symptomatic and interventional radiology or operative intervention indicated	—	—
Phlebolymphatic cording	Phlebolymphatic cording	Asymptomatic, clinical findings only	Symptomatic; medical intervention indicated	Symptomatic and leading to contracture or reduced range of motion	—	—
Lymphatics – Other (Specify, __)	Lymphatics – Other (Specify)	Mild	Moderate	Severe	Life-threatening; disabling	Death

METABOLIC/LABORATORY

Adverse Event	Short Name	Grade				
		1	2	3	4	5
Acidosis (metabolic or respiratory)	Acidosis	pH <normal, but ≥7.3	—	pH <7.3	pH <7.3 with life-threatening consequences	Death
Albumin, serum-low (hypoalbuminemia)	Hypoalbuminemia	<LLN – 3 g/dL <LLN – 30 g/L	<3 – 2 g/dL <30 – 20 g/L	<2 g/dL <20 g/L	—	Death
Alkaline phosphatase	Alkaline phosphatase	>ULN – 2.5 x ULN	>2.5 – 5.0 x ULN	>5.0 – 20.0 x ULN	>20.0 x ULN	—
Alkalosis (metabolic or respiratory)	Alkalosis	pH >normal, but ≤7.5	—	pH >7.5	pH >7.5 with life-threatening consequences	Death
ALT, SGPT (serum glutamic pyruvic transaminase)	ALT	>ULN – 2.5 x ULN	>2.5 – 5.0 x ULN	>5.0 – 20.0 x ULN	>20.0 x ULN	—
Amylase	Amylase	>ULN – 1.5 x ULN	>1.5 – 2.0 x ULN	>2.0 – 5.0 x ULN	>5.0 x ULN	—
AST, SGOT (serum glutamic oxaloacetic transaminase)	AST	>ULN – 2.5 x ULN	>2.5 – 5.0 x ULN	>5.0 – 20.0 x ULN	>20.0 x ULN	—
Bicarbonate, serum-low	Bicarbonate, serum-low	<LLN – 16 mmol/L	<16 – 11 mmol/L	<11 – 8 mmol/L	<8 mmol/L	Death
Bilirubin (hyperbilirubinemia)	Bilirubin	>ULN – 1.5 x ULN	>1.5 – 3.0 x ULN	>3.0 – 10.0 x ULN	>10.0 x ULN	—

REMARK: Jaundice is not an AE, but may be a manifestation of liver dysfunction/failure or elevated bilirubin. If jaundice is associated with elevated bilirubin, grade bilirubin.

| Calcium, serum-low (hypocalcemia) | Hypocalcemia | <LLN – 8.0 mg/dL <LLN – 2.0 mmol/L | <8.0 – 7.0 mg/dL <2.0 – 1.75 mmol/L | <7.0 – 6.0 mg/dL <1.75 – 1.5 mmol/L | <6.0 mg/dL <1.5 mmol/L | Death |
| | | Ionized calcium: <LLN – 1.0 mmol/L | Ionized calcium: <1.0 – 0.9 mmol/L | Ionized calcium: <0.9 – 0.8 mmol/L | Ionized calcium: <0.8 mmol/L | |

REMARK: Calcium can be falsely low if hypoalbuminemia is present. Serum albumin is <4.0 g/dL, hypocalcemia is reported after the following corrective calculation has been performed: Corrected Calcium (mg/dL) = Total Calcium (mg/dL) – 0.8 [Albumin (g/dL) – 4].[4] . Alternatively, direct measurement of ionized calcium is the definitive method to diagnose metabolically relevant alterations in serum calcium.

METABOLIC/LABORATORY

Adverse Event	Short Name	Grade 1	2	3	4	5
Calcium, serum-high (hypercalcemia)	Hypercalcemia	>ULN – 11.5 mg/dL >ULN – 2.9 mmol/L Ionized calcium: >ULN – 1.5 mmol/L	>11.5 – 12.5 mg/dL >2.9 – 3.1 mmol/L Ionized calcium: >1.5 – 1.6 mmol/L	>12.5 – 13.5 mg/dL >3.1 – 3.4 mmol/L Ionized calcium: >1.6 – 1.8 mmol/L	>13.5 mg/dL >3.4 mmol/L Ionized calcium: >1.8 mmol/L	Death
Cholesterol, serum-high (hypercholesteremia)	Cholesterol	>ULN – 300 mg/dL >ULN – 7.75 mmol/L	>300 – 400 mg/dL >7.75 – 10.34 mmol/L	>400 – 500 mg/dL >10.34 – 12.92 mmol/L	>500 mg/dL >12.92 mmol/L	Death
CPK (creatine phosphokinase)	CPK	>ULN – 2.5 x ULN	>2.5 x ULN – 5 x ULN	>5 x ULN – 10 x ULN	>10 x ULN	Death
Creatinine	Creatinine	>ULN – 1.5 x ULN	>1.5 – 3.0 x ULN	>3.0 – 6.0 x ULN	>6.0 x ULN	Death

REMARK: Adjust to age-appropriate levels for pediatric patients.

ALSO CONSIDER: Glomerular filtration rate.

Adverse Event	Short Name	Grade 1	2	3	4	5
GGT (γ-Glutamyl transpeptidase)	GGT	>ULN – 2.5 x ULN	>2.5 – 5.0 x ULN	>5.0 – 20.0 x ULN	>20.0 x ULN	—
Glomerular filtration rate	GFR	<75 – 50% LLN	<50 – 25% LLN	<25% LLN, chronic dialysis not indicated	Chronic dialysis or renal transplant indicated	Death

ALSO CONSIDER: Creatinine.

Adverse Event	Short Name	Grade 1	2	3	4	5
Glucose, serum-high (hyperglycemia)	Hyperglycemia	>ULN – 160 mg/dL >ULN – 8.9 mmol/L	>160 – 250 mg/dL >8.9 – 13.9 mmol/L	>250 – 500 mg/dL >13.9 – 27.8 mmol/L	>500 mg/dL >27.8 mmol/L or acidosis	Death

REMARK: Hyperglycemia, in general, is defined as fasting unless otherwise specified in protocol.

Adverse Event	Short Name	Grade 1	2	3	4	5
Glucose, serum-low (hypoglycemia)	Hypoglycemia	<LLN – 55 mg/dL <LLN – 3.0 mmol/L	<55 – 40 mg/dL <3.0 – 2.2 mmol/L	<40 – 30 mg/dL <2.2 – 1.7 mmol/L	<30 mg/dL <1.7 mmol/L	Death
Hemoglobinuria	Hemoglobinuria	Present	—	—	—	Death
Lipase	Lipase	>ULN – 1.5 x ULN	>1.5 – 2.0 x ULN	>2.0 – 5.0 x ULN	>5.0 x ULN	—
Magnesium, serum-high (hypermagnesemia)	Hypermagnesemia	>ULN – 3.0 mg/dL >ULN – 1.23 mmol/L	—	>3.0 – 8.0 mg/dL >1.23 – 3.30 mmol/L	>8.0 mg/dL >3.30 mmol/L	Death
Magnesium, serum-low (hypomagnesemia)	Hypomagnesemia	<LLN – 1.2 mg/dL <LLN – 0.5 mmol/L	<1.2 – 0.9 mg/dL <0.5 – 0.4 mmol/L	<0.9 – 0.7 mg/dL <0.4 – 0.3 mmol/L	<0.7 mg/dL <0.3 mmol/L	Death
Phosphate, serum-low (hypophosphatemia)	Hypophosphatemia	<LLN – 2.5 mg/dL <LLN – 0.8 mmol/L	<2.5 – 2.0 mg/dL <0.8 – 0.6 mmol/L	<2.0 – 1.0 mg/dL <0.6 – 0.3 mmol/L	<1.0 mg/dL <0.3 mmol/L	Death
Potassium, serum-high (hyperkalemia)	Hyperkalemia	>ULN – 5.5 mmol/L	>5.5 – 6.0 mmol/L	>6.0 – 7.0 mmol/L	>7.0 mmol/L	Death

METABOLIC/LABORATORY

Adverse Event	Short Name	Grade				
		1	2	3	4	5
Potassium, serum-low (hypokalemia)	Hypokalemia	<LLN – 3.0 mmol/L	—	<3.0 – 2.5 mmol/L	<2.5 mmol/L	Death
Proteinuria	Proteinuria	1+ or 0.15 – 1.0 g/24 hrs	2+ to 3+ or >1.0 – 3.5 g/24 hrs	4+ or >3.5 g/24 hrs	Nephrotic syndrome	Death
Sodium, serum-high (hypernatremia)	Hypernatremia	>ULN – 150 mmol/L	>150 – 155 mmol/L	>155 – 160 mmol/L	>160 mmol/L	Death
Sodium, serum-low (hyponatremia)	Hyponatremia	<LLN – 130 mmol/L	—	<130 – 120 mmol/L	<120 mmol/L	Death
Triglyceride, serum-high (hypertriglyceridemia)	Hypertriglyceridemia	>ULN – 2.5 x ULN	>2.5 – 5.0 x ULN	>5.0 – 10 x ULN	>10 x ULN	Death
Uric acid, serum-high (hyperuricemia)	Hyperuricemia	>ULN – 10 mg/dL ≤0.59 mmol/L without physiologic consequences	—	>ULN – 10 mg/dL ≤0.59 mmol/L with physiologic consequences	>10 mg/dL >0.59 mmol/L	Death
ALSO CONSIDER: Creatinine; Potassium, serum-high (hyperkalemia); Renal failure; Tumor lysis syndrome.						
Metabolic/Laboratory – Other (Specify, ___)	Metabolic/Lab – Other (Specify)	Mild	Moderate	Severe	Life-threatening; disabling	Death

MUSCULOSKELETAL/SOFT TISSUE

Adverse Event	Short Name	Grade 1	Grade 2	Grade 3	Grade 4	Grade 5
Arthritis (non-septic)	Arthritis	Mild pain with inflammation, erythema, or joint swelling, but not interfering with function	Moderate pain with inflammation, erythema, or joint swelling interfering with function, but not interfering with ADL	Severe pain with inflammation, erythema, or joint swelling and interfering with ADL	Disabling	Death

REMARK: Report only when the diagnosis of arthritis (e.g., inflammation of a joint or a state characterized by inflammation of joints) is made. Arthralgia (sign or symptom of pain in a joint, especially non-inflammatory in character) is graded as Pain – *Select* in the PAIN CATEGORY.

Adverse Event	Short Name	Grade 1	Grade 2	Grade 3	Grade 4	Grade 5
Bone: spine–scoliosis	Scoliosis	≤20 degrees; clinically undetectable	>20 – 45 degrees; visible by forward flexion; interfering with function but not interfering with ADL	>45 degrees; scapular prominence in forward flexion; operative intervention indicated; interfering with ADL	Disabling (e.g., interfering with cardiopulmonary function)	Death
Cervical spine-range of motion	Cervical spine ROM	Mild restriction of rotation or flexion between 60 – 70 degrees	Rotation <60 degrees to right or left; <60 degrees of flexion	Ankylosed/fused over multiple segments with no C-spine rotation	—	—

REMARK: 60 – 65 degrees of rotation is required for reversing a car; 60 – 65 degrees of flexion is required to tie shoes.

Adverse Event	Short Name	Grade 1	Grade 2	Grade 3	Grade 4	Grade 5
Exostosis	Exostosis	Asymptomatic	Involving multiple sites; pain or interfering with function	Excision indicated	Progression to malignancy (i.e., chondrosarcoma)	Death
Extremity-lower (gait/walking)	Gait/walking	Limp evident only to trained observer and able to walk ≥1 kilometer; cane indicated for walking	Noticeable limp, or limitation of limb function, but able to walk ≥0.1 kilometer (1 city block); quad cane indicated for walking	Severe limp with stride modified to maintain balance (widened base of support, marked reduction in step length); ambulation limited to walker, crutches indicated	Unable to walk	—

ALSO CONSIDER: Ataxia (incoordination); Muscle weakness, generalized or specific area (not due to neuropathy) – *Select*.

Adverse Event	Short Name	Grade 1	Grade 2	Grade 3	Grade 4	Grade 5
Extremity-upper (function)	Extremity-upper (function)	Able to perform most household or work activities with affected limb	Able to perform most household or work activities with compensation from unaffected limb	Interfering with ADL	Disabling; no function of affected limb	—
Fibrosis-cosmesis	Fibrosis-cosmesis	Visible only on close examination	Readily apparent but not disfiguring	Significant disfigurement; operative intervention indicated if patient chooses	—	—

MUSCULOSKELETAL/SOFT TISSUE

Adverse Event	Short Name	Grade				
		1	2	3	4	5
Fibrosis-deep connective tissue	Fibrosis-deep connective tissue	Increased density, "spongy" feel	Increased density with firmness or tethering	Increased density with fixation of tissue; operative intervention indicated; interfering with ADL	Life-threatening; disabling; loss of limb; interfering with vital organ function	Death

ALSO CONSIDER: Induration/fibrosis (skin and subcutaneous tissue); Muscle weakness, generalized or specific area (not due to neuropathy) – *Select*; Neuropathy: motor; Neuropathy: sensory.

Fracture	Fracture	Asymptomatic, radiographic findings only (e.g., asymptomatic rib fracture on plain x-ray, pelvic insufficiency fracture on MRI, etc.)	Symptomatic but non-displaced; immobilization indicated	Symptomatic and displaced or open wound with bone exposure; operative intervention indicated	Disabling; amputation indicated	Death
Joint-effusion	Joint-effusion	Asymptomatic, clinical or radiographic findings only	Symptomatic; interfering with function but not interfering with ADL	Symptomatic and interfering with ADL	Disabling	Death

ALSO CONSIDER: Arthritis (non-septic).

Joint-function[5]	Joint-function	Stiffness interfering with athletic activity; ≤25% loss of range of motion (ROM)	Stiffness interfering with function but not interfering with ADL; >25 – 50% decrease in ROM	Stiffness interfering with ADL; >50 – 75% decrease in ROM	Fixed or non-functional joint (arthrodesis); >75% decrease in ROM	—

ALSO CONSIDER: Arthritis (non-septic).

Local complication – device/prosthesis-related	Device/prosthesis	Asymptomatic	Symptomatic, but not interfering with ADL; local wound care; medical intervention indicated	Symptomatic, interfering with ADL; operative intervention indicated (e.g., hardware/device replacement or removal, reconstruction)	Life-threatening; disabling; loss of limb or organ	Death
Lumbar spine-range of motion	Lumbar spine ROM	Stiffness and difficulty bending to the floor to pick up a very light object but able to do activity	Some lumbar spine flexion but requires a reaching aid to pick up a very light object from the floor	Ankylosed/fused over multiple segments with no L-spine flexion (i.e., unable to reach to floor to pick up a very light	—	—

[5] Adapted from the *International SFTR Method of Measuring and Recording Joint Motion, International Standard Orthopedic Measurements (ISOM)*, Jon J. Gerhardt and Otto A. Russee, Bern, Switzerland, Han Huber 9 Publisher), 1975.

MUSCULOSKELETAL/SOFT TISSUE

Adverse Event	Short Name	Grade				
		1	2	3	4	5
Muscle weakness, generalized or specific area (not due to neuropathy) – Select: – Extraocular – Extremity-lower – Extremity-upper – Facial – Left-sided – Ocular – Pelvic – Right-sided – Trunk – Whole body/generalized	Muscle weakness – Select	Asymptomatic; weakness on physical exam	Symptomatic and interfering with function, but not interfering with ADL	Symptomatic and interfering with ADL	Life-threatening; disabling	Death
ALSO CONSIDER: Fatigue (asthenia, lethargy, malaise).				object)		
Muscular/skeletal hypoplasia	Muscular/skeletal hypoplasia	Cosmetically and functionally insignificant hypoplasia	Deformity, hypoplasia, or asymmetry able to be remediated by prosthesis (e.g., shoe insert) or covered by clothing	Functionally significant deformity, hypoplasia, or asymmetry, unable to be remediated by prosthesis or covered by clothing	Disabling	—
Myositis (inflammation/damage of muscle)	Myositis	Mild pain, not interfering with function	Pain interfering with function, but not interfering with ADL	Pain interfering with ADL	Disabling	Death
REMARK: Myositis implies muscle damage (i.e., elevated CPK).						
ALSO CONSIDER: CPK (creatine phosphokinase); Pain – Select.						
Osteonecrosis (avascular necrosis)	Osteonecrosis	Asymptomatic, radiographic findings only	Symptomatic and interfering with function, but not interfering with ADL; minimal bone removal indicated (i.e., minor sequestrectomy)	Symptomatic and interfering with ADL; operative intervention or hyperbaric oxygen indicated	Disabling	Death

MUSCULOSKELETAL/SOFT TISSUE

Adverse Event	Short Name	Grade				
		1	2	3	4	5
Osteoporosis[6]	Osteoporosis	Radiographic evidence of osteoporosis or Bone Mineral Density (BMD) t-score −1 to −2.5 (osteopenia) and no loss of height or therapy indicated	BMD t-score < −2.5; loss of height <2 cm; anti-osteoporotic therapy indicated	Fractures; loss of height ≥2 cm	Disabling	Death
Seroma	Seroma	Asymptomatic	Symptomatic; medical intervention or simple aspiration indicated	Symptomatic, interventional radiology or operative intervention indicated	—	—
Soft tissue necrosis – Select: – Abdomen – Extremity-lower – Extremity-upper – Head – Neck – Pelvic – Thorax	Soft tissue necrosis – Select	—	Local wound care; medical intervention indicated	Operative debridement or other invasive intervention indicated (e.g., hyperbaric oxygen)	Life-threatening consequences; major invasive intervention indicated (e.g., tissue reconstruction, flap, or grafting)	Death
Trismus (difficulty, restriction or pain when opening mouth)	Trismus	Decreased range of motion without impaired eating	Decreased range of motion requiring small bites, soft foods or purees	Decreased range of motion with inability to adequately aliment or hydrate orally	—	—
NAVIGATION NOTE: Wound-infectious is graded as Infection – Select in the INFECTION CATEGORY.						
NAVIGATION NOTE: Wound non-infectious is graded as Wound complication, non-infectious in the DERMATOLOGY/SKIN CATEGORY.						
Musculoskeletal/Soft Tissue – Other (Specify, __)	Musculoskeletal – Other (Specify)	Mild	Moderate	Severe	Life-threatening; disabling	Death

[6] "Assessment of Fracture Risk and its Application to Screening for Post-menopausal Osteoporosis," Report of a *WHO Study Group Technical Report Series*, No. 843, 1994, v + 129 pages [C*, E, E, F, R, S], ISBN 92 4 120843 0, Sw.fr. 22.-/US $19.80; in developing countries: Sw.fr. 15.40, Order no. 1100843.

NEUROLOGY

Adverse Event	Short Name	Grade				
		1	2	3	4	5

NAVIGATION NOTE: ADD (Attention Deficit Disorder) is graded as Cognitive disturbance.

NAVIGATION NOTE: Aphasia, receptive and/or expressive, is graded as Speech impairment (e.g., dysphasia or aphasia).

Adverse Event	Short Name	1	2	3	4	5
Apnea	Apnea	—	—	Present	Intubation indicated	Death
Arachnoiditis/meningismus/radiculitis	Arachnoiditis	Symptomatic, not interfering with function; medical intervention indicated	Symptomatic (e.g., photophobia, nausea) interfering with function but not interfering with ADL	Symptomatic, interfering with ADL	Life-threatening; disabling (e.g., paraplegia)	Death

ALSO CONSIDER: Fever (in the absence of neutropenia, where neutropenia is defined as ANC <1.0 x 10⁹/L); Infection (documented clinically or microbiologically) with Grade 3 or 4 neutrophils (ANC <1.0 x 109/L) – Select; Infection with normal ANC or Grade 1 or 2 neutrophils – Select; Infection with unknown ANC – Select; Pain – Select; Vomiting.

Adverse Event	Short Name	1	2	3	4	5
Ataxia (incoordination)	Ataxia	Asymptomatic	Symptomatic, not interfering with ADL	Symptomatic, interfering with ADL; mechanical assistance indicated	Disabling	Death

REMARK: Ataxia (incoordination) refers to the consequence of medical or operative intervention.

Adverse Event	Short Name	1	2	3	4	5
Brachial plexopathy	Brachial plexopathy	Asymptomatic	Symptomatic, not interfering with ADL	Symptomatic, interfering with ADL	Disabling	Death
CNS cerebrovascular ischemia	CNS ischemia	—	Asymptomatic, radiographic findings only	Transient ischemic event or attack (TIA) ≤24 hrs duration	Cerebral vascular accident (CVA, stroke), neurologic deficit >24 hrs	Death

NAVIGATION NOTE: CNS hemorrhage/bleeding is graded as Hemorrhage, CNS in the HEMORRHAGE/BLEEDING CATEGORY.

Adverse Event	Short Name	1	2	3	4	5
CNS necrosis/cystic progression	CNS necrosis	Asymptomatic, radiographic findings only	Symptomatic, not interfering with ADL; medical intervention indicated	Symptomatic and interfering with ADL; hyperbaric oxygen indicated	Life-threatening; disabling; operative intervention indicated to prevent or treat CNS necrosis/cystic progression	Death
Cognitive disturbance	Cognitive disturbance	Mild cognitive disability; not interfering with work/school/life performance; specialized educational services/devices not indicated	Moderate cognitive disability; interfering with work/school/life performance but capable of independent living; specialized resources on part-time basis indicated	Severe cognitive disability; significant impairment of work/school/life performance	Unable to perform ADL; full-time specialized resources or institutionalization indicated	Death

REMARK: Cognitive disturbance may be used for Attention Deficit Disorder (ADD).

Adverse Event	Short Name	Grade				
		1	2	3	4	5
Confusion	Confusion	Transient confusion, disorientation, or attention deficit	Confusion, disorientation, or attention deficit interfering with function, but not interfering with ADL	Confusion or delirium interfering with ADL	Harmful to others or self; hospitalization indicated	Death

REMARK: Attention Deficit Disorder (ADD) is graded as Cognitive disturbance.

NAVIGATION NOTE: Cranial neuropathy is graded as Neuropathy-cranial – *Select*.

Dizziness	Dizziness	With head movements or nystagmus only; not interfering with function	Interfering with function, but not interfering with ADL	Interfering with ADL	Disabling	—

REMARK: Dizziness includes disequilibrium, lightheadedness, and vertigo.

ALSO CONSIDER: Neuropathy: cranial – *Select*; Syncope (fainting).

NAVIGATION NOTE: Dysphasia, receptive and/or expressive, is graded as Speech impairment (e.g., dysphasia or aphasia).

Encephalopathy	Encephalopathy	—	Mild signs or symptoms; not interfering with ADL	Signs or symptoms interfering with ADL; hospitalization indicated	Life-threatening; disabling	Death

ALSO CONSIDER: Cognitive disturbance; Confusion; Dizziness; Memory impairment; Mental status; Mood alteration – *Select*; Psychosis (hallucinations/delusions); Somnolence/depressed level of consciousness.

Extrapyramidal/ involuntary movement/ restlessness	Involuntary movement	Mild involuntary movements not interfering with function	Moderate involuntary movements interfering with function, but not interfering with ADL	Severe involuntary movements or torticollis interfering with ADL	Disabling	Death

NAVIGATION NOTE: Headache/neuropathic pain (e.g., jaw pain, neurologic pain, phantom limb pain, post-infectious neuralgia, or painful neuropathies) is graded as Pain – *Select* in the PAIN CATEGORY.

Hydrocephalus	Hydrocephalus	Asymptomatic, radiographic findings only	Mild to moderate symptoms not interfering with ADL	Severe symptoms or neurological deficit interfering with ADL	Disabling	Death
Irritability (children <3 years of age)	Irritability	Mild; easily consolable	Moderate; requiring increased attention	Severe; inconsolable	—	—
Laryngeal nerve dysfunction	Laryngeal nerve	Asymptomatic, weakness on clinical examination/testing only	Symptomatic, but not interfering with ADL; intervention not indicated	Symptomatic, interfering with ADL; intervention indicated (e.g., thyroplasty, vocal cord injection)	Life-threatening; tracheostomy indicated	Death

NEUROLOGY

Adverse Event	Short Name	Grade				
		1	2	3	4	5
Leak, cerebrospinal fluid (CSF)	CSF leak	Transient headache; postural care indicated	Symptomatic, not interfering with ADL; blood patch indicated	Symptomatic, interfering with ADL; operative intervention indicated	Life-threatening; disabling	Death
REMARK: Leak, cerebrospinal fluid (CSF) may be used for CSF leak associated with operation and persisting >72 hours.						
Leukoencephalopathy (radiographic findings)	Leukoencephalopathy	Mild increase in subarachnoid space (SAS); mild ventriculomegaly; small (+/- multiple) focal T2 hyperintensities, involving periventricular white matter or <1/3 of susceptible areas of cerebrum	Moderate increase in SAS; moderate ventriculomegaly; focal T2 hyperintensities extending into centrum ovale or involving 1/3 to 2/3 of susceptible areas of cerebrum	Severe increase in SAS; severe ventriculomegaly; near total white matter T2 hyperintensities or diffuse low attenuation (CT)	—	—
REMARK: Leukoencephalopathy is a diffuse white matter process, specifically NOT associated with necrosis. Leukoencephalopathy (radiographic findings) does not include lacunas, which are areas that become void of neural tissue.						
Memory impairment	Memory impairment	Memory impairment not interfering with function	Memory impairment interfering with function, but not interfering with ADL	Memory impairment interfering with ADL	Amnesia	—
Mental status[7]	Mental status	—	1 – 3 point below age and educational norm in Folstein Mini-Mental Status Exam (MMSE)	>3 point below age and educational norm in Folstein MMSE	—	—
Mood alteration – Select: – Agitation – Anxiety – Depression – Euphoria	Mood alteration – Select	Mild mood alteration not interfering with function	Moderate mood alteration interfering with function, but not interfering with ADL; medication indicated	Severe mood alteration interfering with ADL	Suicidal ideation; danger to self or others	Death
Myelitis	Myelitis	Asymptomatic, mild signs (e.g., Babinski's or Lhermitte's sign)	Weakness or sensory loss not interfering with ADL	Weakness or sensory loss interfering with ADL	Disabling	Death

[7]Folstein, M.F., Folstein, S.E. and McHugh, P.R. (1975). "Mini-Mental State: A Practical Method for Grading the State of Patients for the Clinician." *Journal of Psychiatric Research*, **12**, 189–198.

NEUROLOGY

Adverse Event	Short Name	Grade				
		1	2	3	4	5

NAVIGATION NOTE: Neuropathic pain is graded as Pain – *Select* in the PAIN CATEGORY.

Adverse Event	Short Name	1	2	3	4	5
	Neuropathy: cranial – *Select* – CN I Smell – CN II Vision – CN III Pupil, upper eyelid, extra ocular movements – CN IV Downward, inward movement of eye – CN V Motor-jaw muscles; Sensory-facial – CN VI Lateral deviation of eye – CN VII Motor-face; Sensory-taste – CN VIII Hearing and balance – CN IX Motor-pharynx; Sensory-ear, pharynx, tongue – CN X Motor-palate; pharynx, larynx – CN XI Motor-sternomastoid and trapezius – CN XII Motor-tongue	Asymptomatic, detected on exam/testing only	Symptomatic, not interfering with ADL	Symptomatic, interfering with ADL	Life-threatening; disabling	Death
Neuropathy: motor	Neuropathy-motor	Asymptomatic, weakness on exam/testing only	Symptomatic weakness interfering with function, but not interfering with ADL	Weakness interfering with ADL; bracing or assistance to walk (e.g., cane or walker) indicated	Life-threatening; disabling (e.g., paralysis)	Death

REMARK: Cranial nerve motor neuropathy is graded as Neuropathy: cranial – *Select*.

ALSO CONSIDER: Laryngeal nerve dysfunction; Phrenic nerve dysfunction.

Adverse Event	Short Name	1	2	3	4	5
Neuropathy: sensory	Neuropathy-sensory	Asymptomatic; loss of deep tendon reflexes or paresthesia (including tingling) but not interfering with function	Sensory alteration or paresthesia (including tingling), interfering with function, but not interfering with ADL	Sensory alteration or paresthesia interfering with ADL	Disabling	Death

REMARK: Cranial nerve sensory neuropathy is graded as Neuropathy: cranial – *Select*.

Adverse Event	Short Name	1	2	3	4	5
Personality/behavioral	Personality	Change, but not adversely affecting patient or family	Change, adversely affecting patient or family	Mental health intervention indicated	Change harmful to others or self; hospitalization indicated	Death
Phrenic nerve dysfunction	Phrenic nerve	Asymptomatic weakness on exam/testing only	Symptomatic but not interfering with ADL; intervention not indicated	Significant dysfunction; intervention indicated (e.g., diaphragmatic plication)	Life-threatening respiratory compromise; mechanical ventilation indicated	Death
Psychosis (hallucinations/delusions)	Psychosis	—	Transient episode	Interfering with ADL; medication, supervision	Harmful to others or self; life-threatening	Death

NEUROLOGY

Adverse Event	Short Name	Grade				
		1	2	3	4	5
Pyramidal tract dysfunction (e.g., ↑ tone, hyperreflexia, positive Babinski, ↓ fine motor coordination)	Pyramidal tract dysfunction	Asymptomatic, abnormality on exam or testing only	Symptomatic; interfering with function but not interfering with ADL	Interfering with ADL or restraints indicated	Disabling; paralysis	Death
Seizure	Seizure	—	One brief generalized seizure; seizure(s) well controlled by anticonvulsants or infrequent focal motor seizures not interfering with ADL	Seizures in which consciousness is altered; poorly controlled seizure disorder, with breakthrough generalized seizures despite medical intervention	Seizures of any kind which are prolonged, repetitive, or difficult to control (e.g., status epilepticus, intractable epilepsy)	Death
Somnolence/depressed level of consciousness	Somnolence	—	Somnolence or sedation interfering with function, but not interfering with ADL	Obtundation or stupor; difficult to arouse; interfering with ADL	Coma	Death
Speech impairment (e.g., dysphasia or aphasia)	Speech impairment	—	Awareness of receptive or expressive dysphasia, not impairing ability to communicate	Receptive or expressive dysphasia, impairing ability to communicate	Inability to communicate	—

REMARK: Speech impairment refers to a primary CNS process, not neuropathy or end organ dysfunction.

ALSO CONSIDER: Laryngeal nerve dysfunction; Voice changes/dysarthria (e.g., hoarseness, loss, or alteration in voice, laryngitis).

Adverse Event	Short Name	Grade				
		1	2	3	4	5
Syncope (fainting)	Syncope (fainting)	—	—	Present	Life-threatening consequences	Death

ALSO CONSIDER: CNS cerebrovascular ischemia; Conduction abnormality/atrioventricular heart block – Select; Dizziness; Supraventricular and nodal arrhythmia – Select; Vasovagal episode; Ventricular arrhythmia – Select.

NAVIGATION NOTE: Taste alteration (CN VII, IX) is graded as Taste alteration (dysgeusia) in the GASTROINTESTINAL CATEGORY.

Adverse Event	Short Name	Grade				
		1	2	3	4	5
Tremor	Tremor	Mild and brief or intermittent but not interfering with function	Moderate tremor interfering with function, but not interfering with ADL	Severe tremor interfering with ADL	Disabling	—
Neurology – Other (Specify, __)	Neurology – Other (Specify)	Mild	Moderate	Severe	Life-threatening; disabling	Death

OCULAR/VISUAL

Adverse Event	Short Name	Grade				
		1	2	3	4	5
Cataract	Cataract	Asymptomatic, detected on exam only	Symptomatic, with moderate decrease in visual acuity (20/40 or better); decreased visual function correctable with glasses	Symptomatic with marked decrease in visual acuity (worse than 20/40); operative intervention indicated (e.g., cataract surgery)	—	—
Dry eye syndrome	Dry eye	Mild, intervention not indicated	Symptomatic, interfering with function but not interfering with ADL; medical intervention indicated	Symptomatic or decrease in visual acuity interfering with ADL; operative intervention indicated	—	—
Eyelid dysfunction	Eyelid dysfunction	Asymptomatic	Symptomatic, interfering with function but not ADL; requiring topical agents or epilation	Symptomatic; interfering with ADL; surgical intervention indicated	—	—

REMARK: Eyelid dysfunction includes canalicular stenosis, ectropion, entropion, erythema, madarosis, symblepharon, telangiectasis, thickening, and trichiasis.

ALSO CONSIDER: Neuropathy: cranial – *Select.*

Adverse Event	Short Name	1	2	3	4	5
Glaucoma	Glaucoma	Elevated intraocular pressure (EIOP) with single topical agent for intervention; no visual field deficit	EIOP causing early visual field deficit (i.e., nasal step or arcuate deficit); multiple topical or oral agents indicated	EIOP causing marked visual field deficits (i.e., involving both superior and inferior visual fields); operative intervention indicated	EIOP resulting in blindness (20/200 or worse); enucleation indicated	—
Keratitis (corneal inflammation/corneal ulceration)	Keratitis	Abnormal ophthalmologic changes only; intervention not indicated	Symptomatic and interfering with function, but not interfering with ADL	Symptomatic and interfering with ADL; operative intervention indicated	Perforation or blindness (20/200 or worse)	—

NAVIGATION NOTE: Ocular muscle weakness is graded as Muscle weakness, generalized or specific area (not due to neuropathy) – *Select* in the MUSCULOSKELETAL/SOFT TISSUE CATEGORY.

Adverse Event	Short Name	1	2	3	4	5
Night blindness (nyctalopia)	Nyctalopia	Symptomatic, not interfering with function	Symptomatic and interfering with function but not interfering with ADL	Symptomatic and interfering with ADL	Disabling	—

OCULAR/VISUAL

Adverse Event	Short Name	Grade				
		1	2	3	4	5
Nystagmus	Nystagmus	Asymptomatic	Symptomatic and interfering with function but not interfering with ADL	Symptomatic and interfering with ADL	Disabling	—
ALSO CONSIDER: Neuropathy: cranial – *Select*; Ophthalmoplegia/diplopia (double vision).						
Ocular surface disease	Ocular surface disease	Asymptomatic or minimally symptomatic but not interfering with function	Symptomatic, interfering with function but not interfering with ADL; topical antibiotics or other topical intervention indicated	Symptomatic, interfering with ADL; operative intervention indicated	—	—
REMARK: Ocular surface disease includes conjunctivitis, keratoconjunctivitis sicca, chemosis, keratinization, and palpebral conjunctival epithelial metaplasia.						
Ophthalmoplegia/ diplopia (double vision)	Diplopia	Intermittently symptomatic, intervention not indicated	Symptomatic and interfering with function but not interfering with ADL	Symptomatic and interfering with ADL; surgical intervention indicated	Disabling	—
ALSO CONSIDER: Neuropathy: cranial – *Select*.						
Optic disc edema	Optic disc edema	Asymptomatic	Decreased visual acuity (20/40 or better); visual field defect present	Decreased visual acuity (worse than 20/40); marked visual field defect but sparing the central 20 degrees	Blindness (20/200 or worse)	—
ALSO CONSIDER: Neuropathy: cranial – *Select*.						
Proptosis/enophthalmos	Proptosis/enophthalmos	Asymptomatic, intervention not indicated	Symptomatic and interfering with function, but not interfering with ADL	Symptomatic and interfering with ADL	—	—
Retinal detachment	Retinal detachment	Exudative; no central vision loss; intervention not indicated	Exudative and visual acuity 20/40 or better but intervention not indicated	Rhegmatogenous or exudative detachment; operative intervention indicated	Blindness (20/200 or worse)	—
Retinopathy	Retinopathy	Asymptomatic	Symptomatic with moderate decrease in visual acuity (20/40 or better)	Symptomatic with marked decrease in visual acuity (worse than 20/40)	Blindness (20/200 or worse)	—

OCULAR/VISUAL

Adverse Event	Short Name	Grade				
		1	2	3	4	5
Scleral necrosis/melt	Scleral necrosis	Asymptomatic or symptomatic but not interfering with function	Symptomatic, interfering with function but not interfering with ADL; moderate decrease in visual acuity (20/40 or better); medical intervention indicated	Symptomatic, interfering with ADL; marked decrease in visual acuity (worse than 20/40); operative intervention indicated	Blindness (20/200 or worse); painful eye with enucleation indicated	—
Uveitis	Uveitis	Asymptomatic	Anterior uveitis; medical intervention indicated	Posterior or pan-uveitis; operative intervention indicated	Blindness (20/200 or worse)	—
Vision-blurred vision	Blurred vision	Symptomatic not interfering with function	Symptomatic and interfering with function, but not interfering with ADL	Symptomatic and interfering with ADL	Disabling	—
Vision-flashing lights/floaters	Flashing lights	Symptomatic not interfering with function	Symptomatic and interfering with function, but not interfering with ADL	Symptomatic and interfering with ADL	Disabling	—
Vision-photophobia	Photophobia	Symptomatic not interfering with function	Symptomatic and interfering with function, but not interfering with ADL	Symptomatic and interfering with ADL	Disabling	—
Vitreous hemorrhage	Vitreous hemorrhage	Asymptomatic, clinical findings only	Symptomatic, interfering with function, but not interfering with ADL; intervention not indicated	Symptomatic, interfering with ADL; vitrectomy indicated	—	—
Watery eye (epiphora, tearing)	Watery eye	Symptomatic, intervention not indicated	Symptomatic, interfering with function but not interfering with ADL	Symptomatic, interfering with ADL	—	—
Ocular/Visual – Other (Specify,__)	Ocular – Other (Specify)	Symptomatic not interfering with function	Symptomatic and interfering with function, but not interfering with ADL	Symptomatic and interfering with ADL	Blindness (20/200 or worse)	Death

PAIN

Adverse Event	Short Name	Grade				
		1	2	3	4	5
Pain – Select: 'Select' AEs appear at the end of the CATEGORY.	Pain – Select	Mild pain not interfering with function	Moderate pain; pain or analgesics interfering with function, but not interfering with ADL	Severe pain; pain or analgesics severely interfering with ADL	Disabling	—
Pain – Other (Specify, ___)	Pain – Other (Specify)	Mild pain not interfering with function	Moderate pain; pain or analgesics interfering with function, but not interfering with ADL	Severe pain; pain or analgesics severely interfering with ADL	Disabling	—

PAIN – SELECT

AUDITORY/EAR
  – External ear
  – Middle ear
CARDIOVASCULAR
  – Cardiac/heart
  – Pericardium
DERMATOLOGY/SKIN
  – Face
  – Lip
  – Oral-gums
  – Scalp
  – Skin
GASTROINTESTINAL
  – Abdomen NOS
  – Anus
  – Dental/teeth/peridontal
  – Esophagus
  – Oral cavity
  – Peritoneum
  – Rectum
  – Stomach
GENERAL
  – Pain NOS
  – Tumor pain

HEPATOBILIARY/PANCREAS
  – Gallbladder
  – Liver
LYMPHATIC
  – Lymph node
MUSCULOSKELETAL
  – Back
  – Bone
  – Buttock
  – Extremity-limb
  – Intestine
  – Joint
  – Muscle
  – Neck
  – Phantom (pain associated with missing limb)
NEUROLOGY
  – Head/headache
  – Neuralgia/peripheral nerve
OCULAR
  – Eye
PULMONARY/UPPER RESPIRATORY
  – Chest wall
  – Chest/thorax NOS

PULMONARY/UPPER RESPIRATORY (continued)
  – Larynx
  – Pleura
  – Sinus
  – Throat/pharynx/larynx
RENAL/GENITOURINARY
  – Bladder
  – Kidney
SEXUAL/REPRODUCTIVE FUNCTION
  – Breast
  – Ovulatory
  – Pelvis
  – Penis
  – Perineum
  – Prostate
  – Scrotum
  – Testicle
  – Urethra
  – Uterus
  – Vagina

PULMONARY/UPPER RESPIRATORY

Adverse Event	Short Name	Grade 1	Grade 2	Grade 3	Grade 4	Grade 5
Adult Respiratory Distress Syndrome (ARDS)	ARDS	—	—	Present, intubation not indicated	Present, intubation indicated	Death

ALSO CONSIDER: Dyspnea (shortness of breath); Hypoxia; Pneumonitis/pulmonary infiltrates.

Adverse Event	Short Name	Grade 1	Grade 2	Grade 3	Grade 4	Grade 5
Aspiration	Aspiration	Asymptomatic ("silent aspiration"); endoscopy or radiographic (e.g., barium swallow) findings	Symptomatic (e.g., altered eating habits, coughing or choking episodes consistent with aspiration); medical intervention indicated (e.g., antibiotics, suction or oxygen)	Clinical or radiographic signs of pneumonia or pneumonitis; unable to aliment orally	Life-threatening (e.g., aspiration pneumonia or pneumonitis)	Death

ALSO CONSIDER: Infection (documented clinically or microbiologically) with Grade 3 or 4 neutrophils (ANC <1.0 x 10^9/L) – *Select*; Infection with normal ANC or Grade 1 or 2 neutrophils – *Select*; Infection with unknown ANC – *Select*; Laryngeal nerve dysfunction; Neuropathy: cranial – *Select*; Pneumonitis/pulmonary infiltrates.

Adverse Event	Short Name	Grade 1	Grade 2	Grade 3	Grade 4	Grade 5
Atelectasis	Atelectasis	Asymptomatic	Symptomatic (e.g., dyspnea, cough), medical intervention indicated (e.g., bronchoscopic suctioning, chest physiotherapy, suctioning)	Operative (e.g., stent, laser) intervention indicated	Life-threatening respiratory compromise	Death

ALSO CONSIDER: Adult Respiratory Distress Syndrome (ARDS); Cough; Dyspnea (shortness of breath); Hypoxia; Infection (documented clinically or microbiologically) with Grade 3 or 4 neutrophils (ANC <1.0 x 109/L) – *Select*; Infection with normal ANC or Grade 1 or 2 neutrophils – *Select*; Infection with unknown ANC – *Select*; Obstruction/stenosis of airway – *Select*; Pneumonitis/pulmonary infiltrates; Pulmonary fibrosis (radiographic changes).

Adverse Event	Short Name	Grade 1	Grade 2	Grade 3	Grade 4	Grade 5
Bronchospasm, wheezing	Bronchospasm	Asymptomatic	Symptomatic not interfering with function	Symptomatic interfering with function	Life-threatening	Death

ALSO CONSIDER: Allergic reaction/hypersensitivity (including drug fever); Dyspnea (shortness of breath).

Adverse Event	Short Name	Grade 1	Grade 2	Grade 3	Grade 4	Grade 5
Carbon monoxide diffusion capacity (DL$_{CO}$)	DL$_{CO}$	90 – 75% of predicted value	<75 – 50% of predicted value	<50 – 25% of predicted value	<25% of predicted value	Death

ALSO CONSIDER: Hypoxia; Pneumonitis/pulmonary infiltrates; Pulmonary fibrosis (radiographic changes).

Adverse Event	Short Name	Grade 1	Grade 2	Grade 3	Grade 4	Grade 5
Chylothorax	Chylothorax	Asymptomatic	Symptomatic; thoracentesis or tube drainage indicated	Operative intervention indicated	Life-threatening (e.g., hemodynamic instability or ventilatory support indicated)	Death

Adverse Event	Short Name	Grade 1	Grade 2	Grade 3	Grade 4	Grade 5
Cough	Cough	Symptomatic, non-narcotic medication only indicated	Symptomatic and narcotic medication indicated	Symptomatic and significantly interfering with sleep or ADL	—	—

PULMONARY/UPPER RESPIRATORY

Adverse Event	Short Name	Grade 1	2	3	4	5
Dyspnea (shortness of breath)	Dyspnea	Dyspnea on exertion, but can walk 1 flight of stairs without stopping	Dyspnea on exertion but unable to walk 1 flight of stairs or 1 city block (0.1km) without stopping	Dyspnea with ADL	Dyspnea at rest; intubation/ventilator indicated	Death
ALSO CONSIDER: Hypoxia; Neuropathy: motor; Pneumonitis/pulmonary infiltrates; Pulmonary fibrosis (radiographic changes).						
Edema, larynx	Edema, larynx	Asymptomatic edema by exam only	Symptomatic edema, no respiratory distress	Stridor; respiratory distress; interfering with ADL	Life-threatening airway compromise; tracheotomy, intubation, or laryngectomy indicated	Death
ALSO CONSIDER: Allergic reaction/hypersensitivity (including drug fever).						
FEV₁	FEV₁	90 – 75% of predicted value	<75 – 50% of predicted value	<50 – 25% of predicted value	<25% of predicted	Death
Fistula, pulmonary/upper respiratory – Select: – Bronchus – Larynx – Lung – Oral cavity – Pharynx – Pleura – Trachea	Fistula, pulmonary – Select	Asymptomatic, radiographic findings only	Symptomatic, tube thoracostomy or medical management indicated; associated with altered respiratory function but not interfering with ADL	Symptomatic and associated with altered respiratory function interfering with ADL; or endoscopic (e.g., stent) or primary closure by operative intervention indicated	Life-threatening consequences; operative intervention with thoracoplasty, chronic open drainage or multiple thoracotomies indicated	Death
REMARK: A fistula is defined as an abnormal communication between two body cavities, potential spaces, and/or the skin. The site indicated for a fistula should be the site from which the abnormal process is believed to have arisen. For example, a tracheo-esophageal fistula arising in the context of a resected or irradiated esophageal cancer should be graded as Fistula, GI – esophagus in the GASTROINTESTINAL CATEGORY.						
NAVIGATION NOTE: Hemoptysis is graded as Hemorrhage, pulmonary/upper respiratory – Select in the HEMORRHAGE/BLEEDING CATEGORY.						
Hiccoughs (hiccups, singultus)	Hiccoughs	Symptomatic, intervention not indicated	Symptomatic, intervention indicated	Symptomatic, significantly interfering with sleep or ADL	—	—
Hypoxia	Hypoxia	—	Decreased O₂ saturation with exercise (e.g., pulse oximeter <88%); intermittent supplemental oxygen	Decreased O₂ saturation at rest; continuous oxygen indicated	Life-threatening; intubation or ventilation indicated	Death

PULMONARY/UPPER RESPIRATORY

Adverse Event	Short Name	Grade				
		1	2	3	4	5
Nasal cavity/paranasal sinus reactions	Nasal/paranasal reactions	Asymptomatic mucosal crusting, blood-tinged secretions	Symptomatic stenosis or edema/narrowing interfering with airflow	Stenosis with significant nasal obstruction; interfering with ADL	Necrosis of soft tissue or bone	Death

ALSO CONSIDER: Infection (documented clinically or microbiologically) with Grade 3 or 4 neutrophils (ANC <1.0 x 10⁹/L) – Select; Infection with normal ANC or Grade 1 or 2 neutrophils – Select; Infection with unknown ANC – Select.

Adverse Event	Short Name	1	2	3	4	5
Obstruction/stenosis of airway – Select: – Bronchus – Larynx – Pharynx – Trachea	Airway obstruction – Select	Asymptomatic obstruction or stenosis on exam, endoscopy, or radiograph	Symptomatic (e.g., noisy airway breathing), but causing no respiratory distress; medical management indicated (e.g., steroids)	Interfering with ADL; stridor or endoscopic intervention indicated (e.g., stent, laser)	Life-threatening airway compromise; tracheotomy or intubation indicated	Death
Pleural effusion (non-malignant)	Pleural effusion	Asymptomatic	Symptomatic, intervention such as diuretics or up to 2 therapeutic thoracenteses indicated	Symptomatic and supplemental oxygen, >2 therapeutic thoracenteses, tube drainage, or pleurodesis indicated	Life-threatening (e.g., causing hemodynamic instability or ventilatory support indicated)	Death

ALSO CONSIDER: Atelectasis; Cough; Dyspnea (shortness of breath); Hypoxia; Pneumonitis/pulmonary infiltrates; Pulmonary fibrosis (radiographic changes).

NAVIGATION NOTE: Pleuritic pain is graded as Pain – Select in the PAIN CATEGORY.

Adverse Event	Short Name	1	2	3	4	5
Pneumonitis/pulmonary infiltrates	Pneumonitis	Asymptomatic, radiographic findings only	Symptomatic, not interfering with ADL	Symptomatic, interfering with ADL; O₂ indicated	Life-threatening; ventilatory support indicated	Death

ALSO CONSIDER: Adult Respiratory Distress Syndrome (ARDS); Cough; Dyspnea (shortness of breath); Hypoxia; Infection (documented clinically or microbiologically) with Grade 3 or 4 neutrophils (ANC <1.0 x 10⁹/L) – Select; Infection with normal ANC or Grade 1 or 2 neutrophils – Select; Infection with unknown ANC – Select; Pneumonitis/pulmonary infiltrates; Pulmonary fibrosis (radiographic changes).

Adverse Event	Short Name	1	2	3	4	5
Pneumothorax	Pneumothorax	Asymptomatic, radiographic findings only	Symptomatic; intervention indicated (e.g., hospitalization for observation, tube placement without sclerosis)	Sclerosis and/or operative intervention indicated	Life-threatening, causing hemodynamic instability (e.g., tension pneumothorax); ventilatory support indicated	Death
Prolonged chest tube drainage or air leak after pulmonary resection	Chest tube drainage or leak	—	Sclerosis or additional tube thoracostomy indicated	Operative intervention indicated (e.g., thoracotomy with stapling or sealant application)	Life-threatening; debilitating; organ resection indicated	Death

PULMONARY/UPPER RESPIRATORY

Adverse Event	Short Name	Grade				
		1	2	3	4	5
Prolonged intubation after pulmonary resection (>24 hrs after surgery)	Prolonged intubation	—	Extubated within 24 – 72 hrs postoperatively	Extubated >72 hrs postoperatively, but before tracheostomy indicated	Tracheostomy indicated	Death

NAVIGATION NOTE: Pulmonary embolism is graded as Grade 4 either as Thrombosis/embolism (vascular access-related) or Thrombosis/thrombus/embolism in the VASCULAR CATEGORY.

Adverse Event	Short Name	Grade				
		1	2	3	4	5
Pulmonary fibrosis (radiographic changes)	Pulmonary fibrosis	Minimal radiographic findings (or patchy or bi-basilar changes) with estimated radiographic proportion of total lung volume that is fibrotic of <25%	Patchy or bi-basilar changes with estimated radiographic proportion of total lung volume that is fibrotic of 25 – <50%	Dense or widespread infiltrates/consolidation with estimated radiographic proportion of total lung volume that is fibrotic of 50 – <75%	Estimated radiographic proportion of total lung volume that is fibrotic is ≥75%; honeycombing	Death

REMARK: Fibrosis is usually a "late effect" seen >3 months after radiation or combined modality therapy (including surgery). It is thought to represent scar/fibrotic lung tissue. It may be difficult to distinguish from pneumonitis that is generally seen within 3 months of radiation or combined modality therapy.

ALSO CONSIDER: Adult Respiratory Distress Syndrome (ARDS); Cough; Dyspnea (shortness of breath); Hypoxia; Infection (documented clinically or microbiologically) with Grade 3 or 4 neutrophils (ANC <1.0 x 10⁹/L) – Select; Infection with normal ANC or Grade 1 or 2 neutrophils – Select; Infection with unknown ANC – Select.

NAVIGATION NOTE: Recurrent laryngeal nerve dysfunction is graded as Laryngeal nerve dysfunction in the NEUROLOGY CATEGORY.

Adverse Event	Short Name	Grade				
		1	2	3	4	5
Vital capacity	Vital capacity	90 – 75% of predicted value	<75 – 50% of predicted value	<50 – 25% of predicted value	<25% of predicted value	Death
Voice changes/dysarthria (e.g., hoarseness, loss or alteration in voice, laryngitis)	Voice changes	Mild or intermittent hoarseness or voice change, but fully understandable	Moderate or persistent voice changes, may require occasional repetition but understandable on telephone	Severe voice changes including predominantly whispered speech; may require frequent repetition or face-to-face contact for understandability; requires voice aid (e.g., electrolarynx) for ≤50% of communication	Disabling; non-understandable voice or aphonic; requires voice aid (e.g., electrolarynx) for >50% of communication or requires >50% written communication	Death

ALSO CONSIDER: Laryngeal nerve dysfunction; Speech impairment (e.g., dysphasia or aphasia).

Adverse Event	Short Name	Grade				
		1	2	3	4	5
Pulmonary/Upper Respiratory – Other (Specify, __)	Pulmonary/Upper Respiratory – Other (Specify)	Mild	Moderate	Severe	Life-threatening; disabling	Death

RENAL/GENITOURINARY

Adverse Event	Short Name	Grade				
		1	2	3	4	5
Bladder spasms	Bladder spasms	Symptomatic, intervention not indicated	Symptomatic, antispasmodics indicated	Narcotics indicated	Major surgical intervention indicated (e.g., cystectomy)	—
Cystitis	Cystitis	Asymptomatic	Frequency with dysuria; macroscopic hematuria	Transfusion; IV pain medications; bladder irrigation indicated	Catastrophic bleeding; major non-elective intervention indicated	Death

ALSO CONSIDER: Infection (documented clinically or microbiologically) with Grade 3 or 4 neutrophils (ANC <1.0 x 109/L) – *Select*; Infection with normal ANC or Grade 1 or 2 neutrophils – *Select*; Infection with unknown ANC – *Select*; Pain – *Select*.

Adverse Event	Short Name	Grade				
		1	2	3	4	5
Fistula, GU – *Select*: – Bladder – Genital tract-female – Kidney – Ureter – Urethra – Uterus – Vagina	Fistula, GU – *Select*	Asymptomatic, radiographic findings only	Symptomatic; noninvasive intervention indicated	Symptomatic interfering with ADL; invasive intervention indicated	Life-threatening consequences; operative intervention requiring partial or full organ resection; permanent urinary diversion	Death

REMARK: A fistula is defined as an abnormal communication between two body cavities, potential spaces, and/or the skin. The site indicated for a fistula should be the site from which the abnormal process is believed to have originated.

Adverse Event	Short Name	Grade				
		1	2	3	4	5
Incontinence, urinary	Incontinence, urinary	Occasional (e.g., with coughing, sneezing, etc.), pads not indicated	Spontaneous, pads indicated	Interfering with ADL; intervention indicated (e.g., clamp, collagen injections)	Operative intervention indicated (e.g. cystectomy or permanent urinary diversion)	—
Leak (including anastomotic), GU – *Select*: – Bladder – Fallopian tube – Kidney – Spermatic cord – Stoma – Ureter – Urethra – Uterus – Vagina – Vas deferens	Leak, GU – *Select*	Asymptomatic, radiographic findings only	Symptomatic; medical intervention indicated	Symptomatic, interfering with GU function; invasive or endoscopic intervention indicated	Life-threatening	Death

REMARK: Leak (including anastomotic), GU – *Select* refers to clinical signs and symptoms or radiographic confirmation of anastomotic leak but without development of fistula.

RENAL/GENITOURINARY

Adverse Event	Short Name	Grade 1	Grade 2	Grade 3	Grade 4	Grade 5
Obstruction, GU – Select: – Bladder – Fallopian tube – Prostate – Spermatic cord – Stoma – Testes – Ureter – Urethra – Uterus – Vagina – Vas deferens	Obstruction, GU – Select	Asymptomatic, radiographic or endoscopic findings only	Symptomatic but no hydronephrosis, sepsis or renal dysfunction; dilation or endoscopic repair or stent placement indicated	Symptomatic and altered organ function (e.g., sepsis or hydronephrosis, or renal dysfunction); operative intervention indicated	Life-threatening consequences; organ failure or operative intervention requiring complete organ resection indicated	Death

NAVIGATION NOTE: Operative injury is graded as Intra-operative injury – Select Organ or Structure in the SURGERY/INTRA-OPERATIVE INJURY CATEGORY.

Adverse Event	Short Name	Grade 1	Grade 2	Grade 3	Grade 4	Grade 5
Perforation, GU – Select: – Bladder – Fallopian tube – Kidney – Ovary – Prostate – Spermatic cord – Stoma – Testes – Ureter – Urethra – Uterus – Vagina – Vas deferens	Perforation, GU – Select	Asymptomatic radiographic findings only	Symptomatic, associated with altered renal/GU function	Symptomatic, operative intervention indicated	Life-threatening consequences or organ failure; operative intervention requiring organ resection indicated	Death
Prolapse of stoma, GU	Prolapse stoma, GU	Asymptomatic; special intervention, extraordinary care not indicated	Extraordinary local care or maintenance; minor revision under local anesthesia indicated	Dysfunctional stoma; operative intervention or major stomal revision indicated	Life-threatening consequences	Death

REMARK: Other stoma complications may be graded as Fistula, GU – Select; Leak (including anastomotic), GU – Select; Obstruction, GU – Select; Perforation, GU – Select; Stricture/stenosis (including anastomotic), GU – Select.

Adverse Event	Short Name	Grade 1	Grade 2	Grade 3	Grade 4	Grade 5
Renal failure	Renal failure	—	—	Chronic dialysis not indicated	Chronic dialysis or renal transplant indicated	Death

ALSO CONSIDER: Glomerular filtration rate.

Adverse Event	Short Name	Grade				
		1	2	3	4	5
Stricture/stenosis (including anastomotic), GU – Select – Bladder – Fallopian tube – Prostate – Spermatic cord – Stoma – Testes – Ureter – Urethra – Uterus – Vagina – Vas deferens	Stricture, anastomotic, GU – Select	Asymptomatic, radiographic or endoscopic findings only	Symptomatic but no hydronephrosis, sepsis or renal dysfunction; dilation or endoscopic repair or stent placement indicated	Symptomatic and altered organ function (e.g., sepsis or hydronephrosis, or renal dysfunction); operative intervention indicated	Life-threatening consequences; organ failure or operative intervention requiring organ resection indicated	Death

ALSO CONSIDER: Obstruction, GU – Select.

Adverse Event	Short Name	1	2	3	4	5
Urinary electrolyte wasting (e.g., Fanconi's syndrome, renal tubular acidosis)	Urinary electrolyte wasting	Asymptomatic, intervention not indicated	Mild, reversible and manageable with replacement	Irreversible, requiring continued replacement	—	—

ALSO CONSIDER: Acidosis (metabolic or respiratory); Bicarbonate, serum-low; Calcium, serum-low (hypocalcemia); Phosphate, serum-low (hypophosphatemia).

Adverse Event	Short Name	1	2	3	4	5
Urinary frequency/urgency	Urinary frequency	Increase in frequency or nocturia up to 2 x normal; enuresis	Increase >2 x normal but <hourly	≥1 x/hr; urgency; catheter indicated	—	—
Urinary retention (including neurogenic bladder)	Urinary retention	Hesitancy or dribbling, no significant residual urine; retention occurring during the immediate postoperative period	Hesitancy requiring medication; or operative bladder atony requiring indwelling catheter beyond immediate postoperative period but for <6 weeks	More than daily catheterization indicated; urological intervention indicated (e.g., TURP, suprapubic tube, urethrotomy)	Life-threatening consequences; organ failure (e.g., bladder rupture); operative intervention requiring organ resection indicated	Death

REMARK: The etiology of retention (if known) is graded as Obstruction, GU – Select; Stricture/stenosis (including anastomotic), GU – Select.

ALSO CONSIDER: Obstruction, GU – Select; Stricture/stenosis (including anastomotic), GU – Select.

Adverse Event	Short Name	1	2	3	4	5
Urine color change	Urine color change	Present	—	—	—	—

REMARK: Urine color refers to change that is not related to other dietary or physiologic cause (e.g., bilirubin, concentrated urine, and hematuria).

Adverse Event	Short Name	1	2	3	4	5
Renal/Genitourinary – Other (Specify, __)	Renal – Other (Specify)	Mild	Moderate	Severe	Life-threatening; disabling	Death

SECONDARY MALIGNANCY

Adverse Event	Short Name	Grade				
		1	2	3	4	5
Secondary Malignancy – possibly related to cancer treatment (Specify, __)	Secondary Malignancy (possibly related to cancer treatment)	—	—	Non-life-threatening basal or squamous cell carcinoma of the skin	Solid tumor, leukemia or lymphoma	Death

REMARK: Secondary malignancy excludes metastasis from initial primary. Any malignancy possibly related to cancer treatment (including AML/MDS) should be reported via the routine reporting mechanisms outlined in each protocol. Important: Secondary Malignancy is an exception to NCI Expedited Adverse Event Reporting Guidelines. Secondary Malignancy is "Grade 4, present" but NCI does not require AdEERS Expedited Reporting for any (related or unrelated to treatment) Secondary Malignancy. A diagnosis of AML/MDS following treatment with an NCI-sponsored investigational agent is to be reported using the form available from the CTEP Web site at http://ctep.cancer.gov. Cancers not suspected of being treatment-related are not to be reported here.

SEXUAL/REPRODUCTIVE FUNCTION

Adverse Event	Short Name	Grade				
		1	2	3	4	5
Breast function/lactation	Breast function	Mammary abnormality, not functionally significant	Mammary abnormality, functionally significant	—	—	—
Breast nipple/areolar deformity	Nipple/areolar	Limited areolar asymmetry with no change in nipple/areolar projection	Asymmetry of nipple areolar complex with slight deviation in nipple projection	Marked deviation of nipple projection	—	—
Breast volume/hypoplasia	Breast	Minimal asymmetry; minimal hypoplasia	Asymmetry exists, ≤1/3 of the breast volume; moderate hypoplasia	Asymmetry exists, >1/3 of the breast volume; severe hypoplasia	—	—
REMARK: Breast volume is referenced with both arms straight overhead.						
NAVIGATION NOTE: Dysmenorrhea is graded as Pain – Select in the PAIN CATEGORY.						
NAVIGATION NOTE: Dyspareunia is graded as Pain – Select in the PAIN CATEGORY.						
NAVIGATION NOTE: Dysuria (painful urination) is graded as Pain – Select in the PAIN CATEGORY.						
Erectile dysfunction	Erectile dysfunction	Decrease in erectile function (frequency/rigidity of erections) but erectile aids not indicated	Decrease in erectile function (frequency/rigidity of erections), erectile aids indicated	Decrease in erectile function (frequency/rigidity of erections) but erectile aids not helpful; penile prosthesis indicated	—	—
Ejaculatory dysfunction	Ejaculatory dysfunction	Diminished ejaculation	Anejaculation or retrograde ejaculation	—	—	—
NAVIGATION NOTE: Feminization of male is graded in the ENDOCRINE CATEGORY.						
Gynecomastia	Gynecomastia	—	Asymptomatic breast enlargement	Symptomatic breast enlargement; intervention indicated	—	—
ALSO CONSIDER: Pain – Select.						
Infertility/sterility	Infertility/sterility	—	Male: oligospermia/low sperm count / Female: diminished fertility/ovulation	Male: sterile/azoospermia / Female: infertile/anovulatory	—	—
Irregular menses (change from baseline)	Irregular menses	1 – 3 months without menses	>3 – 6 months without menses but continuing menstrual cycles	Persistent amenorrhea for >6 months	—	—

SEXUAL/REPRODUCTIVE FUNCTION

Adverse Event	Short Name	Grade				
		1	2	3	4	5
Libido	Libido	Decrease in interest but not affecting relationship; intervention not indicated	Decrease in interest and adversely affecting relationship; intervention indicated	—	—	—
NAVIGATION NOTE: Masculinization of female is graded in the ENDOCRINE CATEGORY.						
Orgasmic dysfunction	Orgasmic function	Transient decrease	Decrease in orgasmic response requiring intervention	Complete inability of orgasmic response; not responding to intervention	—	—
NAVIGATION NOTE: Pelvic pain is graded as Pain – *Select* in the PAIN CATEGORY.						
NAVIGATION NOTE: Ulcers of the labia or perineum are graded as Ulceration in DERMATOLOGY/SKIN CATEGORY.						
Vaginal discharge (non-infectious)	Vaginal discharge	Mild	Moderate to heavy; pad use indicated	—	—	—
Vaginal dryness	Vaginal dryness	Mild	Interfering with sexual function; dyspareunia; intervention indicated	—	—	—
ALSO CONSIDER: Pain – *Select*.						
Vaginal mucositis	Vaginal mucositis	Erythema of the mucosa; minimal symptoms	Patchy ulcerations; moderate symptoms or dyspareunia	Confluent ulcerations; bleeding with trauma; unable to tolerate vaginal exam, sexual intercourse or tampon placement	Tissue necrosis; significant spontaneous bleeding; life-threatening consequences	—
Vaginal stenosis/length	Vaginal stenosis	Vaginal narrowing and/or shortening not interfering with function	Vaginal narrowing and/or shortening interfering with function	Complete obliteration; not surgically correctable	—	—
Vaginitis (not due to infection)	Vaginitis	Mild, intervention not indicated	Moderate, intervention indicated	Severe, not relieved with treatment; ulceration, but operative intervention not indicated	Ulceration and operative intervention indicated	—
Sexual/Reproductive Function – Other (Specify, __)	Sexual – Other (Specify)	Mild	Moderate	Severe	Disabling	Death

SURGERY/INTRA-OPERATIVE INJURY

NAVIGATION NOTE: Intra-operative hemorrhage is graded as Hemorrhage/bleeding associated with surgery, intra-operative or postoperative in the HEMORRHAGE/BLEEDING CATEGORY.

Adverse Event	Short Name	Grade				
		1	2	3	4	5
Intra-operative injury – Select Organ or Structure 'Select' AEs appear at the end of the CATEGORY.	Intraop injury – Select	Primary repair of injured organ/structure indicated	Partial resection of injured organ/structure indicated	Complete resection or reconstruction of injured organ/structure indicated	Life threatening consequences; disabling	—

REMARK: The 'Select' AEs are defined as significant, unanticipated injuries that are recognized at the time of surgery. These AEs do not refer to additional surgical procedures that must be performed because of a change in the operative plan based on intra-operative findings. Any sequelae resulting from the intra-operative injury that result in an adverse outcome for the patient must also be recorded and graded under the relevant CTCAE Term.

Intra-operative Injury – Other (Specify, __)	Intraop Injury – Other (Specify)	Primary repair of injured organ/structure indicated	Partial resection of injured organ/structure indicated	Complete resection or reconstruction of injured organ/structure indicated	Life threatening consequences; disabling	—

REMARK: Intra-operative Injury – Other (Specify, __) is to be used only to report an organ/structure not included in the 'Select' AEs found at the end of the CATEGORY. Any sequelae resulting from the intra-operative injury that result in an adverse outcome for the patient must also be recorded and graded under the relevant CTCAE Term.

AUDITORY/EAR
- Inner ear
- Middle ear
- Outer ear NOS
- Outer ear-Pinna

CARDIOVASCULAR
- Artery-aorta
- Artery-carotid
- Artery-cerebral
- Artery-extremity (lower)
- Artery-extremity (upper)
- Artery-hepatic
- Artery-major visceral artery
- Artery-pulmonary
- Artery NOS
- Heart
- Spleen
- Vein-extremity (lower)
- Vein-extremity (upper)
- Vein-hepatic
- Vein-inferior vena cava
- Vein-jugular
- Vein-major visceral vein
- Vein-portal vein
- Vein-pulmonary
- Vein-superior vena cava
- Vein NOS

DERMATOLOGY/SKIN
- Breast
- Nails
- Skin

ENDOCRINE
- Adrenal gland
- Parathyroid
- Pituitary

ENDOCRINE (*continued*)
- Thyroid

HEAD AND NECK
- Gingiva
- Larynx
- Lip/perioral area
- Face NOS
- Nasal cavity
- Nasopharynx
- Neck NOS
- Nose
- Oral cavity NOS
- Parotid gland
- Pharynx
- Salivary duct
- Salivary gland
- Sinus
- Teeth
- Tongue
- Upper aerodigestive NOS

GASTROINTESTINAL
- Abdomen NOS
- Anal sphincter
- Anus
- Appendix
- Cecum
- Colon
- Duodenum
- Esophagus
- Ileum
- Jejunum
- Oral
- Peritoneal cavity
- Rectum
- Small bowel NOS

GASTROINTESTINAL (*continued*)
- Stoma (GI)
- Stomach

HEPATOBILIARY/ PANCREAS
- Biliary tree-common bile duct
- Biliary tree-common hepatic duct
- Biliary tree-left hepatic duct
- Biliary tree-right hepatic duct
- Biliary tree NOS
- Gallbladder
- Liver
- Pancreas
- Pancreatic duct

MUSCULOSKELETAL
- Bone
- Cartilage
- Extremity-lower
- Extremity-upper
- Joint
- Ligament
- Muscle
- Soft tissue NOS
- Tendon

NEUROLOGY
- Brain
- Meninges
- Spinal cord

NERVES:
- Brachial plexus
- CN I (olfactory)
- CN II (optic)
- CN III (oculomotor)
- CN IV (trochlear)

NEUROLOGY (*continued*)

NERVES:
- CN V (trigeminal) motor
- CN V (trigeminal) sensory
- CN VI (abducens)
- CN VII (facial) motor-face
- CN VII (facial) sensory-taste
- CN VIII (vestibulocochlear)
- CN IX (glossopharyngeal) motor pharynx
- CN IX (glossopharyngeal) sensory ear-pharynx-tongue
- CN X (vagus)
- CN XI (spinal accessory)
- CN XII (hypoglossal)
- Cranial nerve or branch NOS
- Lingual
- Lung thoracic
- Peripheral motor NOS
- Peripheral sensory NOS
- Recurrent laryngeal
- Sacral plexus
- Sciatic
- Thoracodorsal

OCULAR
- Conjunctiva
- Cornea
- Eye NOS
- Lens
- Retina

PULMONARY/UPPER RESPIRATORY
- Bronchus
- Lung
- Mediastinum
- Pleura
- Thoracic duct
- Trachea
- Upper airway NOS

RENAL/GENITOURINARY
- Bladder
- Cervix
- Fallopian tube
- Kidney
- Ovary
- Pelvis NOS
- Penis
- Prostate
- Scrotum
- Testis
- Ureter
- Urethra
- Urinary conduit
- Urinary tract NOS
- Uterus
- Vagina
- Vulva

SYNDROMES

Adverse Event	Short Name	Grade				
		1	2	3	4	5

NAVIGATION NOTE: Acute vascular leak syndrome is graded in the VASCULAR CATEGORY.

NAVIGATION NOTE: Adrenal insufficiency is graded in the ENDOCRINE CATEGORY.

NAVIGATION NOTE: Adult Respiratory Distress Syndrome (ARDS) is graded in the PULMONARY/UPPER RESPIRATORY CATEGORY.

| Alcohol intolerance syndrome (antabuse-like syndrome) | Alcohol intolerance syndrome | — | — | Present | — | Death |

REMARK: An antabuse-like syndrome occurs with some new anti-androgens (e.g., nilutamide) when patient also consumes alcohol.

NAVIGATION NOTE: Autoimmune reaction is graded as Autoimmune reaction/hypersensitivity (including drug fever) in the ALLERGY/IMMUNOLOGY CATEGORY.

| Cytokine release syndrome/acute infusion reaction | Cytokine release syndrome | Mild reaction; infusion interruption not indicated; intervention not indicated | Requires therapy or infusion interruption but responds promptly to symptomatic treatment (e.g., antihistamines, NSAIDS, narcotics, IV fluids); prophylactic medications indicated for ≤24 hrs | Prolonged (i.e., not rapidly responsive to symptomatic medication and/or brief interruption of infusion); recurrence of symptoms following initial improvement; hospitalization indicated for other clinical sequelae (e.g., renal impairment, pulmonary infiltrates) | Life-threatening; pressor or ventilatory support indicated | Death |

REMARK: Cytokine release syndromes/acute infusion reactions are different from Allergic/hypersensitive reactions, although some of the manifestations are common to both AEs. An acute infusion reaction may occur with an agent that causes cytokine release (e.g., monoclonal antibodies or other biological agents). Signs and symptoms usually develop during or shortly after drug infusion and generally resolve completely within 24 hrs of completion of infusion. Signs/symptoms may include: Allergic reaction/hypersensitivity (including drug fever); Arthralgia (joint pain); Bronchospasm; Cough; Dizziness; Dyspnea (shortness of breath); Fatigue (asthenia, lethargy, malaise); Headache; Hypertension; Hypotension; Myalgia (muscle pain); Nausea; Pruritis/itching; Rash/desquamation; Rigors/chills; Sweating (diaphoresis); Tachycardia; Tumor pain (onset or exacerbation of tumor pain due to treatment); Urticaria (hives, welts, wheals); Vomiting.

ALSO CONSIDER: Allergic reaction/hypersensitivity (including drug fever); Bronchospasm, wheezing; Dyspnea (shortness of breath); Hypertension; Hypotension; Hypoxia; Prolonged QTc interval; Supraventricular and nodal arrhythmia – Select; Ventricular arrhythmia – Select.

NAVIGATION NOTE: Disseminated intravascular coagulation (DIC) is graded in the COAGULATION CATEGORY.

NAVIGATION NOTE: Fanconi's syndrome is graded as Urinary electrolyte wasting (e.g., Fanconi's syndrome, renal tubular acidosis) in the RENAL/GENITOURINARY CATEGORY.

| Flu-like syndrome | Flu-like syndrome | Symptoms present but not interfering with function | Moderate or causing difficulty performing some ADL | Severe symptoms interfering with ADL | Disabling | Death |

REMARK: Flu-like syndrome represents a constellation of symptoms which may include cough with catarrhal symptoms, fever, headache, malaise, myalgia, prostration, and is to be used when the symptoms occur in a cluster consistent with one single pathophysiological process.

NAVIGATION NOTE: Renal tubular acidosis is graded as Urinary electrolyte wasting (e.g., Fanconi's syndrome, renal tubular acidosis) in the RENAL/GENITOURINARY CATEGORY.

Adverse Event	Short Name	Grade				
		1	2	3	4	5
"Retinoic acid syndrome"	"Retinoic acid syndrome"	Fluid retention; less than 3 kg of weight gain; intervention with fluid restriction and/or diuretics indicated	Mild to moderate signs/ symptoms; steroids indicated	Severe signs/symptoms; hospitalization indicated	Life-threatening; ventilatory support indicated	Death

REMARK: Patients with acute promyelocytic leukemia may experience a syndrome similar to "retinoic acid syndrome" in association with other agents such as arsenic trioxide. The syndrome is usually manifested by otherwise unexplained fever, weight gain, respiratory distress, pulmonary infiltrates and/or pleural effusion, with or without leukocytosis.

ALSO CONSIDER: Acute vascular leak syndrome; Pleural effusion (non-malignant); Pneumonitis/pulmonary infiltrates.

NAVIGATION NOTE: SIADH is graded as Neuroendocrine: ADH secretion abnormality (e.g., SIADH or low ADH) in the ENDOCRINE CATEGORY.

NAVIGATION NOTE: Stevens-Johnson syndrome is graded as Rash: erythema multiforme (e.g., Stevens-Johnson syndrome, toxic epidermal necrolysis) in the DERMATOLOGY/SKIN CATEGORY.

NAVIGATION NOTE: Thrombotic microangiopathy is graded as Thrombotic microangiopathy (e.g., thrombotic thrombocytopenic purpura [TTP] or hemolytic uremic syndrome [HUS]) in the COAGULATION CATEGORY.

Adverse Event	Short Name	1	2	3	4	5
Tumor flare	Tumor flare	Mild pain not interfering with function	Moderate pain; pain or analgesics interfering with function, but not interfering with ADL	Severe pain; pain or analgesics interfering with function and interfering with ADL	Disabling	Death

REMARK: Tumor flare is characterized by a constellation of signs and symptoms in direct relation to initiation of therapy (e.g., anti-estrogens/androgens or additional hormones). The symptoms/signs include tumor pain, inflammation of visible tumor, hypercalcemia, diffuse bone pain, and other electrolyte disturbances.

ALSO CONSIDER: Calcium, serum-high (hypercalcemia).

Adverse Event	Short Name	1	2	3	4	5
Tumor lysis syndrome	Tumor lysis syndrome	—	—	Present	—	Death

ALSO CONSIDER: Creatinine; Potassium, serum-high (hyperkalemia).

Adverse Event	Short Name	1	2	3	4	5
Syndromes — Other (Specify, __)	Syndromes — Other (Specify)	Mild	Moderate	Severe	Life-threatening; disabling	Death

VASCULAR

Adverse Event	Short Name	Grade				
		1	2	3	4	5
Acute vascular leak syndrome	Acute vascular leak syndrome	—	Symptomatic; fluid support not indicated	Respiratory compromise or fluids indicated	Life-threatening; pressor support or ventilatory support indicated	Death
Peripheral arterial ischemia	Peripheral arterial ischemia	—	Brief (<24 hrs) episode of ischemia managed non-surgically and without permanent deficit	Recurring or prolonged (≥24 hrs) and/or invasive intervention indicated	Life-threatening; disabling and/or associated with end organ damage (e.g., limb loss)	Death
Phlebitis (including superficial thrombosis)	Phlebitis	—	Present	—	—	—

ALSO CONSIDER: Injection site reaction/extravasation changes.

Adverse Event	Short Name	Grade				
		1	2	3	4	5
Portal vein flow	Portal flow	—	Decreased portal vein flow	Reversal/retrograde portal vein flow	—	—
Thrombosis/embolism (vascular access-related)	Thrombosis/embolism (vascular access)	—	Deep vein thrombosis or cardiac thrombosis; intervention (e.g., anticoagulation, lysis, filter, invasive procedure) not indicated	Deep vein thrombosis or cardiac thrombosis; intervention (e.g., anticoagulation, lysis, filter, invasive procedure) indicated	Embolic event including pulmonary embolism or life-threatening thrombus	Death
Thrombosis/thrombus/embolism	Thrombosis/thrombus/embolism	—	Deep vein thrombosis or cardiac thrombosis; intervention (e.g., anticoagulation, lysis, filter, invasive procedure) not indicated	Deep vein thrombosis or cardiac thrombosis; intervention (e.g., anticoagulation, lysis, filter, invasive procedure) indicated	Embolic event including pulmonary embolism or life-threatening thrombus	Death
Vessel injury-artery – Select: – Aorta – Carotid – Extremity-lower – Extremity-upper – Other NOS – Visceral	Artery injury – Select	Asymptomatic diagnostic finding; intervention not indicated	Symptomatic (e.g., claudication); not interfering with ADL; repair or revision not indicated	Symptomatic interfering with ADL; repair or revision indicated	Life-threatening; disabling; evidence of end organ damage (e.g., stroke, MI, organ or limb loss)	Death

NAVIGATION NOTE: Vessel injury to an artery intra-operatively is graded as Intra-operative injury – Select Organ or Structure in the SURGERY/INTRA-OPERATIVE INJURY CATEGORY.

VASCULAR

Adverse Event	Short Name	Grade				
		1	2	3	4	5
Vessel injury-vein – Select: – Extremity-lower – Extremity-upper – IVC – Jugular – Other NOS – SVC – Viscera	Vein injury-vein – Select	Asymptomatic diagnostic finding; intervention not indicated	Symptomatic (e.g., claudication); not interfering with ADL; repair or revision not indicated	Symptomatic interfering with ADL; repair or revision indicated	Life-threatening; disabling; evidence of end organ damage	Death

NAVIGATION NOTE: Vessel injury to a vein intra-operatively is graded as Intra-operative injury – Select Organ or Structure in the SURGERY/INTRA-OPERATIVE INJURY CATEGORY.

Adverse Event	Short Name	1	2	3	4	5
Visceral arterial ischemia (non-myocardial)	Visceral arterial ischemia	—	Brief (<24 hrs) episode of ischemia managed medically and without permanent deficit	Prolonged (≥24 hrs) or recurring symptoms and/or invasive intervention indicated	Life-threatening; disabling; evidence of end organ damage	Death

ALSO CONSIDER: CNS cerebrovascular ischemia.

Adverse Event	Short Name	1	2	3	4	5
Vascular – Other (Specify, __)	Vascular – Other (Specify)	Mild	Moderate	Severe	Life-threatening; disabling	Death

DEPARTMENT OF HEALTH AND HUMAN SERVICES FOOD AND DRUG ADMINISTRATION	Form Approved: OMB No. 0910-0014. Expiration Date: May 31, 2009 See OMB Statement on Reverse.
INVESTIGATIONAL NEW DRUG APPLICATION (IND) *(TITLE 21, CODE OF FEDERAL REGULATIONS (CFR) PART 312)*	**NOTE:** No drug may be shipped or clinical investigation begun until an IND for that investigation is in effect (21 CFR 312.40).

1. NAME OF SPONSOR	2. DATE OF SUBMISSION

3. ADDRESS *(Number, Street, City, State, and Zip Code)*	4. TELEPHONE NUMBER *(Include Area Code)*

5. NAME(S) OF DRUG *(Include all available names: Trade, Generic, Chemical, Code)*	6. IND NUMBER *(If previously assigned)*

7. INDICATION(S) *(Covered by this submission)*

8. PHASE(S) OF CLINICAL INVESTIGATION TO BE CONDUCTED:

☐ PHASE 1 ☐ PHASE 2 ☐ PHASE 3 ☐ OTHER_____ *(Specify)*

9. LIST NUMBERS OF ALL INVESTIGATIONAL NEW DRUG APPLICATIONS (21 CFR Part 312), NEW DRUG OR ANTIBIOTIC APPLICATIONS *(21 CFR Part 314)*, DRUG MASTER FILES *(21 CFR Part 314.420)*, AND PRODUCT LICENSE APPLICATIONS (21 CFR Part 601) REFERRED TO IN THIS APPLICATION.

10. *IND submission should be consecutively numbered. The initial IND should be numbered "Serial number: 0000." The next submission (e.g., amendment, report, or correspondence) should be numbered "Serial Number: 0001." Subsequent submissions should be numbered consecutively in the order in which they are submitted.* SERIAL NUMBER ____ ____ ____ ____

11. THIS SUBMISSION CONTAINS THE FOLLOWING: *(Check all that apply)*

☐ INITIAL INVESTIGATIONAL NEW DRUG APPLICATION (IND) ☐ RESPONSE TO CLINICAL HOLD

PROTOCOL AMENDMENT(S): INFORMATION AMENDMENT(S): IND SAFETY REPORT(S):
☐ NEW PROTOCOL ☐ CHEMISTRY/MICROBIOLOGY ☐ INITIAL WRITTEN REPORT
☐ CHANGE IN PROTOCOL ☐ PHARMACOLOGY/TOXICOLOGY ☐ FOLLOW-UP TO A WRITTEN REPORT
☐ NEW INVESTIGATOR ☐ CLINICAL

☐ RESPONSE TO FDA REQUEST FOR INFORMATION ☐ ANNUAL REPORT ☐ GENERAL CORRESPONDENCE
☐ REQUEST FOR REINSTATEMENT OF IND THAT IS WITHDRAWN, INACTIVATED, TERMINATED OR DISCONTINUED ☐ OTHER _____ *(Specify)*

CHECK ONLY IF APPLICABLE

JUSTIFICATION STATEMENT MUST BE SUBMITTED WITH APPLICATION FOR ANY CHECKED BELOW. REFER TO THE CITED CFR SECTION FOR FURTHER INFORMATION.

☐ TREATMENT IND 21 CFR 312.35(b) ☐ TREATMENT PROTOCOL 21 CFR 312.35(a) ☐ CHARGE REQUEST/NOTIFICATION 21 CFR312.7(d)

FOR FDA USE ONLY

CDR/DBIND/DGD RECEIPT STAMP	DDR RECEIPT STAMP	DIVISION ASSIGNMENT:
		IND NUMBER ASSIGNED:

FORM FDA 1571 (4/06) PREVIOUS EDITION IS OBSOLETE. **PAGE 1 OF 2**

PSC Graphics: (301) 443-1090 EF

| 12. | **CONTENTS OF APPLICATION** |
| | This application contains the following items: *(Check all that apply)* |

☐ 1. Form FDA 1571 *[21 CFR 312.23(a)(1)]*

☐ 2. Table of contents *[21 CFR 312.23(a)(2)]*

☐ 3. Introductory statement *[21 CFR 312.23(a)(3)]*

☐ 4. General Investigational plan *[21 CFR 312.23(a)(3)]*

☐ 5. Investigator's brochure *[21 CFR 312.23(a)(5)]*

☐ 6. Protocol(s) *[21 CFR 312.23(a)(6)]*

      ☐ a. Study protocol(s) *[21 CFR 312.23(a)(6)]*

      ☐ b. Investigator data *[21 CFR 312.23(a)(6)(iii)(b)]* or completed Form(s) FDA 1572

      ☐ c. Facilities data *[21 CFR 312.23(a)(6)(iii)(b)]* or completed Form(s) FDA 1572

      ☐ d. Institutional Review Board data *[21 CFR 312.23(a)(6)(iii)(b)]* or completed Form(s) FDA 1572

☐ 7. Chemistry, manufacturing, and control data *[21 CFR 312.23(a)(7)]*

      ☐ Environmental assessment or claim for exclusion *[21 CFR 312.23(a)(7)(iv)(e)]*

☐ 8. Pharmacology and toxicology data *[21 CFR 312.23(a)(8)]*

☐ 9. Previous human experience *[21 CFR 312.23(a)(9)]*

☐ 10. Additional information *[21 CFR 312.23(a)(10)]*

---

13. IS ANY PART OF THE CLINICAL STUDY TO BE CONDUCTED BY A CONTRACT RESEARCH ORGANIZATION? ☐ YES ☐ NO

   IF YES, WILL ANY SPONSOR OBLIGATIONS BE TRANSFERRED TO THE CONTRACT RESEARCH ORGANIZATION? ☐ YES ☐ NO

   IF YES, ATTACH A STATEMENT CONTAINING THE NAME AND ADDRESS OF THE CONTRACT RESEARCH ORGANIZATION, IDENTIFICATION OF THE CLINICAL STUDY, AND A LISTING OF THE OBLIGATIONS TRANSFERRED.

---

14. NAME AND TITLE OF THE PERSON RESPONSIBLE FOR MONITORING THE CONDUCT AND PROGRESS OF THE CLINICAL INVESTIGATIONS

---

15. NAME(S) AND TITLE(S) OF THE PERSON(S) RESPONSIBLE FOR REVIEW AND EVALUATION OF INFORMATION RELEVANT TO THE SAFETY OF THE DRUG

I agree not to begin clinical investigations until 30 days after FDA's receipt of the IND unless I receive earlier notification by FDA that the studies may begin. I also agree not to begin or continue clinical investigations covered by the IND if those studies are placed on clinical hold. I agree that an Institutional Review Board (IRB) that complies with the requirements set fourth in 21 CFR Part 56 will be responsible for initial and continuing review and approval of each of the studies in the proposed clinical investigation. I agree to conduct the investigation in accordance with all other applicable regulatory requirements.

| 16. NAME OF SPONSOR OR SPONSOR'S AUTHORIZED REPRESENTATIVE | 17. SIGNATURE OF SPONSOR OR SPONSOR'S AUTHORIZED REPRESENTATIVE | |
| 18. ADDRESS *(Number, Street, City, State, and Zip Code)* | 19. TELEPHONE NUMBER *(Include Area Code)* | 20. DATE |

(**WARNING:** A willfully false statement is a criminal offense. U.S.C. Title 18, Sec. 1001.)

Public reporting burden for this collection of information is estimated to average 100 hours per response, including the time for reviewing instructions, searching existing data sources, gathering and maintaining the data needed, and completing reviewing the collection of information. Send comments regarding this burden estimate or any other aspect of this collection of information, including suggestions for reducing this burden to:

Department of Health and Human Services
Food and Drug Administration
Center for Drug Evaluation and Research (HFD-143)
Central Document Room
5901-B Ammendale Road
Beltsville, MD 20705-1266

Department of Health and Human Services
Food and Drug Administration
Center for Biologics Evaluation and Research (HFM-99)
1401 Rockville Pike
Rockville, MD 20852-1448

"An agency may not conduct or sponsor, and a person is not required to respond to, a collection of information unless it displays a currently valid OMB control number."

Please DO NOT RETURN this application to this address.

DEPARTMENT OF HEALTH AND HUMAN SERVICES
FOOD AND DRUG ADMINISTRATION

STATEMENT OF INVESTIGATOR
(TITLE 21, CODE OF FEDERAL REGULATIONS (CFR) PART 312)
(See instructions on reverse side.)

Form Approved: OMB No. 0910-0014.
Expiration Date: May 31, 2009.
See OMB Statement on Reverse.

NOTE: No investigator may participate in an investigation until he/she provides the sponsor with a completed, signed Statement of Investigator, Form FDA 1572 (21 CFR 312.53(c)).

1. NAME AND ADDRESS OF INVESTIGATOR.

2. EDUCATION, TRAINING, AND EXPERIENCE THAT QUALIFIES THE INVESTIGATOR AS AN EXPERT IN THE CLINICAL INVESTIGATION OF THE DRUG FOR THE USE UNDER INVESTIGATION. ONE OF THE FOLLOWING IS ATTACHED.

☐ CURRICULUM VITAE   ☐ OTHER STATEMENT OF QUALIFICATIONS

3. NAME AND ADDRESS OF ANY MEDICAL SCHOOL, HOSPITAL, OR OTHER RESEARCH FACILITY WHERE THE CLINICAL INVESTIGATION(S) WILL BE CONDUCTED.

4. NAME AND ADDRESS OF ANY CLINICAL LABORATORY FACILITIES TO BE USED IN THE STUDY.

5. NAME AND ADDRESS OF THE INSTITUTIONAL REVIEW BOARD (IRB) THAT IS RESPONSIBLE FOR REVIEW AND APPROVAL OF THE STUDY(IES).

6. NAMES OF THE SUBINVESTIGATORS *(e.g., research fellows, residents, associates)* WHO WILL BE ASSISTING THE INVESTIGATOR IN THE CONDUCT OF THE INVESTIGATION(S).

7. NAME AND CODE NUMBER, IF ANY, OF THE PROTOCOL(S) IN THE IND FOR THE STUDY(IES) TO BE CONDUCTED BY THE INVESTIGATOR.

FORM FDA 1572 (5/06)   PREVIOUS EDITION IS OBSOLETE   PAGE 1 OF 2

8. ATTACH THE FOLLOWING CLINICAL PROTOCOL INFORMATION:

☐ FOR PHASE 1 INVESTIGATIONS, A GENERAL OUTLINE OF THE PLANNED INVESTIGATION INCLUDING THE ESTIMATED DURATION OF THE STUDY AND THE MAXIMUM NUMBER OF SUBJECTS THAT WILL BE INVOLVED.

☐ FOR PHASE 2 OR 3 INVESTIGATIONS, AN OUTLINE OF THE STUDY PROTOCOL INCLUDING AN APPROXIMATION OF THE NUMBER OF SUBJECTS TO BE TREATED WITH THE DRUG AND THE NUMBER TO BE EMPLOYED AS CONTROLS, IF ANY; THE CLINICAL USES TO BE INVESTIGATED; CHARACTERISTICS OF SUBJECTS BY AGE, SEX, AND CONDITION; THE KIND OF CLINICAL OBSERVATIONS AND LABORATORY TESTS TO BE CONDUCTED; THE ESTIMATED DURATION OF THE STUDY; AND COPIES OR A DESCRIPTION OF CASE REPORT FORMS TO BE USED.

9. COMMITMENTS:

I agree to conduct the study(ies) in accordance with the relevant, current protocol(s) and will only make changes in a protocol after notifying the sponsor, except when necessary to protect the safety, rights, or welfare of subjects.

I agree to personally conduct or supervise the described investigation(s).

I agree to inform any patients, or any persons used as controls, that the drugs are being used for investigational purposes and I will ensure that the requirements relating to obtaining informed consent in 21 CFR Part 50 and institutional review board (IRB) review and approval in 21 CFR Part 56 are met.

I agree to report to the sponsor adverse experiences that occur in the course of the investigation(s) in accordance with 21 CFR 312.64.

I have read and understood the information in the investigator's brochure, including the potential risks and side effects of the drug.

I agree to ensure that all associates, colleagues, and employees assisting in the conduct of the study(ies) are informed about their obligations in meeting the above commitments.

I agree to maintain adequate and accurate records in accordance with 21 CFR 312.62 and to make those records available for inspection in accordance with 21 CFR 312.68.

I will ensure that an IRB that complies with the requirements of 21 CFR Part 56 will be responsible for the initial and continuing review and approval of the clinical investigation. I also agree to promptly report to the IRB all changes in the research activity and all unanticipated problems involving risks to human subjects or others. Additionally, I will not make any changes in the research without IRB approval, except where necessary to eliminate apparent immediate hazards to human subjects.

I agree to comply with all other requirements regarding the obligations of clinical investigators and all other pertinent requirements in 21 CFR Part 312.

INSTRUCTIONS FOR COMPLETING FORM FDA 1572
STATEMENT OF INVESTIGATOR:

1. Complete all sections. Attach a separate page if additional space is needed.

2. Attach curriculum vitae or other statement of qualifications as described in Section 2.

3. Attach protocol outline as described in Section 8.

4. Sign and date below.

5. FORWARD THE COMPLETED FORM AND ATTACHMENTS TO THE SPONSOR. The sponsor will incorporate this information along with other technical data into an Investigational New Drug Application (IND). INVESTIGATORS SHOULD NOT SEND THIS FORM DIRECTLY TO THE FOOD AND DRUG ADMINISTRATION.

10. SIGNATURE OF INVESTIGATOR   11. DATE

(WARNING: A willfully false statement is a criminal offense. U.S.C. Title 18, Sec. 1001.)

Public reporting burden for this collection of information is estimated to average 100 hours per response, including the time for reviewing instructions, searching existing data sources, gathering and maintaining the data needed, and completing reviewing the collection of information. Send comments regarding this burden estimate or any other aspect of this collection of information, including suggestions for reducing this burden to:

Department of Health and Human Services
Food and Drug Administration
Center for Drug Evaluation and Research (HFD-143)
Central Document Room
5901-B Ammendale Road
Beltsville, MD 20705-1266

Department of Health and Human Services
Food and Drug Administration
Center for Biologics Evaluation and Research (HFM-99)
1401 Rockville Pike
Rockville, MD 20852-1448

"An agency may not conduct or sponsor, and a person is not required to respond to, a collection of information unless it displays a currently valid OMB control number."

Please DO NOT RETURN this application to this address.

FORM FDA 1572 (5/06)   PAGE 2 OF 2

Index

A

Accuracy, 69–70. *See also* Precision
  strategies for
    general strategies, 75
    instrument strategies, 76
    intervention strategies, 77
    observer strategies, 76
    subject strategies, 76
ACE inhibitors. *See* Angiotensin converting enzyme (ACE) inhibitors
Active arm, 96
Active extension designs, 115–116
Adaptive randomization, 89
  balancing, 89–90
  response, 90
Add-on design, 117
Adverse event
  classification of, 354–356
  defined, 137, 353
Agent-based model, 229
Aggregate data, 4, 318, 343–344, 369–370
Allocations, study groups
  allocation concealment, 87–88
  randomization. *See* Randomization
  subject assignments, 87
Analysis of endpoints
  frequency analysis, 126–127
  landmark analysis, 126
  repeated measure analysis, 127
  slope of change, 127
  time-to-event, 127–128
Anecdotal data, 4
Angiotensin converting enzyme (ACE) inhibitors, 3
Approval process
  of drugs. *See* Drug development and approval
  of medical devices. *See* Medical devices, approval process
Associational studies, 79
Assumptions, 305–306
  invalid assumption, 307
Audits
  CRO, 252
  FDA audits, 250–251
  investigator audits, 252–253
  overview, 250
  sponsor, 251–252
Autonomy, of patients, 28–29

B

Bayes' Theorem, 221–222
Beecher, Henry K., 19
Bell-shaped curves. *See* Normal distribution
Belmont Report, 19, 22–27
Beneficence, 27
Biased samples, 45
Biases, 72, 75
Bioequivalence, 352
Blinding
  biases and rationale for, 91–92
  breaking, 94
  techniques, 93–94
  types, 92–93
    double-blind, 93
    single-blind, 93
Blocked randomization, 88–89
Bonferroni correction, 346
Bootstrapping, 227–228

C

Case-controlled study, 6
Categorical variables, 64–65
Categorizing data, 318–319
Central limit theorem, 50–51
Central tendency
  arithmetic mean (average), 45–46
  defined, 45
  median, 46
Chi-square test, 334
Clinical development plan, 237
Clinical operations
  budgets, 263–264
  CRA, 263
  CRO

Clinical operations (*continued*)
managing and monitoring, 265–266
selection, 264–265
CSC, 269
site monitoring and compliance, 267–269
study conduct report, 269
Clinical relevance, of endpoints
determinants of, 124–125
overview, 123–124
Clinical research associate (CRA), 263
Clinical study coordinator (CSC), 269
Clinical trial medicine (CTM)
characteristics, 9–10
defined, 3
as methodological science, 3–4
practice of, 11
Clinical trials
design
principles, 15
variables, 15–16
design principles, 15
limitations of
assumptions, 8
effectiveness, 7
generalizability, 7
performance criteria, 12–15
rationale for
regulatory, 7
scientific, 6–7
Cluster designs. *See* Nested designs
Cluster randomized studies, 379
Cohort study, 6
Comparative statistics, 43–44
Comparators, 80–81
Compartment model, 228–229
Composite endpoints
efficacy of, 131–133
types of, 133–135
Conclusions
endpoint, 387
external validity, 386
patient population, 386–387
relative *vs.* absolute difference, 387
risk-benefit analysis, 388
Concurrent control group, 81
Conditional probability, 213–214
Confidence interval, 54–56, 329–330
Confidentiality, 29
Confounding, 344–345
Construct validity, 78
Content validity, 77–78
Continuous variables, 327
Contract research organizations (CRO)
audits, 252
managing and monitoring, 265–266
selection, 264–265
Control
active control, 86–87
defined, 80
dose control, 86

general considerations, 83–85
comparison groups, 84
early escape, 84
internal *vs.* external control, 84–85
no-treatment control, 86
placebo control, 85–86
sham control, 86
Control group. *See* Control
Controlled experiment or trial, 80–81
Convergent validity, 78
Co-primary endpoints, 130–131
Corrective action, 253–254
Correlation
highly correlated, 51
linearly correlated, 51
negatively correlated, 51
Pearson's correlation, 51–52
poorly correlated, 51
positively correlated, 51
Spearman's rho, 52
Costs and rewards, valuation
intangible, 150–151
tangible, 148–150
CRA. *See* Clinical research associate (CRA)
Criterion validity, 78
CRO. *See* Contract research organizations (CRO)
Crossover study analysis, 351
Crossover trial, 101
Cross-sectional study, defined, 6
CSC. *See* Clinical study coordinator (CSC)
CTM. *See* Clinical trial medicine (CTM)
Cumulative probability, 214–215

D
Data analysis
bioequivalence, 352–353
confounding, 344–345
crossover study, 351
descriptive statistics
comparison of variables, 327–328
single variables, 325–327
factorial analysis, 351
inferential statistics. *See* Inferential statistics
interactions, 345
pharmacodynamics, 352
pharmacokinetics, 352
primary endpoint, 345–348
regression discontinuity analysis, 353
safety analysis. *See* Safety analysis, of data
secondary endpoints, 349–351
sensitivity analysis, 348–349
tests selection, 342–344
Database
design, 270
lock, 271
Data interpretation
aggregate data, 369–370
cluster randomized studies, 379
equivalence studies, 379
erroneous analysis, 367–368

flawed study design, 364–365
instrumental valriable, 381
oncology data, 378–379
overview, 361–362
pharmacodynamics (PD), 380–381
pharmacokinetics (PK), 379–380
primary enpoint, 368–369
p-value assessment, 362–364
safety data, 381–386
statistical common errors, 370–374
study execution, 365–367
subgroup analysis, 374–377
survival data, 377–378
validation, 362
Data management
CRF, 270
database
design, 270
lock, 271
data entry, 270
electronic data capture (EDC), 270–271
listings, 271–273
monitoring, 271
quality, 271
Data quality
aggregating data, 318
categorizing data, 318–319
correction, 318
data validation, 314
data verification, 313–314
deriving data, 318
error detection, 317–318
importance and format, 303
incomplete data, 313
measures, 303–305
missing data, 307–308
dealing with, 309–313
patient dropouts, 308–309
Data Safety Monitoring Board (DSMB), 30
Decision analysis, 224
decision trees, 225
expected values, 224–225
Declaration of Helsinki, 19, 20–21
Degrees of freedom (df), 50
Descriptive statistics, 43
comparison of variables, 327–328
single variables, 325–327
Deterministic model, 227
Digoxin, 5
Discrete event simulation, 229
Discriminant validity, 78
Dispersion. *See* Spread (dispersion or variability)
Dose
components of
administration routes, 197–199
baseline characteristics, 195
flat doses, 194–195
interval and duration, 196–197
titrated or adaptive, 195–196
control, 86

defined, 182–183
escalation, 201–204
within-patient designs, 103
phase I studies
dose escalation, 201–204
starting dose, 199–201
response. *See* Dose-response
response parameters, 204–206
selection
challenges, 184–185
definitions, 183–184
design issues, 185
definitions and objective, 183–184
Dose-response
curve, 190–193
standard model, 193–194
study-design
choosing target dose, 207
trial design options, 208–210
Dosing. *See* Dose
Double-blind, 93
"Drop the Loser" design, 109
Drug development and approval, in US
clinical studies, 34–35
IND application, 33–34
label review, 36
new drug application (NDA), 35–36
overview, 32
post-market surveillance of, 39
pre-clinical development, 32–33
special mechanisms in, 36–37
Drug supply, 278–279
DSMB. *See* Data Safety Monitoring Board (DSMB)

E
Early-escape design, 116–117
Economic analysis
arena, 146–147
audience in, 146
importance, 145–146
incremental analysis, 153–154
perspective, 147
selection of, 152–153
sensitivity analysis, 154
time, 147–148
valuation
costs and rewards, 148–151
externalities, 151
measuring rewards, 151–152
productivity losses, 151
Effectiveness, of clinical trials, 7
Endpoints, 141–144
analysis
frequency analysis, 126–127
landmark analysis, 126
repeated measure analysis, 127
slope of change, 127
time-to-event, 127–128
characteristics of, 121–123
clinical relevance of, 123–125

Endpoints (*continued*)
    composite. *See* Composite endpoints
    co-primary, 130–131
    and measures, 65
    overview, 123–124
    primary, 129–130
    responsiveness, endpoints, 125
        susceptibility to treatment, 129
Epidemiological studies, 79
Epidemiology, 5
    disease outcomes, 218–219
    risk, 216–218
Equivalence studies, 379
Erroneous analysis, in data interpretation, 367–368
Ethical principles
    acceptance, 29
    beneficence, 27
    confidentiality, 29
    freedom of religion and beliefs, 29
    human dignity, 29
    informed consent, 27–28
    justice, 28
    maleficence, 27
    open access, 28
    patient's autonomy, 28–29
    privacy, 29
    tolerance, 29
European Union
    clinical trial directive, 246–247
    data protection directive, 247
Evidence-based medicine, 4
Explanatory studies, 79–80
External control, 84–85

F
Face validity, 77
Factorial analysis, 351
Factorial designs, 104–106
FDA. *See* Food and Drug Administration (FDA)
Financial disclosure regulations, in U.S., 247–248
Fisher's exact test, 334
Flat doses, 194–195
Flawed study design, 364–365
Flexible designs, 96–97
    sequential designs
        group design. *See* Group sequential design
        individual design, 108
Food and Drug Administration (FDA), 244
    audits, 250–251
    CRO, 265–266
    definitions, 279–280
    drug development and approval process, 32–37
    GMP, 31–32
    on informed consent, 256
    internal compliance manual, 389–407
    medical device approval, 37–39
    meetings, 274–277
    pressure-tests by, 362
    site monitoring, 267–268
    TPP, 235

Fraud, 254
Freedom of religion and beliefs, 29
Frequency analysis, 126–127
F-test (ANOVA), 333

G
Gaussian distributions. *See* Normal distribution
GCP. *See* Good clinical practice
Generalizability, of clinical trials, 7
Good clinical practice (GCP), 243–244
    content, 245
Good Manufacturing Practices (GMP), 31–32
Group sequential design
    defined, 108
    dose modification, 109–110
    "Drop the Loser", 109
    "Play the Winner", 109
GXP
    good clinical practice (GCP), 243–244
        content, 244–245
    international data, 249
    overview, 242
    quality system, 249
    regulations, 245–249
    standard operating procedures (SOP), 249
    training, 249–250

H
HDE. *See* Humanitarian Device Exemption (HDE)
Health economics. *See* Economic analysis
Health Insurance Portability and Accountability Act (HIPAA), 30–31, 245–246
Hierarchical designs. *See* Nested designs
HIPAA. *See* Health Insurance Portability and Accountability Act (HIPAA)
Holm correction, 347
Human dignity, 29
Human experimentation
    Belmont Report, 19, 22–27
    Declaration of Helsinki, 19, 20–21
    Nremberg Code, 18–19
    Tuskegee Experiment, 19
Humanitarian Device Exemption (HDE), 38
Humanitarian Use Device (HUD), defined, 38
Hypothesis testing
    confidence interval, 54–56
    null hypothesis, 52–53
    one-tail and two-tail tests, 54
    type I and II errors, 53–54

I
Incremental analysis, in economic analysis, 153–154
IND application. *See* Investigational new drug (IND) application
Induction period, 111–112
Inferential statistics, 44
    background, 328
    comparing multiple samples, 330
    confidence interval, 329–330
    Friedman test, 340
    F-test (ANOVA), 333

multiple measurements, 338–339
nested datasets, 338
nominal variables, analysis
Chi-square test, 334
Fisher's exact test, 334
z -test, 333–334
ordinal variables, analysis
Kruskal-Wallis test, 335–336
Mann-Whitney rank sum test, 335
paired tests, 338
paired t-tests, 339
parametric *vs.* nonparametric tests, 331–332
p-value, 330–331
ratio t-test, 339
regression, 340–342
repeated measures analysis of variance, 339–340
standard error, 329–330
survival curves, 336–337
t-test, 332–333
Wilcoxon signed rank sum test, 340
Informed consent, 27–28, 255–257
Institutional Review Board (IRB), 29–30
Instrumental variable, in data interpretation, 381
Intention to treat (ITT) analyses, 321–323
Interactions, 345
Interactive voice response system (IVRS), 278–279
Interim analysis, 358
Internal control, 84–85
International Conference on Harmonization and Good Clinical Practices (ICH GCP), 31
Intervention, defined, 181–182
Investigational Device Exemption (IDE), 38
Investigational new drug (IND) application, 33–34
Investigator audits, 252–253
Investigator's Brochure, 257–259
IRB. *See* Institutional Review Board

J
Joint probability, 214
Justice, 28

K
Kruskal-Wallis test, 335–336
Kurtosis, 47–48

L
Label review of drugs, 36
Landmark analysis, 126
Latin square design, 101–103
Least-squared regression, 341
Limitations, of clinical trials, 7–8
assumptions, 8
effectiveness, 7
generalizability, 7
Limited data set, 30
Linear programming, 226
Listings, 271–273

M
Maleficence, 27
Mann-Whitney rank sum test, 335

Manufacturing standards
GMP, 31–32
ICH GCP, 31
Masking. *See* Blinding
Measurement errors
biases, 72, 75
instrument variability, 74–75
observer variability, 73–74
random, 72
subject variability, 73
Measures
accuracy. *See* Accuracy
affecting design of trials, 66–67
defined, 61
and endpoints, 65
errors. *See* Measurement errors
obstacles to, 69
Precision. *See* Accuracy
purposes of, 65–66
selection of, 67–69
types of, 62–65
validity, 76–78
Medical devices
approval process, 37
HDE, 38
pre-market approval, 38
pre-market notification 510(k), 38
defined, 37
post-market surveillance of, 39
Medical monitoring, 254–255, 259–260
report writing, 262–263
safety monitoring, 262
Meta-analysis
effect size, 222
steps in
analysis, 223–224
data abstraction, 223
paring down studies, 222–223
Missing data, 307–308
dealing, 309–313
Models
agent-based model, 229
compartment model, 228–229
deterministic, 227
simulation. *See* Simulation
stochastic, 227
validation, 227
Monte Carlo simulation, 227
Multi-center sites, 283
Multiple arm design, 98–99

N
Natural history study, 79
Nested designs, 106–108
New drug application (NDA), 35–36
Nocebo effect, 82
Nominal variables, 325–326
Noninferiority studies, 352–353
Normal distribution
importance of, 48

Normal distribution (*continued*)
    standard, 49
    t-distribution, 49–50
Null hypothesis, 52–53
Numeric variables, 326–327
Nuremberg Code, 18–19

O
Oncology data, 378–379
One-tail tests, 54, 58
Open access, 28
Open-level follow up study, 113
Operator dependency, of intervention, 181–182
Ordinal variables, 326
    Kruskal-Wallis test, 335–336
    Mann-Whitney rank sum test, 335

P
Paired tests, 338
Parallel designs
    multiple arm design, 98–99
    single-arm design, 97–98
Patient recruitment
    screening
        noncompliant subjects, 295–296
        qualifiers *vs.* nonqualifiers, 295
    strategies
        broad strategies, 289–293
        general, 285–287
        selection, 287–289
        targeted, 293–295
Patient reported outcome (PRO)
    collection of, 155–156
    free text, 163–164
    instruments for
        administration, 157–158
        development, 156–157
    questionnaire
        characteristics, 158–160
        closed-ended, 160
        open-ended, 160
    response options
        characteristics of, 160–161
        multiple choice questions, 161–162
        rank order, 162
        response scales, 162–163
    response rate
        nonresponse bias, 164
        strategies for, 165
    roles and uses, 154–155
Patients. *See also* Study group
    autonomy of, 28–29
    characteristics, 168–169
    conditions, 167–168
    discontinuers, 297–298
    diseases, 167–168
    dropouts, 296–297
    judgment to choose, 169–171
    recruitment. *See* Patient recruitment
    response. *See* Patient reported outcome (PRO)

retention strategies, 298–299
sampling
    clinical trial characteristics, 179–180
    process, 176–179
    selection criteria
        defined, 171–172
        patients to exclude, 175–176
        patients to include, 172, 173–175
Pearson's correlation, 51–52
Periods
    defined, 95–96
    induction period, 111–112
    run-in period, 110–111
    screening period, 112
    treatment administration and follow-up. *See* Treatment administration and follow-up
Pharmaceutical approval process, in US. *See* Drug development and approval, in US
Pharmacodynamics (PD), 380–381
Pharmacoeconomics. *See* Economic analysis
Pharmacokinetics (PK), 352, 379–380
    concepts, 185–189
    factors affecting, 189–190
    therapeutic drug monitoring (TDM), 190
Pharmacovigilance, 279–282
Placebos, 116
    challenges with, 82–83
    control, 85–86
    defined, 81
    placebo effect, 81–82
"Play the Winner" design, 109
Population pharmacodynamics (PD), 206–207
Population pharmacokinetics (PK), 206–207
Power
    defined, 56
    determinants of
        between-subject *vs.* within-subject designs, 57–58
        effect size, 56–57
        sample size, 57
        significance level (a), 57
        two-tails *vs.* one tail test, 58
        variance, 57
Precision, 69–70
    measurements, 71–72
    strategies for
        general strategies, 75
        instrument strategies, 76
        intervention strategies, 77
        observer strategies, 76
        subject strategies, 76
Pregnant patients, 210–211
Pre-market approval, of medical devices, 38
Pre-market notification 510(k), 38
Primary endpoint, 345–348
    Bonferroni correction, 346
    hierarchical testing, 347–348
    Holm correction, 347
    multiple comparison, 346
Primary endpoints, 129–130
Privacy, 29

Privacy Rule, 30–31
Probability
  conditional, 213–214
  cumulative, 214–215
  joint, 214
  sequential events, 215–216
Productivity losses, 151
Project management, 233–235
  clinical development program, 237
  flowcharting, 237–239
  key players in, 239–240
  sponsor teams, 240
  TPP, 235–236
Protected health information (PHI), 30
Protection of patients' rights. *See* Rights and welfare protection
Protocol
  compliances, 315–317
  development, 255
  deviations, 314–315
  violations, 260–261, 315
  waivers, 261–262
p-value assessment, in data interpretation, 362–364

Q
Quantitative variables, 62–64

R
Random errors, 72
Randomization
  adaptive, 89
    balancing, 89–90
    response, 90
  blocked, 88–89
  simple, 88
  stratified, 89
Randomized withdrawal designs, 115
Random samples
  simple, 45
  stratified, 45
Range, 46
Rank sum test, 335
Rationale, for clinical trials
  regulatory, 7
  scientific, 6–7
Reed, Walter, 18
Regression discontinuity analysis, 353
Regression lines, 340–341
Regulations
  human experimentation. *See* Human experimentation
  reasons for, 17–18
Regulatory agencies, interaction with, 273–278
Repeated measure analysis, 127
Report writing, medical monitoring, 262–263
Responsiveness, endpoints, 125. *See also* Analysis of endpoints
  susceptibility to treatment, 129
Retention strategies, for patients, 298–299
Rights and welfare protection
  DSMB, 30
  HIPAA, 30–31
  IRB, 29–30

Rules and regulations. *See* Regulations
Run-in period, 110–111

S
Safety analysis
  adverse event
    classification of, 354–356
    defined, 353
  descriptive analysis, 356–358
  goals of, 354
  limitations of, 354
Safety data, 381–386
Safety endpoints
  anticipated safety events, 136
  characteristics of, 135–136
  classification, 137
  collection, 137
  harbinger safety events, 136–137
  special conditions, 137–138
  unanticipated safety events, 137
Samples
  biased, 45
  defined, 44
  random, 45
  size
    calculation of, 59–60
    determinants of, 58–59
Sampling distributions
  central limit theorem, 50–51
  standard error, 50
Scientific rationale, for clinical trials, 6–7
Screening period, 112
Secondary endpoints, 131, 349–350
  subendpoint analysis, 351
  subgroup analysis, 350–351
Semi-interquartile range, 46
Sensitivity analysis, 348–349
  economic analysis, 154
Sequence, defined, 96
Sequential designs
Sequential events, probability in, 215–216
Sham devices, 82
Shape, 46–48
  kurtosis, 47–48
  skew, 47
Simulation
  discrete event, 229
  Monte Carlo, 227
  role of, 226–227
Single-arm design, 97–98
Single-blind, 93
Single site, 283
Single variables
  continuous variables, 327
  nominal variables, 325–326
  numeric variables, 326–327
  ordinal variables, 326
Site selection
  characteristics, 284–285
  international sites, 283–284

Site selection (*continued*)
    multi-center sites, 283
    single site, 283
Skew, 47
Slope of change analysis, 127
Spearman's rho, 52
Special population, 211–212
Spread (dispersion or variability), 46
Staggered start designs, 116
Standard deviation, 46
Standard error, 50
Standard normal distribution, 49
Statistical common errors, in data interpretation, 370–374
Statistics
    comparative, 43–44
    correlation. *See* Correlation
    descriptive, 43
    hypothesis testing. *See* Hypothesis testing
    inferential, 44
    normal distribution, 48–50
    and parameters
        central tendency, 45–46
        shape, 46–47
        spread (dispersion or variability), 46
    power, 56–58
    samples, 44–45
    sample size, 58–60
    sampling distribution, 50–51
    statistical analysis plan, 269–270
Stochastic model, 227
Stratified randomization, 89
Study arm, defined, 96
Study execution, 365–367
Study groups
    allocations
        concealment, 87–88
        randomization. *See* Randomization
        subject assignments, 87
    blinding. *See* Blinding
    comparators, 80–81
    control group. *See* Controls
    placebos. *See* Placebos
    sham devices, 82
Study population. *See* Patients
Subgroup analysis, 350–351, 374–377
Surrogate endpoints
    high quality endpoints, 139
    urgency for, 138–139
    validation of, 139–140
Survival data, 377–378
Systematic errors. *See* Biases

T
Target produce profile (TPP), 236–237
T-distribution, 49–50
Testing
    Bayes' Theorem, 221–222
    test performance, 219–221
Test performance, 219–221
Tests selection, 342

aggregate data, 343–344
assumptions, 343
Time, economic analysis
    predictive analyses, 147
    retrospective analyses, 147
    time frame, 147–148
    and value, 148
Time-to-event analysis, 127–128
Timing, 95
Tolerance, 29
TPP. *See* Target produce profile (TPP)
Traditional designs, 96–97
    factorial designs, 104–106
    nested designs, 106–108
    parallel designs
        multiple arm design, 98–99
        single-arm design, 97–98
    within-patient designs. *See* Within-patient designs
Transformation, of data
    application of, 321
    data sets, 321
    ITT analysis, 321–323
    per protocol analysis, 323
    types of, 319–321
Treatment administration and follow-up
    event-driven studies, 112–113
    open-level follow up, 113
    post-study follow up, 113
Treatment arm, 96
Tuskegee Experiment, 19
Two-tail tests, 54, 58

U
Uncontrolled clinical trial, 79

V
Validity
    construct validity, 78
    content validity, 77–78
    convergent validity, 78
    criterion validity, 78
    definition of, 77
    discriminant validity, 78
    face validity, 77
Valuation, economic analysis
    costs and rewards
        intangible, 150–151
        tangible, 148–150
    externalities, 151
    measuring rewards, 151–152
    productivity losses, 151
    tangible costs and rewards, 148–150
Variability. *See also* Spread (dispersion or variability)
    instrument, 74–75
    observer variability, 73–74
    subject variability, 73
Variables. *See also* Measures
    categorical, 64–65
    comparison of, 327–328
    defined, 65

quantitative, 62–64
single. *See* Single variables
Variance, 46

W
Withdrawal designs, 114–115
Within-patient designs
crossover trial, 101

dose escalation in, 103
Latin square design, 101–103
rationale, 99–101
World Medical Association Declaration of Helsinki, 19, 20–21

Z
Z -test, 333–334

Back Cover

Richard Y. Chin, MD
San Francisco, California, USA

Dr. Chin is currently President and CEO of Oxigene, a biotechnology company. Previously, he was Senior Vice President and Head of Global Development for Elan Corporation, Head of Clinical Research for the Biotherapeutics Unit at Genentech, and adjunct clinical faculty at Stanford Medical School. Dr. Chin is a Board Certified internist with extensive drug development experience across a wide range of specialties. Dr. Chin holds a Medical Degree from Harvard Medical School. He received the equivalent of a J.D. with honors from Oxford University, England under a Rhodes Scholarship. He graduated with a Bachelor of Arts in Biology, magna cum laude, from Harvard University.

Bruce Y. Lee, MD, MBA
University of Pittsburgh
Pittsburgh, Pennsylvania, USA

Dr. Lee is currently an Assistant Professor of Medicine and Biomedical Informatics at the University of Pittsburgh. His previous positions include serving as Senior Manager at Quintiles Transnational, working in biotechnology equity research at Montgomery Securities, and co-founding Integrigen, a biotechnology company. He has authored three books, as well as numerous research publications, review articles, and book chapters. Dr. Lee received his B.A. from Harvard University, M.D. from Harvard Medical School, and M.B.A. from the Stanford Graduate School of Business. Board-certified in Internal Medicine, he completed his residency training at the University of California, San Diego.

- Teaches both the basic and advanced topics in clinical trial design, conduct, analysis, and interpretation.
- Written in an easy-to-understand manner with plenty of analogies and examples.
- Addresses both the theory and practice of clinical trials.
- Written by authors with extensive academic and industry experience.
- Provides a global perspective of the many applications of clinical trial medicine.
- Covers a wide range of topics including statistics, pharmacoeconomics, adaptive trial designs, patient recruitment, regulatory issues, intervention dosing, and data management.

Randomized clinical trials are a cornerstone of the health care industry and patient care today. Many patients' lives depend on the design, conduct, and interpretation of clinical trials. A well-designed trial can protect patients from dangerous medical treatments, and bring important therapies to patients. A poorly-designed trial can break careers, sink a company, bring legal and ethical complications, hinder the advancement of science, and expose patients to considerable danger.

If you use, produce, study, purchase, invest in, or do research in drugs, medical devices, or any other type of health care intervention, understanding the science and operations of formal clinical trials is important. Today, even understanding many major medical news items requires at least some knowledge of clinical trials. Whenever a drug or medical device is recalled, a medical intervention is debunked, or a new therapy hits the market, clinical trial design, conduct, or analysis is at the heart of the evidence or the controversy. Health care is such a major business that even seemingly unrelated industries and professions can be dramatically affected by a successful or unsuccessful clinical trial. If you want a book that comprehensively covers this important subject in an easy-to-read manner, *Principles and Practice of Clinical Trial Medicine* is for you.